DISABILITY IN ANTIQUITY

This volume is a major contribution to the field of disability history in the ancient world. Contributions from leading international scholars examine deformity and disability from a variety of historical, sociological and theoretical perspectives, as represented in various media. The volume is not confined to a narrow view of 'antiquity' but includes a large number of pieces on ancient western Asia that provide a broad and comparative view of the topic and enable scholars to see this important topic in the round.

Disability in Antiquity is the first multidisciplinary volume to truly map out and explore the topic of disability in the ancient world and create new avenues of thought and research.

Christian Laes is Associate Professor of Latin and Ancient History at the University of Antwerp (Belgium), and Adjunct Professor of Ancient History at the University of Tampere (Finland). From 2014–16, he has been a Senior Research Fellow at the Institute of Advanced Social Research, University of Tampere. He has published five monographs, four edited volumes and over seventy international contributions on the human life course in Roman and late Antiquity. Childhood, youth, old age, family, marriage and sexuality as well as disabilities are the main focuses of his scholarly work.

Rewriting Antiquity

Rewriting Antiquity provides a platform to examine major themes of the ancient world in a broad, holistic and inclusive fashion. Coverage is broad both in time and space, allowing a full appreciation of the selected topic rather than an exclusive view bound by a relatively short timescale and place. Each volume examines a key theme from the ancient Near East to late Antiquity, and often beyond, to break down the boundaries habitually created by focusing on one region or time period.

Volumes within the series highlight the latest research, current developments and innovative approaches, situating this with existing scholarship. Individual case studies and analysis held within sections build to form a comprehensive and comparative overview of the subject, enabling readers to view matters in the round and establish interconnections and resonance across a wide spectrum. In this way the volumes allow new directions of study to be defined and provide differing perspectives to stimulate fresh approaches to the theme examined.

Available:

Sex in Antiquity
Mark Masterson, Nancy Sorkin Rabinowitz, James Robson

Women in Antiquity
Stephanie Lynn Budin and Jean Macintosh Turfa

Disability in Antiquity
Christian Laes

Forthcoming:

Childhood in Antiquity
Lesley Beaumont, Matthew Dillon, Nicola Harrington

Globalisation in Antiquity
Konstantin Vlassopoulos

DISABILITY IN ANTIQUITY

Edited by Christian Laes

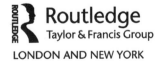

Routledge
Taylor & Francis Group

LONDON AND NEW YORK

First published 2017
by Routledge

2 Park Square, Milton Park, Abingdon, Oxfordshire OX14 4RN
52 Vanderbilt Avenue, New York, NY 10017

Routledge is an imprint of the Taylor & Francis Group, an informa business

First issued in paperback 2020

British Library Cataloguing-in-Publication Data
A catalogue record for this book is available from the British Library

Library of Congress Cataloging-in-Publication Data
Names: Laes, Christian, editor.Title: Disability in antiquity / edited by
Christian Laes.
Description: Abingdon, Oxon ; New York, NY : Routledge, 2016. |
Series: Rewriting antiquity
Identifiers: LCCN 2016013479| ISBN 9781138814851 (hardback : alk.
paper) | ISBN 9781315625287 (ebook)
Subjects: LCSH: People with disabilities--History--To 1500. | People with
mental disabilities--History--To 1500. | Civilization, Classical. | Disability
studies.
Classification: LCC HV1552 .D576 2016 | DDC 305.9/08093--dc23
LC record available at https://lccn.loc.gov/2016013479

ISBN: 978-1-138-81485-1 (hbk)
ISBN: 978-0-367-51804-2 (pbk)

Typeset in Times New Roman
by HWA Text and Data Management, London

CONTENTS

Contents

FIGURES

NOTES ON
CONTRIBUTORS

Richard H. Beal is a senior research associate on the Hittite Dictionary Project of the Oriental Institute of the University of Chicago, a project he has been working on since its inception in 1976. He received his PhD from the same institution after studying with leading Hittitologists Hans Gustav Güterbock and Harry Hoffner. In addition to his lexical work, he is the author of *The Organisation of the Hittite Military* (1992) and has written articles on Hittite political, social and religious history. He co-edited *Hittite Studies in Honor of Harry A. Hoffner* (1993), *In the Wake of Tikva Frymer-Kensky* (2009), and *Creation and Chaos: A Reconsideration of Hermann Gunkel's Chaoskampf Hypothesis* (2013). He is married to Assyriologist JoAnn Scurlock. Together they have travelled widely in the interest of better understanding the cultures that they are studying.

Julia Watts Belser is an Assistant Professor in the Department of Theology at Georgetown University, USA. Her research brings ancient texts into conversation with disability studies, queer theory, feminist thought and environmental ethics.

Hocine Benkheira is Directeur d'étude at the Ecole Pratique des Hautes Etudes, section des sciences religieuses – Groupe Société Religions Laïcités of the CNRS. He has published extensively on Islam and celibacy, Islamic regulations on food, and Islamic views on sexuality and impotence.

Sarah E. Bond is an Assistant Professor of Classics at the University of Iowa (United States). She received her PhD from the University of North Carolina at Chapel Hill in 2011 and was a Mellon Post-Doctoral Fellow in History and Classics at Washington & Lee University in 2011–12. Her monograph, out in October 2016, focuses on the literary, social and legal marginalization of certain artisans in the ancient Mediterranean. Her various articles and scholarly publications focus on perceptions of worker-bodies, the period of late Antiquity, and the disconnect between Roman literature and law.

Martin Claes studied musicology, philosophy and theology, and finished his PhD on Augustine as a pedagogue in 2011 at Tilburg University, Netherlands. He is affiliated to the Centre for Patristic Research of the same university and Free University Amsterdam. The focus of his research is early Christian theology, and especially Augustine's rhetoric and pedagogy. He has lectured on international conferences and published on this topic. He teaches patristics and philosophy at several theological institutes and works as a pastor in a parish.

Omar Coloru is an associate member of the laboratory ArScan HAROC (Nanterre). From 2010 to 2012 he has been a Postdoctoral Researcher and then a Research Assistant to the chair of History and Civilization of the Achaemenid World held by Pierre Briant at the Collège de France (Paris). His main research interests include Hellenistic history, history of Iran and pre-Islamic Central Asia, and the relations between the Greeks and the Iranian world. His scholarly work includes a monograph, an edited book, articles and book chapters on specific aspects of the Hellenistic East.

Rosalie David is Emerita Professor at the University of Manchester (UK), where she formerly held posts as Director of the KNH Centre for Biomedical Egyptology, and Keeper of Egyptology at Manchester Museum. She is the author of over forty books and many articles in peer-reviewed journals, and has acted as consultant and contributor to several television programmes. Her main research interests are the application of bio-scientific techniques to ancient Egyptian human remains, and ancient Egyptian religion. She is Vice-President of the Egypt Exploration Society, and holds Fellowships of the Royal Society of Arts and the Royal Society of Medicine. In 2003, she was awarded the Order of the British Empire (OBE) for services to Egyptology.

Matthew Dillon is Associate Professor of Classics and Ancient History at the University of New England, Australia. He has published on classical Greek religion with special reference to women, children and the nature of the ancient religious experience, as well as working on aspects of Greek society such as disabilities, torture and athletics. Special interests include the iconography and epigraphy of ancient Greek cults. With Lynda Garland, he is the author of *Ancient Greece: Social and Historical Documents from Archaic Times to the Death of Alexander*, 3rd edn (2010), *The Ancient Greeks* (2012), and *The Ancient Romans*, 2nd edn (2014).

Carol Downer retired from a career in Classics teaching in 1991, to study for an MA in Coptic dialects at UCL before acquiring her PhD there in 2004 with the editing of a Coptic martyrdom. From 1998–2011 she was a Sessional Lecturer in Egyptology at Birkbeck, lecturing on the pharaonic and late antique periods, and since then has focused on Coptic language and literature in the Theology Department at KCL, where she is a visiting teacher and convenes an advanced study group. She also teaches Coptic on the London Summer Schools. Recent work has been on the translation of the Coptic fragments of Eusebius' *Quaestiones* on which she has published several chapters and articles, as well as several on aspects of Coptic hagiography which include novelistic features, healing and *martyria*.

Anthony Dupont is Research Professor in Christian Antiquity, and is a member of the Research Unit History of Church and Theology at the Faculty of Theology and Religious Studies, KU Leuven, Belgium. The main focus of his research concerns the interrelated topics of divine grace and human freedom in the writings of Augustine of Hippo (354–430), and in particular in his *sermones ad populum*, on which he has published two monographs and several articles. Currently he is studying the development of the doctrine of sin and grace in North African theology. He is co-organizer and co-editor of *Ministerium Sermonis*, conferences and studies (within Instrumenta Patristica et Mediaevalia, Brepols) devoted to Augustine's sermons and of 'The Uniquely African

Controversy', a conference and anthology on Donatist North Africa (within LAHR). In 2013 he received the Research Council Award in Humanities and Social Sciences KU Leuven.

Stephanos Efthymiadis is a Professor at the Open University of Cyprus. He is the editor of the two-volume *Ashgate Research Companion to Byzantine Hagiography*. He has published numerous studies on Byzantine hagiography, historiography and prosopography. He co-edited the volume *Niketas Choniates: A Historian and a Writer* (with Alicia Simpson, La Pomme d'or, Geneva). A volume of collected articles on Byzantine hagiography appeared in the Variorum Reprint series (2011). He is currently working on a monograph on the history of Hagia Sophia of Constantinople (532–1204) and a book on the hagiography of Byzantine Cyprus.

Robert Garland is Roy D. and Margaret B. Wooster Professor of the Classics at Colgate University. In addition to his thirty years teaching Classics, he has taught English and Drama to secondary school students in England and lectured at the British School at Athens. His research focuses on the social, religious, political and cultural history of both Greece and Rome. He is the author of *The Eye of the Beholder: Deformity and Disability in the Graeco-Roman World,* 2nd edn (2010). His latest book is *Wandering Greeks*: *The Ancient Greek Diaspora from the Age of Homer to the Death of Alexander the Great* (2014). He has recorded *Greece and Rome: An Integrated History of the Ancient Mediterranean, The Other Side of History* and *Living History* for The Great Courses.

Matthew Alan Gaumer is a Commissioned Officer in the US Army. His combat and strategic experience include deployments to Afghanistan and the Horn of Africa as well as tours at US Africa Command and US European Command. In 2012 he completed a PhD in Theology at the University of Leuven. A polymath, he holds degrees in various subjects from Loyola University Chicago, Saint Meinrad School of Theology, American Military University and the University of Oklahoma. His research interests include: epidemiology, philosophy, late antiquity, artificial intelligence applications, geology and conflict theory.

T. H. M. Gellar-Goad is Assistant Professor of Classical Languages at Wake Forest University in Winston-Salem, North Carolina (USA). He works primarily on Roman comic poetry: satire, comedy and elegy, and Lucretius.

Bert Gevaert, Catholic University Leuven, completed his PhD on deformities and disabilities in the epigrams of the Roman author Martial in 2013. He combines his work as teacher in a secondary school with giving lectures on historical subjects, writing articles and books. Recently he saw the publication of first book, *Te Wapen,* dealing with historical European martial arts.

Danielle Gourevitch is Directeur d'études *émérite* at the Ecole pratique des hautes Etudes (Paris). She has published or co-published some thirteen books and 320 articles or chapters on the history of ancient medicine, especially gynaecology and pediatrics, and 19th-century European medicine and medical erudition. She received a volume of Mélanges *Femmes en médecine*, ed. V. Boudon-Millot, V. Dasen and B. Maire. She is *chevalier de la Légion d'honneur* and a member of Princeton Institute for Advanced Studies.

Emma-Jayne Graham is Lecturer in Classical Studies at the Open University (UK). She was Rome Fellow at the British School at Rome (2005–6) and previously taught at the Universities of Cardiff, St Andrews and Leicester. Her research focuses on the archaeology of Roman

Italy, with a particular interest in the body and its relationship with material culture. She has published on mortuary practices, disability, swaddled infant votives, sensory experience and the materiality of religion.

Edgar Kellenberger is Dr.theol. of the University of Basel (Switzerland) and is a retired pastor of the Reformed Church (Presbyterian). He gave lectures about the Old Testament at the European School for officers of the Salvation Army in Basel and at the School for Deacons in Zurich. He has published three monographs and over twenty international contributions on different topics of the Old Testament and Ancient Near East (history and theology).

Jenni Kuuliala is a postdoctoral researcher at the University of Tampere, Finland. Her research interests include disability history as well as medieval hagiography, childhood and folklore. She is the author of *Childhood Disability and Social Integration in the Middle Ages: Constructions of Impairments in Thirteenth- and Fourteenth-Century Canonization Processes* (2016).

Christian Laes is Associate Professor of Latin and Ancient History at the University of Antwerp (Belgium), and Adjunct Professor of Ancient History at the University of Tampere (Finland). From 2014 to 2016, he has been a Senior Research Fellow at the Institute of Advanced Social Research, University of Tampere. He has published five monographs, four edited volumes and over seventy international contributions on the human life course in Roman and late Antiquity. Childhood, youth, old age, family, marriage and sexuality as well as disabilities are the main focuses of his scholarly work.

Lennart Lehmhaus is postdoctoral research associate within the SFB 980 (FU Berlin). As a member of project A03 he enquires into medical discourses in Talmudic traditions in cultural comparison, Jewish epistemologies and their encyclopedic dimensions. His doctoral dissertation (Halle, 2013) on the early medieval tradition Seder Eliyahu Zutah provides a first-time annotated bilingual edition (German/Hebrew) as well as a study of the work's literary, discursive and socio-cultural dimensions. He has published articles on culture and history of rabbinic Judaism, Jewish knowledge cultures and literature, informed by approaches from literary theory, intertextuality and socio-cultural readings of texts.

John W. Martens is Professor of Theology at the University of St Thomas (Minnesota) and Director of the Master of Arts in Theology at the St Paul Seminary School of Divinity. He has published four monographs and has contributed to numerous edited volumes and academic journals on the New Testament, Hellenistic Judaism and early Christianity. His writing focuses on sexuality in early Christianity, the life of children in early Christianity and Judaism, the Apostle Paul, Philo of Alexandria and apocalyptic thought.

Michiel Meeusen (PhD KU Leuven) specialises in ancient science, medicine and the literature and culture of the Greco-Roman Empire. Meeusen is the author of *Plutarch's Science of Natural Problems. A Study with Commentary on Quaestiones Naturales*, published in the Plutarchea Hypomnemata series (2016). He also collaborated on the edition of Plutarch's Quaestiones Naturales for the Collection des universités de France, Série grecque (Budé). As a postdoctoral fellow of the Research Foundation Flanders (FWO), Meeusen published on the broader genre of natural-medical problem literature after the model of the Aristotelian Natural Problems. He is currently working, as a postdoctoral fellow of the British Academy, on a project about the reception of the Problems in the Greco-Roman Empire. He also received a fellowship from the Center for Hellenic Studies (Harvard) for the 2016–17 academic year to work on this project.

Irina Metzler holds a Wellcome Trust University Award at Swansea University, and is a Fellow of the Royal Historical Society. She has published three books in the field of medieval disability studies, including most recently a monograph on intellectual disability, and is working on a fourth volume on the connections between idoneity, health, illness and the later medieval clergy. Her interests in medieval culture extend beyond physical or mental disability to cats, monsters and race, on all of which she has published articles.

Olivia Milburn is an Associate Professor at the Department of Chinese Language and Literature, Seoul National University. Her research focuses on the history of marginalized groups in ancient China and their relationship with dominant groups and power structures, particularly non-Chinese peoples, the elderly and the disabled.

M. Miles worked for twenty years in disability-related services, partly in Pakistan (1978–92). He studied histories of responses to disability in South Asia (PhD, Birmingham University, 1999), then extended his research across East Asia, the Middle East and Africa, with many journal articles. To increase recognition of the contribution of non-western civilizations to the human heritage of knowledge on accommodating disabled or vulnerable people, Miles produced annotated bibliographies available online, with evidence from major regions, impairment categories, historical periods and religious contexts.

Alexandre Mitchell is the director of Expressum Ltd, a translation agency in London, specializing in translations of academic research in classics, archaeology and history from Antiquity to the late Middle Ages. He is an Honorary Associated Researcher at the Institute of Archaeology, Oxford, and a collaborateur scientifique of the University of Fribourg. He has published widely in the fields of classical archaeology and ancient humour, the history of medicine and reception studies, particularly the reception of Antiquity in political cartoons.

April Pudsey is a Lecturer in Ancient History at Manchester Metropolitan University, where she teaches Greek, Roman and Egyptian history, and classical languages and is a core member of the Manchester Centre for Youth Studies. She is author and co-editor of a number of items relating to ancient historical demography, childhood, youth and housing, including a forthcoming monograph on demography in Roman Egypt. She is co-editor of *Demography and Society in the Greek and Roman Worlds: New Insights and Approaches* (with Claire Holleran, 2011), and of a forthcoming volume on ancient housing *Between Words and Walls: Material and Textual Approaches to Ancient Housing* (with Jen Baird). She is co-author of a forthcoming monograph *Growing up in an Ancient Metropolis: Children's Everyday Lives in Roman Oxyrhynchos* (with Ville Vuolanto).

Martha Lynn Rose is Professor Emerita of History. She taught Ancient History and Disability Studies at Truman State University (in Kirksville, Missouri), and internationally as a guest professor, for example as a Fulbright Scholar (2010–11) and at the University of Rostock (Germany). Her current interests include the death-row prison industry in the US.

Evelyne Samama is Professor of Ancient History at the Université de Versailles Saint-Quentin-en-Yvelines. She has published several books on ancient medicine. Having collected Greek inscriptions on medical professions (*Les médecins dans le monde grec,* Geneva: Droz, 2003), she has also published her research on epidemics, poisons, charlatans, ancient pharmacists and dentists as well as disabled persons or medical care during wartime in the Greek world.

Anna Rebecca Solevåg is Associate Professor of New Testament Studies at VID Specialized University in Stavanger, Norway. Solevåg is the author of *Birthing Salvation: Gender and Class in Early Christian Childbearing Discourse* (2013). She is currently working on a monograph about representations of disability in early Christian literature.

Chiara Thumiger is Wellcome Research Associate in Medical Humanities at the University of Warwick (UK) and visiting scholar at the Humboldt Universität zu Berlin. She has published on Greek tragedy, ancient views on animals and ancient medicine. In particular, in recent years she has focused on ancient medical views on mental health (the Hippocratics, Galen and late antique medicine). Her interests include disability studies, literary theory, history of psychology and cognitive studies.

Peter Toohey is Professor of Classics in the Department of Classics and Religion at the University of Calgary in Canada. He was educated at Monash University in Melbourne, Australia, and at the University of Toronto. He is particularly interested in the nature, representation and the history of painful emotional and physical conditions, how people cope with these and how individuals sometimes turn these to their own advantage. His most recent books are *Jealousy* (2014) and *Boredom: A Lively History* (2011). His books have been translated into seven languages.

Lisa Trentin is a Lecturer in Classics in the Department of Historical Studies at the University of Toronto Mississauga (Canada). A specialist in the visual culture and social history of ancient Rome, much of her research has focused on deformed and disabled bodies, and most intensely on the body of the hunchback. Her publications include a monograph, *The Hunchback in Hellenistic and Roman Art* (2015), and book chapters and journal articles on 'Talking about Disability in the Classics Classroom' (2014); 'Exploring Visual Impairment in Ancient Rome' (2013); 'Deformity in the Roman Imperial Court', *Greece and Rome* (2011); and 'What's in a Hump? Re-examining the Hunchback in the Villa Albani-Torlonia', *CCJ* (2009). Lisa is currently the President of the Women's Network of the Classical Association of Canada.

Toon Van Houdt is Associate Professor of Latin and reception studies at the University of Leuven (Belgium). He has written several articles on early modern political, moral and economic thought. In 2015 he published a Dutch book on the reception of classical modes of thought in early modern and modern times: *Mietjes, monsters en barbaren: Hoe we de klassieke oudheid gebruiken om onszelf te begrijpen* which was awarded the Homer Prize of the Classical Association of the Netherlands (NKV).

PREFACE AND ACKNOWLEDGEMENTS

The invitation by Routledge to edit a volume on disabilities in the series Rewriting Antiquity could not have come at a better moment. A first monograph on disabilities in the Roman world appeared in 2014, and in the same year a website brought together scholars from different backgrounds in order to study the ancient world in a broad chronological framework – from 3000 BCE to 800 CE – and consequently take into account quite diverse regional and cultural backgrounds. At the same time, scholars of medieval disabilities were turning their attention to the late ancient and the early medieval times, a period of passages *par excellence*, with the coming of monotheistic religions, changing social and economic conditions, new cultural exchanges and the rise of new empires.

This volume is a major contribution to the field of disability history in the ancient world. Contributions from leading, international scholars examine deformity and disability from a variety of historical, sociological and theoretical perspectives, as represented in various media. The volume is not confined to a narrow view of 'Antiquity' but includes a large number of pieces on ancient western Asia that provide a broad and comparative view of the topic and enable scholars to see this important topic in the round. This multidisciplinary volume is the first to truly map out and explore the topic of disability in the ancient world and create new avenues of thought and research.

This book could only take shape in two research environments which were most stimulating in many ways. A Senior Research Fellowship (2014–16) at the Institute of Advanced Social Research of the University of Tampere generously provided me with opportunities for research, writing and academic travels, as well as for much needed interdisciplinary exchange of thoughts and ideas. The new focus on world history of the History Department at the University of Antwerp also was an incentive for taking up this task.

I am very grateful to the many contributors who kindly put up with an editor being quite insistent, to Lynn Rose for the thorough language revision, as well as to Matthew Gibbons, Elizabeth Thomasson and the Routledge team for the confidence given.

Christian Laes, July 2016

1

INTRODUCTION

Disabilities in the ancient world – past, present and future

Christian Laes

The bridge on the Drina

Be it as a literary device or simply as a commonplace, bridges have always been popular to denote communication and understanding between people of different time periods, places or cultures. A beautiful example is seen in *Na Drini ćuprija* (The Bridge on the Drina), a superb novel in Serbo-Croatian by the Yugoslavian writer Ivo Andrić (1892–1975), winner of the Nobel Prize in Literature in 1961. It tells the story of the town of Višegrad in Bosnia and Herzegovina and its famous Mehmed Paša Sokolović bridge over the Drina river. The story spans about four centuries during the Ottoman and subsequent Austro-Hungarian administrations of the region. In wonderful detail and with a sense of mild humour, it describes the lives, destinies and relations of the local inhabitants, with a particular focus on Muslims and Orthodox Christians living together in Višegrad.

To a historian of disabilities, the book is no less than a goldmine. They are all there. A one-legged, one-eyed and one-eared war veteran had capabilities that were enough to make him the guardsman of the bridge, the monument which was considered the jewel of the town from its building in the early Ottoman years of Mehmed Paša. An impoverished and deaf-mute girl was seen as mentally retarded. Despite this (or rather because of it) she was sexually harassed. She became pregnant and gave birth to twins; the father remained unknown. The mere threat of torture by the Ottoman authorities after an attempt to sabotage the bridge caused a traumatized official to go mad. 'At least I was not tortured' was the only phrase he kept uttering during his rages of madness. Another unnamed deaf-mute and retarded boy was known for his performing tricks on the bridge. One day he was punished by his elder brother with a severe beating 'as if he were a little kid'. Sometimes, disabled people got along well in jobs and daily life. A mullah was known for his severe stuttering, but at the same time he was a great and wise adviser to many who were in need. A skilled blacksmith is described as a giant with the brains of a chicken.

And surely, at least some of these disabled people were taken care of. After the death of his mother, a gypsy boy, whose father was an officer who had left the town soon after the baby was born, took the role of the son of the whole community. He was never given a surname, but he received food that was donated by almost everybody at different moments, and in many ways he functioned as the city's jester or fool. Towards the end of the novel, when Višegrad is living its last days as part of the Austro-Hungarian Empire, we read about a mentally retarded and crippled boy who could hardly stand on his feet. He was born when his mother was already of considerable age. Nevertheless, the bustling Galician Jewish hotel keeper Lottika took care of him in her old age, and in the end she only regretted two things: that she had never been able to send him to a specialized institution such as existed in Vienna, and that God had never helped her or the poor boy.

Andrić's book even describes what we would now call social disabilities, caused by prejudice in society. Gypsies are a telling example of this: their children were rumoured not to have souls, which explained their crude behaviour of putting a cigar in the mouth of the decapitated priest whose head was displayed on the bridge. Another gypsy boy could not resist his own appetites and ate himself to death during a city celebration with a free distribution of food. In the local inn, one could encounter the one-eyed gypsy Corkan, unlucky in love, dancing drunk on the parapet, or Saha, a squint-eyed gypsy virago, who was a better drinker than any other male customer.

There is a risk that a historian of disabilities would promptly lay this volume aside, after reading my first enthusiastic introductory remarks on a novel which was admittedly a literary sensation to me. And also a more general audience might reasonably question my motives for writing these opening paragraphs. Indeed, one does not expect a volume on disabilities in Antiquity to be anything more than an enumeration of 'remarkable' case stories, which either offer a glimpse of recognition, or give way to the self-confident feeling that 'we' surely handle things in a better way than 'the people of the past'. Not that there is nothing to be learnt for an ancient historian from the examples cited by Andrić: some of the anecdotes I selected are indeed illustrative of the *longue durée* and it is not unreasonable to imagine scenarios which were not very different in towns or villages in Antiquity. The *Bridge on the Drina* is also sensitive to the topic of continuity and change over four centuries in Višegrad. Andrić nicely describes how the ceding of Bosnia-Herzegovina to Austria-Hungary in 1878 changed the daily lives of the inhabitants of the town at the river, which came under the Habsburgian protectorate. Streetlights appeared, and the new regime put a great emphasis on cleanliness and personal hygiene. People from all parts of the Austro-Hungarian kingdom arrived, opening their businesses and bringing new customs with them. A railway line was built to Sarajevo which reduced the significance of the bridge. Children now went to Sarajevo for education. Newspapers spread news from all over the world, and at least Lottika was aware of the existence of special asylums for people with mental conditions in the capital of Vienna. On the other hand, inside the walls of the houses of the mixed Serbian, Turkish, Jewish and gypsy population, not too many things changed. When the First World War broke out, the bridge again became of crucial importance. Being on the frontline of the conflict, it was evacuated by the Austrians and eventually partly blown up. Restored, it stands as one of the beautiful tourist highlights of present-day Bosnia-Herzegovina. As the Ivo Andrić foundation proclaims on its website:

> The Bridge on the Drina can be seen as a portrait of history itself. History is made as much by individual personalities as by mass movements ... The clearest implication of the broad time-scale is the predictable one in Andrić's work: that, for all these events and changes, nothing of significance alters.
> *<http://www.ivoandric.org.rs/html/the_bridge_on_the_drina.html>*

I would like to justify these somewhat unusual first paragraphs in four main points.

For many periods and regions, disability studies in the ancient world are only at the very beginning phase. Searching for 'interesting and significant cases' is in this situation the first thing to do. Hopefully, the mere joy of recognizing such particular instances of disabilities as I experienced when reading Andrić's novel will be transferred to the readers who consult this volume.

Secondly, the force of anecdotal evidence often lies in the presenting agency of the people concerned – a virtue which will be demonstrated in at least some contributions of this volume (cf. the recent plea for study of agency by Marx-Wolf and Upson-Saia 2015: 246).

Thirdly, from the very start, this volume was meant to be comparative, by referring to cultures which existed before or were contemporary with Greco-Roman civilization, with an eye open for continuity and change of the classical tradition in later times.

Fourthly and finally, this volume is grounded in the belief that there *is* such a thing as disability, that it is not merely a social construct characterized by perceptions of people living in a specific region or area. As such, the bridge on the Drina not only stands as a symbol of Andrić's views on history and human existence, but also characterizes the present volume which will indeed build bridges between people of different times and civilizations.

A short history of the history of disabilities

By 2010, disability studies had been institutionalized in several countries.[1] Specialized chairs are devoted to the subject. At its best, scholars specializing in the branch are at the intersection of history, educational, political and social science departments, even though the historical and much needed philosophical dimensions are sometimes lacking. There are specialized journals devoted to the subject. Disabled scholars and their allies have stood up for their civil rights, and even such specific genres as disability poetry have developed and been studied. Combining insights from disciplines as sociology, psychology and anthropology, a sophisticated methodology and terminology has come to the fore, especially in literary criticism.

Yet it would be inaccurate to state that scholarly attention to the matter of disability is a recent phenomenon. On the contrary, already by the first decades of the 20th century, both doctors and historians of medicine were eager to 'find' the disabled in historical sources. As a compilation, their studies are still valuable, though they obviously took their own categories of physical and mental 'abnormality' for granted throughout the human past. Also, 'recognizing' diseases or disabilities from historical written records is not as easy as it may seem to be. Here, the problem of retrospective diagnosis comes in. Challenging this medicalized approach in the 1980s, the earliest scholars in the new field studied the complex interactions among cultural values, social organization, public policy and professional practice regarding people with impairments. Instead of a history of medicine, disability studies took the form of social history. By the 1990s, these investigations into disability developed into a new disability history, focused on concepts of otherness. Now, scholars viewed disability on the model of gender, race or ethnicity. As such, disability studies had become able to contribute to our understanding of the way in which western cultures constructed hierarchy and social order. Current disability history, too, often takes into account Foucauldian structures of power and oppression. In the last decade, disability historians have been increasingly interested in memoirs and autobiographies, records left by disabled people themselves. Agency became a matter of crucial importance, though for this approach there is the problem of a nearly complete absence of source material for some periods and civilizations on the one hand, and the strong presence of internalized discriminatory judgement in the surviving records on the other. Indeed, 'normalcy' often seems to be imposed on people. Also, disability studies developed into a multicultural world approach. The five-volume *Encyclopaedia of Disabilities* was a big enterprise involving scholars of many nationalities and including editorial work in New Delhi. For quite a few regions which remain 'exotic' to western scholars, the entries in this encyclopedia provided the first and in some cases still the only access (Albrecht 2006).

Taken all together, the various waves of disability studies have made historians aware that disability is a concept which has been constructed differently in different periods and cultures. They have also changed the vocabulary used in approaching the subject, drawing a distinction between disability – essentially a social and cultural construct – and impairment, which points to physiological and biological characteristics. One can be born impaired, in the sense that one is not able to walk. But it is social forces that either make this person disabled or enables him. Access for wheelchairs and other architectural accommodation means that in some countries users of a wheelchair are much more 'able' than people of other regions who for example may have once broken a leg and consequently experience difficulties in moving around for the rest of their lives (Metzler 2006 has scrupulously discerned between impairment and disability in her study of medieval disabilities). Others have criticized even this model as too constructivist (thereby again pointing to bodily similarities through the centuries) or because it omits the fact that impairment is culturally defined too.[2]

What is disability? The crux of the matter

Before expanding on issues such as content, methodological approaches or organization of this volume, any book approaching the matter of disability in the pre-industrial past should insist on making two crucial points to its readers.

First, disability is a recent term, one which profoundly characterizes attitudes and approaches of modern western civilization. The focus lies on the body's physical and cognitive limitations that render it unable or unfit for work. In any modern state which typically views itself as 'healthy', such a condition is considered undesirable. Pre-modern concepts, on the contrary, focus on bodies being marked or blighted by physical or mental deviance, both in Antiquity and in the early Islamic world (Laes 2014; Richardson 2012). Therefore, infirmity is much more appropriate as a term for pre-modern society. Such infirmity was a highly fluid, differentiating category, often used ad hoc and mostly defined in the context of a person's social role (Kuuliala *et al.* 2015: 5–7). Indeed, it is only the modern states from the 18th century on that focused on the 'hygiene' of their population, and the moral duty of their citizens to keep themselves healthy. State-organized medicine involved rights and duties, and the question of costs entered the equation. Surely, the benefits of the development in health care in the industrial period were considerable, and impaired people were often looked after in a more efficient and professional way. But along with this, the concept of guilt became much more pronounced. Doesn't the modern western condemnation of smokers, alcoholics or obese people stem largely from the idea that 'they cost us a lot', and that with some self-restraint on their part much of these expenses could be lowered? And isn't the whole discussion on abortion and disability – the question of who should and who should not inhabit the world (Hubbard 2013) – very much connected to an utilitarian approach of functioning in human society, enforced by the diagnostic possibilities of pre-natal medicine? Industrialized states divided handicaps and disabilities into categories, entitling people to basic rights and benefits as well as support from social welfare. In the present day, this process is part of a tendency towards social integration. Indeed, categorization need not always imply exclusion. Inclusion, however, is a fairly recent development, and discussions about the desirability of including disabled children in schools, for example, are ongoing in quite a few western countries.

All of these fluctuations are reflected in vocabulary, too. The now somewhat unfashionable term handicap is recent, with the first reference dating from the 17th century in the context of a game of chance (Laes 2014: 14). Two players would place their hands in a cap. An open hand meant that the deal had been accepted, and a closed hand indicated refusal. The first player to withdraw an open hand from the cap would receive the objects, plus the money that had been wagered. If both players revealed an open hand, the referee won the money. The term also appears in the context of horse racing. In order to make races more exciting and balanced, bookmakers in the period after the First World War starting assigning additional weight to stronger horses or allowing a head start to slower animals. The massive amounts of disabled war veterans after the two world wars increased the attention on the phenomenon of what was then commonly called handicaps: the 1948 International Wheelchair Games, which were intended to coincide with the 1948 Olympics, became the forerunner of the Paralympic Games first held in 1960. The Wheelchair Games were originally only intended for Second World War veterans with spinal cord injuries (see Frass 2012 for disabled athletes who took part in the ancient Olympic Games where there were obviously no such categories).

Recognizing the inapplicability of the term disability within the ancient world is one thing. But even more sobering is the second observation that also our present-day use of the term disability is far from equivocal. Here is what the United Nations have to say on the subject:

> The term persons with disabilities is used to apply to all persons with disabilities including those who have long-term physical, mental, intellectual or sensory impairments which, in interaction with various attitudinal and environmental barriers, hinders their full and effective participation in society on an equal basis with others. The drafters of this Convention were clear that disability should be seen as the result of the interaction between a person and his or her environment. Disability is not something that resides in the individual as the result of some impairment. This convention recognizes that disability is an evolving concept and that legislation may adapt to reflect positive changes within society. Disability resides in the Society not in the Person.
>
> *<http://www.un.org/esa/socdev/enable/faqs.htm>*

The definition offered by the World Health Organization is very much along the same lines, and uses *umbrella term* to denote the concept of disabilities.[3] It is exactly this shifting use of the term which makes it a challenge to the historian of disabilities. It only needs a little extension or a slightly broader interpretation to include women in the definition. Indeed, in more than one society, be it from the past or the present, being a woman is an impediment to social functioning (and it is indeed listed on the same level as a deaf or a blind man in a Hittite document, see Beal p. 39 in this volume). Other cases come to the mind: having a colour of skin that is a variant from the majority, or being perceived as belonging to another 'race'; homosexual behaviour in a heteronormative culture; displaying 'other' sexual tastes – which are subsequently classified as 'deviant'. But also other less 'drastic' examples come to the mind: baldness, old age, ugliness or just remarkable bodily features (see Efthymiadis p. 391 on the Byzantine fascination for special features of certains emperors). Also, the line between a disease and a disability is not as sharp as we might imagine it: epilepsy or leprosy are examples of this (Kuuliala *et al*. 2015: 5–7). This makes a dialogue with the past all the more challenging. While we would not automatically think of being blond and blue-eyed, or being twins, as a disability, the former might classify as such in early Islamic culture (Richardson 2012: 27–9), while the elimination of twins or at least one baby of the pair is attested by anthropologists in some cultures (Harris 1994: 5 n. 35; Witt 2011 on Antiquity). And what can we say about our almost endless list of so-called social disabilities, like blushing when talking in public, fear of failure or hypersensitivity? In all likelihood, people from the past would not have noted these phenomena the way present society does. Finally, the line between a disease and a disability is not as sharp as we might imagine it. What about the disabling effects of Parkinsons's disease or epilepsy? The accompanying symptoms of dermatological diseases? The list can easily be expanded.

All this confronts the editor and the contributors of a volume on disabilities in the ancient world with a dilemma, which runs the risk of becoming unresolvable. The term disability is simply unsuitable to describe concepts and conditions of people in the ancient world. At the same time, the very same term appears supremely vague, to the point of allowing inclusion to for example black people in a white majority, women in the historical context of men's dominance and homosexuals in heterosexual normative cultures in the list of oppressed subjects under study. Surely, this is not what one expects to read in a book on disabilities in the ancient world. I therefore propose a practical solution, recurring to the following categories (cf. already Laes 2014: 16–17):

1 physical handicaps/mobility impairment
2 sensory impairment (visual, auditory)
3 speech disorders
4 learning disorders or intellectual disabilities
5 mental conditions
6 multiple impairments (often a combination of the above-mentioned categories).

Comparative anthropological and ethnological studies that have adopted more or less similar frameworks have, tellingly, included additional categories such as deformation of the genitalia, the symptoms of albinism and skin disease, the condition of being twins, left-handedness and so on (Neubert and Cloerkes 1994). More or less similar systematic lists are found throughout the historical record from Mesopotamian and Egyptian diagnostic handbooks to enumerations by St Augustine or the proverbial Latin *a capite ad calcem* – from head to toe (Laes *et al.* 2013b: 1–2). As a *leitmotiv* for the present volume, these six categories will be taken into account by the contributors, not excluding some other 'deviant' or non-normative appearances or conditions as observed by anthropologists. In allowing space for a 'miscellaneous category', we follow trends as they have been observed by evolutionary psychologists such as Steven Pinker. Throughout different times and cultures, human beings' initial reactions towards what is 'strange' – in the sense that they have not seen it before – are mostly dismissive at best, and often fearful, rejecting and defensive. It is ultimately one's culture and education that decides how one copes with this initial feeling of strangeness. When a West European child raised in a remote village in the countryside meets a black person for the first time, it is the reassuring reactions of his parents and the person encountered which ensure that there is actually nothing to fear. One can easily imagine what would happen, instead, if educators were to reinforce the child's initial feeling of anxiety.

Needless to say, the admittance of such a 'miscellaneous category' risks some arbitrariness. The category will appear mostly in the chapters on iconographical representations (by Mitchell and by Trentin), since ancient Greek and Roman artefacts exhibit strong and vivid attention to the exotic and the bizarre: hunchbacks as good-luck charms are just one example of such visual representations of disability (see also Trentin 2015). The chapters on osteology (Graham and to a minor extent Pudsey), in the same way, include observations on giantism, dwarfism or other factors that made the body look strange or notable. The topic of teratology, and the extended ancient and medieval discourse on monsters and monstrous races comes up in the same chapters; as a theme of its own, it could fill another volume (Gevaert and Laes 2013 for a connection with disability history; Mittman and Dendle 2013 for a comprehensive volume on the subject). Dermatological conditions appear in both the contribution on Coptic/Aethiopic disabilities by Downer and the chapter on rabbinic Judaism co-authored by Watts Belser and Lehmhaus. The Semitic chapters on Judaism and early Islam have a strong focus on such sexual disabilities as infertility and impotence. Other miscellaneous categories could have been included. This book has no contributions on multiple births/twins or left-handedness: both have been treated elsewhere exhaustively (respectively Dasen 2005a, b, 2015; Wirth 2010). It surely would not go too far to include being a woman in the ancient world as a disabling factor to some extent and some chapters do touch upon the subject (Thumiger, Beal, Watts Belser and Lehmhaus). Solevåg takes a specifically gendered approach (and see Boehringer 2004 for 'lesbian women' as monsters in ancient thought).

Ancient history, medieval history and disability history

Ancient historians and medievalists have now come to terms with the problem of defining disabilities for their research (Laes *et al.* 2013a; Kuuliala *et al.* 2015). Comprehensive bibliographies of disability in Antiquity are now available online (see the websites of Laes and of Marx-Wolf detailed after the bibliography). In this way, historians of Antiquity and the Middle Ages have finally caught up on a backlog. Indeed, for decades these periods of history significantly lagged behind other branches of history where the study of disabilities is concerned.

Ancient disability history first focused on the case of disabled babies and their chances of survival in a world where exposure and infanticide were rampant (Eyben 1980–1; Harris 1994; Laes 2008: 92–9). Earlier, medical doctors who knew their classics had been fascinated by the theme; as a result, studies on e.g. blindness, deafness or speech impairment in Greco-Roman Antiquity were available as early as the beginning of the 20th century (Ferreri 1906a, 1906b; Werner 1932; Esser 1961 are examples of such approaches which are still invaluable as source books). By paying attention to comparative evidence, the monograph by Robert Garland (1990) was a breakthrough for disability studies of the ancient world. Garland aptly demonstrated that disability was indeed often in 'the eye of the beholder'. Since he mostly concentrated on anecdotal evidence, however, and with special attention towards the bizarre and teratology, the book was never meant to be the authoritative synthesis on the subject. For ancient Greece, a first survey was produced by Martha Lynn Rose in 2003. Her book focuses on classical and Hellenistic Greece (roughly 5th–3rd century BCE), and takes various disabilities as starting points for the division of the chapters: speech impairment, deafness, blindness and – to a less extent – mobility impairment (mental conditions are not considered). Also the question of selection and infanticide is treated. It is Rose's great merit to have introduced both the anthropologically well-known community concept and the difference between disability/impairment into disability studies in ancient history, as well as to have collected a wide range of sources which had barely been considered previously.

For the Roman Empire, the situation has advanced thoroughly only in the last five years. A conference at the University of Antwerp in September 2011 gathered for the first time the small group of scholars dealing with disabilities in Roman Antiquity. The subsequent book volume (Laes *et al.* 2013a) treats the subject of disabilities 'from head to toe': in twelve chapters, a wide range of disabling conditions are for the first time thoroughly treated. The contributors pay much attention to terminology and vocabulary, as well as to intensive reading of the source material. The osteological and the iconographic evidence, too, is given due attention. Though the authors reject excessive constructionism, they treat disability as a concept which may well have been viewed differently in different periods and cultures. Also, the contributors to the volume were alert to the obvious pitfalls of retrospective diagnosis based on modern terminology. Stemming from a conference with a similar range and purpose, Harris's collection (2013) became the first book volume ever to systematically treat the subject of mental conditions in Greco-Roman Antiquity. The first PhD dissertation dealing with deformity and disability with one specific Latin author, in the literary tradition of satire and epigrams, was defended in 2013 (Gevaert 2013). A monograph dealing with disablement in Roman Antiquity came out in April 2014 (Laes 2014, English version forthcoming). Here also, I opted for the *a capite ad calcem* approach, carefully paying attention to terminology (both Greek and Latin) and discourse analysis. I defined ancient disability as an instrumental problem, with the potential to put a person at a disadvantage at certain moments, and in particular situations. I referred to the way ancient writers applied the shifting and fluid category of disability in biographies, physiognomics, political invective, philosophical and medical treatises on disability. Disability was used ad hoc by the ancient writers whenever it seemed appropriate to the literary and rhetorical context.

Too often, scholars of Greco-Roman Antiquity have neglected research on Judaism. This is regrettable, since Jewish thought and culture was integral to the cultural and intellectual tradition of the Roman Empire. In turn, Jewish concepts are crucial to understanding Christian thinking, which also came into being in the Imperium Romanum. In recent decades, some Jewish people themselves – especially students and intellectuals – have taken a newfound interest in their legal heritage – the Bible and the Talmud, the law codes and the rabbinical response literature. How these sources relate to the issue of disability, and the degree to which halakhic attitudes to disability are in harmony with or opposite to contemporary sensibilities, has become an important topic of research. The books by Judith Abrams (1998) and Zvi Marx (2002) are landmark studies in this field, while standard reference works such as the *Jewish Encyclopaedia* go back to a long established tradition and remain invaluable research tools for the matter (Singer and Adler 1901–6). Closely connected to this research tradition is the study of disabilities in both the Hebrew and Christian scriptures, which are goldmines of multiple thoughts and practices concerning the matter (e.g. Schipper 2006).

Despite their high potential as areas of study for disability history (one only has to consider the enormous popularity of miracle and healing stories in various traditions) late Antiquity and the early Middle Ages, periods of 'passage' *par excellence* are still largely understudied (Réal 2001 and Laes 2011b deal with Merovingian times). Yet in this period various religious traditions such as paganism, Christianity, Judaism and Islam – all in multiple forms – came together at a moment when some empires collapsed, others managed to maintain themselves, new states emerged and socio-economic and cultural traditions changed. On the theoretical level, the views of the church fathers on the matter of disability and human suffering have recently been studied in a sourcebook on the Christian tradition up to the 20th century (Brock and Swinton 2012). In studies on families in the Roman Empire, the comparative view and the subsequent attention towards Coptic, Syriac, Armenian and Persian sources have come under question in scholarly research only very recently (several contributions in Laes *et al.* 2015). The interaction of pagan custom and new Christian tradition has been highlighted in the case of the sickness of children affecting their families and the ways in which people coped with this reality (Horn 2009, 2013, 2015). As for early Islam, a new stimulus has been provided in the books by Kristina Richardson (2012) on Mamluk Egypt, and the largely legislative study by Mohammed Ghaly (2009) which gives due attention to the question of theodicy and the explanations of early Islamic theologians on the matter (see Richardson 2015 for an apt overview of the research on disabilities in early Islam). Also for research in this region, disability historians are well served by standard reference works as the *Encyclopaedia of Islam* (Fleet *et al.* 2007) and the *Encyclopaedia of the Qur'ân* (Dammen MacAuliffe 2001–6).

A recent volume of the *Journal of Late Antiquity* exclusively focused on religion, medicine, disability and health in this period, and laid the foundation for most engaging further research in the form of four overarching questions (Marx-Wolf and Upson-Saia 2015). First, one may ask how far and whether 'basic medical logic' permeated the various discourses on disabilities. Such study has the potential of nuancing the idea of an opposition between the Christian religious movement on the one side, and scientific and medical learning on the other side. In fact, humoural theory and self-therapy as found in ancient philosophical treatises, seems to have been very much in the background of for instance John Chrysostom's thinking about etiology of sorrow and its therapeutic benefits (Leyerle 2015). Also, late Antiquity invites further study of the correlation between impairment and asceticism. As 'thorns in the flesh' (Crislip 2013) disabilities could remind ascetics of their humanity and be a test to remain humble. On the other hand, when long life and extraordinary health were interpreted as signs of an extraordinary state of the soul, a connection between bad health and a sinful life is an obvious possibility. Thirdly, late ancient evidence offers ample opportunities to study the correlation between (miraculous) healing and disability. It remains to be studied whether the ancient notion of incurability had an impact on beliefs on the role of the divine in the causation and treatment of health and disease (van der Eijk 2013, 2014). For this, the issue of congenital disabilities might be a special case, as healing of such patients might be considered 'particularly miraculous' (Kelley 2009). Finally, late Antiquity is the period *par excellence* to study the development of new social structures and institutions, which took up the care for the socially vulnerable in general, and more specifically the disabled (Crislip 2005).

Disability studies in the Middle Ages was also a long-neglected area of research. Here, book-length studies by Irina Metzler (2006, 2013, 2016) and edited volumes by Joshua Eyler (2010), Cordula Nolte (2013) and Wendy Turner with Tory Vanderventer Pearman (2010) were a real breakthrough. Fully engaging with the theoretical approaches of disability studies for other periods, Metzler not only succeeded in giving an apt overview of medieval theoretical concepts of the (impaired) body, but also offered a social history of disability in a lengthy chapter on medieval miracles and impairment. Currently, the Homo Debilis project at the University of Bremen under the supervision of Cordula Nolte is the leading world centre for disability studies concerning the High Middle Ages and the Early Modern period, while the diachronically and cross-culturally highly sophisticated research of the contributions in Krötzl *et al.* (2015) brought scholars of Antiquity and the Middle Ages closer together.

In short, this book volume came into being in a period in which the subject of disability history in the ancient world has for the first time gained the attention it has long deserved. The collection aims to fill a gap in an era which has received too little attention and which has high potential to pose challenging new questions.

The structure of this volume

As can be gleaned from the contents pages, this volume is organized in both a chronological and a geographical way.

The section on the Ancient Near East largely deals with the period before the rise of classical Greek civilization, though by their very nature the chapters on Iran, Egypt, India and China also include later periods up to late Antiquity in some cases.

The chapters on the Greek and the Roman world include a wide variety of approaches, corresponding to the different levels of what Michel Vovelle has so aptly called 'the house of the history of mentalities' (see Laes 2011a on the application of this model for the history of disabilities). The theoretical discourse as it is found in philosophers and medical doctors

– Vovelle's upper floor – has been given due attention (Chapters 9, 14, 15, 20 and 21), while legislative sources are also crucial to understand the topic (Chapters 10, 12 and 21). Other contributions dwell on Vovelle's first floor: artistic representation in many ways adds to the picture, be it literary representations of disabled people in comedy and tragedy (Chapter 11), in the satirical tradition (Chapter 16), or in artefacts of common use from the Hellenistic times and in Roman depictions of a 'monstrous' world (Chapters 13 and 17). Vocabulary and terminology very much reflect scientific opinions and popular mentality, and therefore can be described as being located in between the upper floor and the first floor (Chapters 9, 12 and 21). Many Greco-Roman chapters deal with the Vovellian ground level, including instances and snapshots of daily life scenarios. Such case stories are eminently represented by the osteological chapters by Graham (Chapter 18) and the juridic chapters by Dillon (Chapter 12) and Toohey (Chapter 21) – both of these clusters of chapters are remarkable not only for their use of imaginative-empathic approaches, but also in their presentation of the many legal cases or patient encounters as they are narrated by jurists and doctors respectively (see also Chapters 10, 19 and 20).

Also, these Greco-Roman chapters stand out for their interesting and sometimes divergent use of methodology. In Chapter 18, Graham explicitly goes against older top-down approaches, which she finds too generalizing: her preference is that of experience and interactional theory. Bringing together literature, epigraphy, archaeology, iconography, osteology and studies of landscape and environment, she brings us close to the manifold and diverse experiences (expectation, belief, relief) of people who were mobility impaired. In the end, Graham's differentiated approach leads to a study of what she calls 'religious space embodied' in the Italian sanctuaries of the Roman Empire. A similar empathic approach is taken by Garland, in Chapter 12 on disabilities in comedy and tragedy. Here, he explicitly raises questions about identification by the audience, who were confronted with some very cruel forms of disablement in Athenian tragedy. In Chapter 15, Gevaert deals with the Stoic school – a line of thought which possibly introduced a new attitude towards the body and ushered in a culture in which people regarded and defined themselves as bodies susceptible to pain and suffering. Disabilities are surely not the centre of Stoic treatises, but the Stoic remarks on dealing with suffering, and not the least on the science of physiognomy, are revealing for any historian of disabilities. Finally, the contributions by Bond and Gellard-Goad (Chapter 16) and to a lesser extent that of Trentin (Chapter 17) opt for a meta-poetical approach of satire, based on literary theory. Here, foul bodies and physical manifestations of impairment are primarily used as images for the persona of the poet, striving to become 'sane and healthy' – this recuperated health then stands for full poetic mastery and consciousness.

The chapters on the late ancient world again follow a geographical and chronological order. After an essay on the early Christian narrative (Chapter 22), our attention turns to the Latin Christian tradition in sermons and in monastic rules (Chapters 23 and 24), to Coptic and Ethiopic Christianity (Chapter 25), and to the Aramaic-Syriac tradition (Chapter 26), as well as to the rich Byzantine dossier (Chapter 27). Rabbinic Jewish sources as well as those of early Islam are given due attention in three chapters (Chapter 28, 29 and 30).

Finally, the endurance of the 'classical' tradition is studied in two quite different dossiers: canon law with echos from Antiquity and reverberations up to the present day (Chapter 31) and the utopian eugenic tradition of Nazi thinking, which used ancient concepts and imaginary of the body in a peculiar way, to say the least (Chapter 32).

What holds this volume together: the classical perspective and the world approach

Even from this brief description, it should be clear that this volume intends to be both focused and comparative. The way I set out to achieve this was to make Greco-Roman civilization central to the book. Indeed, studying the Greek and Roman worlds means taking into account at least the large Mediterranean area for the former, and territory from Scotland to Iraq for the latter. As such, focusing on the Greeks and Romans inherently involves a strong element of multiculturalism, since I explicitly avoid restricting these worlds in a traditional way to the cities of Athens and Rome. Admittedly, for some subjects and areas we are so limited by our sources that we need to depart from a narrow basis *faute de mieux*. This is painfully true for the history of disabilities in the classical Greek world. What is left of the literary record of the period before 500 BCE is almost completely silent on the matter. Homeric heroes are wounded to a disabling degree, but as true superheroes they continue battle with bodies miraculously cured by the gods, rather than dying of their injuries. There are hardly any disabled war veterans in the Homeric tales, except for Philoctetes who due to his war wounds was suffering from exile, isolation and pain on the island of Lemnos (Edwards 2000). As the antithesis of the aristocracy of the Homeric heroes, Thersites is displayed as a fool with bodily deficiency. His clumsy social behaviour was reflected in his bodily disability (Goodey and Rose 2013: 18 and 26). The lyric poets of the 6th century BCE do not pay any attention to disablement whatsoever, although they lament the harsh sorrows of old age (for age as disability, see Harlow and Laurence 2015). It is only in the extended corpus of the so-called ten Athenian orators of the 5th and 4th century BCE that one can start studying disabilities as they are commonly understood in a systematic way. And already in this period, the material expands geographically. The Corpus Hippocraticum, which came into being in roughly the same period, reflects medical thoughts and practices by various doctors belonging to a school which was influential all over the Mediterranean. From the Hellenistic period on, Greek influence – both in art and in literature – reached from Egypt to India, and this alone ensures a world approach. For Roman Antiquity, testimonia on disabilities go back to the earliest and legendary times of the City of Rome, with such war veterans as Mucius Scaevola, who lost his right hand, or Horatius Cocles, who was deprived of one eye (Van Lommel 2015). The literary sources referring to these war veterans and to other cases of disablement during the times of the Roman Republic (mainly in the form of monstrous births or *prodigia*) only start in the 2nd century BCE. The material for the Roman Empire – a large collection of data in written sources in both Latin and Greek, as well as archaeological and osteological records – from the 1st century BCE on has potential significance for the whole Imperium and exemplifies the world context.

Christianity came into being in the context of the Roman Empire and in many ways could be a potential factor for diversified and changing attitudes towards disabilities and bodily suffering. Indeed, one chapter devotes attention to disabilities as they appear in the Gospels and other early Christian sources, and another treats St Augustine, whose work offers abundant information on the topic and became inspirational for western Christian thought for centuries to come. Regional traditions as they appeared in the Aramaic-Syriac, Coptic, Ethiopic and Byzantine Christian sources are carefully scrutinized in other chapters. Moreover, as Christianity cannot be understood without the context of Hebrew culture and the Old Testament tradition, at least two chapters are devoted to Judaism: one places the Old Testament in the broader context of Akkadian and Sumerian culture, and the other pursues rabbinic and halakhic traditions in the Mishna and Talmud up to late Antiquity. Pharaonic Egyptian and Hittite civilizations are extraordinarily rich in information on disabilities, as well as helpful in contextualizing the Old Testament. Contributions on these periods are included as well.

Ever since the Pirenne Thesis on the origins of the Middle Ages and Peter Brown's foundational work, ancient historians have seen the spread of Islam and the subsequent establishment of Baghdad as the capital of the Abbasid Empire in 800 CE as the end of the ancient world. As early Islam came into being in the ancient world, and incorporated pagan, Jewish and Christian elements, its inclusion in this volume is totally justified, no matter how late it is: the first extended sources for Islam and disabilities, the traditions of the Hadith and the legal sharia material, should be dated to the 9th century at the earliest (Richardson 2015). Fully recognizing these limitations, two chapters have tried to answer questions as to what difference Islam made, and to define impotence, effeminacy and infertility as 'new' disabilities in the context of Islamic history.

A volume that opts for the world perspective, however, should be concerned with more than the Greco-Roman world and the monotheistic traditions of Judaism, Christianity and Islam which came out of it in order to be truly comparative. The comparison with contemporaneous large Iron Age empires is an obvious choice. China, the Akkadian and Hittite kingdoms, the Persian Empire and India, in their various stages, are therefore given due attention. Compared to the Greco-Roman material, the source material seems overwhelming. At the same time, the reader is struck by the lack of studies in these areas. The contributors to these chapters struggle with a variety of languages and texts for which often no adequate editions, let alone search engines exist. More than any others, these chapters should be viewed as pioneering work, in an area where nearly everything still needs to be done. The comparative approach of this volume also extends to the endurance of Greco-Roman tradition, especially canon law, which in many ways continued Roman legal thought and concepts, and ancient viewpoints regarding selection of the weakest, namely infanticide and exposure. No matter what reality behind the ancient concept (dealt with in Chapters 2 and 12), the persistence of the thought is important, as it was used up to the Nazi regime and beyond. Ideologists and doctors of the Nazi regime purposefully used Greco-Roman texts and statements to defend their eugenic programme.

On a final note concerning the comparative world approach, it is good to point out what is not in the volume, and why such choices have been made. There are no chapters on Celtic, Germanic or Scythian approaches to disabilities. Unfortunately these peoples (like the many hundreds of others who were in the Roman Empire) are only known through Greek and Latin writers. In late Antiquity they sometimes evolved into 'funny foreigners' in stereotypical passages describing Burgundian soldiers, Goths or Vandals (Halsall 2002). There is ongoing discussion on whether or not these 'barbarians' were somehow disabled by the way they were conceptualized by the Greco-Roman authors (cf. the debate on the invention of racism by Isaac 2004, an influential and controversial work). But apart from occasional references to Germanic tribes raising all their newborns (Laes 2008: 95), no source material is available to justify a chapter on disabilities as we understand them for the present volume. The Finnish national epic poem, the Kalevalaa, is a goldmine for information on disabilities of all sorts, from bodily to mental and intellectual impairment. Though the compilation dates from the Romantic 19th century, it is commonly believed to have come from a long and even pre-Christian tradition, with the early Finnish-speaking population almost surely being in the region of Finland in the first centuries CE. However, since there were hardly any established contacts with Greco-Roman civilization, this potentially interesting field must be left aside here (de Anna 1988 for disabling depictions of Nordic people as monsters in the medieval tradition). The same goes for the manifold black African cultures with an enormously rich oral tradition, and with very different frames of references as far as disabilities are concerned (Devlieger 1999). Mayan or Aztec cultural views on disability and rehabilitation are nowadays studied and reconstructed by anthropological fieldwork (modern studies on the matter again mostly focus on how 'strange' native people were put on exhibit: Bogdan 1988; Aguirre 2005; Durbach 2010). Although obviously most interesting and belonging within the chronological framework of this book, no contributions will focus on these cultures.

In other words, the world approach does not imply simply placing various cultures next to each other because they happened to exist in the same period. On the contrary, it requires a focused collection which can offer inspiration for a well-based comparative approach.

Continuity between the present and the past, or, bridges again

The classic question of 'continuity or change' is a discussion which brings us back to the image of the bridge as used by Andrić. It will be the focus of the last two sections of this introduction.

There is certainly much in this book which points to a history of disabilities of the *longue durée*. The demographic and ecological conditions as described in Chapter 2 reveal conditions of sensory (visual and aural) handicaps, mobility and even mental impairment, all of which must have been daily reality for a considerable part of the population in the Mediterranean world from roughly 3000 BCE up to late Antiquity. Undoubtedly, specific regional conditions created specific local issues, such as eye problems in marshy regions, environmentally related health risks linked with living in relatively densely populated towns, hereditary factors in closed island communities and resulting from endogamic marriage patterns in Egypt. As such, this volume indeed includes various contributions which take 'hard' demographic and ecological data into account: the sections on osteology in Chapter 18 or the contributions focusing on specific regions, most notably Egypt, India and China (Chapters 6–8) all take this approach. With the aid of the index, readers of this volume will be able to track down almost any affliction that comes close to what we would consider a disability. The same goes for attitudes and reactions, such as mockery, pity, disdain, anxiety and fascination – these seem to be almost universal reactions to non-normative appearances and behaviours though the way they are constructed and represented in literature may differ significantly. For the details of such discussions, I again refer the reader to the index as a guide through these diverse themes.

Other topics are recurrent throughout the collection's chapters. I focus here on what I consider seven outstanding features of the collection.

No matter with which ancient language one deals (the sources in this volume represent about a dozen different tongues), one is struck by the sheer variety of terms to denote impairing bodily or mental afflictions. 'Fascinating philology and defect terms' is the way Miles (p. 95–7 in this volume) describes the linguistic landscape for his chapter on the Indian dossier, and this in fact says it all. However, in the vocabulary list which for some languages easily outreaches a hundred terms (witness the painstaking enumerations in Chapter 9 on the Greek vocabulary), one will search in vain for words which unambiguously connote congenital conditions as distinguished from disabilities acquired in later life. Although doctors and lay persons must have had an idea about certain conditions being more permanent and/or chronic than others, this distinction is rarely if ever made in the terminology, and was surely not the dividing line between what we would call disabilities or illnesses (e.g. the Latin *infirmitas* in no way was opposed to *morbus* or *aegritudo* – it is at best a more general term, cf. Kuuliala p. 349–50 in this volume). On a comparative level, the rich Greek vocabulary studied in Chapter 9 should be compared to the terminology of other ancient languages. It surely seems to be richer than the Latin, which in turn also revealed a multiplicity of terms (Chapter 20). Not withstanding the obvious fact that these ancient civilizations did not know our disability, it shows how they were worried, puzzled, intrigued about the phenomenon of 'different' or marked bodies and/ or behaviour. Some of these worries, anxieties or just questions were reflected in their rich vocabulary for denoting them. The fluidity of terms is particularly remarkable in denoting mental or intellectual conditions (Chapter 20). More often than not madness is used in a metaphoric way: to blame opponents in court (Chapter 10), to satirize insane behaviour or beliefs (Chapter 16), or simply to denote a lack of intellectual and philosophical understanding. In the same way, spiritual blindness or deafness turn up as metaphors in both the Christian and the early Islamic discourse.

Different or somehow vague notions of (in)curability did not exclude the belief in miraculous healing. Almost every tradition dealt with in the present volume has examples of miraculous cures – the Christian 'trinity' of the blind, the deaf and the lame was prepared in the Old Testament tradition and became exceedingly influential in the Christian texts of late Antiquity and in early Islam (cf. Gaumer p. 416 in this volume). There are only very few exceptions to the belief in miracles. No attestations seem to occur in the Hittite dossier, though this may well result from the absence of sources (cf. Beal p. 43 in this volume). The Desert Fathers in Egypt seemed to be extremely reluctant to show off by performing their miracles (cf. Downer, p. 365–7 in this volume), and this attitude might well have been reflected by Muhammed, who is said not to have performed miracles, but only signs which revealed the greatness and power of Allah (cf. Gaumer, p. 415 in this volume). The Byzantine authors seem to have raised the possibility that the healing of the congenitally disabled was the exclusive field of the saint miracle healer (cf. Efthymiadis, p. 396 in this volume).

Physical and mental integrity was a requirement *par excellence* for kings and priests. For the former, the constraints of dynastic succession constituted an extra impediment. The emphasis on purity or integrity for leaders seems to be delineated clearly in the Persian-Iranian sources and in the Semitic traditions of Judaism and early Islam, though without exaggeration one may state that a similar way of thinking was present in all ancient cultures dealt with in this volume. At the same time, there always was the practical ad hoc solution, which rests on the observation that to a certain extent we indeed encounter kings and/or priests with non-normative appearances or behaviour in all periods and regions under study. Here, habituation and securing continuity seem to have been crucial elements to explain the phenomenon: crooked kings indeed existed (Ogden 1997), as did imperfect pharaohs, emperors and other leading figures.

Both in vocabulary and in daily life practice, being 'infirm' often seems to have been understood as not being able to perform or carry out one's duties. Indeed, in the Galenic tradition, full health is defined as having the possibility of functioning in the labour force and not suffering from pain (Laes 2014: 184–8). At the same time, there seems to have existed a constant concern for integrating impaired people into the productive community, be it out of sheer necessity (the constraint of economic conditions), or for practical advantages (the use of deaf – i.e. silent and discreet – servants at court is a well-known example of this situation, as are the so-called fools or jesters). In the Roman legal records, (in)capability to perform tasks became a key issue in defining the worth of a slave, and determined the possible sum of indemnification after fraudulent selling. In the case of the medieval world, the chapter on canonical records even shows striking instances of sick leaves and subsequent return to work by priests with mental conditions, as well as cases which come close to fixed appointment – when it was impossible to remove a priest from his benefice, a helper was called upon to deal with the practical part of the job. In the final analysis, all monastic traditions of late Antiquity seem to have included the possibility of the presence of 'infirm' monks or nuns who were encouraged to participate as much as possible in monastic life. As such, the major part of the contributions in this volume have again confirmed the key importance of the community concept to understand pre-modern notions of disability (Rose 2003).

Closely connected with this is the care for those who dropped out. Throughout the whole period under study, this was first and foremost a family affair – in as much as Solevåg's introduction of the term *kyrarchy* in Chapter 22 enables us to imagine the gendered aspect of being disabled in the context of ancient households. This also brings up the question of institutional care for those who were not supported by families. While the debate on whether or not the city-state of Athens had any sort of state provision for what we would call the disabled is ongoing (Rose and Dillon disagree on this, as can be understood from their Chapters 10 and 12; Penrose 2015 is in favour of the latter), the phenomenon of hospitals indeed seems to have been for the most part a Christian and consequently early Islamic matter. Discussion of institutionalized aid appears in all contributions on late Antiquity in this volume, most markedly in the chapters on Coptic and Ethiopic disabilities, in the Byzantine dossier, and in Gaumer's discussion on the change brought about by the advent of Islam (as well as in the discussion on the late ancient period within Coloru's chapter on Iran). However, readers will do well to take into account a considerable deal of continuity here too: for pharaonic Egypt and Buddhist India, David and Miles respectively have pointed to the presence of similar institutions. While acknowledging their quite diverse nature, given that pilgrims with very diverse wishes and promises of votive gifts and wishes visited, Graham in Chapter 18 has demonstrated how 'hotels' in ancient sanctuaries performed a hospital-like function. Also, the late ancient hospitals were in no way restricted to 'hopeless cases' or particular forms of disabilities. As the chapters by Kuuliala and Efthymiadis – respectively on the western monastic rules and the Byzantine Empire – demonstrate, we are far from being well informed about the practicalities of such infirmaries, but it seems sure that a wide amalgam of patients were treated there.

Another outstanding feature which runs through this volume is the caring attitude as we find it expressed by ancient medical writers. Although we lack much vital information on everyday practice of these doctors (we must presume that most of their patients belonged to the privileged upper class), and although it would certainly be wrong to propose them as role models on how to act nowadays, Thumiger is right in pointing out how Galen's 'reasonable' approach to mental and bodily afflictions might serve as an antidote to normative absolutism in medicine. Gourevitch aptly demonstrates that the ideal of the kind and caring physician (*medicus amicus*) was not a Christian invention after all. Despite the considerable deal of learned pedantry and literary games in Plutarch's oeuvre, Meeusen does well to call the Plutarchean approach 'human after all'.

Finally, reading the human body and giving negative significance to awkward difference runs like a red thread through the volume. The case appears as particularly painful in Ancient (Near) East cultures, where mutilation was a punishment commonly inflicted upon criminals – the equation of bodily mutilation with misbehaviour was consequently easily made. According to Milburn, the scenario became imminently precarious in ancient Chinese culture in which imposing mutilating punishment was a very common practice (the irreversible nature of the punishment made things even more difficult for those who were sentenced unjustly). Byzantine and Islamic tradition too show a strong tradition of punishment by mutilation, while the Greco-Roman world had the habit of linking bodies marked with scars with the status of servile submission. The concept of physiognomy, too, greatly contributed to prejudice; this featured strongly in the Homeric depiction of the anti-hero Thersites. The persistence of negative physiognomical connotations is seen nowhere stronger than in the Stoic school. While Stoic theory ideally singled out such prejudices based on corporal *indifferentia*, more than one Stoic thinker was deeply influenced by physiognomical thought and practice (Chapter 15). Finally, the fear of anomalous and ominous births and the consequent exposure or active elimination of such 'frightening' babies is a recurring reality in many ancient cultures, and treated as such in the chapters on Mesopotamia and the Old Testament, India, Greece (in Chapter 12) and Rome (Chapter 2, see also Chapter 32 for the endurance of the tradition, note that David p. 84

explicitly denies the existence of the phenomenon for pharaonic Egypt). It is well known that the monotheistic traditions emphatically disapproved of the practice, though any account on pre-modern practice will confirm that in practice it persisted in the very *longue durée* (Vuolanto 2011 among a plethora of literature, and Chapter 2 in this volume).

Ruptures or significant change

I now turn to the matter of change, or the crucial question on where one can distinguish breaches in the ancient world, and how these new ways of thinking or acting possibly foreshadow our contemporary western approaches to disabilities.

In discerning ruptures, I refrain from overly generalizing approaches which moreover run the well-known risk of the *argumentum ex silentio*. Surely, the fascination in Hellenistic statuettes with the grotesque, the bizarre or the monstrous points to a new sensibility towards the matter of non-normative bodies on the part of the artisans. In what ways this coincided with changes in society is hard or even impossible to tell (Chapter 13). The same goes for measures of support for disabled people in the Hellenistic city-states after Alexander the Great. The sources are almost completely silent on the matter, and the continuity of the Greek polis was in any case so strong that it survived up to Hellenistic times, and even into the Roman era. Again, it is dangerous to posit that the solidarity of the polis would have disappeared in the times of Hellenistic world empires (Chapter 12). In the same line, a recent article (Van Lommel 2015) has informed the thesis that there would have existed fundamentally different lines of thoughts on war wounds and war veterans in the Greek and the Roman tradition (as stated by Samama 2013). Quite often, such generalizing claims are made to satisfy our basic need to divide and schematize history into periods, though reality is indeed more complex than that (Le Goff 2014).

On the other hand, certain claims on change and difference which are often made seem to be confirmed when we return to the primary sources with renewed attention: the Semitic emphasis on ritual purity stands out as remarkable and deeply influential for the Judaic and Islamic approach regarding the matter of disability (Ghaly 2009; Richardson 2012, 2015; Katz 2014 on Islamic preoccupations with ritual cleanses; cf. Watts Belser and Lehmhaus p. 439 in this volume on the Hebrew concept of *mum* indicating being unfit to do sacrifice, Gaumer p. 414 on ritual cleanliness in early Islam).

It strongly seems that the impact of monotheism (the Jewish, Christian and Islamic traditions in their very diverse forms) can hardly be overstated if one wishes to understand profound and fundamental changes in the ancient approaches and concepts of disabilities. Indeed, some scholars have provocatively explained the rise in popularity of Christianity and early Islam by group formation and solidarity after the so-called plague of Cyprian for the former and the disastrous Justinian plague and the year without sun (536) for the latter (cf. Gaumer p. 408–10 in this volume). Moreover, in monotheistic thought, the theodicy gets all the more poignant. If there is only one God, who is to blame for defects and disabilities? All ancient polytheistic traditions were acquainted with the idea of divine punishment, and the etiology of disablement was well developed in several lines of thinking. But it is in Jewish thought that it is explicitly mentioned that disabilities ultimately come from God, since He was the third party involved at the moment of conception (cf. Watts Belser and Lehmhaus p. 441–2 in this volume; Kellenberger p. 53 and 58 for the matter of theodicy in the Old Testament tradition). The recorded words of Jesus Christ tried to counter this way of thinking, by pointing out that in the case of the congenitally blind man, neither he nor his parents had sinned (John 9: 1–44) – the church fathers repeatedly confirm such statements, though the opposite way of thinking was also present in the Christian tradition (Laes 2008: 113; 2013: 132–3; Kelley 2009). After all, wasn't his blindness caused by God to make God's good works apparent in him? Islamic thought on the matter is again very diverse as different schools interpreted diversely (Ghaly 2009), though there was also the element of divine punishment, that is, Allah's ultimate responsibility for disability (cf. Gaumer p. 413–4 in this volume). Of course, monotheistic traditions have managed to solve the awkward problem of blaming an essentially good God by resorting to agents such as evil spirits and demons, by calling upon help of protecting saints or holy men, and by pointing to free human beings (proof of God's ultimate goodness) who intentionally and malevolently deviate from the right path and from God's good intentions. By bringing forward the importance of 'other powers', these religions faced the ever imminent danger of dualism. But in practice and in everyday life, solutions such as demons and good or evil spirits might have come close to the practices of contemporary fellow pagans – in the sense that it also made the new religions more acceptable to the common people.

On the practical level of daily life, people might indeed have seen things changing with the advent of monotheism. However, such change was not always drastic, and had sometimes been prepared for long before. I have already mentioned the prohibition of child exposure, and the development of the institution of the hospital. Other examples come to mind. Would our rising with perfect bodies mean that in the end infirmity and disability were not quintessential to the understanding of an individual (cf. Solevåg p. 325–6 in this volume)? A same line of thought was already there in pharaonic Egypt (cf. David p. 86 in this volume), and the Stoics largely considered bodily suffering as an *indifferens* (Chapter 15). In ancient Chinese thought, there was the vision of an ideal world without disabilities, though this was not connected to the hereafter (cf. Milburn p. 116 in this volume). The cult of the martyrs and the consequent attention to the Passion of the Christ meant a notable shift of attention towards the mutilated and impaired body. Yet it remains unclear how this would have affected the way people who were suffering were viewed by their contemporaries (Horn 2013; Downer p. 370–1 in this volume; Efthymiadis p. 392). Monotheistic thought and practice laid a new and formerly utterly unknown emphasis on the institution of marriage. As a sacred bond (and in fact the only right and legitimate form for having sex), marriage would not only secure procreation, but it would also ensure the continuity of the belief in the one and only God (Cooper 2007 on the Christianization of marriage). Only in this context can one properly understand the almost painfully painstaking attention to such matters as impotence and infertility with the consequent attention to all sorts of mishaps of the genitalia in the Jewish, Islamic, Byzantine and canonical tradition – though, obviously, sexual malfunctioning has always bothered human beings, and is as such present in many polytheistic traditions too (see e.g. Beal, p. 42–3 for Hittite examples, or the phallic poetry of Roman satire, see Chapter 16). Yet it was only when marriage became a profoundly Jewish, Christian or Islamic matter, to be protected as one of the highest values in society, that sexual disabilities prominently came to the fore (Chapters 26 and 29).

However, monotheism matters for the study of disability in a more profound way, which goes deeper than the problem of theodicy or changes which might be observed and experienced in everyday life. Indeed, in the traditions of Judaism, Christianity and Islam all human beings are equal in the sight of God. This causes a fundamental problem, even a strong contradiction for the matter of dealing with disabled people. Taking care of a disabled fellow human being is one thing; considering him or her as your equal is another. At the same time, equality is an ideal that in many ways is extremely difficult to reach. Of course, the problem of equality in the eyes of God is not restricted to the issue of disabilities: it has raised endless and ever continuing questions on poverty, social injustice and the status and position of non-believers. But it is in no way an exaggeration to state that, in the monotheistic tradition, the issue of equality positioned disability as an *existential* problem. 'If we are all sinners, in the grand scheme of things disability pales into insignificance' (Metzler, p. 465 in this volume). In a way, this poignant phrase says it all, as the categories, distinctions, rules and exceptions for the infirm or disabled which were formed and (re)formulated throughout the centuries prove the opposite – or at least the innate contradiction inherent in the premise. Such an existential approach never existed in pagan thought, where disability was at best an instrumental problem, putting a person at a disadvantage at certain moments and in particular situations (cf. Toohey, p. 298 and 309 in this volume). It was only when the 'caring modern' state in search of 'healthy' citizens took over in the late 18th century (Leven 2008) that the charitable attitude in combination with the existential approach towards the matter gave rise to the modern western concept of disability. However, both approaches have their origin in the ancient world, which makes its study vital and crucial to understanding our concepts and attitudes towards disabled people. It is my hope and intention that this volume may contribute to such understanding

Notes

1 For surveys of the history of disabilities for ancient historians, I refer to Laes *et al.* 2013 and Laes 2014: 31–3 which contain many bibliographical details. Handbooks or introductions to modern disability studies include Albrecht *et al.* 2001; Longmore and Umansky 2001; Jones and Webster 2010; Förhammar and Nelson 2010 and Van Trigt 2011.
2 Eyler 2010: 8 (too constructivist); Hughes and Paterson 1997 and Shakespeare 2006 (impairment as construction). A good summary of this potentially endless debate in Kuuliala *et al.* 2015: 2–3.
3 Disability is an umbrella term, covering *impairments, activity limitations* and *participation restrictions.* An *impairment* is a problem in body function or structure; an *activity limitation* is a difficulty encountered by an individual in executing a task or action; while a *participation restriction* is a problem experienced by an individual in involvement in life situations. Disability is thus not just a health problem. It is a complex phenomenon, reflecting the interaction between features of a person's body and features of the society in which he or she lives. Overcoming the difficulties faced by people with disabilities requires *interventions* to remove environmental and social barriers <http://www.who.int/nmh/a5817/en>.

Bibliography

Abrams, Judith Z., *Judaism and Disability: Portrayals in Ancient Texts from the Tanach through the Bavli* (Washington, DC, 1998).
Aguirre, Robert D., *Informal Empire: Mexico and Central America in Victorian Culture* (Minneapolis, MN, 2005).
Albrecht, Gary L. (ed.), *Encyclopaedia of Disabilities,* 5 vols (Chicago, IL, 2006).
Albrecht, Gary L., Seelman, Katherine D., and Bury, Michael (eds), *Handbook of Disability Studies* (Thousand Oaks, CA, 2001).
Boehringer, Sandra, ""Ces monstres de femmes." Topique des *thaumata* dans les discours sur l'homosexualité féminine aux premiers siècles de notre ère', in O. Bianchi and O. Thévenaz (eds), Mirabilia: *Conceptions et représentations de l'extraordinaire dans le monde antique. Actes du colloque international, Lausanne, 20–22 mars 2003* (Berne, 2004), 75–98.
Bogdan, Robert, *Freak Show: Presenting Human Oddities for Amusement and Profit* (Chicago, IL, 1988).
Breitwieser, Rupert (ed.), *Behinderungen und Beeinträchtigungen/Disability and Impairment in Antiquity* (Oxford, 2012).
Brock, Brian, and Swinton, John (eds), *Disability in the Christian Tradition: A Reader* (Grand Rapids, MI, and Cambridge, 2012).
Cooper, Kate, *The Fall of the Roman Household* (Cambridge, 2007).
Crislip, Andrew, *From Monastery to Hospital: Christian Monasticism and the Transformation of Health Care in Late Antiquity* (Ann Arbor, MI, 2005).
Crislip, Andrew, *Thorns in the Flesh: Illness and Sanctity in Late Ancient Christianity* (Philadelphia, PA, 2013).
Dammen MacAuliffe, Jane (ed), *Encyclopaedia of Qur'ân.* 5 vols plus index (Leiden, 2001–6).

Dasen, Véronique, *Jumeaux, jumelles dans l'Antiquité grecque et romaine* (Zurich, 2005a).

Dasen, Véronique, 'Blessing or Portent? Multiple Births in Ancient Rome', in K. Mustakallio, J. Hanska, H. L. Sainio and V. Vuolanto (eds), *Hoping for Continuity: Childhood, Education and Death in Antiquity and the Middle Ages* (Rome, 2005b), 61–74.

Dasen, Véronique, '*Infirmitas* or Not? Short-Statured Persons in Ancient Greece', in C. Krötzl *et al.* (eds), *Infirmity in Antiquity and the Middle Ages* (Farnham, 2015), 29–49.

de Anna, Luigi, *Conoscenza e immagine della Finlandia e del Settentrione nella cultura classico-medievale* (Turku, 1988).

Devlieger, Patrick, 'Frames of Reference in African Proverbs on Disability', *International Journal of Disability, Education and Development* 46 (1999), 439–51.

Durbach, Nadja, *Spectacle of Deformity: Freak Shows and Modern British Culture* (Berkeley, CA, 2010).

Edwards, Martha Lynn [= Rose, Martha Lynn], 'Philoctetes in Historical Context', in D. A. Gerber (ed.), *Disabled Veterans in History* (Ann Arbor, MI, 2000), 55–69.

Esser, Albert, *Das Antlitz der Blindheit in der Antike* (Leiden, 1961).

Eyben, Emiel, 'Family Planning in Graeco-Roman Antiquity', *Ancient Society* 11–12 (1980–1), 5–82.

Eyler, Joshua R., 'Introduction: Breaking Boundaries, Building Bridges', in J. R. Eyler (ed.), *Disability in the Middle Ages: Reconsiderations and Reverberations* (Farnham, 2010), 1–15.

Ferreri, Giulio, 'I sordomuti nell' antichità', *Atena e Roma* 9 (1906a), 39–47.

Ferreri, Giulio, 'I sordomuti nella letteratura latina', *Atena e Roma* 9 (1906b), 367–78.

Fleet, Kate, Krämer, Gudrun, Matringe, Denis, Nawas, John, and Rowson, Everett (eds), *Encyclopaedia of Islam* (Leiden, 2007).

Förhammer, Staffan, and Nelson, Marie Clark, *Funktionshinder i ett historiskt perspektiv* (Stockholm, 2010).

Frass, Monika, '"Behinderung" und Leistungssport in der Antike? "Mys" der wundersame Ringer', in R. Breitwieser (ed.), *Behinderungen und Beeinträchtigungen/Disability and Impairment in Antiquity* (Oxford, 2012), 57–63.

Garland, Robert, *The Eye of the Beholder: Deformity and Disability in the Graeco-Roman World* (London, 2010).

Gevaert, Bert, *Parcere personis, dicere de vitiis: Deformitas in de epigrammen van Publius Valerius Martialis* (unpublished PhD, Brussels, 2013).

Gevaert, Bert, and Laes, Christian, 'What's in a Monster? Pliny the Elder, Teratology and Bodily Disability', in C. Laes *et al.* (eds), *Disabilities in Roman Antiquity* (Leiden, 2013), 211–30.

Ghaly, Mohammed, *Islam and Disability: Perspectives in Theology and Jurisprudence* (London and New York, 2009).

Goodey, Chris F., and Rose, Martha Lynn, 'Mental States, Bodily Dispositions and Table Manners: A Guide to Reading "Intellectual" Disability from Homer to Late Antiquity', in C. Laes *et al.* (eds), *Disabilities in Roman Antiquity* (Leiden, 2013), 17–44.

Halsall, Guy, 'Funny Foreigners: Laughing with the Barbarians in Late Antiquity', in G. Halsall (ed.), *Humour, History and Politics in Late Antiquity and the Early Middle Ages* (Cambridge, 2002), 89–113.

Harlow, Mary, and Laurence, Ray, 'Age, Agency and Disability: Suetonius and the Emperors of the First Century CE', in C. Krötzl *et al.* (eds), *Infirmity in Antiquity and the Middle Ages* (Farnham, 2015), 15–27.

Harris, William V., 'Child Exposure in the Roman Empire', *Journal of Roman Studies* 84 (1994), 1–22.

Harris, William V. (ed.), *Mental Disorders in the Classical World* (Leiden and Boston, MA, 2013).

Horn, Cornelia B., 'Approaches to the Study of Sick Children and their Healing: Christian Apocryphal Acts, Gospels, and Cognate Literatures', in C. B. Horn and R. R. Phenix (eds), *Children in Late Ancient Christianity* (Tübingen, 2009), 171–98.

Horn, Cornelia B., 'A Nexus of Disability in Ancient Greek Miracle Stories: A Comparison of Accounts of Blindness from the Asklepieion in Epidauros and the Shrine of Thecla in Seleucia', in C. Laes *et al.* (eds), *Disabilities in Roman Antiquity* (Leiden, 2013), 115–43.

Horn, Cornelia B., 'From the Roman East into the Persian Empire: Theodoret of Cyrrhus and the Acts of Mar Mari on Parent–Child Relationships and Children's Health', in C. Laes *et al.* (eds), *Children and Family in Late Antiquity* (Leuven, 2015), 257–87.

Horn, Cornelia B., and Phenix, Robert R. (eds), *Children in Late Ancient Christianity* (Tübingen, 2009).

Hubbard, Ruth, 'Abortion and Disability: Who Should and Who Should Not Inhabit the World', in L. Davies (ed.), *The Disability Studies Reader* (London and New York, 2013, 4th edn), 74–86.

Hughes, Bill, and Paterson, Kevin, 'The Social Model of Disability and the Disappearing Body: Towards a Sociology of Impairment', *Disability and Society* 12/3 (1997), 325–40.

Isaac, Benjamin, *The Invention of Racism in Classical Antiquity* (Princeton, NJ, 2004).

Jones, Daniel, and Webster, Li, *Handbook on Mainstreaming Disability* (London and Bali, 2010).

Katz, Marion Holmes, 'Fattening up in Medieval Caïro', *Annales Islamologiques* 48 (2014), 1–23.
Kelley, Nicole, 'The Deformed Child in Ancient Christianity', in C. B. Horn and R. R. Phenix (eds), *Children in Late Ancient Christianity* (Tübingen, 2009), 199–216.
Krötzl, Christian, Mustakallio, Katariina, and Kuuliala, Jenni (eds), *Infirmity in Antiquity and the Middle Ages: Social and Cultural Approaches to Health, Weakness and Care* (Farnham, 2015).
Kuuliala, Jenni, Mustakallio, Katariina, and Krötzl, Christian, 'Introduction: Infirmitas in Antiquity and the Middle Ages', in C. Krötzl *et al.* (eds), *Infirmity in Antiquity and the Middle Ages* (Farnham, 2015), 1–11.
Laes, Christian, 'Learning from Silence: Disabled Children in Roman Antiquity', *Arctos* 42 (2008), 85–122.
Laes, Christian, 'How does one Do the History of Disability in Antiquity? One Thousand Years of Case Studies', *Medicina nei Secoli* 23/3 (2011a), 915–46.
Laes, Christian, 'Disabled Children in Gregory of Tours', in K. Mustakallio and C. Laes (eds), *The Dark Side of Childhood in Late Antiquity and the Middle* Ages (Oxford, 2011b), 39–62.
Laes, Christian, 'Raising a Disabled Child', in J. Evans Grubbs, T. Parkin, with R. Bell (eds), *The Oxford Handbook of Childhood and Education in the Classical World* (Oxford, 2013), 125–44.
Laes, Christian, *Beperkt? Gehandicapten in het Romeinse Rijk* (Leuven, 2014).
Laes, Christian, Goodey, Chris F., and Rose, Martha Lynn (eds), *Disabilities in Roman Antiquity: Disparate Bodies A Capite ad Calcem* (Leiden, 2013).
Laes, Christian, Goodey, Chris F., and Rose, Martha Lynn, 'Approaching Disabilities *a Capite ad Calcem*: Hidden Themes in Roman Antiquity', in C. Laes *et al.* (eds), *Disabilities in Roman Antiquity* (Leiden, 2013), 1–15.
Laes, Christian, Mustakallio, Katariina, and Vuolanto, Ville (eds), *Children and Family in Late Antiquity: Life, Death and Interaction* (Leuven, 2015).
Le Goff, Jacques, *Faut-il vraiment découper l'histoire en tranches?* (Paris, 2014).
Leven, Karl-Heinz, *Geschichte der Medizin: Von der Antike bis zur Gegenwart* (Munich, 2008).
Leyerle, Blake, 'The Etiology of Sorrow and its Therapeutic Benefits in the Preaching of John Chrysostom', *Journal of Late Antiquity* 8/2 (2015), 338–85.
Longmore, Paul K., and Umansky, Lauri (eds), *The New Disability History: American Perspectives* (New York, 2001).
Marx, Zvi, *Disability in Jewish Law* (London and New York, 2002).
Marx-Wolf, Heidi, and Upson-Saia, Kristi, 'The State of the Question: Religion, Medicine, Disability and Health in Late Antiquity', *Journal of Late Antiquity* 8/2 (2015), 257–72.
Metzler, Irina, *Disability in Medieval Europe: Thinking about Physical Impairment during the High Middle Ages, c.1100–1400* (London and New York, 2006).
Metzler, Irina, *A Social History of Disability in the Middle Ages: Cultural Considerations of Physical Impairment* (London and New York, 2013).
Metzler, Irina. *Fools and Idiots? Intellectual Disability in the Middle Ages* (Manchester, 2016).
Mittman, Asa Simon, and Dendle, Peter (eds), *The Ashgate Research Companion to Monsters and the Monstrous* (Farnham, 2013).
Neubert, Dieter, and Cloerkes, Günther, *Behinderung und Behinderte in verschiedenen Kulturen* (Heidelberg, 1994²).
Nolte, Cordula (ed.), *Homo debilis: Behinderte – Kranke – Versehrte in der Gesellschaft des Mittelalters* (Affalterbach, 2009).
Nolte, Cordula (ed.), *Phänomene der Behinderung im Alltag: Bausteine zu einer Disability History der Vormoderne* (Affalterbach, 2013).
Ogden, Daniel, *The Crooked Kings of Ancient Greece* (London, 1997).
Penrose, Walter D., Jr., 'The Discourse of Disability in Ancient Greece', *Classical World* 4 (2015), 499–523.
Pinker, Steven, *The Blank Slate: The Modern Denial of Human Nature* (New York, 2002).
Réal, Isabelle, *Vies des saints, vie de famille : Représentation du système de la parenté dans le Royaume mérovingien (481–751) d'après les sources hagiographiques* (Turnhout, 2001).
Richardson, Kristina L., *Difference and Disability in the Medieval Islamic World: Blighted Bodies* (Edinburgh, 2012).
Richardson, Kristina L., 'Islam and Disabilities', *Oxford Bibliographies* (Oxford, 2015).
Rose, Martha Lynn, *The Staff of Oedipus: Transforming Disability in Ancient Greece* (Ann Arbor, MI, 2003).

Samama, Evelyne, 'A King Walking with Pain? On the Textual and Iconographical Images of Philip II and Other Wounded Kings', in C. Laes *et al.* (eds), *Disabilities in Roman Antiquity* (Leiden, 2013), 231–48.

Schipper, Jeremy, *Disability Studies and the Hebrew Bible: Figuring Mephibosheth in the David Story* (London and New York, 2006).

Shakespeare, Tom, *Disabilities Rights and Wrongs* (London, 2006).

Singer, Isidore, and Adler, Cyrus (eds), *The Jewish Encyclopaedia* (New York, 1901–6).

Trentin, Lisa, *The Hunchback in Hellenistic and Roman Art* (London, 2015).

Turner, Wendy J., and Vandeventer, Pearman Tory (eds), *The Treatment of Disabled Persons in Medieval Europe: Examining Disability in the Historical, Legal, Literary, Medical, and Religious Discourses of the Middle Ages* (Lewiston, 2010).

van der Eijk, Philip J., 'Cure and the (In)curability of Mental Disorders in Ancient Medical and Philosophical Thought', in w. V. Harris (ed.), *Mental Disorders in the Classical World* (Leiden and Boston, MA, 2013), 307–8.

van der Eijk, Philip J., 'Galen and Early Christians on the Role of the Divine in the Causation and Treatment of Health and Disease', *Early Christianity* 5 (2014), 337–70.

Van Lommel, Korneel, 'Heroes and Outcasts: Ambiguous Attitudes towards Impaired and Disfigured Roman Veterans', *Classical World* 109/1 (2015), 91–117.

Van Trigt, Paul, '*Disability history*: Een vergeten geschiedenis in Nederland? Over het nut van een nieuwe discipline voor het onderzoek naar de geschiedenis van blinde en slechtziende mensen', *Leidschrift* 26/1 (2011), 49–62.

Vuolanto, Ville, 'Infant Abandonment and the Christianization of Medieval Europe', in K. Mustakallio and C. Laes (eds), *The Dark Side of Childhood in Late Antiquity and the Middle Ages* (Oxford, 2011), 3–19.

Werner, Hans, *Geschichte des Taubstummenproblems bis ins 17. Jahrhundert* (Jena, 1932).

Wirth, Henning, *Die linke Hand: Wahrnehmung und Bewertung in der griechischen und römischen Antike* (Stuttgart, 2010).

Witt, Mathias, 'Die "Zwillinge des Hippokrates": Ein antikes Zeugnis von erblich disponierter Erkrankung (Augustinus, *De civitate dei* V, 2), seine mögliche Quelle und Rezeption', in L. Perilli, C. Borckmann, K.-D. Fischer and A. Roselli (eds), Officina Hippocratica: *Beiträge zu Ehren von Anargyros Anasassiou und Dieter Irmer* (Berlin, 2011), 271–328.

Websites

Laes, Christian, 'Disability History and the Ancient World' <http://www.disability-ancientworld.com/bibliography/bibliography.htm>

Marx-Wolf, Heidi, 'REMEDHE. Bibliographic Resources' <http://remedhe.com/bibliographic-resources>

2

DISABILITY AND *INFIRMITAS* IN THE ANCIENT WORLD

Demographic and biological facts in the longue durée

April Pudsey

Introduction: environment, biology and culture

The demography of disability and *infirmitas* is one which is heterogeneous and multi-faceted. Demography concerns itself largely with death, and with age and ageing of individuals and population groups – the influences and interdependence between causes of death and population behaviour. Disability and *infirmitas* are physical in nature, but to some degree also dependent on behaviour and can be observed as social constructs (as borne out by the chapters in this volume), yet frequently bound up in matters relating directly or indirectly to demographic dynamics, and the same factors which influence mortality. They are underpinned by the physical realities of environmental pressures and the process of ageing, on the one hand, and by culturally determined responses to health and ill-health, on the other. In this chapter I aim to outline the key physical attributes of ancient demographics on the body. I provide an outline of the environmental and other factors that would have impacted on long-term (generational) health and *infirmitas*: disease environments; water and food supply; resources for infant-nurture; living conditions and diet. The chapter explains the influence of these factors on a range of examples of ancient bodily health and *infirmitas* across the cities, villages and deserts around the Mediterranean. A comprehensive and medical account of the impact of demography and ageing on health in Antiquity is beyond the scope of this chapter, and of our source material. But it is hoped that this chapter will present, within the framework of environment, biology and culture, a background for the detailed case studies of cultural aspects of disability in Antiquity that follow.

Ecological conditions varied hugely across the Mediterranean, from Egypt's arid deserts and Nile Delta marshlands, to the mountainous infertile lands of rural Attica and the marshlands of Italy and the city of Rome. The population of the Roman world at the height of its empire was over fifty million. The inhabitants of each region lived in a physical environment which shaped not only their day-to-day lives but their very being, and their capacity to survive or to adapt and live within challenging or changing environments. Demographic circumstances, health and wellbeing are in large part a product of such localized environmental features: heat, aridity or humidity, water supply, land fertility and food supply, and disease environment. But they are also in part a function of behavioural responses to life in these environments, and the biological impacts of their features; population density and living conditions are directly correlated with the movements, vivacity and development of particular disease cultures, and practices of infant feeding, animal husbandry and migration and mobility, all have their roles to play. Biology and culture respond to one another, influencing the health and wellbeing of the populations of the ancient Mediterranean over generations (see in particular the work of Hin 2011, 2013, for biology and culture in late Republican Italy).

The impacts of disease, diet and mobility are felt in the short term, but also in the longer term, as bodily health, fitness and promise of longevity depend particularly on human environment in early life. As people grow older, a key determinant in the quality of life is health. In later life health conditions impart to physical capacity some limitations, such as changes in eyesight, hearing, cognitive abilities and lung capacity (Lynch *et al.* 2009). The pathological aspects of health and its deterioration are of course intrinsically biological, but their impact on individuals' lives is also largely a matter of social and cultural context, and the extent to which failing functionality in the body is socially disabling is a matter of definition. Disability can in part be understood in terms of the extent to which a physical impairment or deterioration limits an individual's capacity to perform specific social roles, as well as functional ones (Verbrugge and Jette 1994; Laes 2014: 8–29). Indeed, in modern usage and according to the World Health Organization, a physical or cognitive impairment is typically considered a disability if it operates in such a way as to limit an individual's life in a particular environment; in another environment that same impairment may not have the same impact (Laes 2014: 17). For instance, disability in these terms in Rome was focused on mental and intellectual disabilities, blindness, deafness and an array of speech defects from stuttering to muteness; all of these are important social functions in a society so heavily focused on oratory (see chapters on each of these areas in Laes 2014). But mobility impairment was also markedly disabling, as were medical issues affecting growth and stature, in a pre-modern (and largely agrarian) world where the capacity to work in physical roles was also socially important. All of these observed aspects of disabilities in Antiquity related both to culture and environment.

How were the inhabitants of the ancient Mediterranean subject to environmental conditions influencing their physical health and ability? Can we assess the biological impact of environment on the human body in Greece, Rome and Egypt, beyond the mere risk of death or survival? How did populations typically respond and adapt to their environments, and what were the consequences of these on human health and *infirmitas*?

Ecological factors affecting mortality illustrate the variety in chronological and regional terms that can occur. These are often seasonal: hotter climates are more accommodating for many endemic diseases in certain regions around the Mediterranean. Such heterogeneity of environment is regional, even to the degree of varying across the localized ecological and climatic conditions of one country. For instance, in Egypt the papyrological and archaeological material yield demographic and ecological data in which Scheidel (2001) observes three main patterns of seasonal mortality: in Upper Egypt and Nubia, Lower Egypt, and in Alexandria, respectively. The evidence is also chronologically diverse, and it is by virtue of the tendency of ecological environments to be slow to change (particularly in Egypt, where the environment was essentially the same in antiquity as it was in the 19th century) that patterns and trends observed in later sources are able to be used for our period.

There is much to say about regional diversity when it comes to understanding the impact of environment on life, as the chapters throughout the rest of this volume will demonstrate. Regional ecological studies have been lacking for the ancient world, with the exception of some key and wide-ranging studies (Holleran and Pudsey 2011: 1–13). Sallares's *The Ecology of the Ancient Greek World* outlined important ecological factors in the creation of specific disease environments around Attica, and their impact specifically on mortality (Sallares 1991); Horden and Purcell (2000) also discuss the relationship between environment and disease. In his *Malaria and Rome*, Sallares approached the disease environments of ancient Italy with the same, thorough, approach to understanding mortality (Sallares 2002). The importance of ecological factors in determining the impact of disease on mortality cannot be overstated. Scheidel discusses the mortality regimes of Roman Egypt in his *Death on the Nile: Disease and Demography in Roman Egypt* (Scheidel 2001) and Hin's *The Demography of Roman Italy* (2014) explores aspects of disease throughout the Italian peninsula.

Death, not surprisingly, as the ultimate outcome of ecologically specific disease, is the focus of all of these key studies. And yet overall population size fluctuated only marginally over hundreds of years; if we are to accept WHO figures on the proportion of people living with disabilities in the modern world – 14.2 per cent (Laes 2014: 9) – then it would be fair to presume the major factor altering this figure historically would be in terms of mortality. In any case, this would still mean that, in all likelihood, hundreds of thousands, if not millions, of living people in the Roman world would have been experiencing disability. The impact of environment is felt in mortality of populations in age- and sex-specific ways, but there is much more to be said on both the immediate and the longer term impact of environment, disease, living conditions, diet and outbreaks of, for instance, smallpox, on the general health of a population over generations. And it is towards the disease environments of Antiquity, where we now focus attention.

Plague: seasonal and regional disease environments

The impact of disease on disability is hugely significant, and its impact stretches beyond the lifetime of some of the individuals who experienced the disease. Physical disabilities frequently accompany the diseases found across the ancient Mediterranean and North Africa, and are evidenced in the texts, medical literature and archaeology of human remains (see below, and also Gaumer in this volume). Seasonal mortality rates are a key indicator of certain endemic disease environments, of diseases which are facilitated and often exacerbated by general living conditions; these patterns of seasonal mortality in each region are, perhaps, indicative of certain types of disease. The ancient written and archaeological data support the existence of such diseases as smallpox and their effects on mortality and on health in population groups more widely. The Fayum region of Egypt in the Roman period had a population exceeding 300,000 with an extensive irrigation system, and the transmission of infectious diseases amongst this population was influenced not only by living conditions but also by precipitation and temperature which affect the survival of pathogens. High humidity and flood levels were prominent in the Fayum of Egypt in this period (see Scheidel 2001: 54–60), setting an ecological backdrop which differed from the ecology elsewhere, even of Alexandria.

Greece, Italy and Egypt were all host to smallpox plagues at some point from the first five centuries BCE to the first six centuries CE. Smallpox spread very quickly around the Greco-Roman world in each appearance of it we read of in our sources from over a thousand years; it is – ecologically speaking – one outbreak in a much larger pandemic of smallpox, the second outbreak of which was the Black Death, originating in Central Asia from the 1330s and spreading across Europe until 1772, and the third outbreak of which originated in China in the late 19th century (Little 2007: 1–7). The evidence from documentary and literary sources suggests that smallpox was prominent; this supports the ecological and other evidence of plague and plague-like diseases in Egypt, Greece, Italy, Gaul and the wider Mediterranean. Moreover, plague and similar diseases varied across climates, seasons and regions, and its effects on mortality varied across age-groups. Plague – smallpox, alongside typhus and measles – was widely known in the ancient Mediterranean, and a major pandemic is attested in the sources: the plague of 430 BCE in classical Athens (Thucydides 2.47–51); the 'Antonine' plague of 166–94 CE; and the 'Justinianic plague' of 541–2 in the Eastern Roman Empire (which returned at various periods even into the 8th century). Survivors of plague and their physical impairments are mentioned briefly in some texts, for instance after the Justinianic plague survivors are referred to in discussion of swelling in the groins, thighs, armpits and neck, all inhibiting mobility (*Incerti auctoris* 2.96–7 and 2.187; see also Procopius, *De bello persico* 2.22.39 on incoherence and speech difficulties of survivors; cf. Little 2007: 67–70).

The Antonine plague was first attested in 165 CE at Nisibis and Smyrna, and had reached Rome by 166. In early 167 people fled for their lives from Dacia (*ILS* 7215; Duncan-Jones 1996: 108). The plague in the Roman provinces in 168 affected military recruitment; emergency drafting had to be conducted because of the high mortality rates amongst soldiers as a consequence of the epidemic (Duncan-Jones 1996: 72; see also Sabbatani and Fiorino 2009). The Antonine plague of 166 and its presence across much of the Roman world in the late 2nd century, especially in Egypt, is confirmed by Galen (for instance in Galen, *Definitiones medicae* 153 (19.391–2 Kühn). Evidence suggests a widespread reach for the Antonine plague across the empire (Cartwright and Biddiss 2014, see also Gaumer in this volume on the 'Plague of Cyprian'). Documentary sources from Egypt illustrate its presence and devastating localized effect. In 168/9 we observe a sudden drop in the numbers registered to pay tax in the settlement of Thmouis (in the eastern delta), due to death from plague, or flight to avoid it. Similar large-scale and sudden patterns were recorded in other delta villages in 167/8 and 168/9, and in 179 CE there was a sudden mortality spike in the records at the Fayum village of Soknopaiou Nesos, in fact a reduction by one-third of the tax-paying population in as little as two months, and in the village of Karanis a drop of 33–47 per cent in those registered is recorded between 145/6 and 171–4 (*P.Ryl.* 594; *P.Mich.* 223–5; Rathbone 1990: 103–42; Duncan-Jones 1996: 121 Table 1).

This plague has been identified as smallpox, which peaks from March to May, and is consistent with the observed patterns in data from Upper Egypt. Its presence is, therefore, confirmed not only by the evidence of mummy labels and inscriptions, but also by literary and documentary sources. The environment of Egypt was unchanging and smallpox was present throughout most of the 2nd century CE (Brunt 1971: 611–24; Jackson 1988: 179–84; Scheidel 1994). Malaria, tuberculosis, typhus, leprosy and measles were also all present (see below on malaria, and see Burke 1996). According to ancient writers, the frequency of the threat of smallpox across the whole empire was high (Pliny, *NH* 7.170, Seneca, *De ira* 3.51, *Tranq.* 9.7.4, *QN* 6.27.2, 6.27.4; ages at death were recognized by Thucydides 2.47, Cicero, *Ad fam.* 5.16.4, Dio 53.33.4 and 54.1.2). Using passages from Galen, Littman and Littman have demonstrated that the plague was indeed smallpox, an identification which has assisted in the establishment of a mortality rate of 7–10 per cent of those infected, and the impact on surviving populations (Littman and Littman 1973: 245). Smallpox pandemics tend to result in mortality rates of up to 25 per cent of those infected, the infected often being up to 40–80 per cent of the total population, total mortality rates can therefore result in fatalities of from 10 to almost 20 per cent of the total population (e.g. in 18th-century Europe: Littman and Littman 1973: 254). In 165/6–168 CE then, this could have caused approximately three and a half to five million deaths across the population of the Roman Empire, the majority of which would likely have occurred in crowded urban dwellings and military camps. But it would also have infected, and affected, many more people.

The 'Justinianic' phase of this ancient outbreak of the plague pandemic is the most widely attested of the phases of the outbreak mentioned by our sources, and detailed in terms of the geography of its impact. John of Ephesus wrote of the impact of the outbreak of plague in Egypt on his visit to Alexandria, as it appeared to have travelled (as had he) through Palestine, Syria and Asia Minor (see extended account in John of Ephesus' *Ecclesiatica Historia*, cf. Little 2007: 61–72). He points out the devastation wrought by the disease in terms not only of death, but also of destruction to crops and fields in Syria and Thrace, and ongoing problems in farming the land due to high mortality. The long-term impact of plague would have been felt in indirect ways, beyond its initial and ongoing devastating effects on mortality. The destruction of crops and food supply, and of agriculture and labour through mortality, would of course have exacerbated the impact on surviving local populations. Procopius of Caesarea tells us that this outbreak began at Pelusium in Egypt, in 541 CE and spread rapidly throughout Byzantium within two years (Procopius, *De bello persico* 2.22). It would appear that this plague moved around from Constantinople in 544 and back again in 558 and had been present in Gaul, in the Rhone Valley in 543 (Gregory of Tours, *Hist. Franc.* 4.31, who also notes that in 571 in Clermont the impact of plague was huge, as in Lyons, Bourges, Chalon-sur-Saone and Dijon, and extended to affect the bishop of the port town of Nantes and then across the Atlantic: Gregory of Tours, *Glor. Conf.* 78). In 590 in Rome, reports of an epidemic followed the flooding of the Tiber, see Gregory of Tours, *Hist. Franc.* 10.1). For 565 onwards we also see the impact of plague in the writings of Paul the Deacon, who details the widespread death of adults and children from the plague, and its consequences on farming, viticulture and life in the countryside, especially from the summer occurrence in 680 in Pavia (Paul the Deacon, *Historia Langobardorum* 56–8 and 254–5).

The impact of the plague so rife in our sources is in its decimation of human populations, and its apparently equal disregard for age. It also impacts quite directly, and substantially, on food production, living conditions, labour value and therefore living standards; the consequences of plague on this level were felt throughout urban and rural populations on a catastrophic scale and impact on diet and bodily health and *infirmitas* across generations. Those who survived suffered in terms of physical health and were disadvantaged by its ravaging effect on agriculture, and food and nutrition supply.

Malaria, tuberculosis and typhus were also prominent across the Greco-Roman world. Regional environments played host to them to varied degrees, and it is important to note the relative susceptibilities of populations to the impact of these diseases; seasonal and age- and sex-specific impact varied according to quite localized climate and conditions, even within one country. Egypt, of course is a case in point. Typhus, typhoid and relapsing fever resulted in a death rate of 50 per cent in ages under 50 years old, 100 per cent in those aged 60 years and over. These water-borne diseases were rife from March to August, and are associated with poor living and hygiene conditions. These patterns are consistent with data for the mortality profile of Upper Egypt and Nubia, and very common in parts of Egypt. Diarrhoeal diseases are grouped with entric fevers such as typhoid and paratyphoid, and occur often from food poisoning and rotaviruses of unknown causes (Scheidel 2001: 101). Mortality happens mostly in the cases of infants and young children; adult deaths are rare but occur in the elderly. Tuberculosis affected early adult mortality, especially in the winter seasons, and infant mortality even more so, and urban crowding only served to aid the infection.

Malaria exacerbated other illnesses, and was present in the Nile Delta and its ecology, especially in the Fayum region with its marsh lands and low-flying insects, where biomolecular analysis of ancient bone samples has confirmed the presence of malaria (Sallares 2002). Even within the ecology of Egypt we can observe a case in point regarding the diversity of disease environment. There are three main mortality patterns discernible in Egypt, focused on disease environment in Upper Egypt and Nubia, Lower Egypt and Alexandria. In Upper Egypt, climate and the ecology was reasonably homogeneous (a pattern is observed in a collection of inscriptional evidence from Aswan, and a Coptic monastery at Saqqara, and Sakinva in Nubia – discussed and analysed by Scheidel 2001: 5, table 1 and *passim*). According to Scheidel's analysis of these inscriptions, at Saqqara the death rate peaked two months earlier than in Nubia, in April and May rather than in May, June and July; Aswan's pattern showed an increase in mortality in the month of August (Scheidel 2001: n. 127, tables 1.2–1.4). The Nile valley data are more smoothly distributed, with variation in environmental conditions; the data from Lower Egypt show a 'complex bimodal distribution' with mortality peaking at the end of the year as much as in the spring in Upper Egypt, and another increase in the middle of the year; the data for Alexandria are *a*seasonal and fall between the two (Scheidel 2001: fig. 1.15–1.17). Mortality rates observed in data from the Nile valley varied significantly from those of the Fayum (Scheidel 2001: figs 1.3, 1.4), and we see 54 per cent of funerary inscriptions commemorating those who died between February and April, the late winter/early spring months (Scheidel 2001). Alexandria and the Nile Delta is the third geographic region which is marked out as having a specific disease environment, as illustrated by mortality rates. Mortality data, in the form of funerary inscriptions from fifteen generations of individuals, suggest that mortality in this region does not appear to peak in springtime, as it does in Upper Egypt, but instead from October to January. Data from Leontopolis and other areas in the Delta illustrate more prominent rises in mortality in June and further peaks in cooler months.

Collectively, these patterns in seasonal mortality which are specific to the regions of Egypt demonstrate clearly that the ecological environment of each was responsible for shaping causes of death; the diseases environments varied even within one country, where seasonal spikes in death rates are reflective of the presence of particular diseases: tuberculosis infection struck mostly in the winter months, and mortality tends to result in the late winter/early spring months (Fares 2011). Egypt in Antiquity, then, was a hotbed of disease and infection; the heterogeneous nature of the environment, ecology and climate led to a diverse range of diseases, impacting variously on women and men in different age groups.

Adults and children were usually affected to different degrees by seasonal mortality which is determined by endemic disease: children tend to be more likely to die in hot seasons and the elderly in cold and wet seasons (Ferrari and Livi Bacci 1985: 280 table 5 on Italy in 1869; compare Shaw 1996: 119–21; Scheidel 1996: 158 fig. 4.25). These data illustrate seasonal patterns which are different for children and for adults, as Scheidel demonstrates: for the first twenty years of life, 40.5 per cent of all deaths occur from May to August; for adults this figure is 18.9 per cent. For a sample of 190 deaths (with and without ages) 25.9 per cent can be placed in that period: the divergence between young and adults in the cool season is inverted (Scheidel 2001: 26). Children's mortality peaked around June, with a smaller peak in winter for adults. Though the evidence here relates to death and mortality rates, it does provide us with some clue as to the rates of infection, the speed and reach of the spread of disease and the specific impact of demography and disease on individual health.

The mosquito's curse: malaria

Disease, then, was dependent on ecological environment and pressures, and its impact was felt more harshly in some areas than in others. The smallpox plague was devastating where it struck, and it travelled as populations migrated both short and long distances. Malaria was a disease which affected huge sections of the population, and differently, and served to exacerbate the effects of other diseases. Malaria struck the city of Rome and other areas of Italy throughout the classical period, and beyond (see Burke 1996). The presence of malaria – more specifically, a number of human species of malaria – across the ancient Mediterranean is well-known; its impact, however, is difficult to assess, given the variety in mosquito populations, breeding patterns and limited flight capacity, all of which contributory factors are compounded by human activity, geography, climate and hydrology (Sallares *et al.* 2004: 311). Malaria's impact would have been localized to some degree but its impact not only on mortality, but on health, was substantial. Studies of the molecular evolution of malaria have established four species of human malaria: *P. falciparum*; *P. vivax*; *P. malariae*; and *P. ovale*. The first of these four, *P. falciparum*, is the most dangerous and devastating to human populations, and has a history stretching back at least 100,000 years (Joy *et al.* 2003) and evolved as a human parasite along with the *Anopheles gambiae* mosquito species complex (Coluzzi *et al.* 2002).

Given the range of infectious disease present in Antiquity, in particular malaria, we should expect to find a good deal of mention of its obvious impact on physical health in our sources. The most common reference to any physical infirmity relating to disease is in reference to fever of some kind – typically in relation to malaria. We see much discussion of fever, in relation to populations living in hot climates and around water, in the medical and Hippocratic texts of the 5th and 4th centuries BCE (Celsus, *De medicina* 3.31; Hippocrates, *Aer.* 7, 10–12). These references refer to a tertian fever – which is caused by *P. vivax*, or a quartan fever, caused by *P. malariae*, both of which were endemic at this point in time to Greece, India and China. *P. falciparum* evolved in Africa (Conway *et al.* 2000), and its tertian fever (distinct from semitertian fever of *P. vivax*) was noted by Celsus, among others in the Roman period, as being common and, in fact, known from its presence in Greece (see Sallares *et al.* 2004: 312; Celsus, *De medicina* 3.3.2, 3.3.1; Pliny, *NH* 26.1–9).

The impact of *Plasmodium falciparium* malaria on many of those infected would have been, eventually, fatal, but survivors of malaria in more recent population groups live with longer lasting physical ramifications of the disease. Indeed, contraction of malaria in childhood likely impacts on cognitive and behavioural development as surviving children grow to adulthood; neuropsychological development can be hugely inhibited by severe malarial infection, or in some cases by the effects of chronic infection, illness and malnutrition. Recovery of optimal cognitive function is far from certain, and malarial patients exhibit signs of seizures, particularly febrile seizures, memory impairment and psychotic and depressive episodes, often not fully realized for years after infection (Holding and Snow 2001; Waruiru *et al.* 1996).

Medical texts from across Antiquity refer frequently to physical manifestations of ill-health, particularly in terms of fevers and febrile seizures, and the symptoms of the disease on the physical health of individuals (see Yeo 2005). In some cases the fever itself is seen as the disease rather than a symptom of it:

> For certainly very many, both now and in the past, have sought the causes of fevers, wishing to hear and learn from the sufferers whether the origin of the illness occurs due to cooling, or exhaustion, or repletion, or from some other cause of this kind, seeking the causes of diseases neither according to truth nor usefully. For if cold were the cause of being febrile, the one who is made more cold would be more febrile. This however is not so, but there are those who are saved after coming to extreme danger from cold who remain without fever from this. Likewise, the same is so in exhaustion and repletion.
>
> *(Galen, De causis procatarcticis 14.8.102–3)*

Of course, fever could have been a symptom of more than malaria, and we see discussion of fevers in relation to bacterial infections and to pregnancy and childbirth (see Draycott 2012: 74–6), as well as to diseases including malaria, typhoid and influenza. But Galen appears to have been quite clear on the prominence and nature of different types of fevers, and that fevers of different duration were related to the humours (Galen, *De differentiis febrium* 2.1: phlegm, quotidian fevers; yellow bile, tertian fevers; and black bile, quartan fevers). The descriptions of the fevers by medical writers is helpful in determining their association with disease environment; the species of *P. vivax* is strongly associated with a benign tertian fever, and *P. falciparum* with a malignant version of this fever, the quartan fever being closely linked with *P. malariae*. It is quite clear that individuals described as suffering from fevers of these types and duration, and living in areas with mosquitoes and an environment of low-flying insects and marshes, and river tributaries (such as parts of Italy, and the Nile Delta and Nile Valley in Egypt, and even close by canals in locations quite distant from rivers) were most likely exhibiting the signs of ill-health associated with malaria and malarial fever (Scheidel 2001 *passim*).

Malaria exhibits a distinct pattern in Italy, as Sallares points out, with a series of three stages of northwards movement (Sallares 2001 *passim*; Sallares *et al.* 2004: 313–28, esp. fig. 1). Malaria was rife in what were the marshlands of Syracuse from the 7th century BCE, where it was also present in the nearby Greek colonies along the coasts of southern Italy, from the 9th to the 7th centuries BCE. In the 5th to the 2nd centuries BCE malaria spread to western central Italy, hitting Etruscan cities and the coastal region of Tuscany – where it was present also in the early Modern period – and advanced then into northern Italy over a long period, up to around 1000 CE, its apparent slowness in some phases was typically due to local ecology and the types of mosquito. *P. vivax*, *P. malariae* and *P. fulciparum* were all present in Italy and Greece over this long period and spread widely, even accounting for different mosquito vectors to carry the disease. (See Gaumer in this volume for a discussion of the spread of contagious disease around North Africa in Antiquity, from the Vandal invasion of the Roman provinces in 429 CE, onwards; see also Stannard 1999.)

The impact of malaria in the ancient Mediterranean on child development in physical terms and Africa can be observed through palaeopathology; skeletal remains from cemeteries can yield information on the presence of types of malaria in the population and the impact on individual health. An infant cemetery in Lugnano, Umbria, dating to around 450, has provided evidence of *P. falciparum*. A sudden, seasonal, spike in mortality in the summer months is suggested by the spatial distribution of the burials, of infants (some premature, some neonates) on such a large scale as to have infected most pregnant women of Lugnano; this is a pattern consistent with *P. falciparum* and indeed with the ecology of the town just a short distance from the River Tiber, and the DNA recovered from the remains (Sallares *et al.* 2004: 316–17; Soren and Soren 1999 *passim*).

In Egypt the mummification of human remains (even into the Roman period) preserved soft tissue and, together with skeletal evidence, provides a great deal of palaeopathological information on diseases affecting these individuals. The most notable palaeopathological and skeletal material evidence comes from Egypt, from the Kellis 2 cemetery in the Dakhleg Oasis of the western desert, inhabited over a long period of time (Bowen *et al.* 2005; Hope 1997; Kaper and van Zoest 2006). Malaria appears to have been present even in this region, and its capacity for exacerbating the impact of other diseases appears to have come into play in the women and children buried in the cemetery. Skeletal remains from the Roman period show signs of bone lesions as a consequence of childhood anaemia, made far worse by malarial infection. Disproportionately small foetal skeletal remains are a strong indication of maternal infection, both reducing the weight of infants to a dangerous, often fatal, point, and directly causing local-population-wide increases in infant mortality (Fairgrieve and Molto 2000; Draycott 2012: 73–4).

Similar signs are found in the mummified remains of the deceased of Dush in the Kharga Oasis of the 1st to 4th centuries CE. Signs of illness and malnutrition affected the growth and bone density of these individuals, were accompanied by evidence of internal parasites associated with enteric diseases, malaria, typhoid and other aspects of ill-health (Lichtenburg 1998).

Inherited genetic resistance was present in Italy, in the form of thalassaemia, in some cases which can lead to osteological modifications (e.g. the 3rd-century CE site of Settefenestre skeleton of a boy, Fornaciari and Mallegni 1985) and the skeletons exhibiting signs of porotic hyperstosis – a characteristic of thalassaemia – from the necropolis of the colony of Metapontum of the 5th century BCE (Carter 1998). Sickle-cell resistance is evident in skeletal remains of a young male from the island of Failaka in the Persian Gulf who had clearly survived to adulthood (Maat and Baig 1990).

Living conditions, nutrition and health

As highlighted above, living conditions and rates of urbanization tend to exacerbate the impact of disease on mortality. Disease was rife; it attacked according to age and season, and varied across Egypt. Seasonal mortality patterns illustrate that the relationship between endemic disease and its environmental ecology were extremely influential in determining death in Egypt; such ecological conditions as precipitation, humidity and flooding have remained steady over the millennia. These conditions differ across various regions of Egypt itself, resulting in different patterns of seasonal mortality, as observed in the epigraphic data. These factors would have affected people across various social levels: those who could afford to be embalmed and/ or commemorated, and those living in urban slums. Certain living conditions where water was susceptible to contamination, or overcrowding, exacerbated the infection rates. Diseases which are common to such ecological conditions (smallpox, typhus, malaria and so on) were well-known in the ancient world as causes of fatality and can be traced through the seasonal observations in the data as well as knowledge of the ecological conditions of each region.

Mortality rates and risks varied according to age, sex and environment. Young people's risk of succumbing to infectious disease, malnutrition and general poor health were undoubtedly high by modern standards, yet the standard view has tended to overestimate one key demographic element affecting life in the ancient world – the relationship between infant and adult mortality (Woods 2007; Scheidel 2001: 1–117); moreover, much of the research has underestimated the degree to which culturally and socio-economically driven behaviours influenced overall demographic dynamics. Demographic dynamics relating to infant survival and health are closely tied with cultural responses to actual and perceived risks and particular social behaviours. Infant skeletal remains from the Dakhleh Oasis in Egypt have been the subject of stable nitrogen isotope analysis (a study of the relative proportions of animal/human protein in the bone marrow), which has demonstrated that supplementary foods were introduced at around six months, and that weaning was completed by three years of age. Even more recent archaeological work on similar samples from early Neolithic cemeteries in central and south-east Turkey has enabled ancient historians to explore the relationship between the duration of exclusive breastfeeding and infant mortality rates among infants varied as a function of not just disease and immediate living conditions, but also of weaning practices and the duration of exclusive breastfeeding – broadly speaking, the longer the period of exclusive breastfeeding, the greater the risk of infant death (Dupras *et al.*, 2001; Prowse *et al.*, 2004; Bourbou and Garvie-Lok 2009). The analysis and comparison of archaeological material from these ancient sites, where nutritional information and agricultural practices are understood, demonstrate clearly that, when communities were unaware of the optimal exclusive breastfeeding and weaning periods, the health, and indeed survival, of infants was at risk. It is abundantly clear that socio-cultural behavioural aspects of infant care both contributed directly towards, and were in part influenced by, particular demographic circumstances.

Nutrition and malnutrition in childhood are of course key factors in determining health, and susceptibility to disease and ill-health, in later life. A recent report conducted by UNICEF (2013) highlighted the causal link between children's malnutrition and disability in developing countries, a link which is supported by research with small groups in Kenya, in which the causal link was demonstrated to have worked both ways, children with disabilities were also more likely to be malnourished as a consequence of limited access to food and resources (Kuper *et al.* 2015; see also Yousafzai *et al.* 2003 for a case study of children living in a slum in Mumbai, India). For many of the populations of classical Antiquity, access to resources would have been limited, especially in times of widespread plague and malaria, and nutritional deficits would have left young people susceptible to ill-health, low birth weights, maternal risks, growth stunting and greater susceptibility to infection with tuberculosis, measles and smallpox. Micronutrient deficiencies, such as iodine, vitamin A, iron can lead directly to growth stunting and bone wasting, and this is an issue not just for infants and children, but of course their mothers when pregnant (Groce *et al.* 2014). A maternal severe lack of vitamin A in pregnancy is a common cause of blindness in children in developing countries (Battacharjee *et al.* 2008). An iodine deficiency during pregnancy can frequently lead to slow development in cognitive abilities and motor skills of the foetus, resulting in intellectual disabilities; again, developing world countries where access to resources is limited are a point of comparison (Delange *et al.* 2004).

Conclusions

This chapter has outlined some demographic background to the discussions which follow throughout this book. One chapter cannot possibly aspire toward comprehensive coverage of medical and environmental conditions across the whole of Antiquity, less still of their impact on individual health, ill-health and infirmity, but it can provide valuable context for understanding the cultural and social attitudes towards certain aspects of health. We have seen that two large incidences of smallpox plague across Antiquity constitute part of the three main outbreaks of the pandemic in European history; our sources betray a knowledge of the symptoms and after effects of the disease on localized populations. Migration around the Mediterranean from the classical period of Greece's history up until the late Roman world would have facilitated the travel of smallpox, and its spread between the populations of Egypt, Greece and Italy, and even beyond, and the overall impact over the long-term course of Antiquity was almost incalculable. Mortality rates 'spiked' in the short term in towns and cities, or even wider regions, where plague struck; but death accounted for only one aspect of the devastation caused by smallpox, which revealed itself in the ill-health of infected individuals and groups, and down the generations in their capacity to farm and feed themselves successfully on a large scale. Nutrition suffered, and so did physical health as a result, as malnutrition was the cause of decreased birth weight, damaged bone density and growth arrest, scurvy, infant mortality and maternal sickness; the effects of tuberculosis and other chronic diseases would have hit harder a malnourished population. Moreover, the consequences of agricultural devastation through disease and mortality among agricultural populations often led to large-scale migration in the case of famine or potential famine, and this in turn would potentially have aided the spread of any endemic disease in a vicious circle of cause and impact as people carried pathogens as they migrated.

Living conditions facilitated the spread of smallpox and its development into a pandemic disease; overcrowded cities (see Alston 2001), towns and military camps (e.g. see Baker

2004) created population densities that were a breeding ground for the carrying of infection from person to person, via fleas or mosquitoes. Water supply in overcrowded centres would have been affected by the greater likelihood of its proximity to human waste, and therefore encouraged the spread of water-borne diseases, including cholera and typhoid fever.

We have seen that malaria influenced life and death for high numbers of individuals across Greece, Italy and Egypt, and that malarial fevers and its causes were widely visible to the populations of Antiquity. The ecological environment of a world of agriculture, marshes, rivers and low-flying insects, indeed even irrigation leading to mosquitoes' presence in abundance around canals, was the background to the rise and impact of malaria, a disease which also made worse the physical devastation wrought by other diseases. Types of fevers, impact on growth, bone health and general physical health were all closely related to disease environment. The (often inescapable) living conditions, and culturally and socially driven behaviours, of populations in Antiquity were in large part determining factors for the spread of health-impacting disease, and this can be seen across the Mediterranean.

The purpose of this chapter, however, is by no means to account for disability and *infirmitas* in purely physical or ecological and environmental terms. The natures of physical and cognitive ability, disability and *infirmitas* are, of course, highly culturally constructed, as is to some degree disease itself. The cultural responses to the ill-health resulting from such disease and movement patterns are observed in the wealth of medical texts, historical writings and papyrological material (see Nutton 2007) from around the ancient world. The purpose of this chapter has been to provide some demographic background to the rest of the chapters in this volume: to outline a pattern in the demographic background to health, ill-health, disability and *infirmitas* in the *longue durée*.

Bibliography

Alston, Richard, 'Urban Population in Late Roman Egypt and the End of the Ancient World', in W. Scheidel (ed.), *Debating Roman Demography* (Leiden, 2001), 161–204.

Bagnall, Roger S. (ed.), *The Kellis Agricultural Account Book (P.Kell.IV Gr. 96)* (Oxford, 1993).

Baker, Patty A., *Medical Care for the Roman Army on the Rhine, Danube and British Frontiers from the First through Third Centuries AD* (Oxford, 2004).

Battacharjee, Harsha, Das, K., Borah, R., Guha, K., Gogate, P., Purukayastha, S. and Gilbert, C. 'Causes of Childhood Blindness in Northeastern States of India', *Community Eye Care* 56/6 (2008), 495–9.

Bourbou, Chryssa, and Garvie-Lok, Sandra J., 'Breastfeeding and Weaning Patterns in Byzantine Times: Evidence from Human Remains and Written Sources', in A. Papaconstantinou and M. A. Talbert (eds), *Becoming Byzantine: Children and Childhood in Byzantium* (Dumbarton Oaks, DC, 2009), 65–83.

Bowen, Gillian E., Chandler, Thomas, and Martin, Derrick, 'Reconstructing Ancient Kellis', *Buried History* 41 (2005), 51–64.

Brunt, Peter Astbury, *Italian Manpower 225 BC–AD 14* (Oxford, 1971).

Burke, Paul F., 'Malaria in the Graeco-Roman World: A Historical and Epidemiological Survey', *ANRW* II, 37, 3 (1996), 2252–81.

Carter, Joseph Coleman, *The Chora of Metaponto: The Necropoleis* (Austin, 1998).

Cartwright, Frederick, and Biddiss, Michael, *Disease and History* (London, 2014).

Coluzzi, Mario, Sabatini, A., della Torre, A., Di Deco, M., and Petrarca, V., 'A Polytene Chromosome Analysis of the *Anopheles Gambiae* Species Complex', *Science* 298 (2002), 1415–18.

Conway, D. J. *et al.*, 'Origin of Plasmodium falciparum Malaria is Traced by Mitochondrial DNA', *Molecular and Biochemical Parasitology* 111, 1 (2000), 163–71.

Delange, Francoise, Benoist, B., Pretell, E., and Dunn, T., 'Iodine Deficiency in the World: Where Do We Stand at the Turn of the Century?', *Thyroid* 11/5 (2004), 437–47.

Draycott, Jane, *Approaches to Healing in Roman Egypt* (Oxford, 2012).

Duncan-Jones, Richard P., 'The Impact of the Antonine Plague', *Journal of Roman Archaeology* 9 (1996), 108–36.

Dupras, Tosha L., Schwarcz, H. P., and Fairgrieve, S. I., 'Infant Feeding and Weaning Practices in Roman Egypt', *American Journal of Physical Anthropology* 115 (2001), 204–12.

Fairgrieve, Scott I., and Molto, J. E., 'Cribra Orbitalia in Two Temporally Disjunct Population Samples from the Dakhleh Oasis, Egypt', *American Journal of Physical Anthropology* 111 (2000), 319–31.

Fares, A., 'Seasonality of Tuberculosis', *Journal of Global Infectious Diseases* 3/1 (2011), 46–55.

Ferrari, G., and Livi Bacci, Massimo, 'Sulle relazioni tra temperature e mortalità nell'Italia unita, 1861–1914', in *La popolazione italiana nell'ottocento. Continuità e mutamenti* (Bologna, 1985), 273–98.

Fornaciari, G., and Mallegni F., 'Analisi antropologica paleonutrizionale dei resti scheletrici umani', in A. Carandini (ed.), *La villa romana di Settefinestre* (Modena, 1985), 275–7.

Groce, N., Challenger, E., Berman-Bieler, R., Farkas, A., Yilmaz, N., Schultink, W., Clark, D., Kaplan, C., and Kerac, M., 'Malnutrition and Disability: Unexplored Opportunities for Collaboration', *Paediatrics and Child Health* 34/4 (2014), 308–14.

Hin, Saskia, 'Family Matters. Fertility and its Constraints in Roman Italy', in C. Holleran, A. Pudsey (eds), *Demography and the Graeco-Roman World. New Insights and Approaches* (Cambridge, 2011) 99–116.

Hin, Saskia, *The Demography of Roman Italy: Population Dynamics in an Ancient Conquest Society 201 BCE–14 CE* (Cambridge, 2013).

Holding, P. A., and Snow, R. W., 'Impact of *Plasmodium falciparum* Malaria on Performance and Learning: Review of the Evidence', in J. G. Breman, A. Egan and G. T. Keusch (eds), *The Intolerable Burden of Malaria: A New Look at the Numbers* (supplement to vol. 64, 1, of the *American Journal of Tropical Medicine and Hygiene* (Northbrook, 2001), 68–75.

Holleran, Claire, and Pudsey, April (eds), *Demography and Society in the Greek and Roman Worlds: New Insights and Approaches* (Cambridge, 2011).

Hope, Colin A., 'The Dakhleh Oasis Project', in R. S. Bagnall (ed.), *The Kellis Agricultural Account Book* (Oxford, 1997), 5–14.

Horden, Peregrine, and Purcell, Nick, *The Corrupting Sea: A Study of Mediterranean History* (Malden, MA, and Oxford, 2000).

Jackson, Ralph P. J., *Doctors and Diseases in the Roman Empire* (London, 1988).

Joy, D. A., Feng, X., Mu, J., Furuya, T., Chotivanich, K., Krettli, A. U., Ho, M., Wang, A., White, N. J., Suh, E., Beerli, P., and Su, X. Z, 'Early Origin and Recent Expansion of Plasmodium Falciparum', *Science* 300/5617 (2003), 318–21.

Kaper, Olaf E., and van Zoest, Karolien (eds), *Treasures of the Dakhleh Oasis* (Leiden, 2006).

Kuper, Hannah, Nypera, Velma, Evans, Jennifer, Munyendo, David, Zuurmond, Maria, Frison, Severine, Mwenda, Victoria, Otieno, David, and Kisia, James, 'Malnutrition and Childhood Disability in Turkana, Kenya: Results from a Case-Control Study', *PLOS ONE* 10/12 (2015), DOI: 10.1371/journal.pone.0144926.

Laes, Christian, *Beperkt? Gehandicapten in het Romeinse Rijk* (Leuven, 2014).

Lichtenburg, R., *Life on the Fringe: Living in the Southern Egyptian Deserts during the Roman and Early Byzantine Periods* (Leiden, 1998), 117–27.

Little, Lester K., *Plague and the End of Antiquity: The Pandemic of 541–750* (Cambridge, 2007).

Littman, R. J., and Littman, M. L., 'Galen and the Antonine Plague', *American Journal of Philology* 94/3 (1973), 243–55.

Lynch, S. M., Brown, J. S., and Taylor, M., 'Demography of Disability', in P. Uhlenberg (ed.), *International Handbook of Population Aging* (Chapel Hill, NC, 2009), 567–82.

Maat, G., and Baig, M., 'Scanning Electron Microscopy of Fossilized Sickle-Cells', *International Journal of Anthropology* 5 (1990), 271–6.

Nutton, Vivian, 'Greco-Roman Medicine and the Greek Papyri', in C. E. Römer and H. Froschauer (eds), *Zwischen Magie und Wissenschaft; Ärzte und Heilkunst in den Papyri aus Ägypten* (Vienna, 2007), 5–12.

Prowse, T., Schwarcz, H. P., Sanders, S., Macchiavelli, R., and Bondioli, L. 'Isotopic Paleodiet Studies of Skeletons from the Imperial Roman-Age Cemetery of Isola Sacra, Rome, Italy', *Jars* 31 (2004), 259–72.

Rathbone, Dominic, 'Villages, Land and Population in Graeco-Roman Egypt', *Proceedings of the Cambridge Philological Society* 36 (1990), 103–42.

Sabbatani, S., and Fiorino S., 'The Antonine Plague and the Decline of the Roman Empire', *Le Infezione in Medicina* 17/4 (2009), 261–75.

Sallares, Robert, *The Ecology of the Ancient Greek World* (New York, 1991).

Sallares, Robert, *Malaria and Rome* (Cambridge, 2002).

Sallares, Robert, Bouwman, A., and Anderung C., 'The Spread of Malaria to Southern Europe in Antiquity: New Approaches to Old Problems', *Medical History* 48/3 (2004), 311–28.

Scheidel, Walter, 'Libitina's Bitter Grain: Seasonal Mortality and Endemic Disease in the Ancient City of Rome', *Ancient Society* 25 (1994), 151–75.

Scheidel, Walter, 'Seasonal Mortality in the Roman Empire', in W. Scheidel (ed.), *Measuring Sex, Age and Death in the Roman Empire. Explorations in Ancient Demography* (Ann Arbor, 1996) 139–163.

Scheidel, Walter, *Death on the Nile: Disease and the Demography in Roman Egypt* (Leiden, 2001).

Shaw, Brent D., 'Seasons of Death: Aspects of Mortality in Imperial Rome', *Journal of Roman Studies* 86 (1996), 100–38.

Soren, David, and Soren, Noelle, *A Roman Villa and Late Roman Infant Cemetery: Excavation at Poggio Gramignano, Lugnano in Teverina* (Teverina, 1999), 633–49.

Stannard, Jerry, 'Diseases in Western Antiquity', in K. F. Kiple (ed.), *The Cambridge World History of Human Disease* (Cambridge, 1999), 262–9.

UNICEF, *State of the World's Children* (New York, 2013) <http://www.unicef.org.uk/Documents/Publication-pdfs/sowc-2013-children-with-disabilities.pdf>.

Verbrugge, L. M., and Jette, A. M., 'The Disablement Process', *Social Science and Medicine* 38/1 (1994), 1–14.

Waruiru, C. M., Newton, C. R., Forster, D., New, L., Winstanley, P., Mwangi, I., Marsh, V., Winstanley, M., Snow, R. W., and Marsh, K., 'Epileptic Seizures and Malaria in Kenyan Children', *Transactions of the Royal Society of Tropical Medicine and Hygiene* 90/2 (1996), 152–5.

Woods, Robert I., 'Ancient and Early Modern Mortality: Experience and Understanding', *Economic History Review* 60 (2007), 373–99.

Yeo, In-Sok, 'Hippocrates in the Context of Galen: Galen's Commentary on the Clarification of Fever in Epidemics VI', in P. van der Eijk (ed.), *Hippocrates in Context* (Leiden, 2005), 433–43.

Yousafzai, Aisha K., Filteau, S., and White, W., 'Feeding Difficulties in Disabled Children Leads to Malnutrition: Experience in an Indian Slum', *British Journal of Nutrition* 90 (2003), 1097–1106.

I

The ancient (near) East

3

DISABILITIES FROM HEAD TO FOOT IN HITTITE CIVILIZATION

Richard H. Beal

Introduction

The Hittites flourished in central Anatolia (today Turkey) from about 1800 to 1177 BCE. At least three languages were widely spoken in the kingdom: Hittite and Luwian (both Indo-European) and Hurrian. In the north Syrian part of the empire Hurrian and Semitic Amorite languages dominated. Hittite culture was heavily influenced by the indigenous Hattians and the Assyro-Babylonian culture of Mesopotamia. Hittite civilization survived the destructions at the end of the Bronze Age in the form of Luwian- and West Semitic-speaking petty states in southern Anatolia and north Syria until these were gradually absorbed into the Neo-Assyrian Empire by the early seventh century.

Hittite terms are attested for 'blind' (*dašuwant-*), 'deaf' (*dudumiyant-*) and 'lame' (*ikniyant-*). The same three disabilities are the most frequently mentioned in the Hebrew Bible (Raphael 2008: 13 and Kellenberger in this volume).

A case of (temporary) inability to speak is described in a text. Young king Muršili II was driving across country in his chariot when a violent thunderstorm terrified him. As a result 'the words in my mouth became small'. He soon recovered and forgot about it. Years passed. Then he had a series of terrifying nightmares and worried about what he had done to make the gods so angry. Finally in one nightmare a god touched his mouth and, as a result, he was unable to speak. This was a devastating blow for a king since, being himself illiterate like most other members of society, he would have had to rely on hand gestures to convey his orders and answers. Based on an oracular inquiry, a ritual was put together to cure him. This involved offerings, scapeoxen and sending all items worn and ridden in by the king on the day of the thunderstorm to the temple of the Stormgod of Manuzzi in the distant province of Kummanni (KBo 4.2 iii 40–2 and duplicates; ed. Lebrun 1983 and tr. Kümmel 1987: 289–92). This presumably worked since this king went on to have a long and successful reign, and so the ritual was filed away in the archives in case of future need.

Hittite texts do not mention the birth of any disabled person. An omen text, imported to the Hittite capital from Mesopotamia, predicts: 'If a woman gives birth and (the baby) is blind, the head of the household will not do well' (KBo 6.25 + KBo 13.35 ii 3–4; ed. Riemschneider 1970: 22–3). Eyesight is one of the things one asks the gods for along with 'life, health, vigor and a long life' (KBo 15.25 obv. 9–11, ed. Carruba 1966: 2–3).

Blindness

Intentional or accidental blinding is, however, referenced in our texts. In the Hittite law collection, dating to the early days of the kingdom, we learn that 'If anyone blinds a free man … formerly he paid (him) forty shekels of silver, but now he shall pay (him) twenty shekels of silver' (§7 = KBo 6.2 i 9–10, ed. Hoffner 1997: 21). A later modification of this law pronounces that: 'If anyone blinds a free man as a result of a quarrel he shall pay forty shekels of silver (to him). If it is an accident, he shall pay (him) twenty shekels' (§5 = KBo 6.4 i 14–15, ed. Hoffner 1997: 21). In both cases the penalty for blinding a slave or slave-girl is half of that. For comparison, forty shekels would buy a mule and twenty would buy a draft horse or twenty sheep. One shekel is the wage of a female harvester for three months' work (ed. Hoffner 1997: 7–8). Interestingly, the penalty for knocking out someone's teeth is identical to that for blinding (§7 = KBo 6.2 i 9–10, ed. Hoffner 1997: 21).

Blinding could also be inflicted by the state authorities, particularly in the Middle Hittite Period (for Persian and Byzantine parallels, see Coloru and Efthymiadis in this volume). An edict rules that 'if a slave steals and (the injured party) holds him for theft, if he has been blinded, they shall not hand him over (to the injured party). If he has not been blinded, they shall hand him over.' Presumably the thinking here is that if the master punishes his slave by blinding, thereby reducing his value to the master, the master has also punished himself for negligence in allowing the slave to steal. However, if the master does not punish the slave, that shows that the master is not simply negligent, but perhaps had ordered the slave to steal and so the master is punished by losing the slave. In contrast: 'If some free person steals and [he has] p[aid] compensation for the theft, they do not blind him, and they [do not] ha[nd him over to him (the injured party)]' (KUB 13.9 ii 11–19, ed. Miller 2013: 136–7 and 348). In a passage in a Middle Hittite instruction text for priests and temple officials showing that the gods will act just like humans: 'If a slave angers his master, they (presumably, the master and his household) will either kill him (the slave), or they will maltreat his nose, his eyes or his ears' (KUB 13.4 i 28–30, ed. Miller 2013: 248–9).

A Middle Hittite treaty stipulates that if the treaty partner receives a messenger who attempts to stir up trouble between the Hittite king and the treaty partner, the treaty partner must seize and blind the messenger and send him to the Hittite king (KUB 31.42 ii 10–14, w. dupls. KUB 31.44 ii 8–12 and KUB 26.24 ii 8–12, ed. Miller 2013: 200–1).[1] It is not clear from the text whether the 'messenger' is a Hittite traitor or the emissary of a hostile king attempting to lure away a Hittite subordinate. This blinding clause occurs only in three treaties with small loosely organized polities. Additionally, three more fragments of such treaties mention 'blind-men', one in a line following two paragraphs discussing 'hostages' (KBo 8.35 i 2'; KBo 17.48 obv. 3; KBo 16.27 + KBo 40.330 i 8–16). Internally, a Middle Hittite king uses the threat of blinding to hurry a subordinate, Kaššu, the military chief of the town of Tapigga, to carry out his orders: 'As soon as this tablet reaches you, drive quickly to My Majesty's presence and bring Maruwa of Gagadduwa. If you don't, they will come and blind you where you are' (HKM 14.10–14, ed. Hoffner 2009: 119–20, similarly HKM 16.11–15, ed. Hoffner 2009: 122–3).

An administrative text from Tapigga gives a list of captives and the amount of ransom that is being requested for them. Twenty-three of these high-value captives are said to be blind and two are said to be sighted (HKM 102, ed. del Monte 1995: 103–4). This is a rather high percentage of soldiers to have been accidentally blinded in battle, so presumably most, if not all, of the blinding occurred after these people were captured. It is not entirely clear whether these were people captured by the Hittites, blinded and being held until the enemy pays the demanded ransom or whether these are Hittites captured and blinded by the enemy, whose ransom demands are here enumerated. Letters from Tapigga mention Hittite capture of important enemies. These are said to be bound and sent to the king, but there is no mention of them being blinded (HKM 65, ed. Hoffner 2009: 217, see also Hoffner 2002: 67).

What became of these blind men? A letter from Šarpa in Šapinuwa to the governor in Tapigga records that 'Blind men have fled from the mill house and come to you there. As soon as this tablet reaches you, [seize the blind men and conduct them] safely [back here]' (HKM 59, ed. Hoffner 2009: 210). A letter from Tapigga back to Šapinuwa, perhaps in response, reads:

> Concerning the matter of the blind men that you wrote to me about, they have conducted all of the blind men up to the city of Šapinuwa. They have left ten men here to work in the mill houses. There is no one here by the name you wrote to me. You should ask Šarpa in Šapinuwa. All the (other) blind men are there.
>
> *(HKM 58.1–14, ed. Hoffner 2009: 207)*

So we learn that one important job of the blind was to mill grain, just as we see with the blinded captive Samson in the Hebrew Bible (Judges 16: 21). Among the Hittites this was done using a metate (and was usually women's work). Since some of these blind men have fled from their employment, presumably they were not doing this milling voluntarily, and were probably war-captives. That they managed to flee some considerable distance would imply either that they were only blinded in one eye or, more likely, that they had a sighted conspirator.

A blind man also plays a part in the 'Festival of Kingly Rank(?)', a festival performed for a prince. In this they strip a blind man and beat him before leading him to the charnel house (IBoT 1.29 rev. 39–41, ed. Mouton 2011: 10 and 16). He is not then killed and seems to play no further part in the ritual, at least as far as it is preserved. The reason for this is entirely unclear.

Blindness can be caused by the gods. In successive passages in an oath given to the army, the soldiers are given a demonstration of something and then told that if they break their oath the oath gods will do the same thing to them that they and the oath gods have just seen demonstrated.

> [The officiant blinds a ...] and says 'Because this was living and used to find heaven above. Just now they have blinded him/it in the place of the oath(-taking). Whoever transgresses these oaths, ... and sets his eyes on the land of Hatti as an enemy, let them blind his army, then let them deafen them. Let comrade not see comrade. Let this one not hear [that one.] May they give them an evil death. Below may they fetter their feet. Above may they bind their hands.'
>
> *(KBo 6.34 i 17'-30', ed. Oettinger 1976: 6–7; tr. Collins 1997: 165)*

Another section reads:

> They bring before them a woman, a blind man and a deaf man. You say to them as follows: 'Here are a woman, a blind man and a deaf man. Whoever plots harm against the king and queen, may the oath gods seize him. May they change him from a man into a woman, blind him like a blind man, deafen him like a deaf man and obliterate him, a mortal, together with his wives, and children and family.'
>
> *(KBo 6.34 iii 2–11, ed. Oettinger 1976: 12–13; tr. Collins 1997: 166)*

In this latter passage, it is clear that blindness and deafness, while they can be imposed on evildoers by the gods, are also disabilities, on the same level as being a woman. In the military oaths, blindness and deafness are among many bad fates that an oathbreaker will assuredly suffer.

However, there is no indication that all blindness was caused by the gods, or that all blindness was the result of misbehaviour/sin. In the ancient Near East, magic worked by saying and simultaneously showing the spirits what you wanted to happen, as in the above quoted military oaths. In one passage a blind person and a deaf person are presented as examples:

> In a meadow there stands a *šišiyamma*-tree. Beneath it sits a blind person and a deaf person. Does the blind person see? Absolutely not! Does the deaf person hear? Absolutely not! Does the lame person run? Absolutely not! In the same way let the words of sorcery not see the person for whom the ritual is performed.
>
> *(KUB 12.62 + KBo 53.3 rev. 7–10)*

Note that the people suffering these disabilities are not in anyway considered 'guilty' or 'sinful'. They are simply ordinary people with a disability, whose disability is being used to make a positive point. However, should the gods punish your tormenter as you are requesting, he/she will find themselves blind and/or deaf as punishment.

One magical text asks the gods to cause blindness and deafness:

> [Those who were continually terrifying [him], those who were continually frightening him, take (their) eyes from them, [(as) blind people]; take (their) ears from them (as) deaf people, (saying to them), 'Will you hear with your ears? Certainly not! Will you see with (your) eyes? Certainly not!'
>
> *(KUB 60.157 iii 7–10, ed. Arıkan-Soysal 2000: 220–1)*[2]

Another magical text requests: 'The person who bewitched me … May the apple take out his/her teeth. May the flint cut out his/her [tongue]. May the *šehuwal*-tool blind [his/her eyes]' (KUB 35.145 rev. 18–20, transliterated and tr. Soysal 1989: 183–4).

In a Hittite myth, when the Stormgod, king of the gods, loses his eyes and heart in a battle with a dragon, he is powerless, though still capable of engendering a son, until he underhandedly gets the dragon to return them (KBo 3.7 iii 10–12, 18–19, tr. Hoffner 1998: 13). In a Hurrian myth, a stone monster, born of the union of a god and a rock, is noted as being blind, deaf and without pity. There is no reason to believe these were in any way punishments for his being evil, or that they are anything but birth-defects, although perhaps the miscegenation at his engendering was thought to have had something to do with his disabilities. He is thus insensitive to the seductive allure and music of the goddess. However, he is stronger than all the gods combined (tr. Hoffner 1998: 55–65). It should be noted that none of the Hittite, Hurrian or Luwian gods or goddesses worshipped by the Hittites are described as disabled (unlike the Greek Hephaistos, for example). However, the Hurrian sky god Anu was emasculated by having his genitals bit off by his rival Kumarbi (tr. Hoffner 1998: 42–43).

Medicines and spells to cure clouded eyes and other eye diseases short of blindness are occasionally mentioned (*Hittite Dictionary* s.v. *šakui*- 1 a 3').

Deafness

We have seen the deaf mentioned alongside the blind in a number of the texts above. However, the deaf have another niche in Hittite society. A deaf person or persons, almost invariably male, play a role in a number of Hittite religious festivals. A festival from the early days of the Hittite kingdom reads: 'When it is morning, the deaf man and I go in and we pick up the bread and beverage offerings', that is, they remove the food left for the god to eat the night before (KBo 17.1

iv 24–5//KBo 17.3 iv 21–2, ed. Otten and Souček 1969: 38–9). In a fragmentary festival text a deaf man gives something to the queen. A deaf man performs a number of actions in the festival of the month. 'A deaf man carries a silver *akugalli*-vessel of water, and the king washes his hands' (KUB 2.13 i 8–9). At the end of the festival he is given something (VAS 28.28 iv 2). In the Winter Festival of the Sun 'the prince gives a bread-piece to the Chief of the Palace Servants. He carries it to the inner chamber and gives it to the deaf men' (KUB 2.6 ii 6–9). Here the highest civilian officer of the state carries an offering into the innermost chamber of the temple, where a deaf man is in attendance. In the festival for Underworld Deities, a deaf man and a palace servant prepare an aromatic oil and later the deaf man carries the sacrificed ram outside for cooking (KBo 11.32 obv. 19–27). In a different festival again a palace servant and a deaf man work together, with the latter carrying a sacrificial pig. Again, this time multiple deaf men and multiple palace servants carry sacred implements to the palace gate (KUB 58.52 ii 4–7). 'The deaf men sweep up' (KBo 19.128 vi 7, ed. Otten 1971: 16–17). Finally, again in the Festival of the Month, 'king goes outside to the hearths of the deaf men' (KUB 56.45 + VAS 28.28 ii 14–15). These deaf men are apparently part of an organization since in some festivals a chief or an overseer of the deaf men appears, for example, giving the king a cup to drink (KUB 58.38 ii 2, 8, 15 and KUB 10.21 v 15–16). A listing of professional groups includes 'deaf-men' (IBoT 3.75:5). While it is far from clear, it would appear that deaf men acted as menial servants in a few Hittite temples. It is interesting to note that Hittite gods required absolute ritual purity for those who served them, and since the king and queen were chief priest and priestess, those serving them needed to be ritually pure. The above examples show that deafness was not a bar to ritual purity and close contact with the gods, but perhaps even an advantage. As they could not hear nor reveal 'secrets', they might have been considered as ideal safeguards (see Laes 2011: 470 on expensive deaf slaves in Roman Antiquity).

Another job performed by deaf men involved the closing of the palace gate for the night:

> Then a palace servant goes up to the roof. A deaf man goes before him. The deaf man closes the window shutters and the palace servant throws the door-bolt closed. Then he comes down. The deaf man pulls closed (door at) the top of the ladder. The palace servant throws the bolt.
>
> *(KBo 5.11 iv 13–17, ed. Miller 2013: 96–7)*

As in the festivals, the deaf man works with a palace servant, and so there may have been deaf men as menial servants in the palace as well. Miller speculates (2013: 88) that they are employed so as not to overhear anything the royal family may say in confidence. There is also a town known as 'Deaf-man's Tell' (KUB 25.23 right edge).

Finally there is a curious mention of a deaf woman in an unfortunately broken text. 'Concerning the aforementioned matter of the taboo which [...]. The waiter (and?) the deaf woman lay down on account of [...] In the heart of that very temple [...] them' (KUB 18.40 rev. 9–12). The text is an oracular inquiry. It is not clear whether this involves checking the results of incubation in the temple or a sexual dalliance in the temple, which would be highly polluting, or something else entirely.

Lameness and mutilation

We have seen lame people mentioned above in passing. The laws order: 'If anyone breaks a free man's arm or leg, if he becomes disabled, he shall pay him twenty shekels of silver. If he does not become disabled, he shall pay him ten shekels of silver' (§10 = KBo 6.4 i 27–9, ed. Hoffner 1997: 25). The compensation is half these amounts for a slave (§11 = KBo 6.5 i 30–2, ed. Hoffner 1997: 26). The amount for permanently disabling a person's arm or leg is half the compensation for blinding. Another law requires:

> If someone injures a (free) person and temporarily incapacitates him, he shall provide medical care for him. In his place he shall provide a person to work on his estate until he recovers. When he recovers, (his assailant) shall pay him six shekels of silver and shall pay the medical bill.
>
> *(§10 = KBo 6.2 i 16–19, ed. Hoffner 1997: 23–4)*

Assaults affecting other senses also required compensation. 'If someone bites off the nose of a free person, he shall pay forty shekels of silver' (§13 = KBo 6.2 i 24, ed. Hoffner 1997: 26). Unbelievably, this is the same compensation that, as we saw, was originally paid for blinding. While society did have a use for the blind, one must believe that the high compensation for the loss of one's nose did not simply involve the impairment of smell, but also involved, shall we say, loss of face. The payment for someone whose ear was torn off, a far less disfiguring loss, was twelve shekels (§15 = KBo 6.3 i 37–8, ed. Hoffner 1997: 27) – only three if the victim was a slave (§16 = KBo 6.3 i 30, ed. Hoffner 1997: 28).

State-sanctioned punishments also included harming hearing and smelling.

> If a slave burglarizes a house, he (the slave or the master) must give (the stolen goods) back in full and give six shekels more for the theft. He (the victim?/the slave owner?) shall mutilate the slave's nose and ear, and they shall give him back to his master.
>
> *(§95 = KBo 6.2 iv 44–6//KBo 6.3 iv 42–3, ed. Hoffner 1997: 93–4)*

A slave arsonist was similarly treated (§99 = KBo 6.2 iv 56–7//KBo 19.4 iv 2–4, ed. Hoffner 1997: 96).

Sexual disability

A different sort of disability is impotence. Paškuwatti, a woman of the western Anatolian country of Arzawa, wrote up a treatment for 'If some man has no procreative power or is not a man vis-à-vis a woman'. The patient makes offerings to Uliliyašši, a goddess probably new to him, and probably a goddess of Paškuwatti's homeland. The goddess's name would indicate that she is a goddess of greenery. The patient removes his clothes and bathes and is then led to an uncultivated place in the steppe. He is handed a spindle and distaff (symbols of femininity) and walks through gates of reeds. Once on the other side of the gate the officiant takes away the spindle and distaff and gives him a bow and arrow and explains that she has taken away from him femininity and given him masculinity, taken away the behaviour of a woman and given him that of a man. She explains to the goddess that when this man went to the bedchamber, all he could produce was urine and faeces. She explains to the goddess that if he is able to produce sons and daughters with his wife he will honour and reward the goddess. She summons the goddess to the offerings and tells the patient to sleep beside the offering table. He is to report if he sees the goddess bodily in a dream, and if she looks at him and has sexual intercourse with him (perhaps a reference to a wet-dream). If so, he is cured. If not after three days, the ritual is to be repeated (KUB 9.27 + KUB 7.8 + KUB 7.5, ed. Harry Hoffner 1987).[3]

Obviously barrenness was also a problem. King Hattušili III wrote to his new friend Ramses II asking the Pharoah to send a pharmacist to cure his now elderly sister Matanazi of her barrenness, presumably on the assumption that exotic foreign medicine can cure things that domestic medicine has failed to cure. The Pharaoh informs Hattušili that Egyptian medicine cannot help a woman in her sixties give birth (ed. Beckman 1983: 253–4).

The absence of miracle stories

It is interesting to note that, in contrast to the Bible and later Christian literature, there are no miracle stories of the blind, deaf or lame being cured by divine intervention. The closest Hittites come to this (aside from the ritual for impotence cited above) is when the young prince Hattušili is judged too infirm to survive, and so in an effort to save his life, his father dedicates him to the service of the goddess Šaušga. He not only survives, but thrives in both temple service and in the military and government, eventually usurping the throne, for all of which he thanks Šaušga (KUB 1.1 ++ and duplicates, ed. Otten 1981, tr. van den Hout 1997). In his old age, Hattušili again suffered disabilities of the eyes and legs and feet and the queen asked the gods to cure him, but these requests (e.g. KBo 8.61: 5–7, ed. de Roos 2007: 130–1 and cf. 26–9) fit into the category of deities curing illnesses rather than performing miracles. It should also be noted that, in contrast to Judahite priests (Raphael 2008: 35) there is no indication that Hattušili's infirmities or Muršili's temporary disabilities (see above) in any way made them unfit to act as high priest to all the gods of the Hitttite Empire.

Exclusion and social disability

Thus some blind/deaf people were simply blind/deaf – the fate assigned to them at birth – while others were blinded/deafened as punishment. In no case were they considered impure or outcasts. In either case there were niches that the society found for them to support themselves.

Taggar-Cohen, in a recent article, states: 'The disabled represent the impure. They are not to enter the temple nor participate in festivals. If they do enter a temple, it is referred to as a sin against the gods' (Taggar-Cohen 2010: 119). As we have seen, the blind do not appear to have been particularly impure and those disabled by deafness hand things to the king and queen, whose ritual purity must be particularly guarded and sometimes serve in the holiest parts of temples during religious festivals. So what is Taggar-Cohen's evidence? An oracular inquiry that asks the god if this or that cultic infraction is the cause of the god's anger[4] reads:

> We further asked the temple personnel and they said: 'A dog went into the midst of the temple and knocked over the (offering) table. The thick-breads were thrown down. And they caused much of the daily thick-bread (offering) to be cut off (from the gods)'. Are you, O god, angry on this account? (Answer:) Unfavorable (i.e., Yes.). If you, O god, are angry only on account of those things, which we already know about, let the extispicy be favorable. (Answer:) Unfavorable. We asked the temple personnel and they said: 'two *kukuršant*-men went into the midst of the temple.' (Answer:) unfavorable. If this is all, ditto? *Hurri*-bird oracle: (answer:) unfavorable. We further asked them and they said: '*iškallant*-people went into the midst of the temple'. *Hurri*-bird oracle: (answer:) unfavorable.
>
> *(KUB 5.7 obv. 24–29, tr. Goetze 1969: 497)*

In another oracular inquiry:

> Because it was established that the god was angry because of defilement, we asked the temple personnel: Tīla said: 'One doesn't look at the Stormgod, but a woman

looked in the window. A child went into the midst of the temple. I was *iškalliyant* and we went into the temple.'

(AT 454 obv. 7-11, ed. Gurney 1953: 116–17)

Clearly since *kukuršant* and *iškallant* people entering the temple is of the same order of misdeed as a dog entering the temple and scattering the offerings, and a woman, of all things, breaking a taboo, *kukuršant-* and *iškallant*-people are somehow unclean and/or otherwise forbidden from entering the temple.

But are they disabled people as Taggar-Cohen states? The nominalized participal *kukuršant* appears to be a reduplicated form of the verb *kuer(š)-* 'to cut'. This would therefore appear to mean 'cut multiple times'. In the Old Hittite Laws, one reads:

> If a slave burglarizes a house, he shall give back precisely in full value (what he has stolen). And he shall pay six shekels of silvers for the theft. He (the victim?) shall repeatedly *kukurš-* (the slave's) nose and ears. If he stole much, much shall they impose on him. If he stole little, then little shall they impose on him.
>
> *(§95 = KBo 6.2 iv 44-47//KBo 6.3 iv 42-45, ed. Hoffner 1997: 93–4)*[5]

Presumably it is *kukurš*-ing that is being imposed on the slave's nose and ears. In an Old Hittite anecdote a miscreant is *kukurš*-ed for abandoning his post in the fear of the enemy (KBo 3.34 i 24–5, ed. Dardano 1997: 37 and cf. Beal 1992: 454 w.n. 1688). Finally, someone or something has his eyes blinded and his ears *kurkurš*-ed, but the context is unfortunately still unpublished (Bo 3640 iii 7–8, see Eheloff 1930: 397, and Hittite Dictionary s.v. *šakui-* 1 d 2' s'). Of suggested translations, since it can be done a little or much, 'mutilate' seems to fit best. Although once paired with the seriously debilitating 'blind', *kukurš-* seems more intended to mark out a criminal as a criminal (see Millburn in this volume).

Iškallant is the nominalized participle of the verb *iškallai-*. This verb too occurs in the laws: 'If anyone *iškallai*-s the ear of a free person, he shall pay six shekels of silver ... if anyone *iškallai*-s the ear of a slave he shall pay three shekels of silver' (KBo 6.3 i 37–9, ed. Hoffner 1997: 27–8). Other objects that one can *iškallai-* include garments, boxes, cheese. The translation 'tear-up', 'tear-off' seems to fit the occurrences. Thus the *kukuršant-* are those who have been mutilated, perhaps as a mark of criminality. Are *iškallant*-people those who have been 'torn-up', perhaps missing a body-part? It is curious, however, that in the second oracular inquiry the person committing a misdeed by being *iškallant-* when entering the temple was in fact a member of the temple staff, so was his *iškallant*-status temporary? In his testimony, he uses a past tense verb: 'I was *iškallant-*'. Could **iškallatar* be removed, like normal impurity (*papratar*) by washing and magic? Or does it imply someone with an open wound that could heal and so a person could resume his temple duties?

So it would appear that that those mutilated, perhaps as a sign of criminality and those who are somehow 'torn' could not enter a temple, perhaps due to impurity. However, it does not appear that all those who were disabled were impure. The deaf certainly do not fit into this category; it is far from clear that the blind or the lame are included in those forbidden from entering a temple; and the impotent spend time sleeping beside an offering table awaiting a visit from the goddess.

Notes

1 Cf. Miller 2013: 369 n. 275 where Miller thinks the word 'blind' must mean 'blind-fold'.
2 For both magical texts, see also *The Hittite Dictionary of the Oriental Institute of the University of Chicago* s.v. *lē* e.

3   On the contrary, Jared Miller argues that the purpose of the ritual is 'to cure the patient of his proclivity for passive sexual acquiescence and to replace it with an inclination toward normative male, i.e., penetrative power': see Miller 2010.
4   On oracle questions see Beal 2002.
5   Hoffner's translation has to be corrected. See similarly for a slave committing arson: Law §99 = KBo 6.2 iv 56–7//KBo 6.3 iv 55–6.

Bibliography

Primary sources

Classicists and ancient historians who have plentiful text editions at their disposal should be aware of the totally different situation of the Hittite records. Large and numerous volumes present the Hittite writings on tablets. The following abbreviations refer to volumes of pen and ink copies of the original cuneiform tablets:

IBoT   Istanbul Arkeoloji Müzelerinde Bulunan Boğazköy Tabletleri
KBo   Keilschrifttexte aus Boghazköi
KUB   Keilschrifturkunden aus Boghazköi
VAS   Vorderasiatische Schriftdenkmäler der Staatlichen Museen zu Berlin

However, these volumes do not present transliterations, let alone commentaries or translations. In the present contribution, 'ed.' means 'edited by', i.e. 'transliterated and translated by'. The list of the consulted edited or simply translated texts follows here:

Arıkan-Soysal, Yasemin, 'Hitit belgelerinde körler', *Archivum Anatolicum* 4 (2000), 207–24.
Beal, Richard, *The Organisation of the Hittite Military* (Heidelberg, 1992).
Beckman, Gary, *Hittite Birth Rituals* (Wiesbaden, 1983).
Carruba, Onofrio, *Das Beschwörungsritual für die Göttin Wišurijanza* (Wiesbaden, 1966).
Collins, Billie Jean, 'Canonical Compositions (Hittite), 3. Rituals', in W. W. Hallo (ed.), *The Context of Scripture: Canonical Compositions, Monumental Inscriptions and Archival Documents from the Biblical World*, I (Leiden, 1996), 160–8.
Dardano, Paola, *L'aneddoto e il racconto in eta' antico-Hittita: La cosiddetta 'cronaca di Palazzo'* (Rome, 1997).
del Monte, Giuseppe, 'I testi amministrativi da Maşat Höyük/Tapika', *Orientis Antiqui Miscellanea* 2 (1995), 89–138.
de Roos, Johan, *Hittite Votive Texts* (Leiden, 2007).
Ehelolf, Hans, 'Zum hethitischen Lexikon', *Kleinasiatische Forschungen* 1 (1930), 137–60.
Goetze, Albrecht, 'Oracles and Prophecies', in J. Pritchard (ed.), *Ancient Near Eastern Texts Relating to the Old Testament* (Princeton, NJ, 1969), 497.
Gurney, Oliver, 'A Hittite Divination Text', in D. J. Wiseman, *The Alalah Texts* (London, 1953), 116–18.
Hoffner, Harry, 'Paskuwatti's Ritual Against Sexual Impotence (CTH 406)', *Aula Orientalis* 5 (1987), 271–87.
Hoffner, Harry, *The Laws of the Hittites* (Leiden, 1997).
Hoffner, Harry, *Hittite Myths* (Atlanta, GA, 1998²).
Hoffner, Harry, *Letters from the Hittite Kingdom* (Atlanta, GA, 2009).
Kümmel, Hans Martin, in *Texte aus der Umwelt des Alten Testaments*, II/2. *Rituale und Beschwörungen* 1 (Gütersloh, 1987), 289–92.
Lebrun, René, 'L'aphasie de Mursili II (CTH 486)', *Hethitica* 5 (1983), 103–37.
Miller, Jared, *Royal Hittite Instructions and Related Administrative Texts* (Atlanta, GA, 2013).
Mouton, Alice, 'Réflexions autour de la notion de ritual initiatique en Anatolie hittite. Au subject de la fête Haššumaš (CTH 633)', *Journal of Ancient Near Eastern Religions* 11 (2011), 1–38.
Oettinger, Norbert, *Die Militärischen Eide der Hethiter* (Wiesbaden, 1976).
Otten, Heinrich, *Ein hethitische Festritual* (Wiesbaden, 1971).

Otten, Heinrich, *Die Apologie Hattusilis III* (Wiesbaden, 1981).

Otten, Heinrich, and Souček, Vladimir, *Ein althethitisches Ritual für das Königspaar* (Wiesbaden, 1969).

Riemschneider, Kaspar, *Babylonische Geburtsomina in hethitischer Übersetzung* (Wiesbaden, 1970).

Soysal, Oğuz, 'Die Apfel möge die Zähne nehmen', *Orientalia* NS 58 (1989), 172–91.

van den Hout, Theo, 'The Apology of Hattušili (I.B.3.b)', in W. W. Hallo (ed.), *The Context of Scripture: Canonical Compositions, Monumental Inscriptions and Archival Documents from the Biblical World*, I (Leiden, 1997), 199–204.

Secondary sources

Arıkan, Yasemin, 'The Blind in Hittite Documents', *Altorientalische Forschungen* 33 (2006), 144–54.

Beal, Richard, 'Gleanings from Hittite Oracle Questions on Religion, Society, Psychology and Decision Making', in P. Taracha, *Silvia Anatolica: Anatolian Studies Presented to Maciej Popko on the Occasion of his 65th Birthday* (Warsaw, 2002), 11–37.

Hoffner, Harry A., 'The Disabled and Infirm in Hittite Society', *Hayim and Miriam Tadmor Volume. Eretz-Israel* 27 (2003) 84*–90*.

Hoffner, Harry A., 'The Treatment and Longterm Use of Persons Captured in Battle', in K. A. Yener and H. A. Hoffner, Jr. (eds), *Recent Developments in Hittite Archaeology and History* (Winona Lake, IN, 2002), 61–72.

Laes, Chr., 'Silent Witnesses: Deaf-Mutes in Graeco-Roman Antiquity', *Classical World* 104/4 (2011), 451–73.

Miller, Jared, 'Paskuwatti's Ritual: Remedy for Impotence or Antidote to Homosexuality', *Journal of Ancient Near Eastern Religions* 10 (2010), 83–9.

Milles, M., 'Hittite Deaf Men in the 13th Century BC: Introductory Notes with Annotated Bibliography' (2008–9) <www.independentliving.org/docs7/miles200809.html> and <www.independentliving.org/docs7/miles200809.pdf>.

Raphael, Rebecca, *Biblica Corpora: Representation of Disability in Hebrew Biblical Literature* (London, 2008).

Siegelová, Jana, 'Blendung als Strafe', *Anatolia Antica: Studi in memoria di Fiorella Imparati.* (Florence, 2002), 735–7.

Taggar-Cohen, Ada, 'The Prince, the KAR.KID Women and the *arzana*-House: A Hittite Royal Festival to the Goddess *Kataḫḫa* (CTH 633)', *Altorientalische Forschungen* 37 (2010), 113–31.

4

MESOPOTAMIA
AND ISRAEL

Edgar Kellenberger

Introduction

As early as the end of the third millennium BCE, Mesopotamian texts mention the topic of disability. There is a rich variety of excavated cuneiform documents demonstrating different perceptions of disabilities. These documents include myths, lexical lists, provision lists, medical and magic literature, omina (systematic collections of omens), curses (in inscriptions), prayers, royal inscriptions, letters, proverbs and wisdom literature. This wide spectrum is important for our understanding of disability. Less important are geographic and political differences (the city-states and proto-empires including Assyria in the upper part of Mesopotamia and Babylonia in the lower part competed for supremacy).

The chronological spectrum of more than 2,000 years is negligible in the face of the strongly traditional textual culture, the scribes of which were occupied with the process of collecting and reproducing texts, which ranged from many centuries to a millennium in age. The majority of extant texts are in the Akkadian language. In the 2nd millennium BCE, only the few literate Mesopotamian scholars could understand the older Sumerian language. After the conquest of the area by the Persian Empire in the 6th century the use of Akkadian, too, became more and more restricted to scholars, but the cuneiform clay tablets, on which both languages were recorded, were produced until late Hellenistic times.

For several reasons, disability scholars of Mesopotamian studies have better research opportunities than those who study ancient Israel. The few excavated Hebrew (and Aramaic) texts do not mention disabilities; we are, therefore, restricted to the limited corpus of the Old Testament. These texts were collected, copied and canonized in the context of a much narrower religious interest than is the case for our sources about everyday life in Mesopotamia. Extrapolating information about Mesopotamia to Israel is often plausible but always risky. Fixing the date of origin of most Old Testament texts is impossible, because they were reworked and actualized over many centuries, within a living religious tradition. As opposed to the course of Mesopotamian history, furthermore, the Old Testament has no break-off of tradition; instead, after Hellenism, there is a twofold continuation of Jewish-rabbinic and Christian literature. This chapter includes some notes on the New Testament as well as the Mishna and other rabbinic sources, though both these traditions are the subject of separate chapters in this volume (see Chapters 22 and 30).

The author of this chapter is the father of a son with an intellectual disability[1] (resulting in a different world than that shaped by physical impairment). The author is privileged as compared with many parents, historically. He and his wife had the free choice to foster and adopt this child. Other parents have been routinely deprived of such a choice.

Attempts of systematization

A general term 'disabled' is missing in the records of the ancient cultures in Mesopotamia and Israel. But the designations of many concrete disabilities are formed by the same noun pattern. Semitic language is structured by semantic roots of (mostly) three consonants (paradigma: *PRS*). In Akkadian, many disability designations follow the noun pattern *PuRRuSu*; Renger (1992: 125–6) lists seventeen examples from a wide spectrum of physical as well as mental impairments. In Hebrew, the pattern *PaRRiS* (also with doubling the middle consonant) designates common variations in seeing, hearing and walking; we find, in addition, references to mute people, the condition of hunchback, and two different designations for bald-headed people (Schipper 2006: 65–9; Olyan 2008: 145–6). Strikingly, neither mental impairments nor impairments of the psyche are referred to by this Hebrew pattern.

Mesopotamia

Early human efforts at systematizing their chaotic world gave rise to the Mesopotamian 'lists'.[2] Various lexical lists (mostly bilingual Sumerian-Akkadian) organize the vocabulary, either by cuneiform signs or by content-related context. In the latter case, nearly synonymous lexemes appear in a row, reflecting the structure of the Mesopotamian worldview. The collection series *Malku* successively brings expressions for 'poor/weak/stupid/crippled' (Hrůša 2010: 12 and 381; further texts e.g. in Reiner *et al.* 1969: 228–9; Civil *et al.* 1979: 278). From such associative combinations we can conjecture how disability was perceived in Mesopotamian thought.

Particularly significant for this inquiry are the systematizing collections of omens. More than 2,000 conceivable birth anomalies (in humans and animals) are collected in *Šumma Izbu* ('if a birth anomaly ... '). Each anomaly is noted with an indication of the effect that is expected in the future (for the family, the country or the king). The following sequence provides an example ([+] signifies a positive consequence, [–] a negative, and the absence of a sign indicates a textual gap):

> If a woman gives birth to wind ... / ... body[–] / idiot (*lillu*)[–] / female idiot / dwarf (masc.[–] / fem.[–]) / cripple (m.[–] / f.[–]) / shape (m.[+]/f.[+]) / blind[–] / contorted[–] / deaf[+] / ... / epileptic[–] / ...
> *(Leichty 1970: 36–7)*

We find a different range of portents in the omen collection *Šumma Alu*, which indicates over 10,000 observations about life in a city:

> If many ... in a city are: ... lame (m./f.[+]) / idiots (m.[+]/f.) / soft men[–] / wise men[–] / men with warts[–] / red men[+] / pockmarked men[–] / deaf men[+] / blind men[–] / cultic performers[–] / openers (?)[–] / cripples[–] / disabled men[–] / runners[–] / ecstatics (m.[–]/f.[–]) / weaklings[–] ...
> *(Freedman 1998: 33)*

The wide range of observations is surprising. Unfortunately, the respective logic of a positive or negative effect is inscrutable to us, even though we can assume that dealing with omens was a science with rational rules.

The so-called *kudurru* inscriptions are land ownership certificates which were usually recorded on a small stele in a sanctuary. In order to protect these important stone documents from theft and malicious destruction, long curse formulations were written and posted. Towards the end of the curse-section we often find the following formulations (in different sequence and detail; see Paulus 2014: 223–5):

> Whoever because he fears these curses causes either a simpleton (*ulālu; saklu*), a person with stopped-up ears, a convictionless person, a powerless, a brutish, a babbler, a weakling ... to take away the stele ...

whereupon follow new curses, expressly directed against the coward commissioner who instrumentalized for his selfish purposes people with (predominantly mental) disabilities. The wide spectrum of the people in the *kudurru* inscriptions appears realistic, even if the precise meaning of some terms remains unclear to us.

In literary texts, references to physical and mental disabilities appear in combination, such as the complaint by a senior official who lost his job position and social contacts by an incurable disease: 'A cripple (*kuṣṣudu*) rises above me, a fool (*lillu*) is ahead of me' (Hallo 1997: 493; further examples in the Assyrian Dictionary under *lillu*). Already in the Sumerian myth 'Enki and Ninmah' (early 2nd millennium BCE), the mother goddess creates seven human beings with physical and mental disabilities (Lambert 2013: 339; Ceccarelli 2016; Pittl 2015). The types of disability include trembling hands, blindness, lame feet, intellectual disability, dribbling of urine (or semen), incapability of giving birth, neither penis nor vagina (?). No systematic order is identifiable here, but elsewhere we find the order 'A Capite ad Calcem', starting from the Sumerian epic 'Enki and Ninhursag' and very often in medical texts, which mention exclusively physical deficits (Böck 2014: 46).

Israel

More limited than the noun pattern *PaRRiS* is the Hebrew conceptual term 'blemish' (*mûm*), which is used to designate some physical anomalies. The etymology is unclear. The Septuagint translates the term as μῶμος, which is used to indicate 'blame' or 'disgrace' in non-Jewish Greek literature. The criteria for whether an impairment counts as *mûm* or not are not crystal clear. Often it concerns the aesthetic ideal of symmetrical body halves (Olyan 2008); e.g. a knocked-out tooth is considered a blemish (Lev. 24: 20). The bodies of sacrificial animals and of the priests had to be without blemish (Lev. 22: 18–25, 21: 17–23, etc.; for Mesopotamia see Walls 2007: 26). Both lists mention twelve blemishes, e.g. a deformed limb (perhaps innate or from a badly healed fracture), paralysis, visible deformation of an eye (iris discoloration and blindness), but also – hardly visible in a dressed man attending sacrifice – deformed testicles (cf. Schipper and Stackert 2013). Other impairments never appear under the term 'blemish': deafness, muteness, psychic and mental disorders, as well as polluting phenomena like skin diseases, seminal discharges and menstruation, are absent.

The ministry of sacrifice was forbidden to blemished priests, though such persons kept all other priestly rights (Lev. 21: 21–2: 'he shall eat the bread of his God, both of the most holy, and of the holy'). This allowed a sort of social security in the case of later acquired impairment. Presumably the stewards of the sanctuary had to ensure that families did not donate those animals (for sacrifice) and sons (as priest candidates) that they could not use for themselves (Hieke 2014). More severe preconditions for priests are mentioned at Qumran (Dorman 2007) and in the Mishna, enumerating even more blemishes.

Other lists of disabilities are more associative than systematic. Most frequent are the word pairs 'blind and lame' and 'deaf and blind'. Some enumerations mention people with physical disabilities together with others who suffer from misery or poverty such as widows, orphans and strangers (in Jer. 31: 8 together with pregnant women and women in childbed). Such people were vulnerable socially: infertile women and men, too, belonged to the margins of society and as such appear on the lists (Ps. 113: 7–9; Job 24: 21; Bereshit Rabba 53: 8; cf. Isa. 56: 3–7).

We find no enumeration of combined physical and mental disabilities. This could be due to the limited corpus of the Old Testament, since one occasionally finds such intermingling at Qumran and in rabbinic texts (Kellenberger 2011: 57; also Bammidbar Rabba 13: 8 and Bereshit Rabba 58: 8). However, the above-discussed Hebrew noun pattern *PaRRiS* never seems to have been used for mental disabilities.

Medical concepts

In contrast to the sparse information for ancient Israel (Beyerle 2008), Mesopotamian medicine is lavishly documented. From a period of over a thousand years we have at our disposal countless symptom observations, reaction tests, diagnoses (often attributed to divine or demonic responsibility), treatments, recipes (from 250 different substances!) and prognoses. In these texts, we find both a strange closeness and a distance when compared to today's medical efforts. While many Mesopotamian medical conventions make immediate sense to us, religious considerations and magical incantations can seem strange, though it is often the very same medically skilled person who performs both magical and rational medicine on the same patient. Behind the magical activities there is the same strictness of rationality and empiricism expressed in modern pharmaceutical practice (Maul 2004; Scurlock 2006: 75–83; but cf. Geller 2010, who separates medicine and magic as different entities). Not all of the Mesopotamian diseases can be identified without difficulty in our modern terms. Philological uncertainties make absolute identification problematic, and the danger of retrospective diagnosis and imposing modern ideas on the ancient texts also keeps us from being able to make definite medical correlations.

Admittedly, today's (however blurred) distinction between illness and disability cannot be transferred uncritically to Mesopotamia. But it is interesting to study which types of disability were perceived and treated, which remained without treatment (annotation: 'he will die') and which are absent in the sources. Particularly striking is the intense engagement with epileptic phenomena, some of which are represented as treatable. The same applies to different types of paralysis. Blindness and deafness are hardly ever mentioned, and the therapeutic magic rarely deals with either, though eye and ear diseases are often mentioned. In the category of untreatable conditions, we see – if these modern identifications apply – cerebral palsy, spinal muscular atrophy, floppy baby syndrome, Huntington's disease, spina bifida and hydrocephalus (Scurlock and Andersen 2005: 331–6, 398, 412). Intellectual disability was also outside Mesopotamian medical interest, so designations such as *lillu* are absent from these texts. Only once the 'protruding tongue' of a person with mental deficits (*la ṭêmu*) is mentioned, possibly indicating a typical symptom of trisomy 21; but this observation is immediately set in opposition to the same, but temporary and treatable symptom (Scurlock and Andersen 2005: 442).

'Hopeless' cases

The frequent prognosis 'he will die' does not mention what the physician was to do in such cases. It probably belongs to the rationality of Mesopotamian medicine that, in some cases, neither incantations nor other therapeutic activities were recommended.

In the cases of a birth anomaly (*izbu*) and its interpretation as an unfavorable omen, we are informed about its consequences (Leichty 1970: 7–14). Letters of the royal staff indicate that birth anomalies were reported. A *barû*-priest decided whether or not a birth merited reporting on the basis of the collection *Šumma Izbu,* and gave an oral or written recommendation, whereupon a complicated *namburbû* ritual was carried out in order to expiate the evil. In a time-consuming and expensive process, the animal or the human newborn (some of which may have been stillbirths) was thrown into the river and so disposed of (Maul 1994: 336–42). Since this expensive procedure was feasible only in the upper classes, there were perhaps also simpler solutions (prayers, amulets). In addition, it must be asked whether all birth anomalies were reported by the parents. We do not know if an anomalous birth carried the same weight among common people.

Many impairments listed in *Šumma Izbu* as unfavourable omens are detectable only long after birth (e.g. blindness, intellectual disability), which demonstrates that children with disabilities were reared and remained alive. Texts mention the existence of many children and adults with disabilities (e.g. Freedman 1998: 33). No judgement is possible, however, of these people's quality of life.

In some rare cases, the anxiety over a particularly significant disability was so great that medical texts advised their eradication 'root and branch' (Scurlock and Andersen 2005: 332–6): A newborn with spastic symptoms who 'wails, twists and is continually rigid' should be buried 'like a stillbirth' so 'the evil will be carried away (with him)'. In another case, an infant who since birth 'does not wail (or) cry or stiffen up' (floppy baby syndrome?) should be thrown away into the water, 'and the evil will be carried away'. In both cases, the unusual procedure is necessary because otherwise 'the destruction of the house of his father' was imminent. That could mean that the family integrity was strained by childcare which demanded too much of the parents. There are also repeated instances in *Šumma Izbu* of the prognosis that the father's house will collapse (*sapahu*) after an extreme birth anomaly, which could refer to the breakup of the family unit.

An unusual procedure was advised for people even of an advanced age. The following text detailed the symptoms that merited this exceptional procedure:

> When a mournful cry roars to him and he continually answers it, he continually cries out 'my father (and) mother or my brothers and my sisters will die' [without] recognizing anybody, [he continually wails] (and) when he has wailed goes to sleep and does not get up (and) when his affliction has left him, he does not know what he wailed.
>
> *(Scurlock and Andersen 2005: 335, supposing Huntington's disease with motor and depressive suffering)*

In such a case, the god Šulpae is responsible, and they shall 'burn (the patient) by fire'. In another case, a patient is to be buried alive:

> If an affliction afflicts him while he is going along the road and when it afflicts him he makes his hands and feet writhe in contortion against the earth, his eyes are dark, his nostrils are contracted, (and) he eats his garments.
>
> *(Scurlock and Andersen 2005: 335)*

Again, the god Šulpae is responsible, and 'destruction of the house of his father' is a threatening possibility. Then follows the advice: 'In order not to approach (the parents) you bury him alive in the earth; its evil will be dispelled.'

Observations about the hereditary character of an illness may be the cause of such extreme 'solutions'. This would explain why the perceived evil had to be eradicated in such an unusual way. The perceptions of diseases that carried hereditary evil could have had the consequence of thinking it necessary to eliminate more than one member of the same family.

Despite these exceptional cases we should keep in mind that Mesopotamian medicine was generally characterized by deep and long-time commitment to the patient.

Blindness

Blindness is the most mentioned disability in the ancient Near East. This condition, which could be perceived as evil, is mentioned frequently also in curses, pronounced against private enemies or made as a threat, in the case, for example, of a breach of a contract. Also often mentioned in curses are dropsy and leprosy, but rarely deafness, paralysis or epilepsy, although these conditions frequently occurred and might have been equally fit to act as a threat deterrent.

Conditions of life for ordinary people were difficult, as is evident from Sumerian texts of the temple economy. Provision lists mention food rations for people who were donated to the sanctuary (or 'gave' themselves) and then worked there. This happened often because of poverty, as is clear from the social characteristics of these workers: 'widows, orphans, old people, especially old women, sterile and childless women, cripples, especially blind and deaf persons, beggars and vagabonds' (Gelb 1972: 10). The lists document many dead, sick or fugitive workers: life as a temple worker was no paradise. The monarchy, which was an important economic power, also set to work people with significant disabilities. Texts mention visually impaired plantation workers, reed weavers, grain grinders, musicians and singers (Fincke 2000: 63–8; cf. Heimpel 2009). The latter are also mentioned in the Sumerian myth 'Enki and Ninmah'; serving as a musician was a typical vocation for people with visual impairments.

But there are also statements in prayers that a deity can give sight to the blind (Assyrian Dictionary under *naṭilu*, in the Old Testament Psalm 146:8). In the same way as the Old Testament promises (Isa. 35: 5, 42: 7–23, etc.), this begs the ultimately unanswerable questions: what could visually impaired people gain from such words, if anything? These words were probably metaphors, addressed to sighted people. To blind or deaf people, it could have seemed especially irritating that Israel's prophets metaphorically use blindness and deafness in their accusations and announcements of judgement, for polemical purposes, and in a negative rating. But jumping to conclusions about the prophet's understanding of disability would be just as problematic as when one accused Jesus of glorification of capitalism by the argument that in several parables (e.g. Matt. 25: 14–30) the main figure is a cynical capitalist.

The law to put no obstacle in the way of a visually impaired person (Lev. 19:14) and not to lead him down the wrong way (Deut. 27: 18) clearly was addressed to sighted people. Deuteronomy 27 is a series of curses against twelve clandestine offences that cannot be avenged in the absence of witnesses (two examples are incest and clandestine adoration of an idol); these misdeeds (e.g. leading a blind person down the wrong path) are to be prevented prophylactically by a spoken 'amen' of the whole congregation. Such prohibitions are missing in the rest of the ancient Near East, except for the prohibition of mocking (in Egypt: Amenemope 25). However, anyone who starts from the modern construct of equal autonomous individuals must criticize such protection provisions (cf. also Job 29: 15) as paternalistic (Raphael 2008: 36).

To Moses, who pretends to be speech impaired and therefore incapable of following God's call, God answers with a counter-question (Exod. 4: 11): 'Who made man's mouth? Or who makes one mute, or deaf, or seeing, or blind? Isn't it I, Yahweh?' God's mention of blindness exceeds Moses' argument and aligns Moses' commission with tasks of both able and (variously) disabled people. Contrary to earlier praise of divine sovereignty elicited by this passage, today it seems to degenerate into a cynical consolation, because ever since the Enlightenment, the biblical statement does not fit into the Procrustean bed of a God who is always benevolent.[3]

In Mesopotamia, as among the Greeks, there was awareness of congenital blindness and other disabilities (Kellenberger 2013 with note 5). In addition, there are records of people who acquired blindness later, and references to gouging out somebody's eyes (e.g. Samson, by the Philistines), which was a standard punishment in Mesopotamia. The Hellenistic (?) story of Tobit's total blindness, healed by fish liver, is exceptional in the Old Testament, but such a therapy is also documented in Mesopotamia and Greece (Fitzmyer 2003: 208–9).

Impairments of the extremities

The Akkadian language has many expressions for 'crippled, maimed, lame', the precise meaning of which cannot always be determined. The Sumerian myth 'Enki and Ninmah' describes the third person in the myth as 'paralysed on his feet' (so most editions, e.g. Hallo 1997: 518; sceptical Lambert 2013: 339; cf. supra p. 49). Enki made him a silversmith, which is reminiscent of the Greek Hephaestus myth.

In the Old Testament, the pairing 'blind and lame' is familiar in various contexts. However, the exact meaning of the saying 'the blind and the lame will (should?) not come into the house' (2 Sam. 5: 8) is unclear. It remains controversial whether the context refers to the temple (Olyan 2008) or to the palace (Schipper 2006). In 2 Samuel we see mention of Saul's son Mephiboshet, whose legs were paralysed by an accident, in which the nurse dropped the 5-year-old child in her hasty flight (4: 4). Schipper (2006) made a subtle study of Mephiboshet, who was allowed to eat at the royal table thanks to David's grace (other interpretations in Hentrich 2013). Schipper eschews contrastive value judgements, but sees statements about disability within a differentiated network of figures related to each other. While he understands paralysis as an obstacle for becoming king, it must be recalled that some Egyptian and Assyrian kings did suffer from significant disabilities. Esarhaddon (7th century), recorded as suffering heavily from a visible chronic and incurable disease, reigned successfully over the mighty Assyrian Empire (Radner 2006).

God is responsible for Jacob's limping after his wrestling at the Jabbok River (Gen. 32) and for the multiply maimed 'suffering servant' (Isa. 53). Valuable studies come from Wynn (2007a) and Schipper (2011), emphasizing the autonomous view of the Old Testament representation which was opposite to modern constructs of disability (and possibly also to popular views of its time); Isaiah 53 describes 'a social experience' and a literary procedure, but not a medical diagnosis.

Hearing impairment

The meaning of the Akkadian terms *sakku* and *sukkuku* ranges from 'blocked' to 'deaf' and 'dumb'. Often, the meaning of the lexemes is blurred (e.g. in the *kudurru* inscriptions). The linking of an inability to speak with intellectual deficits appears in many societies. The causes of the inability to speak are not taken into account.

Unlike blindness, deafness appears rarely in curses and imprecations. Deafness – as blindness and paralysis – is occasionally wished upon a demon, to render him unable to harm people (Kellenberger 2013: 457 with note 43). The Old Testament provision not to curse a deaf man (Lev. 19: 14) is missing in the rest of ancient Near East; this provision probably concerns the inability of the accursed person of taking countermeasures against a curse which he would not notice. The function of the goddess Sukkukutu ('numbness') and the god Lillu ('mentally disabled'), documented in cuneiform fragments, remains an open question.

A narrower range of professions was open to deaf people (as well as to people otherwise impaired) than to people without deafness, as suggested in Mesopotamia by 'sheltered jobs' in the royal and the temple economy during the early 2nd millennium. A thousand years later, we see royal alimentation programmes (Kellenberger 2013 with notes 58–9).

Unlike Akkadian, the Hebrew *ḥereš* belongs to the root *ḤRŠ* 'quiet, silent'. Again, the line between deaf and mute (*'illem*) is blurred. Moses' 'heavy tongue and mouth' (Exod. 4: 10–12) may refer to a physiological disability (Schipper 2011: 27), or to his being utterly awed by God's order. And the Psalms use metaphors in which either the supplicants or God Himself are 'mute/deaf' (valuable interpretation by Raphael 2008: 110–19).

Epilepsy and other neurological disorders

Mesopotamia

The precise symptoms and effects of cerebral palsy were observed in Mesopotamia (Scurlock and Andersen 2005: 331). In addition, the physicians practised a diagnostic test for reflexes (today known as the Moro reflex test): the diagnostician holds the infant's head and then withdraws support, allowing the head to fall backward. Most infants quickly flex their extremities and then extend their arms wide open. The absence of this reaction points to cerebral palsy or other neurological disorders (Scurlock and Andersen 2005: 341; also, further tests). Typical phenomena of dyslexia (wrong direction of writing, etc.) could be detected in a pupil's exercise tablet (Foster 2003: 86), then as now.

The very differing views on epilepsy in Mesopotamian medicine are demonstrated particularly well in the diagnostic-prognostic collection *Sakikkû* ('symptoms', around 1000 BCE), where phenomena of epilepsy account for more than one-eighth of a total of 4,000 lines (Heeßel 2000). The density of observation (differentiated according to the stages of life) as well as the variety of diagnoses and treatments are impressive. Even the terminology here (as in other texts) is manifold, including *bennu* (most general term), *antašubba* (Sumerian 'what has fallen from heaven'), *miqtu* ('fall'), *rihut* *ᵈŠulpaea* ('spawn of the god Šulpaea'), *Lugal-urra* (Sumerian 'Lord of the Roof'). Some scholars suggest that not all cases should be interpreted as epilepsy (cf. the maximalist view by Stol 1993 with the minimalist by Scurlock and Andersen 2005).

The reality of epilepsy is demonstrated as early as the law of Hammurabi in the early 2nd millennium, where slave sales needed a waiting period of one month (later, a hundred days), within which a slave who turned out to be epileptic could be sent back to his previous master. A similar practice existed among the Greeks and Romans (Stol 1993: 138–41).

Israel (incl. New Testament)

Given these realities, it is surprising that epilepsy is never mentioned in the Old Testament, in deuterocanonical writings or in the Qumran scrolls (Bendemann 2008).[4] The Mishna has one single mention of epilepsy (a prohibition of priestly ministry in Bekhorot 7: 5). Talmud passages discuss some consequences regarding people with epilepsy, who are designated *nikpeh* (passive participle of 'overthrow'). Striking is the sober-mindedness of the Jewish scholars who are primarily interested in prevention, and therefore take seriously the hereditary character of epilepsy. In contrast to other diseases, therapeutic efforts are largely missing. Occasionally epilepsy is discussed in terms of unusual sexual practices (such as seeing one's wife naked or taking unusual positions during copulation) – specifically, whether or not they are the cause of epileptic and otherwise disabled children – but ultimately, all forms of marital intercourse are allowed (Pesachim 112b; Nedarim 20b). Demonological assignations are rare, and ideas of demonic possession are non-existent. As such, Bendemann suggests a deliberately polemical point against both pagan and Christian practices. In contrast to rabbinic writings, the Synoptic Gospels stressed demonology, and they give detailed descriptions of epileptic symptoms.

However, instead of presuming a somewhat unexpected innovation by the New Testament, I prefer to see a continuity between the evangelists and the age-old Mesopotamian tradition, where gods and demons were important agents of epilepsy. The demon's name 'Lord of the roof' is documented from the Sumerian texts up to the Syriac translation of Matthew 17: 15 (Stol 1993: 16–19) and to late antique and medieval Jewish incantations against epilepsy found in the Cairo Geniza (see Kellenberger 2013 with note 46; Naveh and Shaked 1993: 140, and 1998: 179; Kwasman 2007). Thus, if a *longue durée* is detected, the cause for the striking Old Testament and rabbinic reserve is to be sought elsewhere. This could be explained by a class-specific attitude of elites against universal popular religious ideas. The latter led a life of their own outside the canonical and rabbinic tradition and are visible in magical incantations and in the pseudepigraphic Testament of Solomon 18: 21. The Gospel of Mark and his successors, with their descriptions of epilepsy and with reports of exorcisms, are closer to the popular religious ideas than to those of the intellectual elites. But Mark now integrated these exorcisms into the new context of Jesus' crucifixion and resurrection, which are prefigured in Jesus' work on the epileptic boy, who becomes like a dead person and is brought to new life (cf. Mark 9: 26–7 with Luke 7: 15). In spite of the clear description of epilepsy, the root ἐπιλημπ- is missing in the New Testament. Matthew only speaks of σεληνιάζεσθαι (4: 24 and 17: 15).

Early Christianity will view epilepsy as a genuine ecclesiastical task with exorcism and prayer, taking it away from the ancient physicians. Based on our modern values, Bendemann interprets this treatment as social exclusion (2008: 42), but source evidence of anyone›s experience with epilepsy, for example by slaves or other persons, is lacking.

Intellectual disability

Mesopotamia

Because of the sparse source material the detection of people with intellectual disabilities is still in its infancy (Kellenberger 2011, 2013). A passage in the Gilgamesh epic, which paints a detailed portrait of such a man (*lillu*) sheds some light on the issue:

> What is given to the fool (*lillu*) is [beer] sludge instead of [...] ghee,
> [he chews] bran and grist instead of [...]
> He is clad in a *mašhandu*-garment, instead of [...,]
> instead of a belt, a cord of [...]
> Because he has no advisers [...]
> because he has no words of counsel [.....,]
> have thought for him, Gilgamesh, [......]!
>
> *(George 2003: 695)*

This somewhat unpleasant portrait presents a contrast to the privileged Gilgamesh. The *lillu* lacks intelligence, and he depends on waste, 'given' to him by other people. He is recommended to the care of King Gilgamesh. This corresponds with the view in the older Sumerian myth 'Enki and Ninmah' where Enki brings the *Lú.LIL* under the protection of the King (Lambert 2013: 339).[5] Strikingly, this figure is referred to as a foreigner from Subartu (north-west of

Mesopotamia), suggesting a negative association. What else does the myth depict, which ends by praising Enki? If Enki boasts of having given bread (i.e. work) to all seven persons with a disability, he essentially restores what Ninmah bungled by creating these disabled humans. This description is often interpreted as demonstrating an admirably inclusive society (e.g. Walls 2007). But we must consider the farcical context of a competition of creating humans between the drunken deities Enki and Ninmah. When we take the dramaturgy seriously, it seems that Ninmah, by creating such humans, deliberately aggravates Enki's task of finding for them a place in society. Enki succeeds in securing three of the seven persons a position with the king, but a question arises: is this a parody of a management suffering from too many ineffective workers doing 'sheltered jobs' (summary of interpretations in Ceccarelli 2016)? The records from the royal administration at Mari (first half of the 2nd millennium) document a female *lillatu* (Kellenberger 2013 with note 57); and the two anonymous 'deafs' (*sukkuku*) who appear among the royal employees – who as a rule are always referred to by their names – may have had a mental disability (Kellenberger 2013, note 58). This responsibility of the king (concerning all disabilities) is typical in royal ideology (see Assyrian Dictionary under *akû* A and B).

The spectrum of meanings of *lillu* (a possible onomatopoeia for 'babbling'?) is not precisely determinable. Even if an intelligence deficit (in Akkadian *la ṭemu*) is repeatedly mentioned, it is not possible to exclude the possibility of a mental illness. Modern medicine, too, cannot always draw a sharp dividing line in all cases. In addition, it must be noted that *lillu* often refers to a non-disabled person who occasionally does something stupid, despite his usual intelligence. The Gilgamesh epic, early composition as it is, already plays with both meanings of *lillu* (Kellenberger 2011: 20–1). However, today's 'vocabulary of respect' demands the use of different lexemes for these two irreconcilable human categories; we can possibly observe here a modern 'social racist' construct leading to new exclusion. It provides ample food for thought, if the historian Laes makes up the balance for the situation of children with (any) disability in classical antiquity:

> The majority of impaired were perhaps more fully integrated into daily life than in present-day Western countries, where, set apart by terminology, legal protections, and medical categorization, they are classified as special case. Paradoxically enough, in the ancient world these 'permanent outsiders' sometimes turn out to be 'outsiders within'.
>
> *(Laes 2013: 140)*

Israel

The double meaning of Akkadian *lillu* makes probable an analogy to the fools in the Old Testament (especially *petî* and *kᵉsîl*). Like *lillu*, also a *kᵉsîl* can be so from birth (Prov. 17: 21.25; cf. Sir 22: 3 LXX). As any reproach to the parents is missing here, it is difficult to think that this term refers to a badly educated son. That this *kᵉsîl* is causing 'grief and bitterness' for his parents, should be related to the vital interests of the intellectuals who were the tradents of Proverbs. Jobs passed down within the family as an economic base to the next generations, but a *kᵉsîl* was unable to perform intellectual tasks. In contrast, such people would have been proficient in agriculture. Because such a phenomenon – an intellectually deficient person performing agricultural tasks – would have passed almost unnoticed, the sources are silent about these instances. Conversely, men and women with certain physical disabilities had much more difficulty in being integrated, and the sources do not remain completely silent. This could also be the reason why the Gospels often report Jesus' healings of the physically maimed persons who had to live as beggars (πτωχοί), but never mention the intellectually disabled, because the latter came through life as day labourers, belonging to the second lowest class of πένητες.

The second term *petî* may have the same double meaning, designating a slighter foolishness, which rarely is blamed (and then only mildly), although the deficits are clearly named. Characteristically the Septuagint translates the term with three different lexemes, emphasizing in each case one aspect of the *petî*: his innocence (ἄκακος), his childishness or naiveté (νήπιος) and his intellectual (and behavioral?) deficit (ἄφρων). A reference to mental disability may be included in Proverbs 14: 15 (he 'believes every word') and 22: 3 (he does not see the danger, but runs into trouble). In addition, Psalms 116: 6 ('YHWH protects the *petîs*') may also refer to such people (Kellenberger 2011: 128–9). There are in Mesopotamia analogue (hymnal) prayer statements about a deity protecting the *lillu* or (more often) the *ulālu* (the *ulālu* occurs frequently in the *kudurru* inscriptions as persons lacking awareness, tricked into stealing or destroying a landmark document, cf. supra p. 49).

In the Qumran texts *petî* often has positive connotations and refers (metaphorically?) to followers or sympathizers of the community. Even a priest can be a *petî*, and his judgement about a leper must be respected despite his lack of cognitive ability (Damascus Document 13: 6; cf. Abrams 1998: 65 about the tannaitic Midrash Sifra). On the other hand the term *petî* heads the list of disabled persons who are not allowed to enter the congregational assembly; the restriction – strangely for us – was explained by the presence of holy angels (15: 15–17).

The rabbinic literature used – instead of *petî* and *kᵉsîl* – the previously uncommon term *šôtê*, which includes all mentally incompetent persons, making no distinction between psychic and intellectual impairments. Three categories of Jews are exempt from many halachic obligations: 'the hearing impaired (*hereš*), the mentally incompetent (*šôtê*) and the minors (*qāṭān*)' (Abrams 1998). The lexemes *petî* and *kᵉsîl* are used only in biblical quotations; but now the significance of *petî* must be explained by non-Hebrew languages, because the word apparently is missing in the actual vocabulary (Sanhedrin 110b, Shemot Rabba 3: 1).

Citations of Psalm 116: 6 ('YHWH protects the *petîs*') demonstrate a surprising post-history of *petî*, exclusively used in the context of birth risks. This psalm verse legitimates the dispensation for using a contraceptive during sexual activities of girls who were too young, who could die during delivery because of their narrow birth canal (Nidda 45a and four other passages in the Tosefta and Talmud). And magic texts use this verse for fighting off the risk of a premature birth (Naveh and Shaked 1993: 102 and 202–3). It seems that here, *petî* is understood as the innocence and naiveté of babies and young girls.

Conclusions

Specialists of Greek and Roman Antiquity will find here much that is well known to them and testifies to a *longue durée*. In the same way, readers of this volume will recognize links between deafness and intellectual disability; blindness as the most frequent occurrence; *A Capite ad Calcem* categorization; fear of bad omens and subsequent elimination; disabled workers and the community concept; and the medical acknowledgement of 'hopeless cases'. There are also parallels in phenomena which are not treated in the present contribution, as the use of personal names designating a physical or mental disability (cf. Waetzoldt 1996). To date, no satisfactory explanation for this has been given, and the effect on the (unfortunate?) namebearer – analogous female names are rarely used – is unknown. Mockery of people with a disability also can be observed in all periods and we see that it was documented already in Sumerian school texts (Hallo 1997: 590).

But it may be worth pointing to other perceptions of disability, too. Throughout the ancient Near East and in the rabbinic and early Christian tradition, epilepsy was always considered an evil. Greek voices proclaiming a 'sacred' disease are missing. In addition, Mesopotamian medicine appears to have been managed more by empiricism than the Hippocratic doctrine of four humours. Scurlock (2006: 81) dares to make the judgement that Mesopotamian physicians produced fewer therapeutic failures than the Greeks.

All historians are tempted to project their own modern experiences onto the ancient texts, especially when the topic is as particularly sensitive topic as disability. Notions about the relation of sin to sickness and disability are lurking in the archaic depths of the human soul and therefore will be sought (and found?) in the ancient texts. The Mesopotamian and Old Testament texts offer less material than expected (Scurlock 2006: 74; Heeßel 2007: 126; but cf. Stol 2000: 166–70). In John 9, Jesus denies the question about a sinful cause of a man born blind, so answering the question uttered by his disciples, the assumption behind which is still resonating in many souls: 'Neither he nor his parents sinned, but the works of God should be made manifest in him' (cf. Wynn 2007b). Jesus' response is challenging,[6] like the above-mentioned theocentric passage (Exod. 4: 11) by evading a moralistic ideology.

In the human soul slumbers also the (often unconscious) dream of a world without disability. The exemplary healing stories in the Gospels (documenting only a small minority of affected people), especially, are to this day often misused to legitimize this idealistic dream of the healing of imperfect bodies and minds here on earth. But the Old and New Testament took into consideration the permanent character of disability. The Apostle Paul famously dealt with his own permanent disability (2 Cor. 12). And the systematic theologian Amos Yong (2011), based on Jesus' nail wounds, which remained after his resurrection (John 20: 20–7), drafts a view of the kingdom of God where disabilities are not eliminated (or 'healed away'), and where people with disabilities are making their genuine contributions to the community of God's children – now and in the future.

Notes

1 Terminology is an insoluble problem: 'Intellectual disability' and 'learning disability' are much too narrow designations, concealing other deficits and a different character of intelligence of these people. Also inaccurate is 'cognitive disability', which includes intelligent people with sight and hearing problems. The same is true for 'mental retardation': 'Retardation' is a euphemism, since the expected normative development is most definitely missed; and 'mental' blurs with predominantly psychic impairments which mostly are missing in these people. Such problems have to be accepted when we want to explore the confusing world of disabilities.
2 It is a striking phenomenon that our son with a severe intellectual disability, after his arduous learning of writing, first wrote long lists (either personal or place names or food) spontaneously during years.
3 I have the impression that personally affected scholars, like Raphael (2008) with hearing impairment, may be especially overwhelmed by this massive and challenging text.
4 Taking into account that epilepsy was not seen as a neurological phenomenon in ancient thought, but was valued as awful, we can say that Israel's priests engaged extensively with another repulsive phenomenon, namely the consequences of various skin diseases (Lev. 13–14).
5 These lines are missing in some of the cuneiform sources (see Lambert 2013: 333). – Enki's subsequent own creation of a disabled person is, due to textual gaps, difficult to understand (see Stol 2000; Ceccarelli 2016).
6 Some Christian texts relapse to interpret this blindness as caused by a personal guilt, see e.g. the Pseudoclementine Homilies 19: 22 (3rd cent.).

Bibliography

Abrams, Judith Z., *Judaism and Disability: Portrayals in Ancient Texts from the Tanach through the Babli* (Washington, DC, 1998).
Assyrian Dictionary of the Oriental Institute of the University of Chicago, vols 1–21 (Chicago, IL, 1956–2010).
Bendemann, Reinhard von, 'Heilige Krankheit? Epilepsie im Spannungsfeld physiologisch-sozialer und religiöser Deutungen im Neuen Testament und im rabbinischen Judentum', in M. Roth and J. Schmidt

(eds), *Gesundheit: Humanwissenschaftliche, historische und theologische Aspekte* (Leipzig, 2008), 11–44.

Beyerle, Stefan, '"Medizin": Phänomene im Alten Testament und im antiken Judentum', in M. Roth and J. Schmidt (eds), *Gesundheit: Humanwissenschaftliche, historische und theologische Aspekte* (Leipzig, 2008), 45–78.

Böck, Barbara, *The Healing Goddess Gula: Towards an Understanding of Ancient Babylonian Medicine* (Leiden, 2014).

Ceccarelli, Manuel, *Enki und Ninmaḫ: Eine mythologische Erzählung in sumerischer Sprache* (Tübingen, 2016).

Civil, Miguel, et al., *MSL XIV: Materials for the Sumerian Lexicon* (Rome, 1979).

Dorman, Joanna, 'The Blemished Body: Disability and Deformity in the Qumran Scrolls' (unpublished PhD, Groningen, 2007). <http://dissertations.ub.rug.nl/faculties/theology/2007/j.h.w.dorman>

Fincke, Jeanette, *Augenleiden nach keilschriftlichen Quellen: Untersuchungen zur altorientalischen Medizin* (Würzburg, 2000).

Fitzmyer, Joseph A., *Tobit* (Berlin, 2003).

Foster, Benjamin R., 'Late Babylonian Schooldays: An Archaizing Cylinder', in Gebhard J. Selz (ed.), *Festschrift für Burkart Kienast zu seinem 70. Geburtstag* (Münster, 2003), 79–87.

Freedman, Sally M., *If a City is Set on a Height: The Akkadian Omen Series* Šumma Alu ina Mēlê Šakin, I (Philadelphia, PA, 1998).

Gelb, Ignace J., 'The Arua Institution', *Revue d'Assyriologie* 66 (1972), 1–32.

Geller, Markham J., *Ancient Babylonian Medicine: Theory and Practice* (Oxford, 2010).

George, Andrew R., *The Babylonian Gilgamesh Epic: Introduction, Critical Edition and Cuneiform Texts* (Oxford, 2003).

Hallo, William W. (ed.), *The Context of Scripture*, 3 vols (Leiden, 1997–2002).

Heeßel, Nils, *Babylonisch-assyrische Diagnostik* (Münster, 2000).

Heeßel, Nils, 'The Hands of the Gods: Disease Names, and Divine Anger', in I. L. Finkel and M. J. Geller (eds), *Disease in Babylonia* (Leiden, 2007), 120–30.

Heimpel, Wolfgang, 'Blind Workers in Ur III Texts', *Kaskal* 6 (2009), 43–8.

Hentrich, Thomas, *'Abgestempelt': Religion and People with Disabilities in the Ancient Near East* (Saarbrücken, 2013).

Hieke, Thomas, *Levitikus 16–27,* Herders Theologischer Kommentar zum AT (Freiburg, 2014).

Hrůša, Ivan, *Die Synonymenliste malku = šarru,* Alter Orient und Altes Testament 50 (Münster, 2010).

Kellenberger, Edgar, *Der Schutz der Einfältigen: Menschen mit einer geistigen Behinderung in der Bibel und in weiteren Quellen* (Zürich, 2011).

Kellenberger, Edgar, 'Children and Adults with Intellectual Disability in Antiquity and Modernity: Toward a Biblical and Sociological Model', *CrossCurrents* 63 (2013), 449–72.

Kwasman, Theodore, 'The Demon of the Roof', in I. L. Finkel and M. J. Geller, *Disease in Babylonia* (Leiden, 2007), 160–86.

Laes, Christian, 'Raising a Disabled Child', in J. Evans Grubbs and T. Parkin (eds), *The Oxford Handbook of Childhood and Education in the Classical World* (Oxford, 2013), 125–44.

Lambert, W. G., *Babylonian Creation Myths* (Winona Lake, IN, 2013).

Leichty, Erle, *The Omen Series Šumma Izbu* (Locust Valley, NY, 1970).

Maul, Stefan M., *Zukunftsbewältigung: Eine Untersuchung altorientalischen Denkens anhand der babylonisch-assyrischen Löserituale (Namburbi)* (Mainz, 1994).

Maul, Stefan M., 'Die "Lösung vom Bann": Überlegungen zu altorientalischen Konzeptionen von Krankheit und Heilkunst', in H. F. J. Horstmanshoff (ed.), *Magic and Rationality in Ancient Near Eastern and Graeco-Roman Medicine* (Leiden, 2004), 79–95.

Naveh, Joseph, and Shaked, Shaul, *Magic Spells and Formulae: Aramaic Incantations of Late Antiquity* (Jerusalem, 1993).

Naveh, Joseph, and Shaked, Shaul, *Amulets and Magic Bowls: Aramaic Incantations of Late Antiquity* (Jerusalem, 1998³).

Olyan, Saul M., *Disability in the Hebrew Bible: Interpreting Mental and Physical Differences* (Cambridge, 2008).

Paulus, Susanne, *Die babylonischen Kudurru-Inschriften von der kassitischen bis zur frühneubabylonischen Zeit: Untersucht unter besonderer Berücksichtigung gesellschaftlich- und rechtshistorischer Fragestellungen* (Münster 2014).

Pittl, Simone, 'Some Considerations on Disabled People in the Sumerian Myth of Enki and Ninmah', *Kaskal* 12 (2015), 467–83.

Radner, Karen, 'König Asarhaddon in Bedrängnis', *Damals* 38/2 (2006), 64–71.

Raphael, Rebecca, *Biblical Corpora: Representations of Disability in Hebrew Biblical Literature* (New York, 2008).

Reiner, Erica, *et al.*, *MSL XII: Materials for the Sumerian Lexicon* (Rome, 1969).

Renger, Johannes, 'Kranke, Krüppel, Debile: Eine Randgruppe im Alten Orient?', in V. Haas (ed.), *Aussenseiter und Randgruppen: Beiträge zu einer Sozialgeschichte des Alten Orients*, (Konstanz, 1992), 113–26.

Schipper, Jeremy, *Disability Studies and the Hebrew Bible: Figuring Mephiboshet in the David Story* (New York, 2006).

Schipper, Jeremy, *Disability and Isaiah's Suffering Servant* (Oxford, 2011).

Schipper, Jeremy, and Stackert, Jeffrey, 'Blemishes, Camouflage, and Sanctuary Service: The Priestly Deity and his Attendants', *Hebrew Bible and Ancient Israel* 3 (2013), 458–78.

Scurlock, JoAnn, *Magico-Medical Means of Treating Ghost-Induced Illnesses in Ancient Mesopotamia* (Leiden, 2006).

Scurlock, JoAnn, and Andersen, Burton R., *Diagnoses in Assyrian and Babylonian Medicine: Ancient Sources, Translations and Modern Medical Analyses* (Urbana, IL, 2005).

Stol, Marten, *Epilepsy in Babylonia* (Groningen, 1993).

Stol, Marten, *Birth in Babylonia and the Bible: Its Mediterranean Setting* (Groningen, 2000).

Walls, Neal H., 'The Origin of the Disabled Body: Disability in Mesopotamia', in H. Avalos, S. Melcher and J. Schipper (eds), *This Abled Body: Rethinking Disabilities in Biblical Studies* (Atlanta, GA, 2007), 13–30.

Waetzoldt, Hartmut, 'Der Umgang mit Behinderten in Mesopotamien', in M. Liedtke (ed.), *Behinderung als pädagogische und politische Herausforderung: historische und systematische Aspekte* (Bad Heilbrunn, 1996), 77–91.

Wynn, Kerry H., 'Johannine Healings and the Otherness of Disability', *Perspectives in Religious Studies* 34 (2007a), 61–75.

Wynn, Kerry H., 'The Normate Hermeneutic and Interpretations of Disability within the Yahwistic Narratives', in H. Avalos, S. Melcher and J. Schipper (eds), *This Abled Body: Rethinking Disabilities in Biblical Studies* (Atlanta, GA, 2007b), 91–101.

Yong, Amos, *The Bible, Disability and the Church: A New Vision of the People of God* (Cambridge, 2011).

5

ANCIENT PERSIA AND SILENT DISABILITY

Omar Coloru

A matter of evidence

Did disability ever exist in ancient Persia? This provocative question is justified by the scarcity of the documentary evidence the historians face when dealing with the pre-Islamic societies of the Iranian world. As a matter of fact, the traditions of these populations have always been pre-eminently oral. The rock inscription of Darius I at Behistun, which represents the first text written in the Old Persian language (Briant 2002: 126–7), was only composed in the 6th century BCE, when the nearby Mesopotamian world could boast a diverse textual tradition dating back three millennia. In fact, the habit of carving inscriptions was not as widespread as in the Greco-Roman world. On the other hand, the documents of the administration such as the Persepolis Fortification Tablets (Briant 2002: 422–5, 440) offer little information on subjects other than economic and administrative matters. What is more, a number of documents were not written on clay tablets but on perishable materials like parchment or wax-covered wooden tablets. Nor do we know about the composition of books or historical works. The existence of royal chronicles recording the deeds of the kings is still debated (Posner 1972: 126; Briant 2002: 889; Stronk 2007: 114; Llewellyn-Jones and Robson 2010: 55–65). Some historical traditions about Persian history survive in epic poems, a genre which was without doubt very popular; still, it was orally transmitted by wandering minstrels. Even religious traditions did not receive a written systematization until the Sasanian period. Likewise, Achaemenid, Parthian and Sasanian art only provide models of health and beauty and seem to exclude anything that may suggest bodily imperfection or illness. Given the nature of the evidence, it is easy to feel discouraged about the possibility of having a clear and definite picture of the condition of the disabled in the Persian world. Nevertheless, we can try to explore the issue by surveying the available documents and comparing and contrasting them with external evidence from the classical world.

The place of disability in ancient Zoroastrianism

A few references to disability can be found in the *Avesta*, the collection of sacred texts of the Zoroastrian religion. Those texts had been orally transmitted for centuries by trained priests, but they were written down in twenty-one parts (*nask*) only under the late Sasanian period. The oldest parts of the *Avesta* were organized in a corpus in the late 2nd millennium BCE, while the other compositions were probably gathered under the Achaemenids. The events following the Muslim invasion of Persia brought the loss of most of the books composing the *Avesta* so that today we possess just a quarter of the total. Within this corpus, there is a compendium called *Videvdad* or *Vēndidad* 'Laws/regulations to keep the demons away', which deals with rituals of purification or preservation of purity against the demons (*daēwa*) (De Jong 1999: 304; Skjaervø 2012: 103–5). The *Videvdad* also includes cosmogonical myths explaining the reason why evil made its appearance in the perfect world created and ordered by Ahura Mazda, the supreme deity of the Zoroastrian pantheon. In fact, the Evil Spirit Angra Mainyu had created 99,999 illnesses to counter the good creation of Ahura Mazda (*Videvdad* 22.1). In addition, the *Bundahishn*, a medieval compendium of Zoroastrian cosmogony and cosmology, ascribes to the Evil Spirit the diffusion of illnesses and noxious animals such as scorpions and snakes (*Bundahishn* 4.10). Therefore, all the creatures that at the beginning of time had been created good by Ahura Mazda had become polluted by Angra Mainyu and the demons, which were his agents. Although evil had entered the world, the story goes that Ahura Mazda entrusted Yima, the first ruler on the earth, to reign over the creation and make it prosper (*Videvdad* 2.4–5). Under his rule, mankind lived a golden age where disease and death did not exist, and Yima made the earth expand three times its original size in order to hold all the living beings whose numbers increased because of their immortality. However, a natural catastrophe put an end to the overpopulation of the earth: after an extremely cold winter, the melting snow caused a huge flood which covered all the lands. To save the living beings for the next repopulation of the earth, Ahura Mazda told Yima to build a *vara*, an underground enclosure where he would house selected specimens of every species so that individuals not contaminated by the evil creation of Angra Mainyu would inhabit the world again:

> There shall be no humpbacked, none bulged forward there; no impotent, no lunatic; no poverty, no lying; no meanness, no jealousy; no decayed tooth, no leprous to be confined, nor any of the brands wherewith Angra Mainyu stamps the bodies of mortals.
>
> *(Videvdad 2.29, tr. Darmesteter 1880)*

Thus, people with disabilities or presenting bodily imperfections were excluded from this version of Noah's Ark. From this passage, it appears clear that disability and, more generally speaking, diseases were not caused by 'natural' factors; they were generated by Angra Mainyu and the demons. Illness, therefore, was the consequence of a demonic possession which was best cured through exorcism. In fact, the health of the body was strictly connected with that of the soul (Gignoux 2004: 102). According to *Videvdad* (7.44) a Zoroastrian physician could cure an individual with the medicine of the knife (Av. *kareta-*), i.e. surgery, or by having recourse to the officinal properties of the plants (Av. *urvara-*). There was a third kind of medicine based on the Sacred Word (Av. *mānthra*) which consisted of the recitation of a 'spell' (if we have to use a loose translation of the term). By virtue of the interrelation between physical condition and soul illness, the medicine of the *mānthra* was thought to be the most effective, as stated also in the hymn in praise of the Zoroastrian deity Airyaman:

> One may heal with the knife, one may heal with herbs, one may heal with the Holy Word: amongst all remedies this one is the healing one that heals with the Holy Word; this one it is that will best drive away sickness from the body of the faithful: for this one is the best-healing of all remedies.
>
> *(Yasht 3.6, tr. Darmesteter 1882)*

The sick and the disabled were not allowed to take part in the sacrifice in honour of Ahura Mazda and the other divine entities because they would have polluted it. This was particularly true for those who were afflicted by deformity, as they showed in their own bodies the 'mark' of evil in a more visible way. As Ahura Mazda had created all that was good and beautiful in the world, a deformity, whether congenital or acquired, could not be anything but the work of Angra Mainyu. In the sight of the *Avesta*, even if an individual was not directly responsible for the illness or disability from which he was suffering, responsibility had no importance. What mattered was that a disabled person displayed a visible sign of demonic action regardless of his innocence or his condition of 'sinner': in both cases, he would be excluded from the sacrifices and, accordingly, from the benefits that the gods might bestow on their worshippers. The hymn in honour of the goddess of the waters Anāhita (*Yasht* 5) clearly states this:

> Of this libation of mine let no foe drink, no man fever-sick, [...] no leper to be confined. I do not accept those libations that are drunk in my honor by the blind, by the deaf, the epileptic [...], nor any of those stamped with those characters which have no strength for the Holy Word. Let no one drink of these my libations who is hump-backed or bulged forward; no fiend with decayed teeth.
>
> *(Yasht 5.92–3, tr. Darmesteter 1882)*

Those who managed to recover from an illness had to perform the *barashnūm*, a ritual of purification in order to cleanse the body from a serious form of pollution (Choksy 1989: 23–52; De Jong 1997: 242–3; 1999: 302–29). The Byzantine historian Agathias of Myrina (*Historiae* 2.23) provides the only description of this ritual that can be found in the Greek literature. Even if this source dates back to the Late Antiquity, it is safe to assume that the ritual could have existed in a much earlier period. Correspondingly, one should suppose that individuals affected by irreversible disability could not participate in the sacrifices for the rest of their lives. In the Sasanian period, the deaf and the blind were excluded from attending the Hērbedestān, a religious school (Macuch 2009: 263).

Although the authors of *Avesta* attribute to the Evil Spirit and the demons the responsibility for illness, sometimes the gods could inflict diseases on their enemies, as we see in *Yasht* 14.47 where the warlike god Verethragna declares that he can bring illness and destruction to the enemy. The god Mithra, who was the personification of the covenant and guaranteed social order by protecting pacts between humans and gods, could make his enemies blind and deaf (*Yasht* 10.48). On the other hand, Ahura Mazda seems not to have ever had recourse to this kind of punishment (Mendoza Forrest 2011: 49). The contrast with the story told in the *Videvdad* is apparent, where death and sickness are still the work of the Evil Spirit, but the gods can use them as a weapon to fight their opponents or to inflict a punishment on them. It is interesting to note that according to the Achaemenid royal ideology the king was the human agent of the divine world who guaranteed order by acting as protector of the good and punisher of the evil (Skjaervø 1999: 50–5). For instance, in the Behistun inscription, which records how Darius I (522–486 BCE) took his power thanks to the protection of Ahura Mazda, the king punishes his opponents by gouging out their eyes and having their nose, ears and tongue cut off. During the Parthian period, Mithradates II (123–88/7) inflicted the penalty of blinding on the Elamite rebel Pittit (Diodorus of Sicily, *Bibliotheca historica* 34/35.19; Shayegan 2011: 118–20). Similar mutilations began to be prescribed in late Roman law as a punishment for a number of crimes (Lascaratos and Dalla-Vorgia 1997: 51–6). Furthermore, disfiguring the face of a ruler in order to disqualify and depose him became a common practice in Byzantium from the 7th century CE (Paradiso 2005: 313–14). However, it is not necessary to argue an Eastern origin for such disfigurements (see Beal and Kelleberger in this volume for the Hittite and Mesopotamian evidence), as the integrity of the face and the body is an important feature in Greco-Roman culture, and several cases of mutilation are attested as well (Laes 2014: 109–10 and index s.v. 'verminking').

In the dualistic vision of the fight between Truth/Good and Lie/Evil, Darius is bringing justice against individuals who 'lied' by pretending to be kings, thus compromising the order Ahura Mazda wanted to give to the world when he chose Darius as sovereign. On the other hand, it is also important to keep in mind that the Achaemenid world was not an isolated entity but had assimilated several cultural and religious elements from the Near East. The literary motif of the lie was a common topos in the narration of acts of disloyalty against a ruler, as shown, for example, by the textual evidence from the Neo-Assyrian Empire (Pongratz-Leisten 2002: 227–43; Llewelyn-Jones 2013: 48, 139). The punishment for that impious action usually consisted of mutilation and/or infliction of a permanent disability before being put to death, as appears clearly in the fate of two of the rebels against Darius, Fravartish the Median (also known as Phraortes in Greek documents) and Ciçantakhma the Sagartian:

> Phraortes, seized, was led to me. I cut off his nose and ears and tongue, and put out one eye.
>
> *(DB 2.32, tr. Kent 1950)*

> By the favour of Ahuramazda my army smote that rebellious army and took Ciçantakhma prisoner, (and) led him to me. Afterwards I cut off his ears and nose and tongue, and put out one eye.
>
> *(DB 2.33, tr. Kent 1950)*

This kind of punishment is echoed in Herodotus (*Historiae* 3.69), who relates that Cyrus the Great had punished the magus Gaumata, the future usurper of the Persian throne, by having his ears cut off after a serious mistake he had made. It has been observed (Kellens 1999–2000: 693; 2002: 443) that the mutilations ordered by Darius correspond closely to the punishment inflicted by Mithra on his enemies:

> Thou bringest down terror upon the bodies of the men who lie unto Mithra; thou takest away the strength from their arms, being angry and all-powerful; thou takest the swiftness from their feet, the eye-sight from their eyes, the hearing from their ears.
>
> *(Yasht 10.23, tr. Darmesteter 1882)*

> And when Mithra drives along towards the havocking hosts, towards the enemies coming in battle array, in the strife of the conflicting nations, then he binds the hands of those who have lied unto Mithra, he confounds their eye-sight, he takes the hearing from their ears; they can no longer move their feet; they can no longer withstand those people, those foes, when Mithra, the lord of wide pastures, bears them ill-will.
>
> *(Yasht 10.48, trs. Darmesteter 1882)*

By depriving an individual of his sensory and movement faculties, the king is inflicting on earth the same fate that the evildoers will suffer after death by Mithra. In other words, those who are punished are damned in both life and death, as the loss of sight, hearing and mobility will prevent them from entering the heaven (Kellens 2002: 443–4). Those who perform evil deliberately put themselves in a condition of blindness and deafness to the precepts of Ahura

Mazda. Despite the religious justification advanced by the king, the final aim of this mutilation was to get rid of his rivals. Parallel motivations may be found in the Byzantine world when dealing with dynastic problems, but with a substantial difference as far as criminal law is concerned: in this case, mutilations were somehow perceived as a compassionate act in order to avoid the infliction of the death penalty (Lascaratos and Dalla-Vorgia 1997: 51–6). Likewise, Islamic law advises the infliction of mutilation in order to induce the criminal to repent and avoid a punishment in the hereafter (Dzhansarayeva *et al.* 2014: 735–6). On the other hand, it must be stressed that according to the teachings of Muhammad transmitted by tradition (*hadith*), which are also a jurisprudential tool for Islamic law, mutilation is prominently prohibited, especially that disfiguring the human face (Lange 2010: 702; for a selection of texts showing the attitude towards the disabled in the classical Muslim world see Miles 2002: 77–88).

Sometimes mutilations were instigated by influential women of the Persian court. If we have to rely on the anecdote recorded by Ctesias of Cnidus (*Persica* F 9.6), the queen Amytis, wife of Cyrus the Great, obtained orders from her husband that the eunuch Petisacas would have his eyes gouged and his skin flayed because he was responsible for the death of her father, the king of the Medes Astyages.

A 10th-century compendium of materials concerning the Zoroastrian religion, the *Dēnkard*, 'Acts of the Religion', relates a tradition about the wonders which circulated around the birth of Zarathustra. It is said that when a *karapan* (a member of the priestly class which opposed the religious message of Zarathustra) by the name of Dūrāsraw saw Zarathustra surrounded by divine glory (*xwarrah*), he tried to kill the infant by crushing the head with his hands. However, he was not able to accomplish the crime because his hands suffered instant paralysis which prevented him even from feeding himself (*Dēnkard* 7.4).

As we have seen so far, the *Avesta* mentions several forms of disabilities, such as blindness, deafness and curved spine, as well as invalidating diseases such as epilepsy and leprosy. As for the latter, the authors of the *Avesta* accompany the term for leper (*paesa-*) with the expression *vītərətō.tanu*, which means 'whose body is isolated'. As a matter of fact, isolation due to conditions of impurity was also applied to women in menses, who had to undergo a ritual of purification (Mendoza Forrest 2011: 75–6, 79–80; De Jong 1997: 241). The Greek historians confirm that, among the Persians, being a leper entailed the social status of pariah, although this was a form of exclusion common to other civilizations of the Ancient Near East. Ctesias of Cnidus, who practised the medical profession at the court of Artaxerxes II, says that the Persians define people affected by leprosy as *pisagas* (*Persica* F 14.43) which is actually the Greek rendering of Old Persian *pēsag*, i.e. 'leper'. Describing the customs of the Persians, Herodotus states that individuals afflicted by leprosy or by *leuke* (a skin disease resembling leprosy) keep themselves outside the towns and avoid any contact with the other Persians. In fact, the Persians thought that this illness was the direct consequence of an offence against the Sun (*Historiae* 1.138). As we can see, the informants of Herodotus relate only one aspect of the aetiology of leprosy, that is, the result of divine punishment, while the demonic activity is not mentioned at all. This omission could be interpreted as a simplification of a more complex matter by Herodotus or his sources; in addition, one should take into account the parallel provided by Babylonian religion, where leprosy was considered the punishment for perjuring against Sin, the Moon-god, and Shamash, the Sun-god (Stol 1993: 128). The god of the Sun mentioned by Herodotus is sometimes understood as the Greek interpretation of Mithra. Although we have proof of an association of Mithra with the sun (see e.g. *Yasht* 10.13), the Persian sources do not assimilate the two, but rather this process will occur only in a much later period (Briant 2002: 251–2; Boyce 1975: 69). On the other hand, *Yasht* 14.48 states that the faithful who do not lie to Mithra and who sacrifice to Verethragna will receive protection from leprosy and other plagues.

Herodotus' information about the condition of social exclusion endured by the lepers is confirmed also by Ctesias, when he recounts an anecdote about Megabyzus (*Persica* F 14.43). This Persian nobleman and general had been sent into exile to a town on the Red Sea by Artaxerxes I (465–424). After five years, Megabyzus was able to come back to Persia by disguising himself as a leper so that nobody would approach him along his journey. Once he arrived, he was barely recognized by his wife Amytis, which brings one to wonder if Megabyzus inflicted mutilation on himself in order to make his disguise more credible and to avoid the attention of the secret agents of the king (Tuplin 2004: 332). For both men and women in a state of uncleanliness the *Videvdad* (9.33–5) prescribes isolation in a building called *armēshtgāh*, 'house of seclusion', whose original function was that of isolating individuals afflicted by serious diseases:

> He shall sit down there in the place of infirmity, inside the house, apart from the other worshippers of Mazda. He shall not go near the fire, nor near the water, nor near the earth, nor near the cow, nor near the trees, nor near the faithful, either man or woman. Thus shall he continue until three nights have passed. When three nights have passed, he shall wash his body, he shall wash his clothes with gômêz and water to make them clean.
> *(Videvdad 9.33, tr. Darmesteter 1880)*

On the other hand, the existence of a hospital (*bimārestān*) is attested in the Sasanian period: it was founded in the city of Gondēshāpur (Khuzistan region) possibly under the order of Khusro I Anushirvān (531–79). This hospital also had a medical school which received philosophers from the Eastern Roman Empire after Justinian had closed the School of Athens in 529. In order to populate the city, the institution hosted Syrian-speaking professionals who had been deported. The School of Gondēshāpur soon became one of the most important scientific centres of the period where Greek and Indian medical traditions were studied and developed (Gignoux 2014).

An exception to the negative attitude towards lepers and other skin diseases may be witnessed by Plutarch (*Artaxerxes* 23.4–5). The story has it that Atossa, wife of king Artaxerxes II (405–358), had contracted *alphos*, a form of non-contagious leprosy which can be identified as vitiligo. Artaxerxes loved his wife so much that he was not disgusted by her disease, but prayed to the goddess Hera to obtain healing for Atossa. If the story is not a mere invention by Plutarch, Hera might represent another Greek interpretation of Anāhitā (Munn 2006: 231; Chaumont 1958: 165–6; a different interpretation in Boyce 1982: 220). We know that Artaxerxes was a fervent worshipper of Anāhitā and favoured her cult in several cities of the Empire (Panaino 2000: 36). According to *Yasht* 5.92–3 a leper could not receive the libations offered to Anāhitā; however, the hymn addresses the goddess as 'health-giving'. As a divinity of the waters, Anāhitā was connected to concepts of purity and fertility, so it is likely that from a certain historical moment onwards she was also given a healing faculty, as her epithet would lead us to suppose. Whether or not Plutarch's anecdote is reliable, it assumes that at least during the reign of Artaxerxes II, healing from diseases was one of the benefits that Anāhitā could bestow on her worshippers. If this is the case, it becomes easier to see the reason that brought Plutarch or his source to assimilate Anāhitā into Hera, as the latter provided help to women afflicted by illness (Chaumont 1958: 166). Thus, it is possible that the story reported by Plutarch describes an act of affection towards the queen in a framework of religious practice. Artaxerxes was asking Anahita for Atossa's recovery because the disease had put her in a condition of ritual pollution and consequently she could not take part in the sacrifice. Nevertheless, we are ignorant of Atossa's fate and whether or not she was prohibited from having contact with other persons. Was there a different treatment for a member of the royal family in such particular conditions? The fact that Artaxerxes opted for a supernatural intervention in order to obtain his wife's healing does not rule out the possibility that Atossa was also being treated by one of the many physicians in the service of the court, as we will see in more detail.

Disability at court

The situation of disability at court brings us to investigate the relation of the Achaemenid kings to their disabled family members. The official image of the royal body in both artwork and inscriptions is marked by the exaltation of health, beauty and strength (Briant 2002: 225–32; Llewellyn-Jones 2015). This form of representation was not new at all; it was a customary portrayal of the ideology of kingship in the ancient Near East civilizations (Llewellyn-Jones 2015: 216–18; see also Kellenberger in this volume). Actually, the beauty of the royal body mirrored the perfection of the god who had bestowed kingship upon the monarch and proved his right to rule. In the two inscriptions carved on his tomb at Naqsh-e Rustam Darius I declares:

> I declare: Ahuramazda, when he saw this earth in commotion, thereafter bestowed it upon me, made me king; I am king. By the favour of Ahuramazda I put it down in its place; what I said to them, that they did, as was my desire.
>
> *(DNa 4.30–7, tr. Kent 1950)*

> This indeed my capability: that my body is strong. As a fighter, I am a good fighter [...]. I am skilled both in hands and in feet. As a horseman, I am a good horseman. As a bowman, I am a good bowman, both on foot and on horseback. As a spearman, I am a good spearman, both on foot and on horseback. These are the skills that Ahuramazda set down upon me and which I am strong enough to bear, by the will of Ahuramazda, what was done by me, with these skills I did, which Ahuramazda set down upon me.
>
> *(DNb 8.31-47, tr. Kent 1950)*

In the same way, Plato (*Alcibiades* 121d) records that, from childhood, the body of the royal prince was the object of particular care in order to make it as handsome as possible and strong in the limbs. Therefore, the royal body had to be represented with all appearances of physical health. As has been pointed out (Briant 2002: 225–6), some classical sources would let us understand that the Persian king was chosen on the basis of his physical appearance, but the reality was that an individual was considered handsome and strong on the basis of the simple fact that he had managed to become king. While official Achaemenid sources are usually silent about health issues, Greek and Roman historians have transmitted some information on the diseases of the Great King. After all, the presence of physicians from both Egypt and Greece in the service of the royal family is well attested by the sources: for the Greek world, we know of Apollonides of Cos, Democedes of Croton, the above-mentioned Ctesias of Cnidus, and Polycritus of Mende. As for Egypt, our sources mention Semtutefnakht, Udjahorresnet and Wenen-Nefer (Briant 2002: 264–6; Tuplin 2004: 318–21; Llewellyn-Jones 2013: 35–6). Nevertheless, data about potential disabilities suffered by the Achaemenid kings are very few and do not always lend themselves to easy interpretation. Among the available evidence there is the 'madness' of Cambyses. In a long passage (*Historiae* 3.25–38), Herodotus describes the alleged foolish behaviour adopted by Cambyses after he had conquered Egypt (Laes 2014: 75). This madness manifested as profane acts against Egyptian religion and its priests, by organizing a military expedition against the Ethiopians, and by murdering members of the Persian nobility as well as his own family. He also adds that Cambyses had suffered ever since his birth from the Sacred Disease, i.e. epilepsy (*Historiae* 3.33). Herodotus concludes the list of Cambyses' crimes by saying that, in his opinion, the only viable justification for such actions was that Cambyses was definitely mad. However, modern scholarship has shown that the 'madness' attributed to Cambyses is nothing but a supernatural explanation of a behaviour that Herodotus failed to understand but which was justified by particular political reasons (Briant 2002: 55–7). What is more, the hypothesis that Cambyses was struck by epilepsy has also been refuted on medical grounds (York and Steinberg 2001: 1702–4). Another anecdote whose reliability is dubious, because it provides a justification for the heirless death of Cambyses, records that the king's wife Rhoxane gave birth to a headless baby, which the Magi interpreted as a bad omen for the reign of Cambyses (Ctesias of Cnidus, *Persica* F 13.14)

A more plausible form of temporary disability, experienced by Darius I, is once again reported by Herodotus (*Historiae* 3.129–30). Due to a fall from his horse, the king twisted his ankle, which had resulted in a tarsal dislocation. The Egyptian physicians in his service were not able to treat the injury properly; on the contrary, they made the situation worse by twisting and overstretching the ankle. As a result, Darius could not move nor sleep for a week because of the intense pain. Eventually, the Great King was successfully cured thanks to the treatment provided by the physician Democedes of Croton. Although this anecdote is clearly a pretext for exalting the medical competence of the Greek doctors compared to that of the Egyptians, there is no compelling reason to doubt the reliability of the story of Darius' accident. It seems that the same Democedes cured Darius' wife Atossa of a breast abscess (Herodotus *Historiae* 3.130). On the other hand, Amytis, the daughter of Xerxes (486–465), died from a disease of the uterus which had become malignant because it was improperly treated by Apollonides of Cos. The latter had taken advantage of his position of physician to start a relationship with the princess on the pretext that sexual intercourse would heal her illness. When the conditions of Amytis worsened, Apollonides stopped the sexual relations, but the dying princess asked her mother Amestris to avenge the outrage. As a result, Apollonides was imprisoned, tortured and buried alive (Ctesias, *Persica* F 13.44; Tuplin 2004: 333–5).

The situation changes when we come to Artaxerxes I (465–425). This king was nicknamed *Macrocheir* (*Macrochir* and *Longimanus* in Latin sources), i.e. 'Long-Hand'. Ancient historians have offered a variety of explanations for this curious epithet: the Roman historian Cornelius Nepos (*De regibus* 21.1) reports that Artaxerxes was distinguished by his imposing and beautiful figure along with his military prowess. Alternately, Plutarch (*Artaxerxes* 1.1) offers a literal interpretation by stating that the king had this nickname because his right hand was longer than his left. Finally, the lexicographer Pollux (*Onomasticon* 2.151) explains the term as a metaphor, saying that *Macrocheir* alludes to the fact that Artaxerxes' power was far-reaching. The same epithet is recurrent in Persian and Arabic sources (New Persian, *derāz-dast*; Arabic, *ṭawīl-al-yadayn*), but is attributed to Bahman, a mythical king of the Persian national epic whose characters are in part influenced by those of the historical Artaxerxes, so that sometimes Bahman is even named Ardashir (Artaxerxes). Like the Greco-Roman authors, these later sources offer a literal or symbolic interpretation for the title. More recently, the attempt has been made to explain the term by positing that the king suffered from a form of unilateral limb gigantism caused by neurofibromatosis (Ashrafian 2011: 557). However, given the ambiguity of the term and the lack of any historical information about a possible limb disorder affecting Artaxerxes, I make any conclusion based on medical analysis too speculative. In fact, this is one of the pitfalls of retrospective diagnosis, in which the scholar tries to apply modern medical concepts to the diseases suffered by historical personalities, the efficacy of which has been debated in recent years (Karenberg 2009: 140–5). A symbolic interpretation of *Macrocheir* seems preferable because in many Iranian languages the word *dast* is used in the meaning of 'authority' and 'power' (Tafażżolī 1994: 320). In addition, *Yasht* praises the prophet Zarathustra in these terms: 'thou art well-shapen, O Spitama! strong are thy legs and *long are thy arms*' (Yasht 17.22 Darmesteter 1882). As a result, it is likely that the epithet may be a Greek translation of a Persian title whose original meaning was related to the sphere of royal ideology and religion (Von Gall 1990: 110) rather than to physical deformity.

A group of permanently disabled individuals operated at the Achaemenid court: the eunuchs (Briant 2002: 268–77; Lenfant 2012: 257–97; Llewellyn-Jones 2013: 38–40). Most of the information that we have about eunuchs in the service of the Achaemenids comes from the classical sources, while at the same time we do not even know the Old Persian term for this royal servant. Only in the Sasanian period do we learn that eunuchs were designated by the Middle Persian term *shābestān*, a title which etymologically means 'women's sleeping quarter', and which in the Shapur I trilingual inscription at Naqsh-e Rustam is translated as the Greek term *eunuchos*. In fact, the title of *shābestān* was understood as man without genitals (Lerner and Skjaervø 2006: 115; Skjaervø 2007: 39). The eunuchs of the Achaemenids are always portrayed as unmarried, whether or not this means that they could never marry. Evidence from other civilizations shows that, as rare as marriage might have been, it may have been a possibility (Lenfant 2012: 285). Indeed, the legend reported by Ctesias of Cnidus (*Persica* F 8d.6) on the ascent of Cyrus the Great attests that the latter had been adopted by the eunuch Artembares, the cupbearer of King Astyages.

Generally speaking, eunuchs could arrive at the court of the Great King through several routes: the slave trade, the tribute from the subject countries or war booty. Do these routes suggest that the eunuchs were usually not Persians? We see that the vast majority of the eunuchs mentioned by the classical sources have Iranian names, a point which can be explained by the assumption that they were given new names once they began their service for the royal household. After all, a precedent for this phenomenon is already attested in the Neo-Assyrian period (Lenfant 2012: 283). It is not too far-fetched to think that even an Iranian might have been castrated, even if we have only one example of a eunuch whose Iranian origin is explicitly stated: Mithridates, who was Xerxes' powerful chamberlain and a relative of Artabanus, a Hyrcanian chief of the bodyguards (Diodorus of Sicily *Bibliotheca Historica* 11.69). But then again, we do not know if, and how, religious principles were overcome concerning the preservation of bodily wholeness and the promotion of procreation. Although it is a very late and isolated piece of evidence, *Denkard* 9.21.5 attests that the emasculation of an individual was perceived as a condition of evil fortune without remedy, as it prevented the castrated man from having a lineage of his own (Skjaervø 2007: 39). However, statements on how eunuchs were perceived in Achaemenid Persia are often contradictory, sometimes attesting repugnance and sometimes great respect. Indeed, there was a hierarchy among the eunuchs: most of them were nothing but domestic workers specializing in one of the many tasks associated with the attendance of the king and his family. According to the record of Ctesias of Cnidus, the guardian of the women did not appear among the duties of the eunuchs. Rather, they were servants of queens and princesses, not their guardians. In addition, they are described as being more often in the service of the king and men in general rather than of women (Lenfant 2012: 269–70). In yet another capacity, a few held the highest positions at court and became very influential; some even attempted to ascend the throne, as shown in the case of Artoxares, who plotted against Darius II (423–405) to become king in his place (Ctesias of Cnidus, *Persica* F 15.54). It seems that being castrated did not prevent the eunuchs from assuming military functions, as did Natakas, who was sent with an army to plunder the shrine of Delphi (Ctesias of Cnidus, *Persica* F 13.31). This phenomenon is not extraordinary and is also attested at the Sasanian court, where eunuchs served in the administration and as members of the Zoroastrian clergy (Lerner and Skjaervø 2006: 114–15). Once in a while, eunuchs occupying the lowest echelons of the hierarchy could rise to a condition of considerable power: Hermotimos of Pedasa, for instance, was enslaved and castrated in Ionia, then sold to the Persians and sent to Darius I as a gift. During the reign of Xerxes he managed to win the confidence of the king. Then, he accompanied Xerxes on his military campaign against Greece and was also entrusted with the task of caring for some of the king's illegitimate sons (Herodotus *Historiae* 8.104–6).

Among the Iranian dynasties that ruled after the fall of the Achaemenids, an interesting case for the study of ancient disabilities is represented by the Arsacids of Parthia. From the mid-3rd century BCE this dynasty of nomadic origin had started to occupy the East Iranian territory of the Seleucids, and by the 2nd century BCE it had become master of an empire stretching from Mesopotamia to eastern Iran. Analysis of royal portraiture on coins has shown that several kings of the dynasty, from Mithridates II onwards, portrayed a nodule on the forehead, the nose or the cheek which was generally described as a wart (Wroth 1903: pp. xlviii, lii, lxxvi, 72–4, 87, 89–90, 93, 95, 99–101, 103, 105, 110, 125–6, 131, 135, 153, 180, 182–3). This particular feature was first analysed from a medical point of view by Gerald Hart (Hart 1966: 547–9) who assumed that the nodule could be a hereditary form of trichoepithelioma, a benign tumour of the skin. However, a more recent study (Todman 2008: 140–6) pointed out that the size as well as the shape of this cutaneous lesion better matches the rounded nodules caused by neurofibromatosis Type I. The main feature of this skin disorder consists in the formation of benign tumours around nerves in the skin as well as in other organs such as the brain. Complications caused by neurofibromatosis include the risk of developing malign tumours, blindness caused by tumours in the retina, learning disabilities, hypertension, and musculoskeletal disorders such as macrocephaly and scoliosis. It seems that in a few cases the lesion was concealed cosmetically by a lock of hair (Hart 1966: 548–9). The possibility of a hereditary feature is plausible, but even in this circumstance the lack of documentation about the conditions of the Parthian kings' health should signal caution in attributing to any of them any specific disease. The question must remain open until more evidence is available for study.

The need to show physical fitness for the sake of maintaining royal ideology remained of paramount importance in the official representation of the Sasanians, as any deformity, mutilation or mental illness would have portrayed an individual as unfit to rule (De Jong 2004: 356). In continuity with traditional practice, the sources witness the recourse to disfiguration in order to get rid of potential rivals or to disqualify a sovereign. This is what happened, for example, to King Hormozd IV (579–90), who was blinded following a palace coup set up to depose him and put his son Khusro II (591–628) on the throne (Pourshariati 2008: 124, 127, 409, 413). The importance of preserving bodily wholeness in order to sit on the throne was noted by the Byzantine historian Procopius of Caesarea when he observed that 'it is not lawful for a one-eyed man or one having any other deformity to become king over the Persians' (*De bello persico* 1.11, tr. Dewing 1914). In the Middle Ages the historian al-Ṭabari was still aware of the tradition that among the Persian customs there was 'the practice of not raising anyone to kingly power who had a physical defect' (Bosworth 1999: 42). The health of the Sasanians was also a topic used in Christian apologia and hagiography: the kings and their families are described as suffering from serious skin diseases like leprosy, or other forms of invalidating illnesses such as heavy headaches, all of which are healed by miracles performed by Christians living at the Sasanian court. In other cases, this literature shows the Zoroastrian clergy plotting against the Christians and blaming them for casting evil spells which caused an illness in a member of the royal family. Those false accusations were made against them in order to obtain their death, thus, from a Christian perspective, martyrdom (De Jong 2004: 350).

Conclusions

In a recent article dealing with the potential to develop disability studies in Iran, Negin Goodrich observed that:

> Iran was mentioned only twice in the Encyclopedia of Disability 2006, and Persia was completely absent in the chronology (pages C1 to C27 in each volume), as well as the volume on the Ancient World (vol. 5). It is necessary to investigate the status of Iran in the global disability studies to explore the reasons for ignoring this country in the international trend of disability studies.
>
> *(Goodrich 2014)*

While this statement should be nuanced as far as medieval and modern Persia are concerned, one cannot deny that in that work the ancient Iranian world is almost absent from the discussion, which, on the contrary, is focused on Mesopotamia. Indeed, this area is geographically close to Persia and some mutual influences are attested between these civilizations, but this fact does not imply that the two should be presented as part of the same system of values as they belong to different worlds, both from a cultural and religious point of view. As for the pre-Islamic period, this chapter has tried to present the difficulty but also the challenge that the nature of the available evidence poses to historians of ancient Persia. It is not possible to draw conclusions on the issue of disability among the Persians and we have to be aware of the fact that, because of this dearth of documentation, many questions are bound to remain open for a long time, maybe forever. What we can do is to make some general observations, which will raise as many questions.

The perception of disability in the ancient Iranian civilizations was undoubtedly influenced by religious beliefs. Being disabled was considered the result of an evil possession regardless of the responsibility of the disabled individual. His condition would have polluted the sacrifices to the divinities. Therefore, the disabled were excluded from an important part of the social life of the Zoroastrian community. But was this always the case? Were the prohibitions expressed in the *Avesta* always applied to the letter in the whole of the ancient Iranian world and in every period of its history? Common sense would suggest a negative response, but we lack data to appreciate the impact of the ritual prohibitions prescribed by the priestly class on the everyday life of the worshippers.

The study of disabilities from the Achaemenid period onwards is problematic as well. To this point, official documents from the court and the administration have been of little help in answering our questions: the importance of depicting a healthy image prevents us from having a first-person narration of the experience of illness. Most of the information on the health of the sovereigns and their families comes from sources outside Persia, and they are often fragmentary. Additionally, any information might have been distorted to fit the ancient authors' agendas. If we exclude the anecdote of Artaxerxes and Atossa, we get the impression that the kings relied more on medical science than the *manthra* of the Zoroastrian religion. Was this the reality, or are we looking through the filter of the classical sources?

Especially in light of all of the dangers of literary evidence, palaeopathological studies seem to be more promising. For instance, the discovery in the Chehrābād salt mine of the mummified remains of six individuals dating from the Achaemenid to the Sasanian period provides interesting data. Among these bodies, the so-called Salt-Man 4, an adolescent who lived between 410 and 350 BCE, was affected by frontal sinus aplasia, and 'butterfly vertebra' a rare congenital anomaly of the spine (Öhrström et al. 2015: 811-821). Hopefully, these and other future findings will improve our knowledge on illness and disability among the ancient Iranian populations.

Bibliography

Primary sources

Boyce, Mary, *Textual Sources for the Study of Zoroastrianism* (Chicago, IL, 1984).
Darmesteter, James, *The Zend Avesta. Part I–II* (Oxford, 1880–2).
Dewing, Henry B., *Procopius, History of the Wars, Books I and II – The Persian War* (London and Cambridge, MA, 1914).
Mills, Lawrence H., *The Zend Avesta, Part III* (Oxford, 1887).
Kent, Roland G., *Old Persian. Grammar Texts Lexicon* (New Haven, 1950).
Lenfant, Dominique, *Ctésias de Cnide. La Perse. L'Inde: Autres fragments* (Paris, 2004).
Llewellyn-Jones, Lloyd, and Robson, James, *Ctesias' History of Persia: Tales of the Orient* (Abingdon and New York, 2010).
Malandra, William W., *An Introduction to Ancient Iranian Religion: Readings from the Avesta and the Achaemenid Inscriptions* (Minneapolis, MN, 1983).
West, Edward W., *Pahlavi Texts, I–V* (Oxford, 1880–97).

Secondary sources

Ashrafian, Hutan, 'Limb Gigantism, Neurofibromatosis and Royal Heredity in the Ancient World 2500 Years Ago: Achaemenids and Parthians', *Journal of Plastic, Reconstructive and Aesthetic Surgery* 64/4 (2011), 557.
Bosworth, Clifford E. (ed.), *The History of al-Ṭabari*, V. *The Sāsānids, the Byzantines, the Lakmids, and Yemen* (Albany, NY, 1999).
Boyce, Mary, *A History of Zoroastrianism I: The Early Period* (Leiden, 1975; 1989²).
Boyce, Mary, *A History of Zoroastrianism II: Under the Achaemenians* (Leiden, 1982).
Briant, Pierre, *From Cyrus to Alexander: A History of the Persian Empire* (Winona Lake, 2002).
Chaumont, Marie-Louise, 'Le culte d'Anāhitā à Staxr et les premiers Sassanides', *Revue de l'histoire des réligions* 153/2 (1958), 154–75.
Choksy, Jamsheed K., *Purity and Pollution in Zoroastrianism: Triumph over Evil* (Austin, TX, 1989).
De Jong, Albert, *Traditions of the Magi: Zoroastrianism in Greek and Latin Literature* (Leiden, 1997).
De Jong, Albert, 'Purification *in absentia*: On the Development of Zoroastrian Ritual Practice', in J. Assmann and G. G. Stroumsa (eds), *Transformations of the Inner Self in Ancient Religion* (Leiden, 1999), 301–29.
De Jong, Albert, '*Sub specie maiestatis*: Reflections on Sasanian Court Rituals', in M. Stausberg (ed.), *Zoroastrian Rituals in Context* (Leiden and Boston, MA, 2004), 345–65.
Dzhansarayeva, Rima, Turgumbayev, Marlen, Malikova, Sholpan, Taubayev, Baurzhan, and Bissenova, Meruert, 'The Concept and Signs of Punishment in Islamic Law', *Middle-East Journal of Scientific Research* 19/5 (2014), 734–9.
Gignoux, Philippe, 'Health in Persia: I. Pre-Islamic Period', *Encyclopaedia Iranica* 12/1 (2004), 102–4.
Gignoux, Philippe, 'Greece xvi: Greek Ideas and Sciences in Sasanian Iran', *Encyclopaedia Iranica* (2014). <www.iranicaonline.org/articles/greece-16-ideas-sciences-sasanian>
Goodrich, Negin H., 'A Persian Alice in Disability Literature Wonderland: Disability Studies in Iran', *Disabilities Studies Quarterly* 34/2 (2014). <http://dsq-sds.org/article/view/4255>
Hart, Gerard D., 'Trichoepithelioma and the Kings of Ancient Parthia', *Canadian Medical Association Journal* 94 (1966), 547–9.
Karenberg, Axel, 'Retrospective Diagnosis: Use and Abuse in Medical Historiography', *Prague Medical Report* 110/2 (2009), 140–5.

Kellens, Jean, 'Promenade dans les Yašt à la lumière des travaux récentes', *Annuaire du Collège de France* (1999–2000), 721–51.

Kellens, Jean, 'L'idéologie religieuse des inscriptions achéménides', *Journal Asiatique* 290/2 (2002), 417–64.

Laes, Christian, *Beperkt? Gehandicapten in het Romeinse Rijk* (Leuven, 2014).

Lange, Christian, 'Crime and Punishment in Pre-Modern Islamic History: A Framework for Analysis', *Religion Compass* 4/11 (2010), 694–706.

Lascaratos, John, and Dalla-Vorgia, Panagiota, 'The Penalty of Mutilation for Crimes in the Byzantine Era (324–1453 A.D.)', *International Journal of Risk and Safety in Medicine* 10/1 (1997), 51–6.

Lenfant, Dominique, 'Ctesias and his Eunuchs: A Challenge for Modern Historians', *Histos* 6 (2012), 257–97.

Lerner, Judith A., and Skjaervø, Prods Oktor, 'The Seal of a Eunuch in the Sasanian Court', *Journal of Inner Asian Art an Archaeology* 1 (2006), 113–18.

Llewellyn-Jones, Lloyd, *King and Court in Ancient Persia 559 to 331 BCE* (Edinburgh, 2013).

Llewellyn-Jones, Lloyd, '"That My Body is Strong: The Physique and Appearance of Achaemenid Monarchy": The Body of the Achaemenid Monarch', in D. Boschung, F. Wascheck and A. Shapiro (eds), *Bodies in Transition: Dissolving the Boundaries of the Embodied Knowledge* (Paderborn, 2015), 211–48.

Macuch, Maria, 'Disseminating the Mazdayasnian Religion: An Edition of the Pahlavi Hērbedestān Chapter 5', in W. Sundermann, A. Hintze and F. de Blois (eds), *Exegisti Monumenta: Festschrift in Honour of Nicholas Sims-Williams* (Wiesbaden, 2009), 251–77.

Mendoza Forrest, Satnam, *Witches, Whores and Sorcerers: The Concept of Evil in Early Iran* (Austin, TX, 2011).

Miles, M., 'Some Historical Texts on Disability in the Classical Muslim World', *Journal of Religion, Disability and Health* 6/2–3 (2002), 77–88.

Munn, Mark, *The Mother of the Gods, Athens, and the Tyranny of Asia: A Study of Sovereignty in Ancient Religion* (Berkeley, CA, 2006).

Öhrström, Lena M., Seiler, Roger, Böni, Thomas, Aali, Abolfazl, Stöllner, Thomas, and Rühli, Frank J., 'Radiological Findings in an Ancient Iranian Salt Mummy (Chehrābād ca. 410–350 BC)', *Skeletal Radiology* 44 (2015), 811–21.

Panaino, Antonio, 'The Mesopotamian Heritage of Achaemenian Kingship', in S. Aro and R. M. Whiting (eds), *The Heirs of Assyria: Proceedings of the Opening Symposium of the Assyrian and Babylonian Intellectual Heritage Project. Held in Tvärminne, Finland, October 8–11, 1998* (Helsinki, 2000), 35–49.

Paradiso, Annalisa, 'Mutilations par voie de justice à Byzance', in J.-M. Bertrand (ed.), *La violence dans le monde grec et roman* (Paris, 2005), 307–20.

Pongratz-Leisten, Beate, '"Lying King" and "False Prophet": The Intercultural Transfer of a Rhetorical Device within Ancient Near Eastern Ideologies', in A. Panaino and G. Pettinato (eds), *Ideologies as Intercultural Phenomena: Proceedings of the Third Annual Symposium of the Assyrian and Babylonian Intellectual Heritage Project. Held in Chicago, USA, October 27–31, 2000* (Milan, 2002), 215–43.

Posner, Ernst, *Archives in the Ancient World* (Cambridge, 1972).

Pourshariati, Parvaneh, *Decline and Fall of the Sasanian Empire: The Sasanian-Parthian Confederacy and the Arab Conquest of Iran* (London and New York, 2008).

Shayegan, Rahim, *Arsacids and Sasanians: Political Ideology in Post-Hellenistic and Late Antique Persia* (New York, 2011).

Skjaervø, Prods Oktor, 'Avestan Quotations in Old Persian? Literary Sources of the Old Persian Inscriptions', *Irano-Judaica* 4 (Jerusalem, 1999), 1–64.

Skjaervø, Prods Oktor, 'A Postscript to the Seal of a Eunuch in the Sasanian Court', *Journal of Inner Asian Art an Archaeology* 2 (2007), 39.

Skjaervø, Prods Oktor, 'Avestan Society', in T. Daryaee (ed.), *The Oxford Handbook of Iranian History* (New York, 2012), 57–119.

Stol, Marten, *Epilepsy in Babylonia* (Groningen, 1993).

Stronk, Jan, 'Ctesias of Cnidus: A Reappraisal', *Mnemosyne* 60 (2007), 25–58.

Tafażżolī, Aḥmad, 'Derāz-dast', *Encyclopaedia Iranica* 7/3 (1994), 319–20.

Todman, Don, 'Warts and the Kings of Parthia: An Ancient Representation of Hereditary Neurofibromatosis Depicted in Coins', *Journal of the History of the Neurosciences: Basic and Clinical Perspectives* 17/2 (2008), 141–6.

Tuplin, Christopher, 'Doctoring the Persians: Ctesias of Cnidus, Physician and Historian', *Klio* 86 (2004), 305–47.

Von Gall, Hubertus, 'The Figured Capitals at Taq-e Bostan and the Question of the So-Called Investiture in Parthian and Sasanian Art', *Silk Road Art and Archaeology* 1 (1990), 99–122.

Wroth, Warwick W., *Catalogue of Coins in the British Museum: Parthia* (London, 1903).

York, George K., and Steinberg, David A., 'The Sacred Disease of Cambyses II', *Archives of Neurology* 58 (2001), 1702–4.

6

EGYPTIAN MEDICINE AND DISABILITIES

From pharaonic to Greco-Roman Egypt

Rosalie David

Sources of evidence

The availability of palaeopathological as well as textual and iconographic evidence from Egypt provides an unequalled opportunity to study one ancient society's perception and attitude towards deformity and disability. Unique geographical features and burial customs have ensured the survival of a wealth of source material. The annual Nile inundation created fertile land required for agriculture and everyday existence, but because this was scarce, burials had to be accommodated on the edges of the desert. The contents of these tombs included the body of the deceased owner, and a funerary assemblage, which provided for everyday needs in the afterlife. The heat and dryness of the desert location created the ideal conditions for preserving the tomb (with its carved and painted wall scenes) and its contents.

Mummification is a process in which natural or artificial preservation prevents putrefaction of bodily tissues. Burial conditions in Egypt produced natural (unintentional) mummies, and from at least 2600 BCE, an enhanced process, artificial (intentional) mummification, was introduced for royalty. This was soon adopted by the elite, and ultimately by all who could afford the procedure, although natural mummification was retained for the poor; both methods were discontinued in the 7th century CE. These skeletal and mummified remains offer unique opportunities for studying disease and medical treatments, and over the past forty years, various diagnostic techniques have been developed for this purpose (David 2008). The true potential of scientific studies, which provide researchers with unbiased evidence, is only now being properly recognized (Aufderheide 2003).

Evidence of deformity in religious art is less specific. This is because the primary aim was not to produce a realistic image of the owner but one which sympathetic magic could 'bring to life' for use in the afterlife (Schäfer 1986). Whatever their physical condition in this world, people hoped that they would be provided with idealized, perfect bodies after death, and to achieve this, royalty and the elite were almost always represented as young, healthy adults. However, peasants, servants and attendants, who could be portrayed realistically, are sometimes shown with various physical anomalies.

On very rare occasions, disability was depicted in a person of high status, but the explanation for this remains unclear. It may not always be possible to provide a literal interpretation of physical anomalies observed in the images: for example, some instances of obesity may represent prosperity rather than excessive weight, and dwarfism may be used as a convention to indicate a generic type of humanity rather than deformity (Nunn 1996: 67–77).

In iconographic evidence, the king is traditionally represented as a perfect, idealized figure, but images of Amenophis IV (Akhenaten) provide a notable exception. Hermaphrodite and other distinctive features observed in Akhenaten's statues and reliefs have been variously attributed to liver disease, hydrocephalus, acromegaly or Frölich's or Klinefelter's syndrome (Aldred and Sandison 1962; Burridge 1993). However, these images may not have been realistic portraits of the king, but symbolic representations of him as a universal, all-encompassing creator-god. Some reliefs and sculptures of this period also portray Akhenaten's daughters with grossly deformed skulls. In all these cases, it is impossible to verify the facts, since none of these bodies has yet been conclusively identified. In other words, the problem of retrospective diagnosis turns up again.

Deformities and disabilities encountered in Ancient Egypt

Available source material provides information about a wide range of deformities and disabilities. Some infirmities are the result of a single specific factor, such as genetic inheritance, congenital abnormality, disease or physical degeneration, whereas others may be due to a variety of causes.

Genetic factors

Dwarfism, a growth disorder mainly arising from genetic mutations, is well-attested in all source material from predynastic times through to the Greco-Roman period (Dawson 1938). Most examples represent the commonest form of dwarfism, achondroplasia (short limbs, a normal trunk, and a disproportionately large head), which is sometimes accompanied by osteoarthritis, deafness, limping, scoliosis and kyphosis (Dasen 1993: 9–11). However, constitutional dwarfism (pygmyism), a genetically transmitted condition found in some central African tribes, also occurs in the record. A letter from the child-king Pepy II to his official, Harkhuf (inscribed on the latter's tomb at Aswan), expresses his eagerness to see the pygmy whom Harkhuf is bringing back for him from Africa (Lichtheim 1975: 26–7). Osteogenesis imperfecta, a rare inherited bone disorder, characterized by multiple fractures as a response to minor stress, usually leads to early death (Aufderheide and Rodriguez-Martin 1998: 365–6). The condition has been identified in an infant in the British Museum collection (41603) (Dawson and Gray 1968: 13–14, 42; Gray 1969) and possibly in a specimen from Nubia (Brothwell 1967; Lowenstein 2009), although another study attributes these findings to spina bifida (Rowling 1960).

Cleft palate, the result of arrested development during embryogenesis, is associated with various genetic and congenital factors. It can cause respiratory and feeding problems which, in antiquity, doubtless led to the death of many infants. Presumably their skeletons have not survived, since only a few examples of the condition have been identified in adult human remains from Egypt and Nubia (Aufderheide and Rodriguez-Martin 1998: 58).

Congenital anomalies

Spina bifida, characterized by the failure of the lower end of the spine to close around the spinal column during foetal development, is a common congenital defect. It is known that this condition occurred in ancient Egypt (Rabino Massa 1978; Molto 1989), although evidence relating to the Nubian specimen discussed above is inconclusive (Cockburn *et al.* 1998: 48). Studies of two female foetuses found in the tomb of Tutankhamun have reported the presence of multiple congenital conditions including Sprengel's deformity and severe spinal conditions (Harrison *et al.* 1979); however, the most serious of these anomalies have not been confirmed by recent CT-scans (Hawass and Saleem 2011).

Any woman with an abnormal pelvic skeletal structure faced the possibility of birth obstruction and consequent death in childbirth. During his examination of the mummy of Princess Hehenit (c.2133–1991 BCE), Derry noted that her death soon after childbirth was probably caused by an abnormally small pelvis (reported by Williams 1929); an associated vesicovaginal fistula may have been the result of a protracted delivery (Janssens 1970: 118). In another case reported by Derry (1909), a Nubian woman's death was caused by an obstructed delivery in her narrowed birth canal (the result of congenitally absent sacroiliac joints).

Researchers have tentatively identified congenital club foot (*talipes equinovarus*) in several mummies. Elliot Smith diagnosed this condition, in which the foot is twisted out of shape or position, when he unwrapped the mummy of King Siptah (c.1209–1200 BCE) and found a shortening of the left leg and gross deformity of the ankle (Smith 1912: 71). Later studies have either supported this diagnosis (Dzierzykray-Rogalski and Prominska 1994) or attributed the condition to poliomyelitis (Harris and Weeks 1973). More recently, club foot has been identified in the mummy of Tutankhamun (1361–1352 BCE) (Hawass *et al.* 2010: 191); however, others dispute this claim (Marchant 2013: 191–4), suggesting instead that the slightly twisted position of the foot is probably due to the embalmers' bandaging techniques. The original investigation of the Two Brothers identified this condition in the left foot of Khnum-Nakht (Murray 1910), but later studies have refuted this, attributing the foot's appearance to tight bandaging (Brothwell 1967; David 1979: 29).

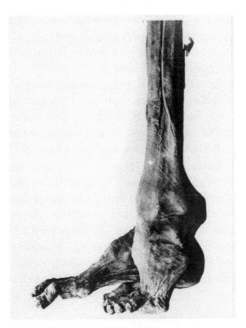

Figure 6.1 When the mummy of King Siptah (1206–1198 BCE) was unwrapped in 1905, the deformity evident in the left leg and foot was identified as a case of congenital club foot (talipes equino-varus). More recent radiological studies indicate a neuro-muscular disease, possibly poliomyelitis. Cairo Museum. Smith 1912: pl. LXII, fig. 2. © Robert B. Partridge/Peartree Design.

Other bone anomalies include a case of Klippel-Feil syndrome, observed in a Ptolemaic skeleton (Wells 1964), and an identical hip deformity (perhaps due to a familial relationship) observed in five women who lived in the same district (Smith and Jones 1910). A mummy in the Oriental Museum, Durham (UK), presents another anomaly: the lower part of the left forearm was absent in the owner's life, and was replaced with a prosthetic arm and hand during mummification. Possible explanations for the missing limb include disease, trauma, surgical amputation, or genetic, congenital or developmental disorders, but results of studies so far remain inconclusive (Gray 1966a; Finch 2012/13).

Acquired infirmities

Some deformities and disabilities were the result of trauma. Fractures, wounds and dislocations, which could lead to permanent joint changes (traumatic arthritis), were the outcome of warfare, domestic or interpersonal conflict, accidents (especially at building sites), and legal punishments such as beatings, fracturing offenders' arms and legs, and punitive amputations. Medical treatments also included intravital therapeutic amputations.

The Edwin Smith Surgical Papyrus (which possibly records a surgeon's work at a royal building site) is the most complete treatise on the treatment of trauma and wounds in ancient Egypt (Breasted 1930). Palaeopathology also contributes information about trauma injuries, and sometimes preserves evidence of the treatments applied to conditions such as head injuries, and simple and multiple fractures of the long bones; these often healed successfully when the bones were correctly aligned and set.

Insight into the incidence of fractures and treatments in one community is provided by a survey of the physical remains of the high officials and workers at the Giza pyramid site (c.2613–2494 BCE) (Hussien *et al*. 2010). This radiological and macroscopic study of 271 skeletons (including 125 females) reveals that treatments included joint manipulation to reduce fractures and dislocations, sometimes aided with pads and splints, and surgical amputations. Good-quality medical care, provided equally for men and women, and for both social groups, ensured that a high rate of success was achieved.

Evidence of healing in skeletal and mummified remains has confirmed that other intravital amputations were also successful (Nerlich *et al*. 2010a). Three individuals from Deir el-Bersheh apparently lost their feet as the result of traumatic amputation (Dupras *et al*. 2008), and a forearm belonging to another body (c.2300 BCE) may be a similar example of traumatic or intravital amputation (Brothwell and Moller-Christensen 1963; Finch 2012/13). A female mummy discovered in a tomb at Thebes (c.1070 BCE) provides evidence of intravital amputation of a big toe, undertaken because it was gangrenous due to arteriosclerosis; the missing toe was replaced with a wooden prosthesis (Nerlich *et al*. 2000) worn by the owner during life (Finch *et al*. 2012).

Surgical removal of the complete forefoot of an isolated, disarticulated foot (c.1100 BCE) has also been confirmed (Nerlich *et al*. 2010a). The lower parts of the legs of Mummy 1770 in the Manchester collection may also have been amputated during life (David 1979: 83–93). In both the Manchester and Durham mummies, embalmers replaced the missing limbs with prostheses to give the owner a complete and functioning body in the afterlife (Gray 1967b).

Pathological conditions

Critical surveys of pathological and artistic evidence have been the traditional ways of identifying the presence of disease processes, but these are now augmented by new methods which can detect antigens or bacterial DNA in ancient physical remains. Bacterial infections

Egyptian medicine and disabilities

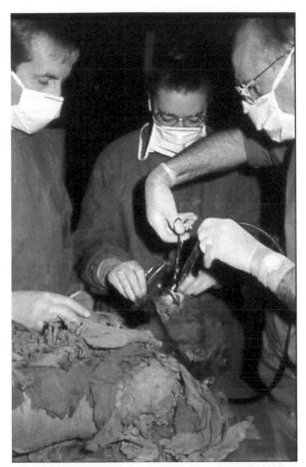

Figure 6.2 Members of the Manchester Mummy Team use endoscopic equipment to investigate the mummy of a priest (the Leeds Mummy). Biomedical research on mummies provides ample evidence of disease and disability in the ancient Egyptian population. © The University of Manchester.

were presumably commonplace, but conditions such as septic arthritis, sepsis following bone fracture, and osteomyelitis are rarely encountered, and in fact, there is ample evidence that in many cases broken limbs healed well with no indication of infection (Smith and Jones 1910; Raven and Taconis 2005: 62; Cockburn *et al.* 1998: 46–8; Hussien *et al.* 2010).

A skeleton in the British Museum (Brothwell 1981: 124, pl. 5.1C) and a mummy in the Boston Museum of Fine Arts (Worth Estes 1989: 44, n. 39) provide good examples of a physical anomaly that can be attributed to a specific disease process. They exhibit enlarged facial bones, a recognizable symptom of a fairly rare endocrine condition, acromegaly, caused by a tumour of the pituitary gland. This disease is characterized by abnormal thickening of all the bones and leads to major changes in an individual's appearance.

Similarly, a rare example of gout (a metabolic disease) was identified in the skeleton of an elderly man who lived near the Temple of Philae (Smith and Dawson 1924: 157). Chemical evidence from tests undertaken on white concretions deposited in many of his bones and joints provided support for this diagnosis.

The physical remains of Geheset, the wife of a high-court judge (c.1786–1633 BCE), have provided the earliest-known evidence of cerebral palsy (Nerlich *et al.* 2010b). This severe neurological disease, often present at birth, is sometimes accompanied by paralysis, poor

79

physical coordination and strange body movements. Although Geheset had a comparatively long lifetime (between 50 and 60 years), her appearance was marred by gross asymmetry of her facial bones (she would have experienced difficulty in swallowing) and she suffered from various postural deformities in her neck and hands. She surely is an example of the survival of the weakest who were not eliminated right after birth (Pudsey and Lepicard in this volume).

Lack of available evidence sometimes makes it difficult to determine an exact pathological explanation for some conditions. For example, three possible cases of poliomyelitis have been identified, but the diagnoses remain uncertain. The deformity observed in the left foot of King Siptah, and the associated atrophied leg, have been variously attributed to *talipes equinovarus* (see above), an inborn defect of the spine, or poliomyelitis.

On his funerary stele, Roma, a temple door-keeper and priest of Astarte, is represented with a foot deformity and a grossly wasted and shortened leg which have been differentially diagnosed as club foot with secondary wasting and shortening of the leg, or poliomyelitis contracted in childhood (Nunn 1996: 77). Poliomyelitis has also been tentatively identified in a skeleton from Deshasha (Harris and Wente 1980: 69; Mitchell 1900).

References to intellectual impairment and malfunction are generally missing from ancient Near Eastern literature (Kellenberger 2013). The Egyptian medical papyri are no exception: there are no titles of physicians specializing in mental illness, nor any reference to severe psychiatric disorders such as schizophrenia. However, these texts do describe some psychic or mental symptoms, but perhaps surprisingly they attribute their origin to organic disease rather than demoniac possession (Ghalioungui 1963: 128–9). Epilepsy is not mentioned as a specific disease in the papyri, but descriptions of seizures may indicate that physicians were aware of epileptic symptoms, although the underlying causes of the disease were not understood (Worth Estes 1989: 107–8). Cognitive disorders form part of a current study which addresses the possible impact that ancient Egyptian consanguineous unions (between individuals biologically related as second cousins or closer) may have had upon genetic and congenital abnormalities (Robinson in progress). Some conditions can be due to a variety of different causes. For example, hydrocephalus (an abnormal accumulation of fluid in parts of the brain) can be the result of congenital factors, trauma, infections or tumours. Until now, only three cases have been identified from ancient Egypt and Nubia (Aufderheide and Rodriguez-Martin 1998: 58; Derry 1913) but doubtless numerous other examples existed. However, without appropriate surgical intervention, most infants with this condition would have died at birth or in early childhood, and presumably their physical remains have simply not survived.

Scoliosis (lateral curvature of the spine with rotation of the vertebrae) or kyphosis (backwards curvature of the upper spine), which sometimes occur together in the same person, can be the outcome of congenital, pathological or degenerative factors. Angular kyphosis (humpback) is often caused by Pott's disease, a progression of tuberculosis, a disease which was probably quite widespread in Egypt (Morse *et al.* 1964; Buikstra *et al.* 1993). Various examples of spinal curvature are represented in tomb scenes, statuary, and collections of human remains (David 1979: 29; Worth Estes 1989: 44; Dawson and Gray 1968: 38–9; Raven and Taconis 2005: 63). Blindness and deafness can be the result of genetic inheritance, birth defects, accidents or disease. Artistic representations and inscriptions provide most information about blindness, although occasionally, histological evidence of disease has been obtained from the examination of intact eyes found *in situ* in mummies (David and Tapp 1992: 147). Trachoma, an infection still common in Egypt and North Africa, was probably the most common cause of blindness (Sandison 1967). Other identified conditions included cataracts, and onchocerciasis ('river blindness') which resulted from worm infestations such as filariasis. A tomb relief showing a harpist with a prominent, tortuous temporal artery may illustrate thrombosed ocular arteries, another cause of blindness (Jantzen 1968).

Treatments for blindness and deafness were prescribed in the medical papyri. Some cases of deafness probably arose from pathological conditions which can still be observed in skeletal and mummified remains, such as otitis media (infection of the middle ear), perforated eardrum (Benitez 1988), or mastoiditis (Smith and Jones 1910: 284; Leek 1986: 191). However, deafness and blindness were also recognized as indicators of old age.

Although there are no conclusive statistics regarding average life expectancy in dynastic Egypt (Wente 1980: 234–85), the available inscriptional and palaeopathological evidence indicates that, apart from some notable exceptions, half the adult population probably died in their mid-thirties, and 90 per cent did not survive much beyond 50. Therefore, 'old age' in ancient Egypt can probably be defined as the period stretching from the mid-thirties to the early fifties, although the concept was associated not so much with a person's actual age as with a set of physical and functional limitations.

The Egyptians approached old age with some trepidation. Unlike some ancient civilizations, no particular role was envisaged for the elderly as repositories of wisdom (Janssen and Janssen 1996: 3); however, society was acutely aware of the many disadvantages associated with ageing, as graphically illustrated in a famous wisdom text, the Instruction of Ptah-hotep (Lichtheim 1975: 62–3). Archaeological and inscriptional sources contain references to arthritis, rheumatism, breathlessness, giddiness, deafness, baldness, deteriorating eyesight, forgetfulness and senility, and provide magico-medical treatments to alleviate some of these ailments.

Some age-related conditions are also amply demonstrated in the palaeopathological record. Osteoarthritis, a disease associated with cartilage degeneration, has often been observed in the weight-bearing joints – spine, knees and hips – of mummified and skeletal remains (Dawson and Gray 1968: 41; Raven and Taconis 2005: 64; Gray 1966b, 1967a, 1973). Identification of other degenerative diseases of the spine commonly found in old age include spondylosis (Aufderheide and Rodriguez-Martin 1998: 96–7) and, spanning the period from predynastic to Roman times, well-documented instances of ankylosing spondylitis, a form of arthritis which results in fusion of the spine (Aufderheide and Rodriguez-Martin 1998: 102–4). Osteoporosis (loss of bone minerals and organic matrix) also occurs widely; one radiological study has reported its presence in equal numbers of male and female mummies, unlike the modern pattern where the disease is most frequently observed in women (Raven and Taconis 2005: 64).

Peripheral vascular disease and aneurysm formation, customarily regarded as products of modern living, were almost certainly present in antiquity (David *et al.* 2010). Early scientific studies of mummies identified atherosclerosis (plaques of calcification in the walls of the large arterial blood vessels) and arterial calcification in the vessels of the upper and lower extremities (Ruffer 1921; Smith 1912; Shattock 1909; Long 1931), while a recent radiological survey of twenty-two mummies in the Cairo Museum has revealed vascular calcification in the hearts and arteries of nine mummies (Allan *et al.* 2009).

However, these conditions mainly occur in royal and elite mummies, especially those belonging to priests and their families, rather than in the general population, an incidence which can probably be explained by the significant difference in the diet of the two groups. Whereas most Egyptians ate a mainly vegetarian diet, derived from the land, the priests' food – provided by offerings removed from the temple-gods' altars at the conclusion of the daily rituals – was rich in saturated fat.

Diabetes mellitus may have been responsible for the extensive vascular calcification observed in the lower extremities of some mummies, and may also have caused some instances of blindness, as well as being a possible cause of peripheral neuritis (David and Tapp 1992: 147) Microscopic evidence found in the tissue of several mummies has indicated cerebrovascular disease, a causative factor in 'strokes' (Worth Estes 1989: 46).

Attitudes towards deformity and disability

Treatment and care

Medical treatment in dynastic Egypt included pharmaceutical and surgical therapies, as well as spells and incantations (Nunn 1996; David 2012/13). New medical practices introduced to Egypt in the Greco-Roman period were largely retained for the exclusive treatment of the Hellenic elite while the indigenous population continued to use traditional methods (Lang 2013). However, these systems also display some level of interaction and adaptation: for example, temple incubation, which combined Egyptian and Greek concepts to treat certain types of physical and mental illness, was apparently available throughout the wider community (Daumas 1957).

Specific diseases or malfunctions are not generally discussed in the medical papyri which concentrate on symptoms associated with ill-health, and relevant therapeutic treatments. This probably explains why no examples of deformity (e.g. dwarfism) can be identified in the texts, although symptoms sometimes associated with disability, such as arthritis, blindness, deafness, paralysis and joint pain, are considered. Several papyri prescribe cosmetic treatments to arrest symptoms associated with old age – wrinkled skin, baldness and loss of hair colour – and the Edwin Smith Papyrus (verso) lists remedies to rejuvenate an old man.

Deformity is not recorded as a specific condition in the medical documents, perhaps because so few texts have survived, or many afflicted individuals did not live long enough to present for treatment, or no effective cures were available (Dasen 1993: 158). However, the latter seems unlikely since the papyri mention palliative care for other incurable afflictions (Breasted 1930: 206). Some deformities may not even have been perceived as medical conditions requiring treatment; for example, dwarfism was probably regarded simply as a form of divine manifestation or spiritual and physical 'otherness'.

Pragmatic solutions for disabilities included walking sticks and staves, as well as prosthetic limbs (Finch 2011). People also used magic to protect themselves against disability, or to restore and maintain good health. They carried amulets, either manufactured in the form of perfect body parts whose completeness would be transferred to the owner's body (Pinch 1994: 108) or as containers which could hold inscribed spells to cure afflictions such as blindness (Pinch 1994: 142–3). The sick and deformed also deposited model limbs and organs as votive offerings at temples and tombs with a reputation as places of healing.

The sick, disabled and elderly were supported by a system of medical and social care. Substantial numbers of healed fractures, and individual cases of recovery provide evidence of effective nursing regimes. One elderly man, comatose for four days after a severe beating, owed his survival to nursing care (Worth Estes 1989: 74), and presumably Geheset was able to manage an important household, despite severe neurological disease and postural abnormalities, because she received considerable family support (Nerlich *et al.* 2010b). Paraplegic patients, exemplified by a male burial at Shurafa (Derry 1913) and a case study in the Edwin Smith Papyrus, could only have survived if they received intensive care.

In some instances, the state or workplace was responsible for medical treatment. Doctors attended the sick and injured in royal necropolis towns such as Giza, where high officials and workers received equal treatment, and amputees were evidently retained and supported in the community (Hussien *et al.* 2010). A scene in the tomb of the architect Ipy shows workmen receiving treatment at a building site for a dislocated shoulder, and eye and foot injuries (Ghalioungui 1963: 82–3).

The king and the government may have provided some 'pensions' in the form of grain rations, land allotments or honorary priesthoods with attached sinecures for royal workmen and soldiers. No provision is made in any legal document for the disabled, but each family was expected to fulfil a moral duty to attend to its own sick, disabled and elderly members (Janssen and Janssen 1996: 87–104). Elderly parents were supported by their children, and traditionally appointed a 'Staff of Old Age' (usually a son) to act as helpmeet, heir and successor.

Employment opportunities

There is no evidence that disability barred Egyptians from holding religious or public office; indeed, inscriptions and tomb reliefs demonstrate that some disabled people held significant positions. The blind were accorded a special status: they performed as choir singers in religious events at tombs and temples, and were engaged as harpists and singers in elite households. Representations of harpists usually show them with closed or blindfolded eyes (Jantzen 1968; Fuchs 1964) and this probably indicates that many musicians were blind. However, some examples may be symbolic (Manniche 1978) or simply depict an occupation that was considered especially appropriate for the blind. Other employment opportunities included land measuring and recording, and positions as door-keepers and herdsmen.

Dwarfs were highly regarded, perhaps because of their rarity value, intelligence and dexterity. They were employed in royal and elite households, as nurses, midwives and male and female personal attendants. The men also produced, maintained and supervised the owner's clothing and jewellery; entertained his household with singing, dancing and music; and looked after domestic pets, as well as assisting with bird-catching and other activities on the master's estate. Their accredited magical powers of rebirth and regeneration enabled them to participate in temple festivals; the dwarf Djeho, a renowned sacred dancer in the bull cults at Memphis, may also have performed at funerals (Dasen 1993: 151–3).

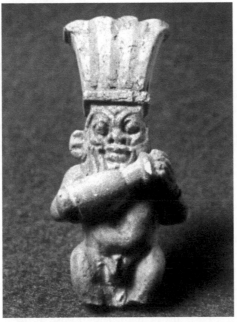

Figure 6.3 The Egyptians accepted dwarfism as a normal, if unusual, condition of humanity, and even represented some of their deities in this form. This amulet of the dwarf-god Bes depicts his characteristic feather head-dress. Believed to use music, singing and dancing to drive away evil forces, he is shown here playing a drum. Late Period (c.900 BCE). The Manchester Museum. © The Manchester Museum, The University of Manchester.

Occasionally, dwarfs are depicted alongside those afflicted with a hunchback or club-foot. It has been suggested that the nature of employment assigned to these groups gave them only a liminal role in society, and that, although the Egyptians expressed affection and respect for dwarfs and pygmies, they probably treated them as lovable curiosities rather than full adults (Dasen 1993: 156–7).

However, ample evidence demonstrates that some individuals with physical anomalies held high office and probably enjoyed complete social acceptance. Seneb is perhaps the best known example of several dwarfs who attained high-ranking status. Initially 'Overseer of dwarfs in charge of linen' and 'Overseer of weaving in the palace', he later held several priesthoods (Junker 1941: 3–6). Seneb's tomb-statue depicts him as an achondroplastic dwarf, accompanied by his normal-sized wife (a high-ranking priestess) and two children. Similarly, lameness did not prevent Siptah from ruling Egypt, or Roya from holding office in the cult of Astarte; and although severely disabled, Geheset managed a large household. Dwarfs and others with physical anomalies were buried in the normal way, and some, including the dwarfs Seneb and Djeho, had particularly fine funerary assemblages (Dasen 1993: 150–1).

Social acceptance of disability

Documentary evidence suggests that the Egyptians had complex, even ambivalent attitudes towards deformity. On one hand, they treated the sick and disabled with kindness and humanity. The Edwin Smith Surgical Papyrus clearly infers that physicians were required to examine and treat all patients, even if they could only recommend palliative care.

The Instruction of Amenemope – one of the wisdom texts, which provided youngsters with a moral and ethical code, and represented society's core values – gives precise advice on how to treat the disabled. It warns against ridiculing a blind man, teasing a dwarf, causing difficulties for the lame, and mocking or criticizing the sick or insane. It affirms that, since these people were the god's creation, they should be given proper respect (Lichtheim 1976: 160). Nevertheless, the very fact that the Egyptians found it necessary to give this advice suggests that, in some circumstances, treatment of the disabled fell short of the ideal.

Other ancient civilizations regarded beauty and physical completeness as indications of divine blessing, and deformity as a mark of the gods' anger. Here, one may think of the earliest references to deformity which occur in Mesopotamian lists (cf. Kellenberger in this volume) or the Romans who regarded inauspicious births as warnings of divine retribution (cf. Trentin in this volume). In contrast, the Egyptians apparently did not feel threatened by such conditions, and their oracular decrees, designed to protect women against birth complications, never included them (Dasen 1993: 99).

Some societies exposed their deformed infants (cf. Pudsey and Lepicard in this volume and Finch 2012/13). There is no evidence of infant exposure in pharaonic Egypt, when deformity was viewed neither as a disease to be cured nor a sign of divine retribution: legal documents are silent on this matter, and medical papyri, while prescribing tests to assess the viability of neonates, contain no criteria for deciding the fate of deformed infants.

The first mention of infant exposure in Egypt dates to the Greco-Roman period, and refers to a member of the resident Greek population, Hilarion, a soldier, who sent a letter to a woman living in his house (West 1998), instructing her to dispose of the baby if it should be a girl (P.Oxy. 4.744). Infant exposure, especially of females, continued in Roman Egypt. However, when Rome's wars decreased in the first two centuries CE, the number of adult captive slaves was greatly reduced, and the state now encouraged Egyptians to rescue exposed infants and bring them up as slaves (Lewis 1983: 58).

Mesopotamian texts and biblical sources (Lev. 21: 16–24) emphasize that physical anomalies were regarded as signs of cultic impurity; only unblemished persons could become priests, enter the temples, or present divine offerings (cf. Kellenberger in this volume; Beal for the more 'relaxed' Hittite attitude). In Egypt, however, there is ample evidence that disability was no bar to holding priestly office at any level; cultic purity, a condition of entry to the god's presence, was attained through the regular performance of rituals.

Whereas some societies believed that physical anomalies were divine retribution for personal sin, the Egyptians did not generally make this association. The only exception are the votive stelae, mainly originating from Deir el Medina, which attribute the petitioners' blindness to divine punishment, inflicted for impiety and blasphemy (Gunn 1916). No other examples of prayers asking gods to intervene and heal a disabling condition have ever been found (Dasen 1993: 159).

A religious context for disability

A unique concept of the world, underpinned by distinctive religious beliefs, may help to explain why the Egyptians' perception and treatment of deformity and disability differed so much from attitudes seen in some contemporary societies. Many aspects of Egyptian civilization demonstrate that they had an inclusive, multi-faceted view of life, in which different, sometimes apparently conflicting ideas and concepts, were retained and pursued simultaneously. For example, their medical treatments embraced complementary systems of care and healing; lawcourts used oracular pronouncements alongside conventional methods of obtaining evidence; and some gods worshipped by foreign residents were incorporated into the Egyptian pantheon.

Religion accommodated a multiplicity of gods and mythologies, and worshippers could approach a variety of gods (Hornung 1983). Some divine powers were attributed to particular animals, and many deities took human, animal or hybrid forms. A god's spiritual power was immanent in his cult-statue, cult animal or in all animals of the species associated with his worship. This encompassing, complex approach greatly facilitated the Egyptians' general acceptance of 'otherness'.

Egyptians and Greeks both believed that the human body was designed in the gods' own images. However, with the exception of lame Hephaestus, the Greeks attributed physical perfection to all their deities. Wholeness and beauty in humans were regarded as blessings that indicated not only moral and intellectual supremacy, but also divine recognition; conversely, deformity, weakness and ugliness were marks of the gods' rejection.

However, the Egyptian pantheon did not demonstrate a similar uniform perfection. It included examples of 'otherness', encompassing not only gods with perfect human physiques and their animal variations, but also dwarf gods, and deities who had suffered and overcome physical injuries. This may have led the Egyptians to believe that every human, whether malformed or whole, had a divine origin; this concept occurs in an astrological calendar from Oxyrhynchus (late 2nd century CE) which attributes creation of various types of deformity to the gods (P.Oxy. 3.465). Indeed, non-fatal conditions such as dwarfism, blindness and mental illness may have been viewed as particular signs of divine favour, and caring for the disabled was probably regarded as a religious duty (Jeffreys and Tait 2000: 87–95).

The most important dwarf-gods, Bes (Romano 1980) and Ptah-Pataikoi (Dasen 1993: 84–98) were associated with solar worship, fertility, birth, sleep, music, entertainment and protection of the dead, women and children. The fact that dwarf deities held such important roles may have encouraged people to accept and even celebrate deformity. Both deities are represented as achondroplastic dwarfs; some Bes-figures also display features, such as a protruding tongue, which may indicate other complex birth anomalies (Dasen 1993: 42; Kellenberger 2013).

Many of the god's images show him playing a musical instrument, and in the Greco-Roman period, he appears as a warrior, fighting the forces of evil. These gods were not associated with any temple cults in dynastic times, although Bes acquired this status in the Greco-Roman period (Frankfurter 1998: 128).

Finally, Egyptian attitudes to death and the afterlife undoubtedly influenced their perception of physical anomalies. They were probably more willing to accept and tolerate deformity and disability because of the belief that no one could achieve perfection in this world. This state was only attainable after death, when a life of piety, divine worship, and good deeds, followed by correct burial procedures, guaranteed a person's rebirth into the kingdom of Osiris, god of the dead. With the doctrine of the perfect resurrected body, Christianity adhered to a similar kind of faith, and it is perhaps no coincidence that, also in the Christian faith, the prevailing ancient attitudes towards disability were not followed (cf. Solevag in this volume).

Although the landscape of Osiris' kingdom recreated the environment of Egypt, perfect conditions prevailed there: eternal springtime, ample food and the company of family and friends. Most importantly, the Egyptians expected to be reborn with idealized, youthful bodies that were free from disease, deformity and the effects of old age. It was essential to ensure that the deceased's corpse was intact so that this transformation could be achieved, and the owner would continue existence in the next world with unimpaired physical functions. Thus, the embalmers went to considerable lengths to restore and preserve the body, even replacing missing limbs with prostheses; this imitated the mythical reassembly of Osiris' body parts, in preparation for his triumphant resurrection as king of the dead.

In Antiquity, enough people with physical anomalies survived to force their communities to consider and address issues associated with deformity and disability. Some societies found religious reasons to reject the deformed and disabled. However, the Egyptians had no religious context for stigmatizing those with physical anomalies: on the contrary, Osirian theology promoted the worship of a physically damaged god who nevertheless attained eternal perfection, and it offered everyone the hope of an idealized afterlife. Against this background, the Egyptians readily integrated the disabled into their society, and developed effective responses to meet many of their practical needs.

Bibliography

Aldred, Cyril, and Sandison, Andrew T., 'The Pharaoh Akhenaten: A Problem in Egyptology and Pathology', *Bulletin of the History of Medicine* 36 (1962), 293-316.
Allan, A. H., Thompson, R. C., Wann, L. S., Miyamoto, M. I., and Thomas, G. S., 'Computed Tomographic Assessment of Atherosclerosis in Ancient Egyptian Mummies', *Journal of the American Medical Association* 302 (2009), 2091–4.
Aufderheide, Arthur C., *The Scientific Study of Mummies* (Cambridge, 2003).
Aufderheide, Arthur C., and Rodriguez-Martin, Conrado, *The Cambridge Encyclopaedia of Human Paleopathology* (Cambridge, 1998).
Benitez, J. T., 'Otopathology of Egyptian Mummy PUM II: Final Report', *Journal of Laryngology and Otology* 102 (1988), 485–90.
Breasted, James H., *The Edwin Smith Surgical Papyrus*. 2 vols (Chicago, 1930).
Brothwell, Don, 'Major Congenital Anomalies of the Skeleton. Evidence from Earlier Populations', in D. Brothwell and A. T. Sandison (eds), *Diseases in Antiquity* (Springfield, IL, 1967), 423–43.
Brothwell, Don, *Digging up Bones* (Ithaca, NY, 1981).
Brothwell, Don R., and Moller-Christensen, Vilhelm, 'A Possible Case of Amputation Dated to 2300 BC', *Man* 244 (1963), 192–4.
Buikstra, Jane E., Baker, Brenda J., and Cook, Della C., 'What Diseases Plagued the Ancient Egyptians? A Century of Controversy Considered', in W. V. Davies and R. Walker (eds), *Biological Anthropology and the Study of Ancient Egypt* (London, 1993).

Burridge, Alwyn L., 'Akhenaten: A New Perspective; Evidence of a Genetic Disorder in the Royal Family of 18th Dynasty Egypt', *Journal of the Society for the Study of Egyptian Antiquities* 23 (1993), 63–74.

Cockburn, Aidan, Cockburn, Eve, and Reyman, Theodore A. (eds), *Mummies, Disease and Ancient Cultures* (Cambridge, 1998²).

Dasen, Véronique, *Dwarfs in Ancient Egypt and Greece* (Oxford and New York, 1993).

Daumas, Francois, 'Le Sanatorium de Dendara', *Bulletin de l'Institut Française d'Archéologie Orientale* 56 (1957), 35–57.

David, Rosalie, 'Introduction. Ancient Medical and Healing Systems: Their Legacy to Western Medicine', in R. David (ed.), *Ancient Medical and Healing Systems: Their Legacy to Western Medicine* (Bulletin of the John Rylands University Library of Manchester 89, Supplement 2012/2013), 7–24.

David, Rosalie (ed.), *Egyptian Mummies and Modern Science* (Cambridge, 2008).

David, Rosalie (ed.), *The Manchester Museum Mummy Project* (Manchester, 1979).

David, Rosalie, and Tapp, Edmund (eds), *The Mummy's Tale* (London, 1992).

David, Rosalie, Kershaw, Amie, and Heagerty, Anthony, 'The Art of Medicine. Atherosclerosis and Diet in Ancient Egypt', *The Lancet* 375 (27 Feb. 2010), 718–19.

Dawson, Warren R., 'Pygmies and Dwarfs in Ancient Egypt', *Journal of Egyptian Archaeology* 24 (1938), 185–9.

Dawson, Warren R., and Gray, Peter H. K., *Catalogue of Egyptian Antiquities in the British Museum. I. Mummies and Human Remains* (Oxford, 1968).

Derry, Douglas E., 'Anatomical Report', *Archaeological Survey of Nubia*, Bulletin 2 (Cairo, 1909).

Derry, Douglas E., 'A Case of Hydrocephalus in an Egyptian of the Roman Period', *Journal of Anatomy and Physiology, London* 47 (1913), 436–58.

Dupras, Tosha, Mathews, Stevie, De Meyer, Marleen, Peeters, Christoph, and Vanthuyne, Bart, 'Just Cut it off: Amputation in Ancient Egypt', *Paleopathological Association 35th Meeting, Abstracts* (2008), 6.

Dzierzykray-Rogalski, Tadeusz, and Prominska, Elzbieta, 'A Further Report on Pharaoh Siptah's Handicap (XIXth Egyptian Dynasty)', *HOMO* 45 (Supplement) (1994), 45.

Finch, Jacqueline, 'The Art of Medicine: The Ancient Origins of Prosthetic Medicine', *The Lancet* 377 (12 Feb. 2011), 548–9.

Finch, Jacqueline, 'The Durham Mummy: Deformity and the Concept of Perfection in the Ancient World', in R. David (ed.), *Ancient Medical and Healing Systems: Their Legacy to Western Medicine* (Bulletin of the John Rylands University Library of Manchester 89, Supplement 2012/2013), 111–32.

Finch, Jacqueline, Heath, F. L., David, A. Rosalie, and Kulkarni, J., 'The Biomedical Assessment of Two Artificial Big Toe Restorations from Ancient Egypt and their Significance to the History of Prosthetics', *Journal of Prosthetics and Orthotics* 24/4 (27 Sept. 2012), 181–91.

Frankfurter, David, *Religion in Roman Egypt* (Princeton, 1998).

Fuchs, Johannes, 'Physical Alterations which Occur in the Blind and are Illustrated on Ancient Egyptian Works of Art', *Annals of the New York Academy of Sciences* 117 (1964), 618–23.

Ghalioungui, Paul, *Magic and Medical Science in Ancient Egypt* (London, 1963).

Gray, Peter H. K., 'A Radiographic Skeletal Survey of Ancient Egyptian Mummies', *Excerpta Medica. International Congress Series* 120 (1966a), 35–8.

Gray, Peter H. K., 'Radiological Aspects of the Mummies of Ancient Egyptians in the Rijksmuseum van Oudheden, Leiden', *Oudheidkundige Mededelingen uit het Rijksmuseum van Oudheden te Leiden* 47 (1966b), 1–30.

Gray, Peter H. K., 'Radiography of Ancient Egyptian Mummies', *Medical Radiography and Photography* 43 (1967a), 34–44.

Gray, Peter H. K., 'Embalmers' Restorations', *Journal of Egyptian Archaeology* 52 (1967b), 138.

Gray, Peter H. K., 'A Case of Osteogenesis Imperfecta Associated with Dentinogenesis Imperfecta, Dating from Antiquity', *Clinical Radiology* 20 (1969), 106–8.

Gray, Peter H. K., 'The Radiography of Mummies of Ancient Egyptians', *Journal of Human Evolution* 2 (1973), 51–3.

Gunn, Battiscombe, 'Religion of the Poor in Ancient Egypt', *Journal of Egyptian Archaeology* 3 (1916), 81–94.

Harris. James E., and Weeks, Kent R., *X-Raying the Pharaohs* (New York, 1973).

Harris, James E., and Wente, Edward F. (eds), *An X-Ray Atlas of the Royal Mummies* (Chicago, IL, and London, 1980).

Harrison, Ronald G., Connolly, Robert C., Ahmed, Soheir, Abdalla, A. B., and el-Ghawaby, M., 'A Mummified Foetus from the Tomb of Tutankhamun', *Antiquity* 53 (1979), 19–21.

Hawass, Zahi, and Saleem, Sahar N., 'Mummified Daughters of King Tutankhamun', *American Journal of Roentgenology* (Nov. 2011), 829–36.

Hawass, Zahi, Gad, Yehia Z., Ismail, Somaia, Khairat, Rabab, Fathalla, Dina, Hasan, Naglaa, Ahmed, Amal, Elleithy, Hisham, Ball, Markus, Gaballa, Fawzi, Wasef, Sally, Fateen, Mohamed, Amer, Hany, Gostner, Paul, Selim, Ashraf, Zink, Albert, and Pusch, Carsten M., 'Ancestry and Pathology in King Tutankhamun's Family', *Journal of the American Medical Association* 303/7 (17 Feb. 2010), 638–47.

Hornung, Erik, *Conceptions of God in Ancient Egypt: The One and the Many.* 2nd edn. tr. and rev.John Baines (London, 1983²).

Hussien, Fawzia, El-Banna, Rokia, Kandel, Wafaa, and El-Din, Azza Sarry, 'Similarity of Fracture Treatment of Workers and High Officials of the Pyramid Builders', in J. Cockitt and R. David (eds), *Pharmacy and Medicine in Ancient Egypt* (Oxford, 2010), 85–9.

Janssen, Rosalind, and Janssen, Jac J., *Getting Old in Ancient Egypt* (London, 1996).

Janssens, Paul A., *Palaeopathology: Diseases and Injuries of Prehistoric Man* (London, 1970).

Jantzen, Gunter, 'Der blinde Harfner auf dem Grabrelief Paatenemheb', *Materia Medica Nordmark* 20 (1968), 689–94.

Jeffreys, David, and Tait, John, 'Social Exclusion in Dynastic Egypt', in J. Hubert (ed.), *Madness, Disability and Social Exclusion: The Archaeology and Anthropology of 'Difference'* (London, 2000), 87–95.

Junker, Herman, *Giza,* V. *Die Mastabas des Snb und die umliegenden Gräber* (Vienna, 1941).

Kellenberger, Edgar, 'Children and Adults with Intellectual Disability in Antiquity and Modernity: Toward a Biblical and Sociological Model', *CrossCurrents: Association for Religion and Intellectual Life* (Dec. 2013), 449–72.

Lang, Phillipa, *Medicine and Society in Ptolemaic Egypt* (Leiden and Boston, MA, 2013).

Leek, Frank F., 'Cheops' Courtiers: Their Skeletal Remains', in R. A. David (ed.), *Science in Egyptology* (Manchester, 1986), 183–99.

Lewis, Naphtali, *Life in Egypt under Roman Rule* (Oxford, 1983).

Lichtheim, Miriam, *Ancient Egyptian Literature,* 2 vols (Berkeley and Los Angeles, CA, 1975–6).

Long, Allen R., 'Cardiovascular Renal Disease: Report of a Case 3000 Years Ago', *Archives of Pathology* 12 (1931), 92–6.

Lowenstein, Eve J., 'Osteogenesis Imperfecta in a 3,000-Year-Old Mummy', *Child's Nervous System* 25/5 (May 2009), 515–16.

Manniche, Lise, 'Symbolic Blindness', *Chronique de l'Égypte* 53/105 (1978), 13–21.

Marchant, Jo, *The Shadow King* (Boston, MA, 2013).

Mitchell, John K., 'Study of a Mummy Affected with Anterior Poliomyelitis', *Philadelphia Medical Journal* 6 (1900), 414–15.

Molto, J. Eldon, 'Spina Bifida Occulta in Skeletal Samples from the Dakhleh Oasis'. Paper Presented at the 16th Annual Meeting of the Paleopathology Association, San Diego. *Paleopathology Newsletter* (abstract) 66 (supplement) (1989), 8.

Morse, Daniel, Brothwell, Don R., and Ucko, Peter J., 'Tuberculosis in Ancient Egypt', *American Review of Respiratory Diseases* 90 (1964), 524–41.

Murray, Margaret A. *The Tomb of Two Brothers* (Manchester, 1910).

Nerlich, Andreas, Zink, Albert, Szeimies, Ulrike, and Hagedorn, Hjalmar, 'Ancient Egyptian Prosthesis of the Big Toes', *The Lancet* 356 (2000), 2176–9.

Nerlich, Andeas G., Panzer, Stephanie, and Lösch, Sandra, 'Surgery in Ancient Egypt: Palaeopathological Evidence for Successful Medical Treatment by Surgery', in J. Cockitt and R. David (eds), *Pharmacy and Medicine in Ancient Egypt* (Oxford, 2010a), 117–21.

Nerlich, Andeas G., Panzer, Stephanie, Hower-Tilmann, Estelle, and Lösch, Sandra, 'Palaeopathological-Radiological Evidence for Cerebral Palsy in an Ancient Egyptian Female Mummy from a 13th Dynasty Tomb', in J. Cockitt and R. David (eds), *Pharmacy and Medicine in Ancient Egypt* (Oxford, 2010b), 113–16.

Nunn, John F., *Ancient Egyptian Medicine* (London, 1996).

Pinch, Geraldine, *Magic in Ancient Egypt* (London, 1994).

Rabino Massa, Emma, 'Two Cases of Spina Bifida in Egyptian Mummies.' Paper Presented at the 2nd European Meeting of the Paleopathology Association, Turin. *Paleopathology Newsletter* (abstract) 25 (supplement) (1978), 13.

Raven, Maarten J., and Taconis, Wybren K., *Egyptian Mummies: Radiological Atlas of the Collections in the National Museum of Antiquities at Leiden* (Turnhout, 2005).

Robinson, Joanne M., 'Close-Kin Marriage and Congenital Abnormalities in Ancient Egypt: The Incidence, Impact and Perception of Disability in Non-Royal Families' (forthcoming).

Romano, James F., 'The Origin of the Bes-Image', *Bulletin of the Egyptological Seminar* 2 (1980), 39–56.

Rowling, J. Thompson, 'Disease in Ancient Egypt: Evidence from Pathological Lesions Found in Mummies' (unpublished PhD, Cambridge, 1960).

Ruffer, Marc A., 'On Arterial Lesions Found in Egyptian Mummies', in R. L. Moodie (ed.), *Studies in the Palaeopathology of Egypt* (Chicago, IL, 1921), 20–31.

Sandison, Andrew T., 'Diseases of the Eyes', in D. Brothwell and A. T. Sandison (eds), *Diseases in Antiquity* (Springfield, IL, 1967), 457–63.

Schäfer, Heinrich, *Principles of Egyptian Art*, tr. and rev. John Baines. (Oxford, 1986).

Shattock, Samuel G., 'A Report upon the Pathological Condition of the Aorta of King Menephtah, Traditionally Regarded as the Pharaoh of the Exodus', *Proceedings of the Royal Society of Medicine, London,* Pathology Section 2 (1909), 122–7.

Smith, Grafton E., *The Royal Mummies: Catalogue Général des Antiquités Égyptiennes du Musée du Caire, Nos. 61051-61100* (Cairo, 1912).

Smith, Grafton E., and Dawson, Warren R., *Egyptian Mummies* (London, 1924).

Smith, Grafton E., and Jones, Frederick W., *The Archaeological Survey of Nubia: Report for 1907–1908, II. Report on the Human Remains* (Cairo, 1910).

Wells, Calvin, *Bones, Bodies and Diseases: Evidence of Disease and Abnormality in Early Man* (London, 1964).

Wente, Edward F., 'Age of Death of Pharaohs of the New Kingdom, Determined from Historical Sources', in J. E. Harris and E. F. Wente (eds), *An X-Ray Atlas of the Royal Mummies* (Chicago, IL, and London, 1980), 234–85.

West, Stephanie, 'Whose Baby? A Note on P. Oxy. 744', *Zeitschrift für Papyrologie und Epigraphik* 120 (1998), 167–72.

Williams, Herbert U., 'Human Palaeopathology', *Archives of Pathology* 7 (1929), 839–902.

Worth Estes, Joseph, *The Medical Skills of Ancient Egypt* (Canton, 1989).

7

INDIA

Demystifying disability in Antiquity

M. Miles

Introduction: whose snatch of India's history?

Before starting on disability history, it will be useful to recognize that the literature of India's general history continues to be a series of bitterly contested battlegrounds. The question has variously been raised whether Indians (or Hindus) have any 'sense of history', or are somehow deficient in what western and other critics count as an obvious accomplishment of a major civilization. The enquiry may then be reversed, with vigorous denunciations by Hindus (and other Indians) suggesting that the critics are playing the usual Eurocentric, racially biased games. These may be based on discredited notions of 'history' as a mono-directional process in which the supposed moral and technological superiority of the 'white man' inevitably triumphs over the feeble-minded muddling of the 'non-white' races. Within India, the mass media have called academic historians before the bar of public opinion, to give authoritative statements on 'facts', such as whether a centuries-old mosque (which had recently been destroyed) was built on the site of an earlier Hindu temple. On territory that was historically India (though now mostly known as Pakistan), the battles concern the 'Indo-Aryan Invasion' theory (or perhaps the hypothesis of migration by users of Indo-European languages). It has been argued that the remarkable early civilization of Harappa and Mohenjadaro from perhaps 2500 to 1500 BCE, and the literary heritage of the Vedic texts from c.1700–1200 BCE, were brought into India by invaders (or migrants). A vigorously advocated riposte is that both the genesis and the genius of that civilization and subsequent religious texts were entirely Indian, and were peacefully and generously sent forth from India to enlighten the savage tribes living to the west, even as far west as England![1]

Amidst these battles, the dating suggested for the completion of the Vedic texts may vary from as early as 4000(!?) BCE to 1200 BCE. The life of such a major teacher as the Buddha Gautama is thought to cover eighty years somewhere between 623 and 355 BCE, and the number of people interested in his life and teachings increased steadily for a thousand years. The origins of great Indian epics such as the *Mahabharata* and the *Ramayana* may also be dated with wide variation. Other recognizably great figures of Antiquity such as the grammarian Panini, the medical pioneers Susruta and Caraka, and the ruler Ashoka, have remained little known to the vast majority of Indians through most of historical time, though their lives (or their myths) might now be reconstructed or embellished for school textbooks.[2] Histories of disability, or of apparent responses to disabled people in earlier ages, have begun to be constructed so recently, and are perhaps so marginal to the general public's interest in history, that they are not yet covered in the smoke and flames of battle. Yet in so far as efforts are being made to discover and verify early records of disability and social responses to it, some of the confusion, anger and competing theories mentioned above will inevitably influence the development of this field. (Kindly be patient ...)

Ancient Indian texts: strong in size, weak on critique

Compared with Europe and the Middle East, South Asia has a larger population and range of languages, a similar land mass, and probably a vaster literature of religious diversity, stretching back through several millennia. Yet the absence of critical textual editing is underlined by seasoned western scholars, reviewing the field of Vedic Hinduism:

> The shocking truth is that even for Vedic texts, not to speak of other Sanskrit texts, there hardly exists any truly critical edition. What we have are the generally reliable standard editions, largely of the last [i.e. the 19th] century by European and American Indologists (Whitney, Bloomfield) which, however, in reality are editions with the variae lectiones more or less diligently recorded. They all lack a stemma of the MSS. In some cases, such as Roth-Whitney's Atharvaveda, it is extremely difficult to get even a vague idea of the distribution of the MSS at a certain passage.
>
> *(Jamison and Witzel 2003: 25)*

These experts further note that 'There is no complete modern English translation, though there are unsatisfactory and outmoded ones', among which is that by Ralph Griffith (*Rig Veda* from 1926). Volumes of a new critical edition and translation of the Rig Veda to German by Witzel and colleagues have slowly been appearing (Witzel and Goto 2007; Witzel *et al.* 2013) with several more volumes to come. A long-awaited new edition and translation to English finally appeared from Oxford University Press in June 2014, in three volumes (*Rig Veda*, Jamison and Brereton 2014). These fresh translations with copious critical apparatus can be expected to encompass the major findings of modern scholarship; yet it was known long before publication that the new English version would be quite obscure for the general literate reader (Thomson 2009: 8–9). Such readers may also take into account Karen Thomson's energetic critique of Witzel and many other western Veda experts, for their (alleged) inability to differentiate and disentangle Ancient Sanskrit from the serious muddle caused by using later materials and assumptions to try to interpret the original language. Thomson (2009) suggests that most of the problems and supposedly 'barbaric syntax' found by the standard methods disappear when using the incoming paradigm.

Similar strictures come from Wendy Doniger O'Flaherty who translated 10 per cent of the Rig Veda hymns. She opens jauntily, 'This is a book for people, not for scholars' (*Rig Veda*, O'Flaherty 1981: 11), while providing for each hymn an introduction and notes that are mostly as long as the hymn, plus forty-four pages of appendices, concordances, bibliographies and indexes. Of the existing English translations she notes that 'some are complete, but unsound (Wilson, Griffith), some incomplete and unsound (Max Müller, P. Lal), some incomplete but sound (Macdonnell, Panikkar), but only Panikkar could be called readable, and his is a strongly slanted selection and rendition' (O'Flaherty 1981: 12). Yet O'Flaherty recognizes that some 'people', who are neither Sanskritists nor Indologists, but are interested in ancient India, will 'fight their way through' the German, French, Russian or other translations, and will pore over the journal articles and dictionaries, in search of meanings (*Rig Veda*, O'Flaherty 1981: 11), without settling down to learn Sanskrit to the point (ten or fifteen years down the line) where they might credibly argue with existing translations and produce their own.

Disability history and ancient India

When searched for, disabilities show up in literary and religious records from the 1st millennium BCE, and there is no shortage of classifications and categorizations of human beings into classes, castes, ranks and appearance. Yet writing on 'disability history' has been comparatively a late starter. The present brief chapter on 'India' can hardly equal the erudition and field maturity displayed by teams of scholars in classical western Antiquity; yet it may suffice to show that India does not lack material evidence depicting social responses to disability through long stretches of Antiquity, and in a variety of disciplines.

For India, a benefit of starting later is that some successes and errors of western disability history are already visible, and something may be learnt from them. One identifiable plague is that people keenly interested in disability history often 'read back' modern agendas into the past. There is a tendency to 'raid the junk rooms' of history, wrenching odds and ends out of context, which might seem to support modern campaigns for greater attention (with some money or privilege attached) to be paid to this or that minority group. Enforcement of disciplinary barriers may also offer an excuse to exclude useful evidence. For example, scholars within western 'Disability Studies' may try to rule out 'medical history', on the grounds that the (so-called) 'medical model' has caused oppression and misunderstanding toward people with disabilities down the ages. Yet such an exclusion would hamper the identification of most historical disabled persons, who tend to show up with a 'defect label' (e.g. blind, deaf, crippled, etc.). Some would argue that the history of women, disabled people, oppressed castes or classes, can properly be studied only by historians personally suffering the same oppression now. Others would be happy to read any author who assures their nation of a 'golden age' (before the 'brutal British imperialists' ruined everything; or the 'brutal Aryan hordes' poured down from the north and wiped out the cultures and languages of a beautiful southern civilization). These temptations or pitfalls can be seen in existing historical writings, and are obstacles to Indians wishing to develop resources for a mature field of disability history. Yet South Asians certainly have much to discover and share from the riches of their ancient cultures. (There is much to be learnt by Westerners too; but it is predictable that scholars familiar with disability in Mediterranean Antiquity will hasten to snatch this or that event, law or person and compare or contrast them with what they know from their own 'home ground' – regardless of any cautions about difficulties and fuzziness of present South Asian texts, translations and knowledge.)

Some useful ground has been reviewed by distinguished Asian scholars such as the late D. P. M. Weerakkody, professor of Western Classics, who was born blind, obtained his doctorate in classical languages at Hull University, became the first blind Sri Lankan to gain a full professorship, and sometimes wrote on historical blindness (e.g. Weerakkody 2008); and Dr Ajit Dalal, Professor of Psychology at the University of Allahabad, whose substantial physical impairments never stopped him being a driving force both in modernizing psychology teaching in India, and retrieving the ancient roots of 'Indian Psychology' (Dalal and Misra 2010). It has been a privilege for the present author to work with Asian colleagues like these and others who shared a concern that 'modernization' should not neglect to build on the richest conceptual roots or rhizomes available in historical South Asia. That a younger Indian generation of researchers in 'critical disability studies' may tackle the complexity of reconfiguring 'corporeality' in historical Asian conceptual terms is indicated recently by Shilpaa Anand (2015).

Evidence from archaeology, geography, agriculture, medicine

Glimpses of these disciplines will be treated first, having some overlap and possessing elements of scientific evidence.

Power knapping?

Recent research in India suggests a link between measurable evidence of hominoid brain growth and differentiation of skills in making fine stone-cutting tools, and in social skills including imitation, possibly also linked with a switch from iconic gestural language to post-iconic sign language and the slow development of spoken language. Such ambitious claims, as for example by Shipton (2013: esp. 79–87), may at times resemble the thoughts of a circus acrobat spinning plates with her toes as she balances upside down on one hand resting on the head of a gibbon riding a donkey round the ring. Yet Ceri Shipton's work acknowledges the more solid basis of forty years' excavations and analysis at Hunsgi, Karnataka, by Professor K. Paddayya and colleagues, beginning in 1975 and probing more deeply into the life and mind of humankind's presumed ancestors. During the past two decades, using new technical tools and arguments of considerable complexity (e.g. Petraglia *et al.* 2005), the show might prove stronger than a circus act. A glance at another Stone Age Indian site adds further spin, e.g. evidence of 'handedness', with a small but recognizable proportion of 'left-handed' tools at Meghalaya in North-East India (Ashraf 2010: 128; cf. Humer 2012, on handedness in Mediterranean Antiquity).

If these scholars' analyses of evidence are even approximately correct, it might be reasonable to spin one more 'plate': that (some of) the ancestors would have become conscious of a spectrum from higher skills to average skills and weaker skills, with (possibly) a slow development of enhanced survival for groups having members with higher physical strength and hand control, fine finger movement skills, sharper visual abilities, clearer hearing for activities needing discussion of strategies (Malafouris 2010). At the weaker end of the perceived spectrum they may have 'discovered' impairments and disabilities as less desirable states, a response generated by the increasing demands of more complex communities and requirements for accurate communication. (Alternatively, or additionally, might some have discovered an increase in 'caring capacity', prolonging the life and comfort of those impaired from infancy, or injured later in life by large, hungry animals?) These few snatches of archaeological evidence hardly give a fair representation of many decades of painstaking work at hundreds of Indian sites. As updated techniques become more widespread, it is likely that evidence bearing more directly on impairments and disabilities may appear.

Iodine deficiency disorders

Ancient Indian geographical events have some links with disabling conditions such as goitre, cretinism, deafness and other outcomes of iodine deficiency, probably lasting through several thousand years (Miles 1998; Stewart 1990), and still capable of disabling significant proportions of local populations. There is a possible visual representation of goitre in ancient Gandhara, in one of the Buddha's tormenters or distractors (Blumberg 1964).

Paralysing lathyrism

More than forty archaeological sites have shown evidence of lathyrus sativus among the oldest legumes of ancient India, dating as far back as 2000 BCE (Fuller and Harvey 2006). While being used at some periods as a resilient fodder crop, and in famine periods as a staple for poorer people across large areas, members of the lathyrus species may cause permanent paralysis in some consumers whose diet lacks adequate micro-nutrients. Evidence of crippling 'lathyrism' is suggested in the ancient Indian medical/surgical text *Susrutasamhita*, (Singhal *et al.* 1972: 28–29): 'When there is trembling in taking the first few steps with limping and when organization of the joint gets loose, it is known as Kalayakhanja [footnote: Kalaya – Khesari pulse].' However, the identification is considered unproven by the Sanskrit medical authority Dominik Wujastyk (*Susrutasamhita*, 1998: 168–9). Wujastyk has made formidable contributions in seemingly conflicting ways: his 'popular' translation of carefully selected ancient and medieval 'Ayurvedic' medical texts mentions some disabling conditions, while also emphasizing the pitfalls in such translations since very little critical textual work has been done to establish reliable authenticity. 'In the absence of such editions we cannot really say we know the foundations of Ayurveda. Our impression of the tradition is partial, fuzzy, out of focus' (*Susrutasamhita*, Wujastyk 1998: 21).

Disabling medical conditions in Vedas and Jatakas

Whether, how and when there was an effective system of Ayurvedic treatment, Kenneth Zysk has shown medicine and medical classification to have a significant presence in the Vedas, while emphasizing that 'The medicine of the Vedic Indians is inextricably connected with their religion and must not be considered in isolation from it'(*Vedas*, Zysk 1998: p. xvii). His detailed, scholarly studies include disability-related conditions such as blindness and eye disease, deafness and ear disease; epilepsy; foot problems and various fractures; insanity or mental disorders; leprosy and other skin disorders; hydrocephalus (with possible treatment by trepanation) (Zysk 1998), found mostly in the Atharva Veda, Rig Veda, Caraka, Susruta, plus many other classical texts and commentaries. (Trepanation as an ancient practice is confirmed by Sankhyan and Weber 2001, and Sankhyan and Schug 2010, though not necessarily for hydrocephalus.) A substantial amount of Sanskrit text is transliterated and translated by Zysk, with corresponding detailed textual annotations (*Vedas*, Zysk 1998: 104–256). Diligent comparison of the indexes of Sanskrit text locations, Sanskrit words and general index will facilitate the path of the reader not equipped with Sanskrit. The bibliographic history and specialized bibliography of primary texts and translations (Zysk 1998: 261–90) usefully show how successive generations of scholars and amateurs played roles, mostly facilitating one another's work, during two 'slow' centuries of pre-electronic work. The seminal contribution of Jean Filliozat (1964), a French medical doctor who became a Sanskrit specialist, is particularly recommended.

Jataka stories

The earliest extant materials showing expressions of interest in disability may be the depictions of dwarf figures and of the *Jataka* (lives of the Buddha) stories (*Jataka*, ed. Cowell, 1895–1907) in cave art of Gandhara, possibly dating back to a period from 3rd century BCE to 2nd century CE. The standard 547 Jataka stories include encounters with blindness (No. 499, Sivi J.; No. 540, Sama [or Shyama] J.); leprosy (No. 516, Mahakapi J.); devoted wifely care of leprosy sufferer (No. 519, Sambula J.); learning difficulties (Nangalisa J.), simulated deafness and mental vacancy (Muga-Pakkha [or Muka-Pangu] J.), and other impairments (No. 536, Kunala J.), some of which are represented also in the Ajanta caves of Maharashtra (Jamkheda 2009: 16, 22–5, 48, 50–1, 71, 75), and in Gandharan cave art at Jamal-Garhi in the Peshawar valley (Foucher 1915: 19–20).

Among many tales casually mentioning disability, two Jataka stories relate to special education or childhood disability. Nangalisa-J. (No. 123; *Jataka*, ed. Cowell I: 271–2) tells of efforts to teach a slow learner using activity methods and a practical curriculum. However, the efforts fail: 'This dullard will never learn'. In Muga-Pakkha-J. (No. 538; *Jataka*, ed. Cowell VI: 1–19), the Bodhisatta appears as a baby prince. Horrified by the harshness of the king, he pretends to be a 'deaf and dumb cripple'. Nurses and courtiers, unconvinced by the pretence, try various tests based on established norms and audiological principles. They watch him closely while causing a conch to be blown suddenly under his bed. They shine lights on him suddenly in the night, but by mental concentration the prince keeps still. They tempt him with milk, fruit or toys and try to surprise him with animals, according to the ages at which children normally responded to such stimuli. Further examples may be found in the Cowell (1895–1907) edition (which is outdated, but has the merit of being freely available online), such as Nos. 80, Bhimasena-J. (Bodhisatta as crooked dwarf); 107 Salittaka-J. (cripple on a little cart); 184, Giridanta-J. (lame horse-trainer, limping horse); 202 Keli-Sila-J. (cruel treatment of elderly people, among whom was the small-statured teacher Lakuntaka). The life of that saintly Buddhist teacher Lakuntaka Baddhiya has recently been assembled from various sources, as one of the most important documents on responses to disability in early Theravada Buddhism (Hartl 2012).

Junko Matsumura (*Jataka*, 2012) gives details of Chinese manuscripts from the 4th and 5th centuries CE, recounting the Jataka story in which the Bodhisattva let himself be eaten by a starving tiger and her cubs. One manuscript was translated by the monk Fasheng (c.406–79 CE), from Turfan. A stupa had been built at the location, and Fasheng travelled through Gandhara to see this stupa, 'two days journey towards east from Taxila'. Fasheng reported that there were 'monks' apartments, a preaching hall and a cloister', and several thousand monks present. Further:

> people from all countries who have illnesses of various kinds like leprosy, mental disease, deafness, blindness or lameness in hand or foot, came to this *stupa*. They burnt incense, lit lamps, spread scented mud, repaired and swept; and [when] they kowtowed and confessed, all diseases were become cured. Immediately after the one that had come earlier left, the next one came and did in the same manner. There were always more than a hundred people without distinction of rank and who all did in the same way, [and thus] there was no interruption.
>
> *(Matsumura 2012: 54)*

This glowing account by Fasheng followed one by Faxian (Fa-hien) about twenty-five years earlier, who had passed through Gandhara on the way to Pataliputtra (modern Patna) in Maghada, a thousand miles south-east. Faxian reported that 'houses for dispensing charity and medicines' were widely established in cities of the region (*Travels of Fa-hien*, Legge 1886: 79). In a detailed history of early medicine and healing in Buddhist monasteries, Zysk (1991: 46–7, 54–6) notes the pre-eminence of Taxila as a centre of medical education, from the 1st century CE until early in the 5th century. Ancient copper surgical instruments have also been discovered in the ruins, from the same period (Naqvi 2003). Eye diseases were prominent on the treatment agenda at Taxila (Zysk 1991: 57, 66, 88–91).

Fascinating philology: words for disabilities

The aggregate vocabularies of Sanskrit and later Indo-Aryan languages, described in Sir Ralph Turner's massive dictionary, display an impressive range of 'defect' terms, varying by vowel change, rhyme, double consonants and other deformations (Turner 1966: pp. ix–xi). The feelings associated with these terms may have evoked some 'audible underlining'. Colin Masica (1989: 183) refers to 'spontaneous nasalization, spontaneous retroflexion, spontaneous aspiration, and spontaneous gemination – "spontaneous" in the sense of not clearly motivated by the preexisting sequence of sounds'. Masica further suggests that defect terms may involve 'other motivations, such as emphasis ... deformation or special treatment of taboo words and words referring themselves to deformities (a category noted by Turner), or contamination with semantically related words' (1989: 471). Reasons for such graphic doublings and 'special treatment' are hard to disentangle centuries later. Consequently it is hard to discern, in the evolution of these languages, just where the descriptive and comparative uses may slyly become abusive. Meanings of the group of Indo-Aryan words given by Turner around *manthara* and *manda* range through 'slow, lazy, dull, bent, hunchbacked, idle, weak, dull-witted, bad, simple, stupid, tardy, thick, corpulent, dim, dwarfish, short, slow, little, base, unprofitable, wicked, evil-speaking, slight, faint, vile', plus other shades of meaning. Further, the *manthara* and *manda* group are part of larger groups with ramifications of meaning in some 200 languages across 3,000 years. See, for example, the 'blockhead' vocabulary formed from Turner's headwords (most diacritical marks removed): baggha- / bajja- / bukka- / butta- / bussa- / bobba- / bhakkha- / bhadrá / bhukkhara- / bhucca- / bhutta- / bhulla- / bhekka- / bheda- / bhela- / matta- / mattá- / matthara- / midda- / mitta- / mugdhá / mutta-. These suggest the luxuriant Indo-Aryan taxonomy of defect. A rough comparison of 'blindness' in Turner's dictionary shows similar variation, with slightly less headwords. It would probably be wrong to make direct comparison between these lists, which seem to display some similar features, and suggest some embarrassment, guilty enjoyment or diffidence in the usage. It would require deeper study even to hazard a guess that 'blindness' might evoke less mirth than 'foolishness'.

The Vedic Index (MacDonell and Keith 1912) seems to show surprisingly few words for blindness, compared with what could be expected from the (supposed) conditions of life in the geography of ancient North India. In warmer regions one could anticipate much dust-related damage to sight; and in cooler regions, more smoke-related damage from cooking fires in enclosed spaces. Whether hunting animals, or chipping rock to form cutting tools, or fighting to defend a tribal patch of ground, there would have been many hazards to eyes, both male and female; yet the fields of Vedic medicine (reviewed above by Zysk) and the Vedic texts seem rather short of visual impairment terms, as compared with the later Ayurvedic studies. Might this merely reflect a different purpose and era in the texts, i.e. of early religious ritual as against medical treatment? Or is it more likely that the vocabularies of Antiquity did not conceptualize or express 'disability' within the semantic range familiar to literate modern readers?

Some 'defect' terms are probably borrowed from agriculture and animal husbandry for application to humans: the crops may come up with good grain and fruit, or may be withered, misformed or worm-eaten. Well-formed and docile sheep or cattle will be contrasted with the deformed or ill-tempered ones. Such 'defect' terms, and coarser ones, would be ready in the mouths of farm workers, as well their superiors. Brian Smith (1992) offers a wide-ranging study of ancient Indian classification of humans and animals for various purposes, some being 'politically incorrect' on the grand scale. He translates briefly from the *Aitareya Aranyaka*, possibly c.500 BCE, some important human versus 'other animal' differences in terms of 'intelligence':

> In the human, the self (*atman*) becomes more manifest, for he is most perfected with intelligence (*prajnanena sampannatamo*). He articulates what he knows (*vijnatam vadati*); he observes what he knows (*vijnatam pasyati*); he knows (that there is) the future; he knows (the difference between) what is in the world and what is otherworldly. He desires the obtainment of the immortal through the mortal – thus (is his) perfection. Now among the other animals, they perceive only hunger and thirst. They do not articulate what they know; they do not observe what they know; they do not know (that there is) the future; they do not know (the difference between) what is in the world and what is otherworldly. They become only so much, according to their intelligence and capacity.)

> (*Aitareya Aranyaka* 2.3.2, Smith 1992: 546)

This kind of intelligence-based differentiation of course raises questions on the available terminology in the period. Olivelle (*Upanisads* 1996: 198, 364) offers a kind of parallel or response from the Aitareya Upanishad, enquiring about 'the self':

> Is it that by which one sees? Or hears? Or smells odours? Or utters speech? Or distinguishes between what is tasty and what is not? Is it the heart and the mind? Is it awareness? Perception? Discernment? Cognition? Wisdom? Insight? Steadfastness? Thought? Reflection? Drive? Memory? Intention? Purpose? Will? Love? Desire? But these are various designations of cognition.
>
> *(Aitareya Upanishad 3.2)*

An earlier translator, Ernest Hume (*Upanishads* 1931: 300) usefully gives the transliterated Sanskrit, on the cognitive features:

> that which is heart (*hridaya*) and mind (*manas*) – that is consciousness (*samjnana*), perception (*ajnana*), discrimination (*vijnana*), intelligence (*prajnana*), wisdom (*medhas*), insight (*dristi*), steadfastness (*dhriti*), thought (*mati*), thoughtfulness (*manisa*), impulse (*juti*), memory (*smriti*), conception (*samkalpa*), purpose (*kratu*), life (*asu*), desire (*kama*), will (*vasa*). All these, indeed, are appellations of intelligence (*prajnana*) [accents omitted].
>
> *(Aitareya Upanishad 3.2)*

Most of these features would seem to provide evident difference between animals in the wild and humankind in community – yet the aspects and features making up intelligence and cognition would also serve to pick out some people having significantly less cognitive speed and capacity.

Evidence from cosmic myths

Among the earliest Upanishads, perhaps from the 6th century BCE but drawing on earlier sources (*Upanisads*, Olivelle 1996: p. xxxvi), *Brihad-aranayaka Upanishad* portrays a detailed Sanskrit cosmology in the modern idiomatic translation of Patrick Olivelle. After descriptions of gods and demons in battle, and the uses of speech, breath-in-the-mouth, smell, hearing, mind and breath-as-vitality (*Upanisads* Olivelle 1996: 8–12, 293–5), humankind arrives on the scene and starts to realize some basic facts of life.

> In the beginning this world was just a single body (*atman*) shaped like a man. He looked around and saw nothing but himself. The first thing he said was, 'Here I am!' Pretty soon the man felt lonely, so he divided himself down the middle, making a husband and a wife.
>
> *(Upanisads Olivelle 1996: 13–14)*

Things gradually got sorted out, with some interconnections of speech, mind and breath, which all play a prominent part in figuring out the universe. Eventually, the various senses or 'vital functions' (*prana*), like breath, speech, sight, hearing, etc., argue about which of them is most important. The competition between them is most clearly expressed in *Chandogya Upanishad* 5.1 (*Upanisads* Olivelle 1996: 137–8, 343), where each sense takes a year's leave, then returns to see how the others fared. For most, the outcome is summarized in *Kausitaki Upanishad* 3, here further abbreviated:

A man continues to live after his speech leaves him, for we see people who are dumb. A man continues to live after his sight leaves him, for we see people who are blind. A man (...) hearing leaves him (...) deaf. A man (...) mind leaves him (...) imbeciles. A man (...) arms are cut off and legs are cut off, for we see such people.

(Upanisads Olivelle 1996: 216–217, 370)

In each account, the punch-line comes when breath prepares to leave: the other vital forces all recognize that the absence of breath will blow them all away.

The point emerges that major categories of impairment or disability are known and listed as everyday illustrations: 'we see such people'. Those people continue their lives with whatever capacities they have. No doctor's certificate is required; it's clear that they have one sense missing. Yet the philosophy school of the Upanishads is not discussing such matters exactly the way most modern philosophy students would tackle them. There is a background of gods and demons, slaughter of horses, fire, thunder and mysterious forces. Translators' explanatory endnotes bridge across the different conceptualization of the Sanskrit terms – or sometimes admit that scholars remain unsure of the meanings, or cannot find equivalents for the double-puns and word-plays embodied in the subtleties of Sanskrit verse. Connections of disability with notions of blame or causality, moral responsibility or *karma* are a further important complex, tackled cautiously by the Sanskritist Julia Leslie (1999), with examples from Antiquity to the television era.

Impairment and disability in the Rig Veda

The case of Dirghatamas (or Durghatamas) is interesting. It is quite possible that there really was a man known as Dirghatamas Mamateya (meaning something like 'utter darkness', son of Mamataa) and traditions suggest that he composed twenty-five hymns of the *Rig Veda* (numbers I: CXL to CLXV, see Griffith 1926: 96). There appear to be references to Dirghatamas in CXLVII; CXLVIII; CLVIII (see Griffith 1926: 100–5); CLXIV (see Griffith 1926: 111); and IV: IV (see Griffith 1926: 203); also in the *Atharva-Veda* (Griffith 1916, II: 448). Dirghatamas reportedly lived to a great age (nominally '100'), had a son, Kaksivant by a female servant named Usij, and this son also became a Rishi (a recognized sage or teacher). Some centuries later the life of Dirghatamas had acquired further detail, as gathered up in the encyclopedic epic *Mahabharata* (Ganguli 1970, I: Adi Parva, CIV, 224–6), whether legendary or having some credible basis in fact. The wife of Dirghatamas, pragmatic Pradweshi, complains during a connubial tiff that her blind husband has not supported her as he ought; on the contrary, she has been obliged to support him. As the quarrel develops, Pradweshi instructs her sons to throw their father into the Ganges. They set him adrift on a raft. Eventually he is rescued by King Vali, who lacks children, so invites the venerable Rishi to beget sons for him, with queen Sudeshna. But Sudeshna, knowing the Rishi is blind and old, sends her Sudra nurse to him, with whom he has eleven children. Dirghatamas has been noted above, as a singer and author of some Rig Veda hymns. However, Macdonell and Keith (1912: I: 366) express doubts about the later Dirghatamas legends.

Comparisons of mental ability and stability, or lack of it, also appear in the *Rig Veda*, though precise meanings have been hard for translators to decide, or to convey across cultural gulfs. *Rig Veda* 10.71 sings of the origins of the personified Word, Wisdom, Spiritual Knowledge, Speech or Expression, and its appropriation by some more than others and by some not at all. These differences caused divergence between fellow Brahmins; and also between translators. Raimundo Panikkar (*Rig Veda* 1977: 95) translates thus:

Friends, though endowed alike with sight and hearing, may yet in quickness of mind be quite unequal. Some are like ponds that reach to mouth or shoulder while others resemble lakes deep enough for bathing. When Brahmins sacrifice together in friendship, forming within their hearts inspirations of the spirit, their wise resolves may leave one man behind, while others, though reckoned as Brahmins, stray away.

(Rig Veda, 10.71.7–8)

An historian addressing ancient education applied the Vedic comparison directly to the world of school, citing the *Rig Veda* with Sayana's medieval commentary.

As the Rigveda itself points out [10.71.7]: 'Class-mates [sakhas, i.e. those of same knowledge ... or who have studied the same Sastras ...] may have equality in the possession of their senses like the eye and the ear, but betray inequality in respect of their power or speed of mind [... or the knowledge or wisdom which is attained by the mind (Sayana)]. Some are like tanks which reach up to the mouth ("unfathomable, i.e. minds whose depths cannot be reached", as explained by Durgacharya), others up to the breast only (i.e. "shallow, whose bottom is within sight"). Some are fit for bath, others are to be seen only'. As Sayana points out, this passage refers to three grades of students, the Mahaprajñañ, the Madhyamaprajñañ, and the Alpaprajñañ, students of high, medium, and low ability.

(Mookerji 1947: 25–6)

Studying these alternative translations, it is not hard to see how different phrases have been picked up to different effect. As Mookerji expatiated on the merits of ancient Indian education, this particular hymn came in for detailed exegesis, underlining the mental poverty of the 'blockhead' who merely chants the vedas without understanding, who is 'fit only for the plough or the loom' (Mookerji 1947: 30–3). Apparently Mookerji countenanced the inclusion of blockhead with egghead in primary school, 'marked by noisy recitation and repetition of texts by pupils in the manner of frogs lustily croaking after rain'. However, in secondary education 'the collective work of the pupils in a class ceased, and their individual work commenced'. Soon the bright stood out from the dim, and 'The more unfit were weeded out, sent back to the plough or the loom [10.71.9]' (Mookerji 1947: 36–7).

Law and legal status

The law code of Manu

The weighty critical edition and translation of Manu, probably 'composed during the first couple of centuries CE' (*Manava-Dharmasastra* Olivelle 2005: 18–25, 37), places this major law code on a new footing. After more than a century during which European translations had too narrow a manuscript base, Olivelle has now collated fifty-three manuscripts (the earliest dates shown are 1182, 1451(?), 1503, 1538 and 1540 CE), noting thirty-eight more manuscripts, and using nine early commentaries, the earliest of the latter probably dated in the 9th century CE (Olivelle 2005: 353–79). Olivelle's interest in disability extends to detailed indexing of pertinent terms, e.g. assault (physical), bald-headed, blind, body, castrate, consumption, crippled, deaf, dumb, ear, epilepsy, eunuch, eye, feet, foot, finger, fool, ghoul, hand, heal, hermaphrodite, idiot, insane, knee, lame, lazy, leprosy, leukoderma, limb, mad, massage, mental retardation, mouth, mute, neck, nose, organs, palm, punishment (corporal), senses, sick, skin, speech, teeth, tongue, women (barren); while 'club-footed' appears in Manu 3.165, on p.117, which escaped the indexer. Apart from some metaphorical use, these words are associated with legal enactments or exhortations, reflecting many centuries of legal and social background and practice, primarily as a 'Hindu' or Brahminical legal code. Manu offers a number of rules and references to disability, in the context of avoiding pollution or detriment in the performance of religious rites. They appear e.g. in a long list of people 'unfit' (through unwholesome means of earning a living, wrong behaviour, ill association, corporeal deficiency, etc.) to be invited to an ancestral rite (standard textual reference: chapter 3: 122–82; translation Olivelle 2005: 114–17, with notes on pp. 262–5; see also his notes on critical edition of Sanskrit: p. 927, where Olivelle discusses alternative readings for a particular term, and shows the reasoning behind his selection).

Some of Manu's remarks seem pejorative toward disabled people, e.g. in lists of those whose presence vitiates the benefit of a religious ritual (as in 3: 176–7). However, some different interpretations are possible, and many further disability-related items appear. Ariel Glucklich (1984) takes Manu's disability-related laws in the context of other Hindu writings and commentaries on law, disability and sickness, bringing out some positive elements, such as exemption from taxes (Manu, 8: 394) and some protection of property (8: 148). He recognizes that many of the rules are restrictive and seem to discriminate against disabled or chronically ill people: 'Handicapped and sick people are, in effect, denied status as legal agents.' Glucklich notes, however, that 'the notion of individuality implicit in the analysis of particular categories of persons could be misleading'. Individuals were seen in the context of the joint family where matters of property and inheritance were concerned, and the family was responsible for maintenance of sick or disabled members.

Arthasastra

This handbook of law, statecraft and politics has been attributed to Kautilya, and perhaps accumulated somewhere between 300 BCE and 200 CE. Kautilya's detailed, sophisticated proposals on statecraft and diplomacy, political economy and such topics as brothel regulation and the best way to run a spy network have a certain flavour and brisk pace, as in the robustly chauvinist batting order for suitors at the king's court: 'gods and deities, hermits, heretics, Brahmins learned in the Vedas, cows, sacred places, minors, the aged, the sick, the handicapped, the helpless and women' (*Arthasastra*: 1.19.29; Rangarajan 1987: 415). The legal incapacities of disabled people were similar to those recorded in Manu: they could neither inherit, nor make a valid contract, nor act as witnesses in court. Women employed in municipal brothels could decline to serve clients with physical defects; but on the positive side, sex workers were discouraged from adding to disfigurement, e.g. 'cutting off a client's ear' in the heat of the fray (Rangarajan 1987: 352, 354). (Could 'biting off' be more plausible?) A man should not insult his wife by calling her a cripple, and there were penalties for defamation involving disability terminology, whether true, false or ironic (Rangarajan 1987: 400, 470–1). The state organized a home-worker scheme by which women with disabilities, widows and similar persons could earn their living from textiles. Severe punishment was promised to the official running this scheme if he tried to frolic with the workforce, outside his proper duties. The latter in turn were encouraged not to skimp their work, under threat of digital amputation (Rangarajan 1987: 60, 332–4). Some disabled people might find employment in the spy network; but spies were sometimes able-bodied people disguised as 'deaf, dumb, blind, or idiotic'. The guise of simple-mindedness was sometimes recommended for entrapment of dishonest artisans, i.e. giving a valuable item into their safekeeping, to test whether they returned it on demand (Rangarajan 1987: 506, 509, 540, 463–4). It is not clear how far, when, or where, these propositions and regulations were actually effected, nor how great may have been the gap between prescription and practice.

Strange behaviour

David Kinsley discusses many episodes of 'madness' or strangeness among the Hindu deities, where frenzied, intoxicated, manic behaviour was exhibited. Similar behaviour also characterized devotees: 'it is abundantly clear that one of the traditional marks of a Hindu saint is madness' (Kinsley 1974: 286). The devotee of Krishna 'plays like a child, behaves like a dolt, and talks like a maniac' (Kinsley 1974: 287). Ramakrishna is quoted suggesting that 'A perfect knower of God and a perfect idiot have the same outer signs' (Kinsley 1974: 294). The major deity Shiva was sometimes portrayed as 'surrounded by idiots, epileptics' and crowds of frightful ghouls. In the *Kavitavali* of Tulsi Das, Shiva was also sometimes known as 'Master Simpleton' while at the same time being celebrated as the saviour of the universe (*Kavitavali* Allchin 1964: 190–3, 222). The gods are gods. They are not bound by human conventions. These points about the varied and curious representations of deities do, however, raise difficult issues for modern Governments of India, as they apply laws supposedly to protect citizens from finding their religious beliefs offended or ridiculed, at least within mass media using the major Indian languages. In many Western countries, 'freedom of speech' is supposed to be a sacred right, yet in practice it is everywhere bounded by laws against conduct liable to evoke violent responses; and such considerations exist no less in South Asia. Thus there is arguably some protection, e.g. for worshippers of Shiva in modern India, against having derogatory material thrust upon them in everyday life; or in Pakistan, for Muslims, against encountering whatever might be considered insulting to the prophet Muhammad.

Epic literature

Mahabharata

This vast 18-book epic poem, in some three million words, probably reached its final form 'between approximately 300 BCE and 300 CE, after the Mauryas and before the Guptas' (Doniger 2009: 261–3). The frame story of this encyclopedic work hinges on the disability of Dhritarashtra, who took the throne after his brother Pandu died. His legitimacy was disputed because he was born blind. The blindness surfaces in various ways. It is given as a reason why he could not prevent the dispute between his sons and nephews. The blind king grumbles to his chariot driver that, because of his inability to exert himself actively, his 'wretched son believes me to be a fool, and listens not to my words' (*Mahabharata*, Ganguli 1970, Vana Parva, XLIX: 108). Dhritarashtra informs this (eldest) son, Duryodhana, that even his own great-grandfather Devapi, eldest of three princes, could not inherit a kingdom because 'The gods do not approve a king that is defective' (Ganguli 1970, Udyoga P., CXLIX: 287–8). Yet Dhritarashtra is not always feeble. When Bhima has defeated Duryodhana in single combat, Pandu's sons go to meet Dhritarashtra: their ally, Krishna, tricks the blind monarch by introducing him to an iron statue in place of Bhima. The king seizes the statue and crushes it in his embrace, suffering much bruising and vomiting blood. He believes he has killed Bhima. After the rage has passed, they tell him he has destroyed an iron statue! (Ganguli 1970, Stree P., XII: 17–18). Late in the epic, after colossal slaughter on all sides, Dhritarashtra and his meek wife Gandhari (who voluntarily blindfolded herself throughout her marriage, to avoid 'seeing more than' her husband, Adi Parva, CX: 235) move across the stage. Sighted Kunti walks ahead, with Gandhari's hand on her shoulder; blind Dhritarashtra follows with hand on his wife's shoulder: an enduring moment of pathos (Ganguli 1970, Asramavasika P., XV: 25).

Ramayana

Originating perhaps in the 4th century BCE, with subsequent evolution through many centuries and multiple translations and locally variant dramatizations, Valmiki's *Ramayana* is the best known and loved of the Indian epics. Originally the story tells of a heroic man, Rama, who should inherit his father's throne, but through some trickery he is instead banished to become a forest dweller, and then suffers the kidnap of his wife Sita. With much anguish, he sets out to regain his wife, with the aid of an inspired band of monkeys. (But is Rama only a human hero, or is he an emissary of the gods, sent to earth to combat some evil powers?)

The story has only a modest disability content, mainly focused on Queen Kaikeyi's crafty hunchback servant Manthara, who plots the banishment of Rama. Valmiki's version has Queen Kaikeyi reflecting aloud to Manthara (= Kubija or Kubja, i.e. a hunchback or deformed person) that 'Deformed women are usually sinful and perverse, but thou, O Kubija, are unique, resembling a lotus bending to the breeze' (*Ramayana*, Shastri 1952: 171). Kaikeyi suggests that 'thy hump protruding like the hub of a wheel is surely filled with wisdom, diplomacy and understanding' (ibid. 171), an early connection of a 'hunch' with crafty wisdom. In some versions, however, Manthara is depicted as *mandamati* or dull witted. She is thus easily duped by an envoy of the gods into precipitating Rama's banishment, the cosmic purpose being to ensure that Rama is not distracted from his undercover mission to clear the earth of demons.

Developments and investments

Of the mass of (translated) Indian literature in which many kinds of disability appear, and responses are limned, the paragraphs above offer barely a glimpse. Given that there are considerable problems of dating and of identifying authors in many cases, and critical textual work is often weak, much of the fun of literary criticism must be postponed. Impatient readers might dismiss such 'evidence' as merely 'legendary' because it is not yet convincingly pinned in time and space recognizable to sceptical scholars. (Kindly be patient!) Yet this would certainly be to their loss. If the quantities of historical literature are vast, the power of modern computing tools is now equal to digitizing and managing even vaster quantities, comparing manuscripts and evoking new ripples in the renowned Indian talent for classification and categorization. If the epics can be turned into films, making new 'gods' out of film stars, perhaps the government can find a revenue stream to tackle the more scholarly study of Indian Antiquity. The great quantities of regional or provincial language material can also be expected to contribute to filling gaps of dating and background. And if disability can be searched for and found, everything else will be there too – because people with disabilities live complete human lives, as everyone else does. They merely do some things differently.

Notes

1 Amidst a vast literature, a few 21st-century items are here 'snatched' for useful reading. Arvind Sharma 2003 cannily titled an article 'Did the Hindus Lack a Sense of History?', and discusses the mistaken assumptions behind this widespread belief. Wendy Doniger (2009: 85–102) analyses the major battles as a series of 'Guesses'. While Doniger is among the liveliest contributors to critical Indian historiography, her meanings and nuances require a strong grasp of Anglo-American slang, punning and irony: the style owes much to the comedies of P. G. Wodehouse. Vinay Lal (2005 with updating) pursues historiography with an impressive range of reference and a talent for balanced portrayal of fellow writers even when differing sharply from their views. Meera Nanda 2009 tackles the 'Voice of India' writers, including Konrad Elst, who wish India to become the world's acknowledged spiritual leader – by power and domination, not mildness and humility.

Steve Farmer, Richard Sproat and Michael Witzel 2004 provide a far-reaching scholarly survey and robust demolition of 'Indus script' studies. Earlier work by Romila Thapar 1978 is also good value in its coverage of many little-known primary sources for deep Indian social history.

2 Thapar (2009) is an interesting update on much earlier work. She notes magnanimous features which might appeal to modern liberal thinkers – with the curious exception of Ashoka's view of the *atavikas* (forest-dwellers), who 'were at the receiving end of a fierce threat by the king of being killed – without any ostensible reason' (Thapar 2009: 32). To be non-persons was (and still is) their *disability*, in the original, legal sense. Dates for Buddha Gautama's life: the Sri Lankan tradition suggests 623–543 BCE; a conservative western dating might be 566–486 BCE; and some modern scholars would settle around 480–400 BCE. Recently, following exhaustive surveys and the 3-vol. compilation by Heinz Bechert (1991–7) of a 1988 conference proceedings on the topic, some support has grown for a 'Short Chronology' closing between 375 and 355 BCE (see e.g. *Upanisads*, Olivelle 1996: p. xxxvi).

Bibliography

Translations, editions and commentaries of primary sources

Arthasastra. Rangarajan, L. N. (ed.), *Kautilya. The Arthashastra. Edited, Rearranged, Translated and Introduced* (New Delhi, 1987).

Atharva Veda. Griffith, Ralph T. H. (tr.) *The Hymns of the Artharva-Veda Translated with a Popular Commentary* (Benares, 1916²).

[*Fa-Hien.*] Legge, James (ed. and tr.), *A Record of Buddhistic Kingdoms, Being an Account by the Chinese Monk Fa-Hien of his Travels in India and Ceylon (A.D. 399–414) in Search of the Buddhist Books of Discipline* (Oxford, 1886).

Jataka. Cowell, E. B. (ed.), *The Jataka, or Stories of the Buddha's Former Births*, tr. R. Chalmers, W. H. D. Rouse, H. T. Francis, R. A. Neil and E. B. Cowell, 6 vols (Cambridge, 1895–1907).

Jataka. Matsumura, Junko, 'A Unique Vyaghri-Jataka Version from Gandhara: The *Foshuo pusa toushen (yi) ehu qita yinytuan jing* [Japanese characters] (T172)', *Journal of the International College for Postgraduate Buddhist Studies* 16 (2012), 48–68 [accents and Japanese characters omitted].

Kavitavali of Tulsi Das, tr. F. R. Allchin (London, 1964).

Mahabharata. Ganguli, Kisari Mohan, *The Mahabharata of Krishna-Dwaipayana Vyasa: Translated into English Prose from the Original Sanskrit Text* (New Delhi, 1970).

Manava-Dharmasastra. Olivelle, Patrick, *Manu's Code of Law: A Critical Edition and Translation of the Manava-Dharmasastra* (New York, 2005).

Ramayana. Shastri, Hari Prasad (tr.), *The Ramayana of Valmiki* (London, 1952).

Rig Veda. Jamison, Stephanie W., and Brereton, Joel P. (eds and tr.), *The Rigveda* (London, 2014).

Rig Veda. Griffith, R. T. H. (tr.), *The Hymns of the Rigveda* (Banares, 1926³).

Rig Veda. O'Flaherty, Wendy D. (ed. and tr.), *The Rig Veda: An Anthology* (London, 1981).

Rig Veda. Witzel, Michael, and Goto, Toshifumi (eds and tr.), *Rig-Veda: Das Heilige Wissen, Erster und Zweiter Liederkreis* (Frankfurt a.M., 2007); Witzel, Michael, Goto, Toshifumi, and Scarlata, Salvatore (*Dritter bis Fünfter Liederkreis*) (Frankfurt a.M., 2007, 2013).

Susrutasamhita. Wujastyk, Dominik (ed. and tr.), *The Roots of Ayurveda: Selections from Sanskrit Medical Writings* (New Delhi, 1998).

Susrutasamhita. Singhal, G. D., Singh L. M., and Singh K.P. (tr.), *Diagnostic Considerations in Ancient Indian Surgery* (Allahabad, 1972).

Upanisads. Olivelle, Patrick, *Upanisads Translated from the Original Sanskrit* (Oxford, 1996).

Upanishads. Hume, Robert E., *The Thirteen Principal Upanishads Translated from the Sanskrit* (London, 1931).

Vedas. Panikkar, Raimundo, Shanta, N., Rogers, M. A. R., Bäumer, B., and Bidoli, M. (eds and tr.), *The Vedic Experience Mantramanjari: An Anthology of the Vedas* (London, 1977).

Vedas. Zysk, Kenneth G., *Medicine in the Veda: Religious Healing in the Veda, with Translations and Annotations of Medical Hymns from the Rigveda and the Atharvaveda and Renderings from the Corresponding Ritual Texts* (Delhi, 1998).

Secondary sources

Anand, Shilpaa, 'Corporeality and Culture: Theorizing Difference in the South Asian Context', in S. Rao and M. Kalyanpur (eds), *South Asian Disability Studies: Redefining Boundaries and Extending Horizons* (New York, 2015), 154–70.

Ashraf, Abdullah A., *Stone Age Traditions of Meghalaya* (Oxford, 2010).

Blumberg, B. S., 'Goiter in Gandhara: A Representation in a Second to Third Century AD Frieze', *Journal of the American Medical Association* 189/13 (28 Sept. 1964), 1008–12.

Bechert, Heinz (ed.), *Die Datierung des Historischen Buddha*, 3 vols (Göttingen, 1991, 1992, 1997).

Dalal, Ajit K., and Misra G., 'The Core and Context of Indian Psychology', *Psychology and Developing Societies* 22 (2010), 121–55.

Doniger, Wendy, *The Hindus: An Alternative History* (New York, 2009).

Farmer, Steve, Sproat, R., and Witzel, M., 'The Collapse of the Indus-Script Thesis: The Myth of a Literate Harappan Civilization', *Electronic Journal of Vedic Studies* 11/2 (2004), 19–57.

Filliozat, Jean, *The Classical Doctrine of Indian Medicine: Its Origins and its Greek Parallels*, tr. Dev Raj Chanana (Delhi, 1964).

Foucher, A., *Notes on the Ancient Geography of Gandhara (A Commentary on a Chapter of Hiuan Tsang)*, tr. H. Hargreaves (Calcutta, 1915).

Fuller, Dorian Q., and Harvey, Emma L. 'The Archaeobotany of Indian Pulses: Identification, Processing and Evidence for Cultivation', *Environmental Archaeology* 11/2 (2006), 219–46.

Glucklich, Ariel, 'Laws for the Sick and Handicapped in the Dharmasastra', *South Asia Research* 4 (1984), 139–52.

Hartl, Wolfgang, 'Lakuntaka-Bhaddiya Ein Verkannter Arahant: Eine Ungewöhnliche "Heiligen-Vita" des Theravada-Buddhismus', in R. Breitwieser (ed.), *Behinderungen und Beeinträchtigungen/ Disability and Impairment in Antiquity* (Oxford, 2012), 119–22.

Humer, Edith, 'Linkshändigkeit in der Antike: Eine Behinderung?', in R. Breitwieser (ed.), *Behinderungen und Beeinträchtigungen/Disability and Impairment in Antiquity* (Oxford, 2012), 123–30.

Jamison, S. W., and Witzel, M., 'Vedic Hinduism', in A. Sharma (ed.), *The Study of Hinduism* (Columbia, SC, 2003), 65–113 <www.people.fas.harvard.edu/~witzel/vedica.pdf>.

Jamkhedar, Arvind P., *Ajanta: Monumental Legacy* (New Delhi, 2009).

Kinsley, David, '"Through the Looking Glass": Divine Madness in the Hindu Religious Tradition', *History of Religions* 13 (1974), 270–305.

Lal, Vinay, *The History of History: Politics and Scholarship in Modern India* (New Delhi, 2003).

Leslie, Julia, 'The Implications of the Physical Body: Health, Suffering and *Karma* in Hindu Thought', in J. R. Hinnells and R. Porter (eds), *Religion, Health and Suffering* (London, 1999), 23–45.

MacDonell, Arthur A., and Keith, Arthur B., *Vedic Index of Names and Subjects* (London, 1912).

Malafouris, Lambros, 'Knapping Intentions and the Marks of the Mental', in L. Malafouris and C. Renfrew (eds), *The Cognitive Life of Things* (Cambridge, 2010), 13–22.

Masica, Colin P., *The Indo-Aryan Languages* (Cambridge, 1989).

Miles, M., 'Goitre, Cretinism and Iodine in South Asia: Historical Perspectives on a Continuing Scourge', *Medical History* 42/1 (1998), 47–67.

Mookerji, Radha Kumud, *Ancient Indian Education (Brahmanical and Buddhist)* (London, 1947).

Nanda, Meera, 'Hindu Triumphalism and the Clash of Civilisations', *Economic and Political Weekly* 44/28 (11 July 2009), 106–14.

Naqvi, Nasim H., 'Surgical Instruments in the Taxila Museum', *Medical History* 47 (2003), 89–98.

Petraglia, M. D., Shipton, C., and Paddayya, K., 'Life and Mind in the Acheulean: A Case Study from India', in C. Gamble and M. Porr (eds), *The Hominid Individual in Context* (London, 2005), 197–219.

Sankhyan, A. R., and Schug, G. R., 'First Evidence of Brain Surgery in Bronze Age Harappa', *Current Science* 100/11 (2010), 1621–2.

Sankhyan, A. R., and Weber, H. J., 'Evidence of Surgery in Ancient India: Trepanation at Burzahom (Kashmir) over 4000 Years Ago', *International Journal of Osteoarchaeology* 11 (2001), 375–80.

Sharma, Arvind, 'Did the Hindus Lack a Sense of History?', *Numen* 50/2 (2003), 190–227.

Shipton, Ceri B. K., *A Million Years of Hominin Sociality and Cognition: Acheulean Bifaces in the Hunsgi-Baichbal Valley, India* (Oxford, 2013).

Smith, Brian K., 'Classifying Animals and Humans in Ancient India', *Man* 26 (1992), 527–48.

Stewart, Alex G., 'For Debate: Drifting Continents and Endemic Goitre in Northern Pakistan', *British Medical Journal* 300 (9 June 1990), 1507–12.

Thapar, Romila, *Ancient Indian Social History: Some Interpretations* (Hyderabad, 1978).

Thapar, R., 'Ashoka – a Retrospective', *Economic and Political Weekly* 44/45 (7 Nov. 2009), 31–7.
Thomson, Karen, 'A Still Undeciphered Text: How the Scientific Approach to the Rigveda Would Open Up Indo-European Studies', *Journal of Indo-European Studies* 37/1–2 (2009), 1–47.
Turner, Sir Ralph, *A Comparative Dictionary of the Indo-Aryan Languages* (London, 1966).
Weerakkody, D. P. M. 'Blindness as a Form of Disability in Pre-Modern South Asia', in C. S. M. Wickramasinghe (ed.), *Philologos: Essays Presented in Felicitation of Merlin Peris, Emeritus Professor of Western Classics, University of Peradeniya* (Colombo, 2008), 125–55.
Zysk, Kenneth G., *Asceticism and Healing in Ancient India: Medicine in the Buddhist Monastery* (Delhi, 1991).

8

DISABILITY IN
ANCIENT CHINA

Olivia Milburn

Introduction

This chapter concerns the perceptions of disability and the treatment of those classified as disabled in ancient China. For the purposes of this discussion, the period in question covers the time from the collapse of the Western Zhou dynasty in 771 BCE, when the regime was ripped apart by a horrific civil war following a series of natural disasters in the capital region, through to the invasions by the Xiongnu (Huns), the Xianbei (a Turkic ethnic group) and other Central Asian peoples in 316 CE, when the whole of northern China came under foreign rule. In the course of this thousand-year period, China underwent massive political and social upheavals. During the Spring and Autumn period (771–475 BCE) and Warring States era (475–221 BCE), the aristocrats who had thrown off any last vestiges of subordination to the Zhou kings fought each other for dominance. In 221 BCE, these realms were unified by the First Emperor, who simultaneously incorporated vast areas of territory inhabited by non-Chinese peoples into the Qin regime. During the Han dynasty (206 BCE–220 CE) yet more lands were conquered in what is now Central Asia, the Korean peninsula and Vietnam. In 220 CE, the territory of the Han was temporarily partitioned among warlords who rose up in the wake of the upheavals caused by the Yellow Turbans Rebellion, a massive uprising provoked by severe flooding along the lower reaches of the Yellow River in 184 CE. China was then briefly reunited by the Jin dynasty in 265–316 CE.

Endemic warfare created a vast number of more or less seriously disabled people, who had suffered injury in battle. These joined the large number of individuals who suffered from congenital conditions, or who had been crippled by disease later in life. Furthermore, Chinese traditional law called for the use of 'mutilation punishments' (*xing*), whereby a wide range of different types of injury were inflicted upon convicted criminals. Such punishments, which included amputation of the feet or the ears, cutting off the kneecaps and so on, created a highly stigmatized group of disabled people, whose injuries were a constant visible reminder of their criminal past. No account of the treatment of the disabled in ancient China can be complete without consideration of the way in which crippling injuries and criminality intersected in the public mind.

Perceptions of disability

Attitudes towards what constituted a disability varied enormously in ancient China. Within mainstream Chinese culture, which developed along the Yellow River, definitions of disability were profoundly affected by the importance accorded to filial piety (*xiao*). Eventually, this concept was codified in the *Classic of Filial Piety* (*Xiaojing*), which argued that it was the duty of every child to maintain their body undamaged as an expression of gratitude towards their father and mother for the gift of life. The link between an intact body and the much prized virtue of filial piety would have major implications for many aspects of Chinese traditional society. First, in direct opposition to the demands of the state for soldiers, it created a mechanism for men (if they could not avoid military service entirely) to refuse to accept front-line positions or dangerous missions which were likely to lead to injury. For example, as a young man Guan Zhong (d. 645 BCE) ran away from the field of battle three times. Accused of cowardice, he escaped criticism by pointing out that he was being filial to his aged mother (*Shiji* 62.2132). His refusal to serve in the army in no way harmed his career, since he eventually became a highly respected statesman.

Secondly, it resulted in an extremely wide definition of disability, encompassing many acts regarded as unproblematic in other cultures: in ancient China cut hair, pierced ears or a tattooed body – while not physically disabling – would have been socially crippling. Finally, filial piety served to create a considerable psychological burden upon those who had suffered any form of injury. In the eyes of society as a whole, they had failed to live up to the ideal form of parent–child relations by allowing their bodies to become damaged. As such, their moral failings could be seen as having assumed physical form. Even those who never experienced injury nevertheless suffered life-long stress at the possibility that they might inadvertently damage their bodies. This explains the remarks of the Confucian philosopher Master Zeng when he was lying on his deathbed, as recorded in the *Analects of Confucius* (*Lunyu*):

> When Master Zeng was terminally ill, he summoned his disciples and said: 'Look at my feet! Look at my hands! The *Book of Songs* (*Shijing*) says: "We should be apprehensive and cautious, as if overlooking a deep gulf, as if treading on thin ice". Now I know I have escaped [all harm]!'
>
> *(Lunyu 79 ['Taibo'])*

The apprehension and caution mentioned in this passage were the result of two main factors, first, the ease with which an individual might fall foul of the law and suffer a mutilation punishment, and secondly, the harsh reality of social exclusion afterwards. Though this is mentioned in many ancient texts, it is expressed most brutally in the Han dynasty *Debates on Salt and Iron* (*Yantie lun*): 'A person who has undergone penal mutilation is no longer classed as a human being' (*Yantie lun* 584 ['Zhou-Qin']). Such a harsh condemnation of this particular group of disabled people was the result of prejudice against the unfilial criminal, combined with the belief that only the physically intact could perform a full social role (Galvany 2009).

In recent years, new studies based upon archaeological material have significantly improved our understanding of the legal position of disabled people in ancient China. From excavated legal texts and census documents, it is clear that, from the perspective of the government, the primary division of the population was between the able-bodied and those belonging to vulnerable groups. The latter included the old and infirm, orphans, the destitute, and the physically impaired. Disabled individuals were described in contemporary records as *pilong* (literally: worn-out and crippled), a term which included both those born with congenital malformations and those who had become disabled through injury, illness or in warfare (Wang 2012). Government officials were responsible for maintaining lists of the *pilong* individuals within their community, and the protection to which they were entitled was clearly set out in legal codes from the Qin and Han dynasty onwards. (It is striking that there was apparently no distinction made between individuals who were disabled as a result of accidents or disease, as opposed to those who had received injuries fighting for their country.) Persons with *pilong* status were further subdivided according to whether their physical health allowed them to perform corvée labour.[1] Even if a *pilong* individual was required to perform labour for the government, they still did significantly less (usually defined as half the workload of an able-bodied person); if their disability was severe, they were exempt, as was the primary care-giver for any person registered as *pilong* (*Zhouli* 12.716 ['Situ']; *Zhangjiashan Hanmu zhujian* 64). Categorization as a *pilong* individual was clearly sufficiently desirable that from the beginning of the Han dynasty onwards the legal code specified the punishment for those who inflicted injuries upon themselves in order to qualify: a person convicted of this offence was tattooed and then sent to perform hard labour (*Zhangjiashan Hanmu zhujian* 12; Feng 2014).

Surviving census records make it clear that the government collected extremely detailed information about the nature of the disabilities suffered by the population under their jurisdiction. These records suggest that many people with *pilong* status were convicted criminals who had suffered mutilation punishment, and that this form of punishment was far from being restricted to the lowest levels of society.[2] The practice of mutilation punishment, which was divided into civil and military systems, was always controversial in China. In the case of civil punishments, there was debate over whether anyone had the right to inflict such a severe penalty on criminals, given that it would lead to life-long social exclusion (*Hanshu* 23.1097–1100; Turner 1999). For those who admitted the use of mutilation punishments, there was a question over who should administer the system; could a ruler punish his people in this way on his own authority, or should the institution of government as a whole be responsible? (This concern seems not to have been raised with respect to the use of mutilation punishments by the military, where the right of the commander-in-chief to issue orders as he saw fit for conditions on the ground was enshrined in Chinese law and custom, without the need to consult the government at home.) As a result of these debates, mutilation punishments were frequently revised and indeed periodically removed from the statute books. Emperor Wen of the Han dynasty (r. 180–157 BCE) was much lauded for his banning of these punishments; however, given that they were replaced by having the convicted criminal beaten to death it is doubtful if any amelioration was intended (Sanft 2005). Mutilation punishments continued to reappear in the Chinese law code during the Han dynasty and indeed through much of the imperial era.

Given the lengthy debates which took place over the use of mutilation punishments it is striking that the issue of wrongful convictions of the innocent seems to have gone entirely unmentioned. In Antiquity, there were some extremely famous miscarriage of justice cases which resulted in mutilation punishments being inflicted on persons innocent of any crime: these cases were well-known but never discussed in this context. Perhaps the single most notorious of these concerns Sun Bin (d. 316 BCE), whose name literally means Sun who-had-his-kneecaps-cut-off. During the Warring States era, Sun Bin was a famous military strategist, said to have been descended from Sun Wu, the putative author of *Master Sun's Arts of War* (*Sunzi bingfa*). Accused of treasonous communication with the enemy while working for King Hui of Wei (r. 370–319 BCE), Sun Bin was crippled for life when his kneecaps were cut off (*Shiji* 65.2162–5). All accounts of these events stress that Sun Bin was innocent; the evidence against him was forged by a jealous rival. After escaping from captivity, Sun Bin devoted the remainder of his life to the destruction of his enemies, though his injuries and the stigma attached to them meant that he very rarely appeared in public. In spite of this and other tales of appalling suffering caused by wrongful convictions, a wide variety of mutilation punishments continued to be used, which inflicted painful and in some cases profoundly disabling injuries on the criminal, and which resulted in social exclusion for the remainder of his or her life.

Perceptions about tattooing are particularly interesting, given that what was for some non-Chinese people an important traditional practice marking the place of the individual within society was for the Chinese an appalling form of mutilation, associated with the punishment of criminals. This divergence of interpretation would cause great conflict with the non-Chinese civilizations located south of the Yangtze River. When the lands of the ancient southern kingdoms of Wu and Yue were incorporated into the Chinese Empire at the time of the unification of China in 221 BCE, the customs of their inhabitants suddenly came under considerable pressure from Chinese norms. There had always been considerable distain for their cultural practices; however, after the unification, the central government became determined to eradicate their 'barbaric' behaviour, which was seen as constituting self-mutilation (Hulsewé 1955: 125). For the peoples living along what is now the southern coast of China, cut hair, blackened teeth, tattooing and other forms of body modification hitherto had been an important part of their cultural identity (*Han Shi waizhuan* 271 [8.1]; Reed 2000). The demands of the central government to cease these practices were no doubt deeply shocking to the people affected; the level of resistance to change may be gauged by the fact that it took nearly a thousand years to persuade the inhabitants of China's southern coastal region to cease practising tattooing.

If penal mutilations were seen as giving physical expression to the moral ugliness of the individual, at the same time Confucian texts such as the *Records of Ritual* (*Liji*) emphasized the 'jade-like countenance' (*yuse*) that came from self-cultivation (*Liji* 567 ['Yuzao']). However, although the Confucian classics and other ancient Chinese canonical texts frequently emphasized the link between physical perfection and moral integrity, this was balanced in wider philosophical discourse by alternative interpretations. In particular, some ancient philosophical texts make reference to traditions that many of the great sages and moral exemplars of earlier times were possessed of strikingly unusual physiques, including 'double pupils' (the sage-king Shun), hemiplegia (the sage-king Yu) and a hunch-back (the Duke of Zhou): the most famous articulation of the idea that a deformed body was a sign of unusual spiritual and intellectual gifts is found in the 'Against Physiognomy' (Feixiang) chapter of the *Book of Master Xun* (*Xunzi* 74–5). Daoist philosophers in particular were sceptical of any claims that physical beauty was linked to virtue; furthermore, they enjoyed pointing out that since disabled persons in ancient China were excused from both military service and corvée labour, it was the able-bodied who suffered lasting damage from the corrupt and bellicose policies of their governments. It is in the works of Daoist philosophers, particularly the *Book of Master Zhuang* (*Zhuangzi*), that the most striking descriptions of disabled persons are to be found, ranging from those who have experienced penal mutilation to those born with severe congenital malformations:

> Disarticulated had his chin hidden in his navel, his shoulders were higher than the top of his head, the bones of his spine pointed at the sky, his five organs were on top, and his thigh-bones had fused to his ribs. By plying his needle and repairing clothes he gained enough to keep himself fed; by shaking a winnowing-basket to separate the wheat [from the chaff] he could feed another ten people. When the government recruited soldiers, Disarticulated could wave his arms and wander around among them; when the government demanded corvée labour, then Disarticulated was disqualified by long-term ill-health. When the government disbursed food to the needy, he would get three measures [of grain] and ten bushels of firewood. Thanks to his appearance Disarticulated could support himself and live out his natural lifespan.
>
> *(Zhuangzi 180 ['Renjianshi'])*

Daoist philosophers stressed that there were great advantages to being crippled or deformed; a viewpoint which must have been shared by many ordinary people, given that otherwise there would have been no need for laws to prevent individuals from mutilating themselves.

The treatment of the disabled

A number of ancient philosophical texts discuss different aspects of social attitudes towards the disabled in early China. It is clear that certain groups of disabled people were able to attain positions of some prestige; the government classified a small number of disability types, as well as dwarfs, as 'talents for government service' (*guanshi zhi suocai*), and such individuals were actively recruited for the court (*Guoyu* 387 ['Jinyu 4']). The presence of dwarves in royal and aristocratic households was considered deeply worrying by the medical profession; an early Han dynasty medical text, the *Book of the Generation of the Foetus* (*Taichan shu*), argues that their abnormal appearance caused unborn babies to mutate in the womb (*Mawangdui Hanmu boshu* 136). Probably the single most prestigious of these positions was that of music master; references to them found in ancient Chinese canonical texts such as the *Book of Songs* describe the magnificent performances of these disabled musicians at state rituals during the Zhou dynasty (*Mao Shi* 730–4 [Mao 280: 'Yougu']). The special treatment that music masters required is the subject of a famous story in the *Analects*, which describes the thoughtful and respectful behaviour that Confucius assumed towards one of these men:

> Music Master Mian paid a visit [to Confucius], and when he reached the steps the Master (Confucius) said: 'There are steps.' When he reached the mats, the Master said: 'There are mats.' When everyone had sat down the Master told him: 'Such and such a person is here; such and such a person is there.' Music Master Mian left, and Zizhang asked: 'Is that the way to speak to a Music Master?' Confucius said: 'Yes. That is definitely the way to guide a Music Master'.
>
> *(Lunyu 170–1 ['Wei Linggong'])*

Music Master Mian, like his colleagues, would have been blind. To reach such a position was the pinnacle of achievement for a disabled individual born into an ordinary family; music masters were members of the official bureaucracy and often performed before the ruler, hence, some music masters are known to have become trusted advisers to their lords. Compared to other kinds of disabled persons, music masters seem to have been treated with respect.

For those disabled persons who were not classified as suitable for government service, the authorities nevertheless retained a considerable interest in seeing them successfully integrated into society, in particular through suitable gainful employment. Although the challenges of finding appropriate employment for the disabled was fully recognized in ancient texts, there was nevertheless some effort made to ensure that they could play a part in the community as a whole. In the *History of the Han dynasty* (*Hanshu*) there is a discussion of suitable employment for those who had suffered mutilation punishment; this may be an idealized account, but it is one that ignores any perceived stigma attached to these convicted criminals and emphasizes that many people not only survived these punishments but needed jobs suited to their disability afterwards. Furthermore, other sources confirm that many disabled people were employed in this way:

> In the past in the laws of the Zhou dynasty ... [there were] five punishments: five hundred crimes [merited] tattooing, five hundred crimes [merited] having the nose cut off, five hundred crimes [merited] castration, five hundred crimes [merited] having

the ear cut off, and five hundred crimes [merited] the death penalty ... Those who were executed were exposed in the market-place, those who had been tattooed were employed to guard the city gates, those who had their noses cut off were employed to guard the borders, those who had been castrated were employed to guard the women's quarters, those who had their ears cut off were employed to guard the hunting parks, and those who remained whole were employed to guard the grain stores.

(Hanshu 23.1091)

It is clear from contemporary records that many disabled persons, particularly those with some kind of congenital malformation, were the subject of considerable humiliating attention from others, and this seems to have been the case regardless of their social background. Numerous stories survive of individuals with some kind of deformity being the subject of invasive curiosity or humiliating mockery by the able-bodied. For example, the Honourable Chonger of Jin (later Lord Wen of Jin, r. 636–628 BCE) was surprised in his bath by Lord Gong of Cao (r. 652–618 BCE), who laughed and joked with his cronies about the Honourable Chonger's deformed ribcage (*Chunqiu Zuozhuan*: 407 [Xi 23]). In another case, a member of the Qi ruling house was overcome with laughter at the sight of a group of visiting ambassadors:

The mother of Lord Qing of Qi (r. 598–582 BCE) was observing [her son's guests] from the upper apartments and laughed at them. The reason for this was that Xi Ke was hunchbacked, and the envoy from Lu was lame, and the envoy from Wei was one-eyed, so that Qi had sent people to them in order to help the guests about. Xi Ke was furious, and on his journey back, above the Yellow River, he said: 'May the River God bear witness, I will revenge myself on Qi!'

(Shiji, 39.1677)

Many of the stories which survive concerning the curiosity and contempt shown by the able-bodied towards the disabled focus specifically – as is the case here – on instances where the able-bodied were eventually punished for the humiliation they had inflicted. Interestingly, there are even stories which concern disabled individuals of more-or-less humble origins being able to avenge the insults heaped upon them by able-bodied members of the elite (*Shiji* 66.2365–6). These stories probably exist because they offered an unusual perspective on a familiar situation; for the vast majority of disabled persons in ancient China, their only option was to endure whatever treatment was meted out to them.

Not surprisingly, most of the information concerning the lives of disabled individuals in ancient China concerns male members of the ruling elite. One aspect of their condition which received a great deal of attention was the issue of inheritance. Could an individual who was disabled (whether by injury or by some congenital problem) be allowed to inherit a hereditary title, with the enormous power that went with it? For the pre-unification period, the evidence on this point is ambiguous. There are some cases where an individual was deprived of his rights due to disability; on the other hand, there are other instances where the disabled person concerned was allowed to inherit their family's honours. The reasons for this flexibility seem to have been twofold. First, before the unification of China, primogeniture was not so strongly established that it overrode all other considerations; most hereditary houses had a plethora of healthy potential heirs, which served to make the risk of appointing a disabled ruler or senior minister even more unattractive. Attempts were made to enforce primogeniture, defined as inheritance by the oldest son of the principal wife, in the pre-unification period; the inter-state covenant at Kuiqiu in 651 BCE was intended to establish this very point (*Chunqiu Guliang jingzhuan* 283 [Xi 9]; *Mengzi* 287 ['Gaozi xia']). However, the evidence of historical texts shows that in many cases favourite sons born to junior wives still inherited their father's titles.

Secondly, a decision seems to have been made on a case-by-case basis; men who were not severely handicapped by their physical disability tended to be allowed to inherit, while those who were considered incapable of government (which seems to have been defined in terms of the ability to travel and interact with peers) were usually dispossessed. Thus for example the Honourable Mengzhi, who was unable to walk, was not allowed to inherit the marquisate of Wei in 535 BCE (*Chunqiu Zuozhuan* 1298 [Zhao 7]). In the context of the treatment of the disabled in ancient China, this incident was marked by the strong prejudices shown by his father's ministers, who described him as being 'not a [fully developed] human being' (*fei ren ye*). At a slightly lower social level, among the hereditary ministerial clans, Cui Shu of Qi dispossessed his son in 546 BCE because he had suffered a crippling illness (*Chunqiu Zuozhuan* 1137 [Xiang 27]). In each case a younger and completely healthy sibling inherited.

Thus in 566 BCE, when a senior minister in Jin announced his retirement, his oldest son, who was disabled, actually refused to inherit his father's honours:

> In the winter in the tenth lunar month Han Xianzi of Jin reported [that he wished to retire due to] his age. The scion of this noble family, [his son] Muzi, had a chronic crippling illness, [nevertheless] they were going to appoint him [to replace his father as minister]. He refused, saying: 'The *Book of Songs* says: "Surely there is not [dew on the roads] in the morning and evening? I shall say that there is too much dew to travel". It also says: "When you do not attend to it yourself, when you do not act in person, ordinary people will not trust you". I have no ability, and so surely it is right for me to give way [for another]? I beg you to appoint Qi (that is Han Muzi's younger brother).'
> *(Chunqiu Zuozhuan 951 [Xiang 7])*

The two quotations from the *Book of Songs* here have traditionally been interpreted as Han Muzi's reflections on the fact of his physical disability: the first an expression of the difficulties he faced in moving from place to place; the second, meaning that his crippling ill-health would alienate him from others. In the end Han Muzi got his wish, and his younger brother inherited their father's position. However, Han Muzi's generosity impressed the ruler of Jin so much that he was appointed as a grandee in his own right, as a result of which he was not able to escape involvement in the government of the country.

The issue of the right of a disabled prince to inherit the throne seems to have been in abeyance during the Han dynasty, thanks to the physical health of the imperial house. Although the mental health of some Han dynasty emperors is open to question, there is no recorded instance of a disabled prince having his right to succeed to the throne called into question. This problem first arose in the Jin dynasty, and would play a key role in determining the fate of the entire country. In 290 CE, Emperor Hui of Jin came to the throne, in spite of severe developmental disabilities. The nature of Emperor Hui's problems has been much debated in modern scholarship. He was apparently not obviously physically disabled – at least this is not mentioned in sources such as the official *History of the Jin dynasty* (*Jinshu*). He seems to have suffered from some form of developmental disability, the nature of which is not sufficiently well-described in contemporary records to make more than a general assessment of what was wrong. Thus Emperor Hui learned to speak, but his recorded remarks suggest serious cognitive difficulties (*Jinshu*, 4:108; Han 2009; Wang 2004). As the oldest surviving son of Emperor Wu of the Jin dynasty (r. 266–90) and his wife, Empress Yang, he had been appointed as Crown Prince in the teeth of considerable opposition, given the extent of his mental problems. That this opposition was entirely well-founded was demonstrated by subsequent events. Emperor Hui's disabilities necessitated a regency, and the fighting between his uncles, cousins and his powerful empress, Jia Nanfeng (257–300), eventually resulted in a civil war: the revolt of the Eight Kings (Dreyer 2009). This internecine conflict so weakened the Jin dynasty that they were unable to withstand the invasion by nomadic and semi-nomadic peoples from Central Asia that occurred in 316, and which eventually resulted in the partitioning of China. By that time, however, Emperor Hui had been dead for some years, poisoned by one of his regents in 307 CE (*Jinshu* 4.108).

The disabled person in the Chinese worldview

In ancient China the theory of 'correspondence' (*ganying*) was enormously influential and had a practical impact on the perception of disabled individuals. According to this theory, there was an intimate connection between events on earth and natural phenomena; any imbalance in the correct and just order on earth would unleash cataclysmic disasters. On the other hand, a humane regime would call forth auspicious omens and the lives of the people would be easy. As a result of this belief, any natural disaster which occurred would be followed by intense efforts on the part of the government to correct the situation – common methods to achieve this included amnesties of people in prison (to disperse the evil auras caused by miscarriages of justice) and disbursal of charitable payments of food and silk to persons in need, including widows and orphans, the elderly, the destitute and those registered as *pilong*. Such gifts occurred at irregular intervals yet remained an important aspect of government policy. As can be seen by comparing examples of this kind of charity which occurred during the reigns of Emperor Guangwu of the Han dynasty (r. 25–57 CE) and his son, Emperor Ming (r. 58–75 CE), charitable gifts were made to the elderly and disabled to respond to a number of different kinds of events:

Emperor Guangwu

6th year (30): grain given to vulnerable groups 'according to the law' following a plague of locusts.
29th year (53): amnesty granted to criminals and grain given to vulnerable groups following a solar eclipse.
30th year (54): grain given to vulnerable groups after severe flooding.
31st year (55): grain given to vulnerable groups following severe flooding; later the same year there was both a solar eclipse and a plague of locusts, but further charitable gifts were not made (*Hou Hanshu* 1.1–194).

Emperor Ming

1st year (57): grain given to vulnerable groups to celebrate Emperor Ming's accession.
3rd year (60): grain given to vulnerable groups to celebrate the appointment of the empress and crown prince.
12th year (69): grain given to vulnerable groups, with no reason recorded.
17th year (74): grain given to vulnerable groups to celebrate the appearance of a series of auspicious omens.
18th year (75): amnesty granted to criminals and grain given to vulnerable groups following a severe drought. (*Hou Hanshu* 2.95–128)

During these two reigns, every serious natural disaster seems to have been met with large-scale disbursal of grain to the needy. Though in some cases this may have been intended to supply relief from want, such widespread donations reached far beyond those actually affected by the disaster to vulnerable individuals across the empire, in the hope that this generosity would provoke a response from the gods. The only occasions when a major disaster or ill-omened astrological phenomenon did not result in such gifts is if such a donation had already been made earlier the same year. In addition to balancing out the injustice which had provoked the natural disaster in the first place, this kind of charity represented an important form of communication between the ruler and the ruled, since by demonstrating his care for vulnerable groups the king or emperor could lay claim to the much-praised virtue of benevolence (*ren*). Benevolence was considered not merely as a good quality in and of itself, but as a key method for legitimizing the power of the dynasty. In 218, at the time of the break-up of the Han dynasty, Cao Cao (155–220), the founder of the Wei dynasty, would move beyond simply offering one-off donations to a system of organized care specifically for the disabled. He enacted legislation whereby disabled people (defined specifically as the blind and those afflicted with injuries or disease affecting the hands and feet), who were in danger of finding themselves destitute, would have the cost of their upkeep devolved upon the state (*Sanguo zhi*, 1.51 [*Weishu*]).

Although individuals registered as disabled in ancient China periodically benefited from the charity given by the government in times of natural disasters, in some cases their very existence was interpreted as an evil omen. In the pre-unification era, a number of accounts (derived particularly from the southern kingdoms of Chu, Wu and Yue) describe the birth of individuals with unusual features as presaging bad luck for their families, and in some cases, for their countries. These accounts are often highly mysterious; the ancient texts compare the features of human beings to those of wild animals and birds, but what this actually meant is unknown. For example in the account given in *Zuo's Tradition* (*Zuozhuan*) for the year 605 BCE, the appearance of a child born to a junior branch of the royal family of Chu is said to have been a great cause for concern:

> Marshal Ziliang of Chu had a son, Yuejiao. Ziwen said: 'You must kill him! This child has the appearance of a bear or a tiger, and the voice of a wolf. If you do not kill him, he will surely destroy the Ruo'ao family (the ruling house of Chu). There is a saying: "A wolfish child has a wild heart". This is a wolf: how can he be tamed?'
> *(Chunqiu Zuozhuan 1492–3 [Zhao 28])*

It is evident from context in this and other similar stories that the animal-like appearance of the individual concerned is intended to be a pejorative description (Milburn 2007: 19–21). In each of these cases, the parents are advised to get rid of the baby concerned. In ancient China, it was legal to abandon children born with major birth-abnormalities – not to mention those unfortunate to be born on an unlucky day – and there seems to have been considerable prejudice against raising such a child (Kinney 2004: 111; *Shiji*, 75.2352). Fortunately for the babies concerned, not everyone believed in the dire consequences threatened:

> The Minister of Education Rui in the state of Song had a daughter, and [she was born] red and covered in hair, so he abandoned her below a dike. A female slave from the household of Lady Ji Gong (wife of Duke Gong of Song, r. 588–576 BCE) found her and took her in [to the palace], and named her Qi (Abandoned).
> *(Chunqiu Zuozhuan 1117 [Xiang 26])*

Qi's story would eventually have a happy ending: Duke Ping of Song (r. 575–532 BCE), the son of her benefactor, fell in love with her and they were married. However, though the ducal family in Song may have been comparatively open-minded about Qi's medical condition, her own family and many others would have considered her disabled – her abnormal appearance meant that she could not be a fully functioning member of society. Later on, during the course of the Han dynasty, thanks to the widespread acceptance of the theory of correspondence, certain kinds of congenital malformation (including the hirsutism that afflicted Qi) came to be considered as portents (*Hanshu*, 27B *xia*: 1419–20). Into this small group of disabled persons come those born with major deformities (in particular with either missing or extra limbs), intersex individuals, conjoined twins and so on. The conditions suffered by disabled persons who were considered as omens are all rare congenital conditions, and usually extremely visible. However, being interpreted as an omen only affected a very small minority of those born with these conditions; in order to come into this category, the birth had not only to be reported to the central government, but it also had to occur within a fairly narrow time-range on either side of a major political upheaval or other kind of disaster. Persons with the right kind of disability born in Han dynasty China within a couple of decades of a significant political crisis might well find themselves classified as a portent; an individual with an identical condition born in an era of unbroken peace would find their existence generally ignored:

> In the second year [of the Guanghe reign era (179 CE)], a woman living outside the Upper West Gate of Luoyang gave birth to a son with two heads. [The baby's heads] had different shoulders but the same torso, and they both faced forward. Since [the mother] considered this an evil omen, she threw him to the ground and abandoned him. From this time onwards, the court became confused and chaotic, and the government was in the hands of a few private individuals, with no proper distinctions being maintained between senior and junior: hence the omen of two heads. Later on [in 189 CE, the tyrant] Dong Zhuo (d. 192 CE) tortured the empress dowager to death, with the excuse that she had not behaved with proper filial piety [towards her mother-in-law]. He deposed the Son of Heaven (Emperor Shao of Han, r. 189 CE) and then afterwards killed him [in 190 CE]. Since the founding of the Han dynasty, there had been no disaster comparable to this.
>
> *(Hou Hanshu 17.3347)*

The significance of this small group of disabled persons from ancient China within the wider discourse on the subject is not clear. In particular, it is well-known that some kinds of congenital abnormalities were interpreted as signs of remarkable intellectual gifts; however, this group was understood as omens of disaster, though not intrinsically evil or disruptive in themselves. The relationship between popular perceptions of these two types of disabled persons is not clear. Likewise, how such an ominous understanding concerning some disabled people affected the wider community is unclear. The records from the Han dynasty which describe those born with congenital abnormalities as evil omens are derived entirely from an extremely small number of court-appointed astrologers and scholars – hence, how widely these opinions were held is not known. In the case cited above: did the unfortunate woman in Luoyang genuinely believe her baby was ill-omened? Or did she abandon her baby because she was unable to provide the necessary care? Furthermore, given that the reporting of the birth of individuals with congenital deformities seems to have been extremely patchy, many of the interpretations as to their significance were made centuries after the persons concerned were dead. (Posthumous interpretations also had the added advantage – from the point of view of astrologers – of being extremely easy, the significance of the historical event which they wished to connect with the birth of a disabled individual having become quite clear in the intervening years.) However, while this may mean that Han dynasty disabled persons were not immediately affected by prejudice attached to their conditions, over time, the belief that those suffering from certain kinds of congenital malformations were harbingers of bad luck became increasingly widespread and began to affect people during their own lifetimes. As the disabled sage-kings of Antiquity retreated further and further into the past, it was the link between disability and misfortune that became ever more entrenched in the minds of ordinary Chinese people.

A world without the disabled

At a very early stage in Chinese history, it was noticed that stressed populations, suffering from the effects of constant warfare and upheaval, had a higher incidence of babies being born with congenital deformities. It was also well-understood that stressed populations had a higher rate of disease, and that any sickness experienced by people in such a situation was liable to be more severe and the effects more lasting, potentially leading to life-threatening consequences, if not to crippling ill-health. Furthermore, the social dislocation caused by warfare was clearly linked to the breaking down of law and order, as increasingly desperate people resorted to criminal activities in order to survive. In the Chinese context, this would lead directly to mutilation punishments, as the law did not take into account the circumstances which had pushed the individual into crime in the first place. As a result of this strong association between war and disability, established on many different fronts, ancient Chinese philosophers regularly expressed the belief that, in a perfect world, there would be no disabled people:

> In an era of peace, there will be no one who is mute, deaf, lame, blind, crippled, dwarfish, or lacking their limbs. Fathers will not have to cry for their sons; older brothers will not have to cry for their younger siblings.
>
> *(Han Shi waizhuan 93 [3.10])*

Given that in a perfect world there would be no disabled people born, and none created, the presence of these individuals within ancient Chinese society was a permanent reminder of the failures of the regime. Looking at the disabled people around them, the able-bodied were constantly reminded of the brutality of war, social and economic injustice, and the inability of their government to deal with these intractable problems. To maintain the body intact may have been considered the duty of a filial child, but people in ancient China were aware that their success in achieving this goal was largely a matter of chance and good luck in a time of unremitting violence.

Notes

1 Figures for Nan Commandery (located in what is now Hubei Province) for the period c.140–129 BCE show that at this date there were 2,708 *pilong* individuals registered in this commandery, of which 480 had received a complete exemption (18%). There was considerable variation between the number of *pilong* individuals recorded and the exemption rate per county (Yuan 2009). Similar documents dating to 171 CE have been found at Dongpailou in the city of Changsha, however, unfortunately they have been badly damaged and are difficult to read (*Changsha Dongpailou Dong-Han jiandu*, 107).

2 For example, the Zoumalou census records (dating from 196–265 CE) provide a wealth of information about individual disabled persons: 'Householder and Grandee of the Eighth Order Li Ping of Fugui Village, aged forty [one illegible character]: blind in the right eye' (strip 9.3075); 'Householder and Grandee of the Eighth Order Lu Kai of Gaoping Village, aged thirty-two: penal amputation of the left hand' (strip 9.3017); 'Married Woman Pa from Leihei [Village], aged thirty-eight: penal amputation of the right foot' (strip 9.2880) (*Changsha Zoumalou Sanguo Wujian*).

Bibliography

Primary sources

Changsha Dongpailou Dong-Han jiandu [Eastern Han dynasty bamboo strips and wooden tablets from Dongpailou in the city of Changsha (168–89 CE)]. Annotated by Changsha shi wenwu kaogu yanjiusuo and Zhongguo wenwu yanjiusuo (Beijing, 2006).

Changsha Zoumalou Sanguo Wujian [Bamboo Strips from the Three Kingdoms era state of Wu, from Zoumalou in the city of Changsha (232–8 CE)]. Annotated by Changsha shi wenwu kaogu yanjiusuo (Beijing, 1999).

Chunqiu Guliang jingzhuan buzhu [*Guliang's Tradition of the Spring and Autumn Annals*, with amendments and commentary (early Han dynasty)]. Annotated by Zhong Wenzheng (Beijing, 1996).

Chunqiu Zuozhuan zhu [*Zuo's Tradition of the Spring and Autumn Annals* with commentary (c.389 BCE)]. Annotated by Yang Bojun (Beijing, 1981).

Guoyu [*Discourses of the States* (431–c.314 BCE)]. Annotated by Shanghai shifan daxue guji zhenglizu (Shanghai, 1978).

Hanshi waizhuan jishi [Collected annotations on *Mr Han's Outer Traditions of the Book of Songs* (c.150 BCE)]. Annotated by Xu Weiyu (Beijing, 1980).

Hanshu [*History of the Han dynasty* (92 CE)]. Compiled by Ban Gu (Beijing, 1962).

Hou Hanshu [*History of the Later Han dynasty* (445 CE)]. Compiled by Fan Ye (Beijing, 1964).

Jinshu [*History of the Jin dynasty* (648 CE)]. Compiled by Fang Xuanling (Beijing, 1974).

Liji zhengyi [Correct meanings of the *Record of Ritual* (early Han dynasty)]. Annotated by Kong Yingda and Zheng Xuan (Shanghai 1990).

Lunyu yizhu [*Analects of Confucius* with translation and commentary (c.473–373 BCE)]. Annotated by Yang Bojun (Beijing, 2008).

Mao Shi zhengyi [Correct meanings of the Mao recension of the *Book of Songs* (3rd–2nd centuries BCE)]. Annotated by Kong Yingda (Shanghai, 1990).

Mawangdui Hanmu boshu [Silk manuscripts from the Han dynasty tomb at Mawangdui (168 BCE)]. Annotated by Mawangdui Hanmu boshu zhengli xiaozu (vol. IV; Beijing, 1985).

Mengzi yizhu [*Mencius* with translation and commentary (late 4th century BCE)]. Annotated by Yang Bojun (Beijing, 2005).

Sanguo zhi [*Records of the Three Kingdoms* (289 CE)]. Compiled by Chen Shou (Beijing, 1959).

Shiji [*Records of the Grand Historian* (91 BCE)]. Compiled by Sima Qian (Beijing, 1959).

Xiaojing zhushu [The *Classic of Filial Piety* with commentary and sub-commentary (c.400 BCE)]. Annotated by Li Longji and Xing Bing (Beijing, 2000).

Xunzi jijie [Collected explanations on the *Book of Master Xun* (c.230 BCE)]. Annotated by Wang Xianqian (Beijing, 2008).

Yantie lun jiaozhu [Collated commentaries on the *Debates on Salt and Iron* (81 BCE)]. Annotated by Wang Liqi (Beijing, 1996).

Zhangjiashan Hanmu zhujian [Bamboo strips from the Han dynasty tomb at Zhangjiashan (c.196–186 BCE)]. Annotated by Zhangjiashan ersiqihao Hanmu zhujian zhengli xiaozu (Beijing, 2006).

Zhouli zhushu [*Rites of Zhou* with commentary and sub-commentary (2nd century BCE)]. Annotated by Zheng Xuan and Jia Gongyan (Beijing, 1980).

Zhuangzi jishi [Collected annotations on the *Book of Master Zhuang* (4th–2nd centuries BCE)]. Annotated by Guo Qingfan (Beijing, 2004).

Secondary sources

Dreyer, Edward L., 'Military Aspects of the War of the Eight Princes', in Nicola Di Cosmo (ed.), *Military Culture in Imperial China* (Cambridge, MA, 2009), 112–42.

Feng Wenwen, 'Qin-Han shiqi canzhang renkou tongji zhidu chutan' [Preliminary studies of the statistics concerning the disabled population of the Qin and Han dynasties], *Gudai wenming* 8/3 (2014), 60–8.

Galvany, Albert, 'Debates on Mutilation: Bodily Impairment and Ideology in Early China', *Asiatische Studien/Études Asiatiques* 64/1 (2009), 67–91.

Han Shufeng, 'Wudi lichu yu Xi-Jin zhengzhi douzheng' [Emperor Wu's appointment of an heir and political struggle during the Western Jin dynasty], *Zhongguo renmin daxue xuebao* 6 (2009), 134–9.

Hulsewé, Anthony François Paulus, *Remnants of Han Law* (Leiden, 1955).

Kinney, Anne Behnke, *Representations of Childhood and Youth in Early China* (Stanford, CA, 2004).

Milburn, Olivia, 'Marked out for Greatness? Perceptions of Deformity and Physical Impairment in Ancient China', *Monumenta Serica* 55 (2007), 1–22.

Reed, Carrie, 'Early Chinese Tattoo', *Sino-Platonic Papers* 103 (2000), 1–52.

Sanft, Charles, 'Six of One, Two Dozen of the Other: The Abatement of Mutilating Punishments under Han Emperor Wen', *Asia Major*, 3rd series 18 (2005), 79–100.

Turner, Karen, 'The Criminal Body and the Body Politic: Punishments in Early Imperial China', *Cultural Dynamics* 11/2 (1999), 237–54.

Wang Wentao, 'Longbing yu Handai shehui jiuzhu' [Disability, disease and social welfare in the Han dynasty], *Hebei shifan daxue xuebao: Zhexue shehui kexue ban* 35/1 (2012), 125–30.

Wang Yongping, 'Jin Wudi lisi ji qi douzheng kaolun – yi Qiwang You duo di wei zhongxin' [Research on Emperor Wu of Jin's appointment of an heir and the subsequent conflict – the case of You, King of Qi's usurpation of power], *Henan keji daxue xuebao (Shehui kexue ban)* 22/3 (2004), 5–11.

Yuan Yansheng, 'Jingzhou Songbai mudu ji xiangguan wenti' [Questions relating to the wooden plaques excavated at Songbai in Jingzhou], *Jianghan kaogu* 112/3 (2009), 114–19.

II

The Greek world

9

THE GREEK VOCABULARY OF DISABILITIES

Evelyne Samama

The perfect theoretical body imagined and created by Hellenic sculptors or painters was certainly not the one Greeks saw in their everyday life. About 10 per cent of the skeletons found in the Greek world (Grmek 1994: 93) show at least one fracture *in vitam*, so that it may be said that a large part of the population suffered from a visible disability (see Graham in this volume). But, as it has been shown elsewhere (Garland 1995; Rose 2003; Samama 2010), the Greeks did not consider disabled persons as different, as long as they could, in one way or another, play a part in socio-economic life. It is interesting to notice that the Greek vocabulary echoes this situation. Obliterating the omnipresent picture of all the persons suffering from any disability, the terms are mostly vague in designating them (for most of the Latin equivalents, see Turner 2013). This can be explained as a logical consequence of their interwoven position inside the society, or of a lack of specific medical vocabulary. The fact that the words are quite numerous proves the widespread existence of disabled people, and it is worth examining what terms the Greek chose to qualify those suffering from any disablement. For this Hesychius of Alexandria, a Greek grammarian and lexicographer from the 5th century CE, is of considerable importance. In his *Collection of All Words*, he lists many words that are not found in surviving texts of the Greek literature; they are called *hapax legomena*, and in this chapter abbreviated as *h.leg.* (for other abbreviations, see the list at the end of the chapter).

The first part of this chapter will examine the different words from a lexical point of view and the second part will point out the difficulty of identifying clearly the different terms, even in the medical treatises.

The vocabulary

Un-abled

Many words express incapacity. As their sense may be amphibolous, the current filing will be based on morphological criteria. Grammatically or, more precisely, lexicologically speaking, a first group of words designating disabilities whatsoever are compound terms, often with the *alpha* (*n-* vowel). Other series present a final in *-los, -bos* and *-sos*.

Alpha privative

Several words, composed with the *alpha* privative, insist on the incapacity to act, or the absence of strength. The *alpha* called privative, or negative, is, in Greek, the most frequent form taken by the nasal, in Latin *in-*, literaly *not, non*, in English *in-* or *un-*.

The term *adunatos* (ἀδύνατος), a verbal adjective in *–tos*, formed after the stem *duna-* (linked with *dunamai* 'I can, I'm able, I have the strength to'), often occurs in Greek literature, meaning 'unable, without strength', as the English dis-abled and comes parallel to the Latin *in-firm-is*. Such a designation stays very general and does not imply any permanent impairment. Although Lysias' text *Huper tou adunatou* shows an Athenian citizen claiming, around 400 BCE, for the amount of money the city grants to any person who needs to be helped, because of an incapacity to earn his living, the speaker himself never qualifies his body as the one of an *adunatos*. The title of the discourse was obviously given afterwards (see Rose in this volume).

In a similar way, the noun *a-rrôs-tia* (ἀρρωστία) 'weakness' (adj. ἄρρωστος, 'weak') is based on the stem *rôs-* meaning 'solid, robust, vigorous',[1] and the noun *a-sthen-eia* (ἀσθένεια) 'without strength' or the adjective *a-sthenes* (ἀσθενής), 'weak, frail, strengthless' are built after *sthen-*, 'strong, powerful' (etymology unclear, cf. *DELG & EDG* s.v.). Both terms indicate a temporary or permanent disorder, or a weakness (e.g. *an-aisthetos* (ἀναίσθητος) which means 'insensible, dumb') which is easily understandable from the presence of the initial negative *alpha*.

Many others are built the same way, as the adjectives *a-guios* (ἄγυιος) 'without limbs, weak' (*CH De muliebrum affectibus* 25; Galen, *Linguarum seu dictionum exoletarum Hippocratis explicatio* [Kühn 19.69]), *a-lalos* (ἄλαλος) 'speechless' (Laes 2011: 461–3), *a-laos* (ἀλαός) 'blind', *an-akoustos* (ἀνάκουστος) or *n-ekoustos* (νήκουστος) 'not hearing', *a-morphos* (ἄμορφος) 'misshapen, ugly' (e.g. Herodotus 1.196 about a woman), *a-kinetos* (ἀκίνητος) 'unable to move', *a-phônos* (ἄμορφος) 'voiceless, mute', *apous* (ἄπους) 'without feet' (Aristotle, *Historia animalium*, for animals, especially birds, cf. 1.1, 487b25 and 9.30, 618a31). The substantives *ablepsia, akinesia, anakoustia, aphonia* and others are derived from those adjectives. To name mental illnesss the Latin usually distinguishes between *amens* (or *amentia*) for a brief and passing crisis, and *demens* (or *dementia*), for a permanent loss of mind (Turner 2013: appendix 1 and Toohey in this volume).

The Greek vocabulary puts the stress on the weakness resulting from any disability, and does not name the impairment from the disabled part of the body or the illness that caused it. The language does not distinguish congenital malformations from a physical defect caused by an accident, or a disease. For the Greek society, a disability, as we perceive it, for instance the deprivation of one of the senses (blindness, deafness, mutity) or the absence of a mutilated limb, is only seen as a permanent (chronic) weakness or inability. Also, there does not seem to be a clear distinction in vocabulary between 'ill' and 'disabled', distinguishing between a temporarily and a lasting condition, as is clear from a word as ἀσθενής. In the same way, the Latin *infirmus* and *aegrotus* do not correspond to our 'disabled' and 'ill', and also the distinction between *vitium* and *morbus* is not that clear-cut (Toohey in this volume).

Final -los-

Many other imprecise terms, mainly adjectives, are characterized by a final in –λος (*-los*), mostly added to a verbal stem (see Chantraine 1979: 237–56). The majority of these words have their tone on the final syllable. In most of them, the pejorative meaning of the suffix is still perceptible (Chantraine 1979: 239). Also used in the building of some appellations designating parts of the body, or technical terms, the suffix was productive for designations of persons with a harmed or diminished body.² It must be said that some of the words showing the final –λος are, in fact, the result of a phonetic evolution and did not present a form in –*los* after their stem, as for instance, κυλλός, from κυλ-νός.

The list follows the Latin alphabet.

- *bat(t)alos* (βάταλος or βάτταλος) 'stammerer' said about Demosthenes (*De corona* 180) whose speech disorder was famous (see Laes 2013: 173–4). Æschines' text (with only one *tau*) and Plutarch (*Vita Demosth.*) refer to the same anecdote. The word is not used by Galen. The term probably derives from *battos* (see infra, p. 128). The word may also be used as an insult with obscene connotation (cf. *LSJ* s.v. and Laes 2013: 174, Batalus referring to the anus, 'the part of the body which is indecent to name', according to Plutarch, *Vita Demosth.* 4.7).

- *chôlos* (χωλός), 'lame, paralyzed, spec. limping' (already in Homer, Chantraine 1979: 238), often because of a lame foot, or hand. The word is very frequent and used in all types of texts; *TLG* lists 1552 instances. The word occurs from the *Iliad* (2.217; 9.503; 18.397) and the *Odyssey* (8.308 and 332) on, to the tragic writers, Aristophanes, philosophers (metaphorically), and to Plutarch, but has no clear etymology. Several nouns and verbs are formed after *chôlos*, as χώλωμα, χώλωσις, χωλεύω, χωλόομαι. The name χωλότης, 'lameness, claudication', appears only during the 2nd century CE and later. The adjective is used for animals as for human beings, or metaphorically, for poetry, in the case of metre. While the prefix *apo-* (*apochôloomai* and *apochôleuô*) diminishes the gravity to 'quite lame', *kata-*, in *katachôlos* (καταχῶλος), 'dead lame', and *pro-*, in *prochôlos* (πρόχωλος), 'very lame' reinforce the word. Limping is, very seldom, also said *skasmos* (σκασμός), from the verb *skazô*, extensively used during the classical period (*DELG* s.v. σκάζω).

- *illos* (ἰλλός), 'squinting', a very rare word, is said of distorted or twisted eyes. Like *strabos* and the verb *illôptein* it is a synonym of *strabizein* and *parablepein* 'to look aside, to squint', according to the grammarians of the 2nd century CE. The etymology is uncertain (from *illô*, 'turn'?, cf. *EDG* s.v., the form *illops* (ἴλλοψ), perhaps parallel to *ellops* (ἔλλοψ) 'mute' and 'dumb'). Before being mentioned by the grammarians of the 2nd century CE and later (Herodian, Pollux and Dionysios), the word appears only one time in Aristophanes, *Thesmophoriazousae* 846 and one time in Galen's *Commentary of the Hippocratic Epidemics*. Lucian (*Lexiphanes* 3), gives *sillos* (σιλλός) as a double of *illos* with the same meaning 'squint-eyed' (cf. *DELG*, s.v. σιλλός). A *sillos* is a satirical poem, but a semantical link, based on the derision aimed at the physical defect, seems difficult, though a mocking connotation cannot be excluded (Masson 1976: 95 recalls a proper name and the verb *silloô* by the 5th-century BCE comic poet Archippus). It seems that the poet Menander had squinting eyes (Grmek 1994: 108–9).

- *kampulos* (καμπύλος), 'curved, bent', is mostly said about objects during the classical period (so as *epikampulos*, of same sense) in relation with *kampsos* (same meaning) and *kamptos* 'flexible' (*DELG* and *EDG* s.v. κάμπτω). Galen uses it more than a dozen times, as synonym of *skolios*, for parts of the body as fingers and eyelids or for letters. The substantive is *kampulotes* (καμπυλότης) 'crookedness' and the derived adjective *prokampulos* 'bent forward'. The influence of *ankulos* (ἀγκύλος), 'crooked, curved' is most probable here.

- *kellas* (κελλάς) 'one-eyed' (probably a feminine of *kellos), is an *h.leg.* quoted by Hesychius, who defines it as a synonym of *monophthalmos* (see Hesychius s.v. *streblos* and *plagios*. The other *hapax*, *kemôn* (κέμων) 'one-eyed', given by Hesychius with the definition *heterophthalmos* is probably mistaken for *kellos* (*DELG* and *EDG* s.v.).

- *kolos* (κολός), 'having a part lopped off, reduced to a stump'. Rare and archaic, challenged by *kolobos*, with the suffix -βος, κολός has the same sense of 'mutilated, lame, shortened'. The adjective is derived from a verbal stem meaning 'to hit' (*DELG*, s.v. and Chantraine 1979: 261). It is used by Herodotus (4.29) to describe the small and distorted horns of the bulls in Scythia, and by Aristophanes about those of a ram. It is not present in the *CH*, using instead *kolobos*, perhaps to avoid the confusion with the substantive *kolon*, the part of the intestine. H.: *kolobos*, *nosôdes* (νοσώδης), 'ill', and *peros*.
- *kullos* (κυλλός) 'deformed, crippled, club-footed and bandy-legged', metaphorically 'distorted, misshapen, deformed', was used since Homer (the compound *kullopodion* as epithet of Hephaistos), Aristophanes and *CH*. Etymology: from *k^wl-nos* related to *k^wel-* ' to turn ' (*DELG* s.v.). H.: *plagios*. With the prefix *epi-*, *epikullôma* (ἐπικύλλωμα), it means 'lameness'.
- *millos* (μιλλός), also *milos* (μιλός) 'flabby, dumb', *h.leg.* in H., who defines the word with *bradus* (βραδύς) 'slow' and *chaunos* (χαῦνος) 'loose'.
- *mullos* (μυλλός), 'crippled, twisted' (H. s.v. accented μυλλός, linked with τὰ μύλλα, 'lips' Masson 1976: 95) and 'swivel-eyed' is rare and posterior to the second century CE. Eustathios of Thessaloniki, a Byzantine scholar (twelfth century) who wrote several commentaries about the Homeric poems and other texts, explains it as ὁ διεστραμμένος τὴν ὄψιν (906.54, see *EDG* and Masson 1976: 94–5).
- *musk(e)los* (μύσκ(ε)λος), 'crippled, hunchbacked' is not present in the texts, but has given the proper name Myskellos. The founder of Croton, during the 7th century BCE, named Myskel(l)os, was said to be hunchbacked (Masson 1989: 64–5; Ogden 1997: 62–72). H.: *musklos* as *skolios*.
- *nenielos* (νενιηλός) 'blinded', appears only one time in the surviving Greek literature, in Callimachus, *In Jovem* 63, explained in the *Scholia in Callimachum* as *mataiophrôn* 'senseless', and by H.: *tuphlos*, *apoplektos*, *anoetos* 'blind, senseless, stupid'. Etymology unknown (*DELG* s.v., possible (?) link with *eneos*, *EDG*).
- *psellos* (ψελλός), 'fastering in speech, speaking inarticulately'. The adjective is used in all periods and all types of texts (*TLG* lists 258 occurrences), mainly comedy, for anyone stummering, typically children inverting letters or syllables. The word is often related with *traulos* (e.g. Galen, *De locis affectis* 4.9 [Kühn 8.272]).
- *siphlos* (σιφλός), 'defect, crippled, maimed', and metaphorically 'mad', was not used before the 3rd century BCE, and appears less than thirty times in Greek literature on whole (e.g. Apollonios of Rhodes, *Argon.* 1.204, about a foot), but is ancient, as the derived verb is already mentioned in the *Iliad* (14.142) with the meaning 'turning mad', with a possible variant *sipalos* (σιπαλός) as *h.leg.* 'blinded (?), maimed (?)'. It expresses an impairment of any kind (Lycophron, *Alexandra* 1134: *siphlos*, *morphès*). H.: *kakos* ('bad'), *pèros*, *aischros* ('shameful'), *môros*, *mômetos* ('to be blamed'), *epimômos* ('blamable'). The etymology is unknown (*DELG* s.v.).
- *skellos* (σκελλός), 'with twisted legs, bandy-legged' is another *h.leg.*, for H., synonym of *raibos*. The word is derived from *skelos*, 'leg', with a probable influence of *kullos*, which explains the expressive geminate. It keeps a vocalism *-e-*, when *skolios* shows the vowel *-o-* (see infra) and has a possible etymological link with the idea of 'twisted, crooked' (see *DELG* s.v. σκέλος).
- *streblos* (στρεβλός), 'twisted, crooked', often used in the classical period in all types of texts, from Aesop to the theatre (Aristophanes, Menander) or the philosophical treatises (Plato, Aristotle); in the *CH*, *Air Water, Places* 14.4 about hereditary strabismus; also metaphorically, meaning 'crooked, cunning'. The connection to the verb *strephô*, 'to

turn, to twist, to whirl', seems evident, but is not phonetically clear. The etymology of στρέφω is unknown (*DELG* and *EDG*). The derived *diastrophos* also means 'twisted, distorted', and the substantive *streblotes* (στρεβλότης), 'crookedness'.

- *traulos* (τραυλός), 'suffering from a speech disorder, with deficient speech, mispronouncing letters, *e.g.* lisping, stammering', as said about Alcibiades, who in his childhood, mixed up the letters R and L (Plutarch, *Life of Alcibiades* 1.6; see Laes 2013: 172). Said by Herodotus 4.155 about Battos, who was *traulos* (also 4.161) and *ischnophonos* (Laes 2013: 170–1) or in the *CH*, *Aphorisms* 6.32, *Epidemics* 1.2, *Epidemics* 2.5.1 and 6.1 in combination with other disorders. The adjective is still used in modern Greek for 'stammerer'. The etymology of it is unclear (perhaps related to *trauma*, *DELG* and *EDG* s.v. τραυλός). The verb *traulizô* (τραυλίζω) 'mispronounce letters, lisp' and the substantive *traulotes* (τραυλότης) 'lisping' are completed with *hupotraulizô* diminishing the disability, like *hupotraulos* (ὑπότραυλος) 'slightly stammering' (*CH*, only in *Epidemics* 7.2.6; 7.3.2; 7.11.9; 7.22.1; 7.43.2).
- *tuphlos* (τυφλός), 'blind, dark' and, metaphorically, 'blocked, clogged', is extensively used in all types of texts (already *Iliad* 6.130, and seven mentions in the *CH*), and is related to the verb τύφομαι 'to stay in smoke, in fog'. The recurrent derived names *tuphlôsis* 'blinding', *tuphlotes* 'blindness', verbs *tuphloô, apotuphloô* (ἀποτυφλόω) and *ektuphloô* 'make quite blind' and adjective *hupotuphlos* (ὑπότυφλος) 'half-blind, weak-sighted' appear within the 2nd century CE (Plutarch and later). Usually translated by 'blind', *tuphlos* designates a person who does not see from birth, or someone who has lost his sight as well as another person who has lost his mind permanently, because he stays 'in a fog'. Again, the vocabulary does not distinguish between a congenital cause, a trauma or a disease which happens later in life, and, in a metaphoric use, about the human mind as strange behaviour. To be blinded, metaphorically, in a 'moral' sense, is said *ateros* (ἀτηρός), based on the word *ate* (ἄτη), 'damage, guilt, blindness, fine'. The adjective and the other words of this family have a common origin based on **dhubh-* (> *tuph-*) expressing the concept of smoke, of fog and darkness, leading to the notion of blindness but also to the idea, as in the English dumb, of deafness, mutism or low mental ability, stupidity. It also expresses the idea of swagger, excessive pride and self-satisfaction (*tuphos*). These words are formed on **dhuH*, 'smoke' (German *Duft*, *DELG* s.v. τύφομαι. Cf. also German *taub*, 'deaf'). The typhus disease takes its name from the lethargy or dullness that strikes the sick.

Many of these terms could be interpreted as mocking, either because of the vowel -*a*- or because of the geminate, often used in the vocabulary of derision. Denigration is a recurrent way of pointing at a physical defect. A rich and variated vocabulary connotes marked and imperfect bodies. But what exactly is an imperfection?

Imperfect

Other groups of adjectives form coherent units, morphologically as well as semantically (Skoda 1991). They are built with prefixes or suffixes that confer on them a sort of intelligible meaning and come to form a series.

Final in -bos

- *bôbos* (βωβός), 'lame, disabled', names a handicap (*EDG* s.v.). *h.leg.* H.: *chôlos* and *peros*.

- *chabos* (χαβός), 'curved', or 'weak', *h.leg.* H.: *kampulos, stenos* 'narrow, painful, cramped' (Skoda 1991: 392).
- *hubos* (ύβός), 'hunchback, hump-backed'; Galen (*Commentary of the Hippocratic Aphorisms* 6.46 [Kühn 18.1.74]) and H.: *kurtos* and *kuphos*. *Hubos* seems to be used by medical authors (Skoda 1988: 253–4) and is not very frequent: only thirty-six occurrences in the *TLG*. Substantives *hubôsis*, 'condition of being humpbacked' and *hubôma* 'hump', verb *huboomai* 'become humpbacked'. The *CH* (*Aphorisms* 6.46) states that becoming humpbacked before puberty is fatal – it has been recognized as a sign of tuberculosis.
- *klambos* (κλαμβός), 'cocked, mutilated' is said of ears, and is related to *skambos* (*DELG* and *EDG* s.v.). *TLG*: only two occurrences in Greek texts (*Hippiatrica*).
- *kolobos* (κολοβός), 'maimed, mutilated, undersized', is common in different kinds of texts (Aesop, Xenophon, Plato, Aristotle) and in the *CH*, related to *kolos* (*DELG* and *EDG s.v.).* The verbs *koloboô* (κολοβόω) and *kolobizô* have the meaning of 'to mutilate', *kolobôsis* 'mutilation', *kolobôma* 'the part taken away in mutilation'.
- *raibos* (ῥαιβός), 'torted, bent inward', is said especially of legs, as synonym of *kullos* (κυλλός) and seems to be an antonym to *blaisos* (βλαισός). H.: *me orthos* ('not straight'), *kampulos, streblos, skambos*. One mention in Lycophron's *Alexandra* (*DELG* and *EDG s.v.*); a compound *raibo-eides* (ῥαιβοειδής), 'of crooked shape' (Skoda 1991: 379). Galen (*De morborum differentiis* 7 [Kühn 6.856] and *Comm. de articulis* 3.407 [Kühn 18.1 604]) brings it together with *roibos* and with *blaisos*. Also used are the derived *huporaibos* 'somewhat crooked', the verb *raiboô* 'bend, make crooked' and the substantive *raibotes* (ῥαιβότης) 'crookedness'.
- *skambos* (σκαμβός), 'crooked, bandy-legged', as *streblos*, said for someone with walking disabilities because of a foot. The word appears in the 1st century CE (Erotian, about distorted wood) and is used by pseudo-Galen as a synonym of *kampulos* (*Introductio seu medicus* 20.2 = Kühn 14.793). The other occurrences are all later than the 5th century CE. The etymology is unclear, perhaps related to *skazô* or *kamptô* (*DELG* s.v. σκαμβός). The word has a derived adjective *huposkambos* 'somewhat crooked' and builds a compound *skambopous* 'with crooked feet' (*EDG* s.v.).
- *skimbos* (σκιμβός), 'lame, crooked' is parallel to the precedent; *h.leg.* H.: *chôlos* and *skambos* (unclear etymology, *DELG*, s.v. σκιμβός).
- *strabos* (στραβός), 'squinting' or *strobos* 'squinting', 'whirling around', is also linked with *streblos*, as *illos* (Pollux 2.51), and used in medical texts after the 1st century BCE (*TLG*: first occurrence in the *Fragmenta* of the grammarian Philoxenus, one occurrence in Soranus and then in Galen's lexical works, e.g. *Hippocratic Glossary* (*Linguarum seu dictionum exoletarum Hippocratis explicatio* [Kühn 19.141]: στρεβλοί, οὓς καὶ στραβοὺς ὀνομάζουσι), as well as Aelius Dionysios and Phrynichos). H.: *streblos* (*DELG* and *EDG* s.v. στρεβλός). *Hupostrabos*, 'squinting a little', *strabizô* 'to squint'.

Even if most of these words show undoubtedly a suffix, the *-b-* in *strabos* belongs to the stem, and the origin of *hubos* stays unclear (Skoda 1991: 368; *DELG* and *EDG* s.v. ύβός). These adjectives may very well have influenced one another, as their semantism converges to a corporeal defect, named in a direct way.

Many of these dissyllabic words indicating a defect or an imperfection of movement or of parts of the body show a vocalism *-a-* said to be colloquial (Chantraine 1979: 434), and/ or the suffix *-sos*, are oxytone, indicating a defect or an imperfection of movement or of parts of the body.

Final in -sos

Many of the adjectives with the final *-sos*, with the accent on the last syllable (oxytone), express the notion of distortion, deviation, or of a defect, lack or imperfection, forming therefore a lexical micro-system (Chantraine 1979: 433–6; Skoda 1991).

- *blaisos* (βλαισός), 'bent, distorted' designates a person with feet turned inward. This word points at the imperfection and not at the impossibility to move. The Latin has *blaesus*, 'stutterer'. Etymology unknown, probably colloquial (*DELG*), but Skoda 1991: 374–80, esp. 379, suggests a stem βλαδ-, stating the idea of 'stunted', or 'flabby'. This adjective is used to name a club-footed person (Xenophon, *De re equestri* 1.3; *CH, De articulis* 53 and 62; Aristotle). Galen uses it in association with *raibos*. About Hephaistos and other clubfeet, see Ziskowski 2012 and Horstmanshoff 2012.
- *gampsos* (γαμψός), 'curved, crooked', so in Aristophanes, *Nubes* 337 (*EDG* and Skoda 1991: 369–71) is also used in the *Iliad* (16.428) for claws of vultures, appears fifty-two times in Greek texts (so *TLG*), and in the *CH* (*De nat. puer.* 31.1), it qualifies a uterus. Substantive *gampsotes* (γαμψότης) 'crookedness'. Related to *skambos* and *chabos* (*DELG*).
- *gausos* (γαυσός), 'crooked, bent outward' stays rare (*TLG* only eleven occurrences), parallel to *blaisos* and *chôlos* in *CH* (*De articulis* 77 and 82 about knees, *Vectiarius* 26; *De fracturis* 20, about thigh bones) and in the commentaries of the physicians Apollonius of Kition (1st century CE) and Galen. H.: *skambos, streblos*. See Skoda 1991: 372–4 and 377.
- *kampsos* (καμψός), also *kamptos* (καμπτός), related to *gampsos* or *gnamptos*, 'crooked, bent', from κάμπτω, means 'to curve, to bend'. H. (*h.leg.*) gives it as a synonym of *kampulos*. Etymology: the stem *kamp-* is used for expressive and often technical terms, with the meaning 'curved, bent' (*DELG* s.v. κάμπτω and Skoda 1991: 371).
- *loxos* (λοξός), 'oblique, slanting, sloping' is used in the medical texts about a misplaced organ, the form of a wound or the orientation of a bandage (*DELG* and *EDG* s.v., Skoda 1991: 389–90). In the literature, it expresses metaphorically ambiguity, ambivalence or obscurity, so Apollo Loxias, the oracular god of ambiguous or enigmatic phrases (Skoda 1991: 390). The adjective is used mainly by poets and astronoms, and physicians (after the first century CE), very often in Rufus of Ephesus and Galen.
- *nusos* (νῦσος) is a Syracusan synonym of χωλός, of unknown etymology (*DELG* and *EDG* s.v. νῦσος). One may add that *Nu-to* (personal name) is already Mycenean (Dubois 2014: 78–9; cf. Landau 1958: 190–3 and Grmek 1994: 38). Is this another instance of a nickname becoming a proper name?
- *rampsos* (ῥαμψός), another *h.leg.* to which H. gives the following definition: *kampulos, blaisos*. The word was probably forged (so *DELG* s.v.) from the combination of *gampsos* and *ramphos* (ῥάμφος) 'beak, bill', leading again to the image of a crooked, bent, distorted or curved form.

It has been noticed that *blaisos* and *gausos* form a pair of quasi-antonyms (the 'real' antonym would obviously be 'straight') both meaning 'distorted ', but the first one ('knock-kneed'), means curved inward and the second one bent outward (Skoda 1991: 377). Other adjectives in *-sos* denote physical imperfections that cannot be considered as disabilities in the present sense of the word, as *phoxos* (φοξός), 'sharp', to qualify e.g. a head, *phrixos* (φριξός), 'hairy, frizzy, fuzzy' for the hair, *rusos* (ῥυσός), 'wrinkled', for the skin. But of course, also these words refer to 'special features' which might have had a disabling effect on the person concerned, in specific situations or contexts.

Final in -aros

Pointing out a frailty, some more adjectives are rather used for objects or organs than for persons; they also form a lexical micro-system, expressing the idea of 'fragile, incapacitated', with the final *-aros*, like *kladaros* (κλαδαρός), 'quivering, invalid', of a lance (Polybius 6.25.5) *pladaros* (πλαδαρός), 'flabby' (of fleshes, *CH, Internal Affections* 40), *psapharos* (ψαφαρός), 'friable, crumbling', *chalaros* (χαλαρός), 'slack, loose', about the skin (*CH, Aphorisms* 5.71) *laparos* (λαπαρός), 'slack, loose, dislocated', of joints (*CH, De articulis* 50), see Chantraine 1979: 227. The final *-aros* often also occurs in pejorative adjectives, like *musaros* (μυσαρός), 'foul, dirty, abominable' or *pinaros* (πιναρός), 'dirty, squalid' (Chantraine 1979: 227 ; Masson 1976: 94, n. 55), which might again point to prejudice or negative connoting of persons experiencing such bodily situations.

- *akaros* (ἄκαρος), 'blind', H.: *tuphlos*. The word is used only in Herodianus (2nd century CE) and H.. Etymology unknown (*DELG* s.v.).
- *asiaros* or *asidaros* (ἀσίαρος or ἀσίδαρος) 'limping upon', *h.leg.* in H. as synonym of *episkazôn*, derived from the verb *skazô* 'to limp'.

Various terms for a variety of ailments

Disparate designations

Many other terms are used to name disabled persons. The majority of these words designate people with eye, speech or walking impairments (blinds, mutes or bent) and some words try to precise the impairment.

- *alaos* (ἀλαός), 'blind', stays rare (*Odyssey* 8.195 and 285; *Odyssey* 10.493 and 12.267. Also in tragedies, Callimachus and all the commentaries of Homeric poems, as well as in Galen's lexical works (*Linguarum seu dictionum exoletarum Hippocratis explicatio* Kühn 19.75); the word is usually replaced by *tuphlos*. The etymology is unknown: an *alpha* privative combined to *laô* 'to see' is not convincing (*DELG* s.v.).
- *anchran* (ἄγχραν), Locrian term for *muops* (μύωψ), means 'short-sighted', *h.leg.* in H. (etymology unknown, so *DELG*, s.v. citing Bechtel 1921).
- *battos* (βάττος), after the name Battos, means 'stammerer, lisper', *h.leg.* in H.[3]
- *blômos* (βλωμός), 'squinting' (probable link with the verb *ballô*, 'to throw'), comes up only (*h.leg.*) in H.: *strabos, illos, streblos*.
- *eneos* (ἐνεός), 'speechless, mute', also means 'stupid' (etymology unknown, so *DELG* and *EDG s.v.; kibon, h.leg.* in H.: *eneon, DELG* s.v. κίβον). Plato (*Cratylus* 422e4) reminds of *eneoi* trying to sign with their hands, their heads and their whole body (cf. also Plato *Alcibiades* 2.140d1 and *Theaetetus* 206d9 and Aristotle, *De sensu et sensibilibus* 437a16 or *Problemata* 899a5). The word progressively specializes in muteness, *kôphos* designating the deaf (Laes 2011: 460–3).
- *grupos* (γρῦπος, γρυπός), 'crooked, hook-nosed', said of nails or nose, is linked to *grups, grupos*, a fabulous bird (*DELG* and *EDG* s.v., cf. Saxon *crumb*, Latin *gryphus*).
- *guros* (γυρός), 'curved, crooked', in H.: *kurtos* and *hubos*. Etymology: from **geu-/*gu-* : 'to turn, to twist' or 'to bend'; some assume a link with *guios* (γυιός) 'lamed' and the verb *guioô* (γυιόω), 'cripple' (*DELG* and *EDG* s.v.).
- *ischnophônos* (ἰσχνόφωνος), 'thin voiced, weak voiced' or 'having an impediment in one's speech' as in Herodotus (4.155) about the Therean Battos, often near *traulos* (e.g.

Hdt, Ps.-Aristotle, *Problemata* 902b22) (Laes 2013: 157 for possible confusion with *ischophonos*).

- *kadamos* (κάδαμος), 'blind', *h.leg.* H.: *tuphlos* in Salamis (very dubious, the text has been contested, cf. *DELG*, s.v.).

- *kôphos* (κωφός), 'blunt, dull, obtuse' is mainly used to designate a mental disorder or a speech impossibility (deafness, mutism). It appears throughout Greek literature, for instance in Herodotus (1.34) about Croisos' boy who is said to be 'deaf and dumb' (Laes 2008; 2011: 453–5). Parallel, the words *dys-kôphos* 'hearing with difficulty' and *hupo-kôphos* 'hard of hearing, rather deaf' (*CH*, *Prorrhetic* 1.95 = *Coa Praesagia* 172) are more specialized and differentiated. *Kophos* it is well attested during the classical period (e.g. in *CH*, Aristophanes, Plato) and has several derivates as *kôphôsis* (*Aphorisms* 4.28; *Coa Praesagia* 165, 186, 187, 191, 205, 206, 207, 328, 413, 525), *kôphôma* and *kôphôtes* (*Epidemics* 3.3.17) 'deafness', verb *kôphoô* (*Coa Praesagia* 178, 192). The term used in modern Greek, *boubos* (βουβός) 'mute', appeared only during the Byzantine period (Dubois 2014: 84). *DELG* s.v. κηφήν, relates it to a non-attested adjective *kephos 'blunt'.

- *kuphos* (κυφός) 'bent forward, hunchbacked' (cf. *CH* sixteen occurrences of which ten in *De articulis*; in *De morbo sacro* 6.1 about patients), from the verb κύπτω, 'to bend for ward, to stoop'; derived are *epikuphos* (ἐπικῦφος) 'bent over' and *hupokuphos* (ὑποκῦφος), 'gibbous, humped' (cf. *DELG* and *EDG* s.v. κύπτω; from the noun *kûphos*, 'hump, hunch', the verb *kuphoomai* 'to be bent, hump-backed, hunchbacked', is used in *Odyssey* 2.16 and in lyric poetry). The name Κύλλαρος proves the existence of a lost adjective *kullaros*. The stem is probably also related to the name Kypselos, tyrant of Corinth (see Ziskowski 2012).

- *kurtos* (κυρτός), 'curved, hunchbacked', or *hupokurtos* (ὑπόκυρτος), 'gibbous, humped', is also quite frequent: *Iliad* (2.218 about shoulders), with scientific writers (Aristotle) and in medical texts. It also occurs in the Latin *curuus* 'curved, convex', as well as in modern Greek (*DELG* and *EDG* s.v.). It was also used as a nickname (Crates); *amphikurteô* 'to be gibbous' and the substantive *kurtotes* (κυρτότης) 'stoop, humped shoulders' are attested as well.

- *lordos* (λορδός), 'bent backward', 'convex', comes as an antonym of *kuphos* (Aristophanes, five occurrences in the *CH* (*Art.* 48; *De fracturis* 16), Aristotle, *De ingressu animalium* 707b18, also with Erotian and Galen).

- *môros* (μωρός) 'dull, sluggish', also 'dumb, silly, foolish' is a very common in Greek literature (from Aesop to the Tragics, ordered chronologically, eighty-two occurrences in the *TLG*; three in the *CH* and eleven in the Galenic texts), but of unclear etymology (*DELG* s.v. μωρός). It corresponds to the English *moron*. How exactly was the word connoted in ancient Greek? This is impossible to find out (the modern Greek vocative μωρε has a very mild connotation and is often used in daily speech).

- *mukos* (μυκός), 'speechless, voiceless, mute' (*DELG* and *EDG* s.v. μυκός), appears in H. (*h.leg.*) with the meaning of *aphônos*. It is also attested with a dental, *muttos* (μυττός), *h.leg.* in H., as a synonym of *eneos*, or *mu(n)dos* (μυ(ν)δός). *Mudos*: *h.leg.* in H., as *aphonos*, *murkos*.

- *muôps* (μύωψ), 'short-sighted', properly 'with eyes getting shut' (*EDG* s.v. μύωψ), commonly used by different authors (Tragics, Xenophon, Ps.-Aristotle, *Problemata* 31.15 and 16, *CH* (*Letter to Ptolemaeus*) and Galen).

- *murkos* (μύρκος) 'completely unable to speak', is again an *h.leg.* in H. and explained as Syracusan for *eneos*, *aphônos*. The word could be influenced by the Latin *murcus* 'mutilated' and was possibly enclosed in the series meaning 'mute' (*DELG*).

- *pèros* (πηρός), 'infirm, invalid, lame or blind' is a most thought-provoking word to the historian of disabilities. It is very frequently used, but stays etymologically isolated and cannot be connected to any other word. Intrestingly, the word is used in a general sense 'paralysed, crippled', but also to name specific disabilities, as 'blind' (in the centuries CE) or 'lame'. It therefore appears to combine the two most common diseases in Antiquity: visual impairment and crippling diseases. Although πηρός seems near to πῆμα 'sorrow', its etymology is unclear (*EDG* s.v. *peros*), as is the origin of most of the adjectives naming disabled persons (Chantraine 1979: 225). The noun *perôsis* (πήρωσις) denotes the action of maiming, so does the verb *peroô*. The derived *ana-pèros*, *em-peros* and *kata-peros* (ἀνάπηρος, ἔμπηρος κατάπηρος) have the same meaning of 'maimed'. Tellingly, ἀνάπηρος is the standard modern Greek term to denote a handicap, though nowadays the politically correct description ἄτομο με ειδικές ανάγκες is far more preferred. However, the adjective has few occurrences in the *CH* (*Diseases* 1.1.1; 1.3; *Diseases* 2, *Diseases of Women* 131), as well as in Galen (*De Usu partium* 2.15 [Kühn 3.146], *De usu partium* 3.5 [Kühn 3.188] and *De usu partium* 8.7 [Kühn 3.653], or *De animi cuiuslibet peccatorum dignotione ...* 2 [Kühn 5.64] about Aesop).
- *pholkos* (φολκός), is an *h.leg.* designating Thersitus (*Iliad* 2.217); the word has sometimes been translated 'squinting', but, as Thersitus is said to be χωλός, it is now preferably understood by philologists as 'curved, crooked', as a developed allusion to his inability to walk, and even to stand straight on his feet. 'Bandy-legged' does seems to be an appropriate translation (uncertain etymology, *DELG* and *EDG* s.v. φολκός).
- *plagios* (πλάγιος), 'oblique, sloping, crooked' meaning 'lopsided, not straight' from the concept of flat (**plag-*). The stem **plH₂g-* (latin: *plaga*, 'expanse, shore', German: *flach*, English: *flat*) means transverse and stretched (cf. *DELG* and *EDG* s.v. πλάγιος). Adjectives in *-ios* do not constitue a group similar to the others; their accentuation is not coherent and their number not sufficient, *plagios* and *skolios*, ev. *balios* (βαλία, ὀφθαλμία, i.e. 'eye-disease', only in H.).
- *riknos* (ρικνός), 'bent, crooked, shrivelled', possibly enhanced with a prefix *kata-riknos*, is used to describe Hephaistos' feet. For H., it is synonym of *skambos* and *skolios*. The etymology stems from 'whirling, rotating, turning around', *DELG* s.v. ρικνός.
- *rôbikos* (ρωβικός), 'unable to pronounce the letter *rhô*' *h.leg.* in Diogenes Laertius, *Vita philosophorum* 1.109, about Demosthenes (where it is used as a comparative).
- *roikos* (ροικός), 'crooked, bow-legged', used for a piece of wood or a distorted leg. It is rarely attested. Galen uses it only on three occasions, in his commentaries of the Hippocratic *De articulis* 3.38 [Kühn 18.1.537], and 3.87 [Kühn 18.1.604–5]; Erotian defines the word as *kampulos*, so does H.: *skolios, kampulos, skambos, rusos* ('wrinkled'), *riknos* (*DELG* s.v. ρικνός). A compound *roiko-eides* meaning 'crooked-looking' also exists.
- *skolios* (σκολιός), 'curved, bent, torted, distorted' is very common (*TLG* lists 1,733 occurrences, from Homer and Hesiod on, to the lyric poets, the tragics and various prose authors. The *CH* has seven mentions and Galen, who gives it as a synonym of *kullos*, brings twelve references). As in modern languages, it is often used metaphorically, to denote 'crooked' laws or methods. Linguistically, it shows a vocalism -o- after *skelos* 'leg'. The Latin *scelus*, 'crime', may be linked to this origin, when interpreted as a 'crooked, distorted act' (*DELG* s.v. σκέλος). Derived words are *huposkoloios* 'somewhat crooked', the substantive *skoliotes* (σκολιότης) 'crookedness', and the compound *skoliôdes* (σκολιώδης), 'crooked-looking'.

Compound words

In composition: dys- / dus-

Greek language disposes of an initial *dus-* 'improper, difficult', which contributes to build many nouns and adjectives expressing a physical lack. So, for instance, and not exhaustively, the abstract feminine substantives *dus-erge-ia* (δυσεργεία), *dus-eid-eia* (δυσειδεία), *dus-morphia* (δυσμορφία) or the epithets *duseides* (δυσειδής) all with connotations of 'unpleasant, ugly', *duskôphos* (δύσκωφος) 'completely deaf', *dus-morphos* (δύσμορφος), 'suffering from a deformity'. The verb *duskopheô* appears only in Galen's time. *Dusergia* (*CH, Ancient Medicine* 10.4) expresses a difficulty or even inability to work, when a person who is used to having lunch, skips the meal and feels weak. The word does not appear in Galen's texts; Soranos (2nd century CE) and Oribasius (c.325–95 CE) use *dusergeia* in the sense of 'disability', based on dysfunction. Given the stress on the impossibility of working and functioning in present-day discussion on disability, these are interesting examples. *Dusmorphia*, absent in the *CH*, comes up only twice in Galen's work. They are easily understood by anyone recognizing the stem and the prefix, and are of common acceptation.

Other compounds

Greek also allows the creation of easily understandable compounds as *ambluôssô* (ἀμβλυώσσω) 'to be short-sighted' (Plato; *CH Prorrhetic* 2.30 and 42; *De morbis* 2.1.15 and 19; *De locis hominis* 10.13; *Epidemics* 5.82 and 7.87; seven occurrences in Plutarch and ten in Galen). It originates from *amblus* 'blunt, dim, faint' and *ops* 'vision'. Other examples include *amphigu(e)eis* (ἀμφιγυήεις, ἀμφιγύεις), 'with both feet crooked', *ommatosteres* (ὀμματοστερής) 'deprived of eyesight, blind', from *omma*, 'eye' and *steromai*, 'to lose, to be deprived of', *peromeles* (πηρομελής) 'disabled in the limbs', from *peros* and *melos*, 'limb', or *skeloturbes* (σκελοτυρβής), 'lameness in the leg' (Ps.Galen, *Definitiones medicae*, [Kühn 19.427]), from *skelos*, 'leg' and *turbe*, 'disorder, confusion', *apôtos* (ἄπωτος), 'deaf', literally with 'far ears', *heterokôphos* (ἑτερόκωφος) 'deaf on one side', *stenophônos* (στενόφωνος) 'with a weak, thin voice'.

To this series must be added three passive voice participles, pointing out the result of a damaging action:

- *paralelumenos* (παραλελυμένος), 'paralyzed', of *paraluô* (παραλύω). In the *CH, Coan Prenotions* 197 it is used about the tongue. In *Epidemics* 7.8.1 it denotes a woman suffering from tetanus. The verb designates a loosening of the tendons (not of the muscles), causing an inability to move (cf. *Epidemics* 5.17.2). Galen has twenty-four occurrences. The prefix *para-* is not elsewhere used to build terms designating physical imperfections or disabilities, because of its meaning 'apart from, beside'. *Para-* is more understandable in the context of mental disorders, as in *paranoia* or *paraphrôn*, literally 'out of his mind', denoting a disordered function or faculty.
- *pepalmenos* (πεπαλμένος), defined by H. as 'disabled, hindered, who got dislocated joints', probably comes from a verb meaning 'to jump off, to be detached of' (*DELG* and *EDG* s.v. πάλέω).
- *tetrômenos* (τετρωμένος), 'wounded, harmed, injured, damaged' (perfect tense) of *titrôskô* (τιτρώσκω) comes up in the entire Greek corpus. The stem τρω- (*terH₃- / *terH₁-) means 'to dig a hole', cf. *trauma* (τρῶμα, τραῦμα or τρῶσις), *DELG* s.v. τιτρώσκω.

Ancient Greeks do not distinguish systematically between physical impairment and mental disorders. The disability itself stays often very hazy to our eyes. The adjectives used do not concern specifically disabled human beings, but apply also to animals, when not to things or concepts. Persons unable to walk or move properly because of disability or injury to their back or legs at different levels were doubtless quite numerous. Many words express the idea of torsion, bent, twisted or distorted shape, that could be a description of a simple physical condition or a defect (about the symbolical interpretation of lameness, cf. Ziskowski 2012: 225 and the quoted bibliography). An important number of the terms expressing disabilities became nicknames, as Aischylos – a diminutive, derived from *aischos* (αἶσχος) 'shame' is only attested in the name of the famous author of tragedies – or Strabon, Στράβων, 'the squinting one' (from *strepho*, 'to turn', like *streblos*), or many others (see e.g. Bechtel 1917 ; Masson 1976; Dubois 2014 ; and, generally, Fraser and Matthews 1987–2010). Some of them may have been used pejoratively, especially in contexts of common language or comic situations, in the Attic comedies for instance, but in the medical texts, their sense stays technical and without any contempt or disapproval. The most frequent *chôlos* has been used as well in medical or scientific texts and in the literature (*TLG*, chronologically ordered, 316 occurrences up to Galen (21), and 1,552 in total; *CH* totals twenty-two occurrences), in the same manner as *traulos*. Of the 166 records in the *TLG*, only thirty-seven appear up to Galen (*CH* seven occurrences; Galen nine occurrences, from which seven in comments on the *CH*).

There is so much we would like to know, but which is beyond our reach, for instance the problem of sociolects: the different ways the words are used are not always clear. Often the antiquarians were just searching for rare words – but what about their context? Would some words appear to be gendered? Unfortunately, this overview cannot reveal it. Would the physicians be more precise ? In a civilization which saw the birth of medical writing, is there, in the medical treatises, any noteworthy lexical specificity ?

The medical texts

The medical texts unfortunately stay quite general in naming the consequences of diseases or wounding which left the persons lame. The different terms are used as well for temporary physical impairments, consequences of an accident or of a disease, as for permanent deficiencies, from birth, or as for mental abnormality. Their medical use is only progressively clear from the context.

The common vocabulary

Many adjectives, especially those ending in *-lo* are common, not only in ordinary life, but also in the technical literature of medical treatises. For instance *kullos* appears in the *CH* about a twisted foot, or a person whose deformed thigh hinders the upright position (*CH, De articulis* 40, 53, 62; *Officina medici* 23; *Vectiarius* 3). Some are said *kulloi* from birth, others after an accident. From the context of this word, one can suppose that to be *chôlos* was worse than to be *kullos*.

Psellos is also a general term. It appears only three times in the *CH*. Linked with a paralysis of the body, the sudden incapacity to utter a word (*psellos*) comes as a symptom of tetanus (*Epidemics* 7.8.1). The Hippocratic *Letter* 21 (To Democritus) joins *pselloi* and *trauloi*, warning the pharmacist to adapt his drug-preparation to the state of the patient. In another case near *traulos*, it only explains the difficulty in speaking during a very hot summer, as the tongue dries because of the heat (*Epidemics* 7.105.2). Some persons with holed chest are said to become *pselloi*, bald (*phalakroi*) and simple-minded (*Epidemics* 2.6.14).

Tuphlos is commonly used in the *CH*, relating blindness with chronic diseases or bad wounds (*Epidemics* 7.1.57; *Precepts* 14; *Epidemics* 4.1.8; *On Breaths* 14; *Prorrhetic* 2.1; *Internal Diseases* 18; *Eight Months' Child* 5). The very common *chôlos* (*CH* twenty-one occurrences in *TLG*) expresses, several times with the verb *gignomai* 'to become', a new state of a patient, resulting from an accident, a disease or a misplacement of a limb after a fracture. The *CH* contains several warnings to avoid becoming χωλός: *Pronostic* (18.5) mentions the risk of limping, because of deposits, in case of inflammation of the articulations, if the urine is not evacuated properly. Galen (*De usu partium* 13.11 [Kühn 4.126]) explains that to be *chôlos* consists in an inability to stand straight on both legs.

Hubos on the other hand is in the *CH* another *h.leg.* (*Aphorisms* 6.46).

It is noticeable, that many of these words are quoted by two or three or even in series (e.g. *Epidemics* 1.2.9 or *Epidemics* 2.5.1), as if they were better understandable together, or, more probably, because they are linked and show multiple consequences of a weakness or a dysfunction, when not a maiming.

Common terms in a 'technical' sense

An interesting group is formed by the family of the verb *plesso* (πλήσσω), 'to hit, to strike'. Several prefixes find their place in the medical vocabulary specifically, as *apo-plesso* (ἀποπλήσσω), 'cripple by a stroke', and the related *apoplegia* (ἀποπληγία) – only in Galen, e.g. *Commentary on the Hippocratic Prorrheticum* 2.84 [Kühn 16.672] – or *apoplexia* (ἀποπληξία) – Ionian *apoplexie* (ἀποπληξίη), e.g. *Aphorisms* 2.42, 3.23; *Coa Praesagia* 500 – *apoplektikos* (ἀποπληκτικός), 'paralysed' (*Coa Praesagia* 161 (whole body), 197 (tongue), 359 (tongue, arm or side) and 361 (jaw and whole body), 400, 401, 467–70; *Prorrhetic* 1.82; *Prorrhetic* 2.14, 38, 39) and *apoplektos* (ἀπόπληκτος), 'disabled by a stroke' so, pertaining to the mind, struck dumb and astounded (Herodotus 2.173 or Tragics as e.g. Sophocles' *Philoctetes*). This sense comes up in the literature in general, as well as the meaning concerning the body, 'paralysed, crippled' (Herodotus 1.167). But a specific medical definition appears as 'stricken with paralysis', involving the whole body (e.g. *Aphorisms* 3.16; 3.31 or 6.57; *Prorrhetic* 2.9) or a part of it (thigh, leg). It has to be noted that, most of the time, the physical sense occurs in the medical texts, whereas the mental affections are used by all the other authors, historians, tragedians and philosophers. For these authors, *apoplexia* is synonym of madness. The same phenomenon is observed with the other group of derivatives of the same stem **pleH$_x$g-/*pleH$_x$k-*, those formed with *para-* 'on the side'. This prefix is very frequent in the words expressing mental illnesses, as it refers to the notion of off-borders, and it is therefore no surprise to find the same meaning 'mad', in the literature (e.g. Sophocles, *Ajax*) for the word *paraplektos* (παράπληκτος). But the medical sense 'paralysed of one side, suffering from *hemiplegia*' is attested in the Hippocratic *Air, Water, Places* 10.6, where *paraplektos* is used as a synonym of *apoplektos* or *paraplex* (παραπλήξ) with several occurrences in the literature of the 5th and 4th century BCE (see *LSJ* s.v.). But some medical vocabulary has to be pointed out, for instance *paraplecktikos* (παραπληκτικός), 'becoming hemiplegic' (*Air, Water, Places* 3.4) or *paraplegikos* (παραπληγικός) 'suffering from *hemiplegia*' or *paraplexia* (παραπληξία), '*hemiplegia*'. It is noteworthy that the name *hemiplegia* (although compounded of Greek words), does not appear in the general Greek vocabulary, with the sense of '*paralysis*', before Paulus of Egina (7th century CE). These terms will be adopted and passed on from one medical treatise to another over centuries.

Conclusion

In medical texts as in general, the majority of words depicting or describing disabilities or imperfections belong to non-specialized terminology and it is, consequently, worth wondering how and why, in a world that has invented rational medical writing, in the form of the *CH*, the distinction between different impairments stays paradoxically imprecise up to the first centuries CE.

For instance, Aesop, the storyteller, who perhaps lived during the 6th century BCE, is said to be *blaisos, kolobos, streblos* and *kuphos*, in one of his many *Lives*, probably written in the 1st century CE. Many of the terms form semantical groups and morphological micro-systems, showing an important interaction between them. If diachronically, we can identify a different origin of the final, for instance for *kullos*, resulting clearly of an assimilation of *-ln-* to *-ll-*, in synchrony, the Greeks certainly perceived the word as belonging to a group of numerous terms used in physical deformations, because of the geminate final. They impacted each other and shaped these groups of words to form micro-systems. As it was already noticed by Galen (*In Hippocratis librum de fracturis commentarii* 3, Kühn 18.2.518) – quoting, in a list, *chôlos, lordos, streblos, kurtos, blaisos, raibos* – most of them are dissyllabic, oxytone, sometimes showing geminate consonants, perhaps sometimes but not systematically, in a comic intention. Many also show the vocalism *-a-* that has been interpreted as the sign of contempt or denigration (*DELG* s.v. ῥαιβός lists several terms in parallel, *klambos, laios* 'left' and *skaios* 'left-handed, unfavourable, inapt', *phaulos* 'mean, common, bad'). It has already been pointed out that they generally stay quite vague, melding mental and physical disorders, and that their abundance does not contribute to offer a real accuracy in the designation of one handicap or the other. Anyway, in general, the disabled persons are considered from their situation of weakness, or from their appearance as cripples, bent, with distorted limbs, and, finally from the consequences of this situation, their hindrance to act or to move. The multitude of words reflect the variety of situations, especially designating people with difficulties in walking or standing upright (certainly the most numerous, 44), followed by the eye complications (19) and the speech disorders (15). This manifold lexical situation, perhaps sometimes also euphemistic, or on the contrary, expressively mocking, is the evident sign of the great number of physical deficiencies in ancient Greek society, or at least for a significant sensibility towards the issue.

Index of mentioned words (following the Latin alphabet)

ablepsia (ἀβλεψία)
adunatos (ἀδύνατος)
aguios (ἄγυιος)
aischos (αἶσχος)
akaros (ἄκαρος)
akinetos (ἀκίνητος) – *akinesia* (ἀκινησία)
alalos (ἄλαλος)
alaos (ἀλαός)
ambluôssô (ἀμβλυώσσω)
amorphia (ἀμορφία)
amorphos (ἄμορφος)
amphigu(e)eis (ἀμφιγυ(ή)εις)
anaisthetos (ἀναίσθητος)

anakoustos (ἀνάκουστος) – *nekoustos* (νήκουστος)
anchran (ἄγχραν)
aphônia (ἀφωνία)
aphônos (ἄφωνος), or *aphônetos* (ἀφώνητος)
apôtos (ἄπωτος)
apous (ἄπους)
arrôstia (ἀρρωστία)
arrôstos (ἄρρωστος)
asi(d)aros (ἀσίαρος or ἀσίδαρος)
astheneia (ἀσθενεία)
asthenes (ἀσθενής)
bat(t)alos (βάταλος or βάτταλος)
battízo (βαττίζω)
battos (βάττος)
blaisos (βλαισός)
blômos (βλωμός)
bôbos (βωβός)
boubos (βουβός)
chabos (χαβός)
chalaros (χαλαρός)
chôlos (χωλός)
duseides (δυσειδής)
duserg(e)ia (or –*e*) (δυσεργ(ε)ία, , -η)
duskôphos (δυσκῶφος)
ellops (ἔλλοψ)
eneos (ἐνεός)
gampsos (γαμψός)
gausos (γαυσός)
grupos (γρυπός)
guioô (γυιόω)
guros (γυρός)
homeros (ὅμηρος)
hubos (ὑβός)
illops (ἴλλοψ)
illos (ἰλλός)
ischnophônos (ἰσχνόφωνος)
kadamos (κάδαμος)
kampsos(καμψός)
kamptos (καμπτός)
kampulos (καμπύλος)
kellas (κελλάς)
kemôn (κέμων)
kibon (κίβον)
kladaros (κλαδαρός)
klambos (κλαμβός)
kolobos (κολοβός)
kolos (κόλος)
kôphos (κωφός)

kullos (κυλλός)
kuphos (κυφός)
kurtos (κυρτός)
laparos (λαπαρός)
lordos (λορδός)
loxos (λοξός)
millos (μιλλός) or *milos* (μιλός)
môros (μωρός)
mukos (μυκός)
mullos (μυλλός)
muôps (μύωψ)
musaros (μυσαρός)
nenielos (νενιηλός)
nusos (νῦσος)
ommatosteres (ὀμματοστερής)
paralelumenos (παραλελυμένος)
paraluô (παραλύω)
pèros (πηρός)
pholkos (φολκός)
phoxos (φοξός)
phrixos (φριξός)
pinaros (πιναρός)
pladaros (πλαδαρός)
plagios (πλάγιος)
psapharos (ψαφαρός)
psellos (ψελλός)
psilos (ψιλός)
raibos (ῥαιβός)
rampsos (ῥαμψός)
roikos (ῥοικός)
rusos (ῥυσός)
sillos (σιλλός)
siphlos (σιφλός)
skambos (σκαμβός)
skimbos (σκιμβός)
skolios (σκολιός)
steromai (στέρομαι)
strabos (στραβός) or *strobos* (στροβός)
streblos (στρεβλός)
tetrômenos (τετρωμένος)
titrôskô (τιτρώσκω)
traulizô (τραυλίζω)
traulos (τραυλός)
trauma (τρῶμα, τραῦμα)
tuphlos (τυφλός)

Abbreviations

CH	*Corpus Hippocraticum* (or Hippocratic Corpus)
DELG	Pierre Chantraine, *Dictionnaire étymologique de la langue grecque* (Paris: Klincksieck, 2009, 2nd edn)
EDG	Robert S. P. Beekes, *Etymological Dictionary of Greek* (Brill Online Dictionaries, 1969)
H.	Hesychius of Alexandria (5th/6th cent. CE, *Lexicon* (*A Collection of All Words*)
h.leg.	*hapax legomenon*
TLG	*Thesaurus Linguae Graecae* online Irving University

Notes

1 The name ῥώμη, built from the same stem, designates physical strength, generally speaking, and also with the sense of acting force, cf. *DELG*, s.v. ῥώννυμι. The verb has the meaning of 'to strengthen, invigorate, to be(come) strong'. For different hypotheses about the etymology, cf. *EDG* s.v.

2 *Psilos* (ψιλός), 'bald, naked', does not, properly speaking, enter in the category of disabilities, as it concerns mainly landscapes and rarely persons (heads), but is belongs to the group of adjectives in *-los* and, in exceptional circumstances, baldness can be felt as an imperfection.

3 Etymology: probably onomatopoetic, so *DELG* s.v., cf. Herodotus 4.155 about the name of the founder and future king of Cyrene, Battos, said to be *traulos*. See also Masson 1976: esp. 92. The adjective *battos* is not present in the *TLG*. The verbs *battarizô* (βατταρίζω), denoting a speech defect, probably "to stammer" and *battologeô* (βαττολογέω) in the same sense are derived from the adjective. The making of an adjective expressing a disability after a proper name, with a sense understandable to all, because of the popularity of its bearer is also attested with the name of Homer: in *Alexandra*, a long poem, v. 422, Lycophron uses the word *homeros* (ὅμηρος) for 'blind' (the noun *homeros* meaning 'hostage'), as a metaphor built after the name of the poet.

Bibliography

Bechtel, Friedrich, *Die historischen Personennamen* (Halle, 1917).

Bechtel, Friedrich, *Die griechischen Dialekte*. 3 vols (Berlin, 1963; 1st edn 1921–4).

Breitwieser, Rupert (ed.), *Behinderungen und Beeinträchtigungen/Disability and Impairment in Antiquity* (Oxford, 2012).

Chantraine, Pierre, *La formation des noms en grec ancien* (Paris, 1979; 1st edn 1933).

Dubois, Laurent, 'Monsieur "Leboitard" en Sicile', in I. Boehm and N. Rousseau (eds), *L'expressivité du lexique médical en Grèce et à Rome: Hommages à Françoise Skoda* (Paris, 2014), 77–85.

Edwards, Martha Lynn [= Rose, Martha Lynn], 'The Cultural Context of Deformity in Ancient Greek World', *Ancient History Bulletin* 10 (1996), 79–92.

Edwards, Martha Lynn [= Rose, Martha Lynn], 'Construction of Physical Disability in the Ancient Greek World', in D. T. Mitchell and A. Snyder (eds), *The Body and Physical Difference: Discourses of Disability* (Ann Arbor, MI, 1997), 35–50.

Fraser, Peter Marshall, and Matthews, Elaine (eds), *A Lexicon of Greek Personal Names* (Oxford, 1987–2010).

Garland, Robert, *The Eye of the Beholder: Deformity and Disability in the Graeco-Roman World* (Ithaca, NY, 1995).

Garland, Robert, 'Deformity' and 'Disability' in R. S. Bagnall, K. Brodersen, C. B. Champion, A. Erskine and S. R. Huebner (eds), *The Encyclopedia of Ancient History* (Chichester, 2013), 1961–2 and 2156–7.

Grmek, Mirko D., *Les maladies à l'aube de la civilisation occidentale* (Paris, 1994; 1st edn 1983).

Grmek, Mirko D., and Gourevitch, Danielle, *Les maladies dans l'art antique* (Paris, 1998).

Horstmanshoff, Manfred, 'Disability and Rehabilitation in the Graeco-Roman World', in R. Breitwieser *Behinderungen und Beeinträchtigungen/Disability and Impairment in Antiquity* (Oxford: 2012) 1–10.

Laes, Christian, 'Learning from Silence: Disabled Children in Roman Antiquity', *Arctos* (2008), 85–122.

Laes, Christian, 'Silent Witnesses: Deaf-Mutes in Graeco-Roman Antiquity', *Classical World* 104 (2011), 451–73.

Laes, Christian, 'Silent History? Speech Impairment in Roman Antiquity', in Chr. Laes, C. F. Goodey, M. L. Rose (eds), *Disabilities in Roman Antiquity. Disparate Bodies A Capite ad Calcem* (Leiden, 2013) 145–180

Landau, Oskar, *Mykenisch-griechische Personennamen* (Göteborg, 1958).

Libero, Loretana de, 'Disability', in H. Cancick and H. Schneider (eds), *Brill's New Pauly: Antiquity* (Brill Online, 2015).

Liddell, Henry George, and Scott, Robert, *A Greek-English Lexicon*, rev. Henry Stuart Jones and Roderick McKenzie (Oxford, 1940).

Masson, Olivier, 'Le nom de Battos, fondateur de Cyrène et un groupe de mots grecs apparentés', *Glotta* 54 (1976), 84–98.

Masson, Olivier, 'Myskellos, fondateur de Crotone, et le nom Muskel(l)os', *Revue de Philologie* 63 (1989), 61–5.

Michler, Markwart, 'Die Krüppelleiden in "De morbo sacro" und "De articulis"', *Sudhoffs Archiv* 45 (1961), 303–28.

Ogden, Daniel, *The Crooked Kings of Ancient Greece* (London, 1997).

Rose, Martha L., *The Staff of Œdipus: Transforming Disability in Ancient Greece* (Ann Arbor, MI, 2003).

Samama, Evelyne, '"Bons pour le service": Les invalides au combat dans le monde grec', in F. Collard and E. Samama (eds), *Handicaps et sociétés dans l'Histoire : L'estropié, l'aveugle et le paralytique de l'Antiquité aux temps modernes* (Paris, 2010), 29–48.

Samama, Evelyne, *La médecine de guerre en Grèce ancienne* (Turnhout, 2016).

Skoda, Françoise, 'Les métaphores zoomorphiques dans le vocabulaire médical en grec ancien', in *Ediston Logodeipnon, Logopedies. Mélanges de Philologie et de linguistique grecques offerts à Jean Taillardat* (Louvain, 1988), 221–34.

Skoda, Françoise, 'Les adjectifs grecs en –ΣΟΣ traduisant des particularités ou des défauts physiques: un micro-système lexical', *Revue des Etudes grecques* 104 (1991), 367–93.

Thumiger, Chiara, 'The Early Greek Medical Vocabulary of Insanity', in W. V. Harris (ed.), *Mental Disorders in the Classical World* (Leiden and Boston, MA, 2013), 61–95.

Turner, Wendy J., *Care and Custody of the Mentally Ill, Incompetent and Disabled in Medieval England* (Turnhout, 2013).

Ziskowski, Angela, 'Clubfeet and Kypselids: Contextualising Corinthian Padded Dancers in the Archaic Period', *Annual of the British School at Athens* 107 (2012), 211–32.

10

ABILITY AND DISABILITY IN CLASSICAL ATHENIAN ORATORY

Martha Lynn Rose

Introduction

An Athenian court case from the late 5th century BCE illustrates several points about the concept of people with physical disabilities in ancient Greek society. Lysias 24, *On the Refusal of a Pension to the Invalid*, as it is conventionally titled, highlights the differences between 'disability' in ancient society and modern, developed society. In order to summarize my findings on physical disability in Greece, I argued in *The Staff of Oedipus: Transforming Disability in Ancient Greece* that one must be aware of the dangers of misinterpreting the critical Greek term, 'unable' (*adunatos*) (Rose 2003). Here, I revisit my thoughts on the vocabulary of ability and disability in Lysias' defence speech, this time with a deeper consideration of Lysias' other speeches and those of his contemporaries, specifically orators of 5th- and 4th-century Athens. In order to provide a summary of Lysias 24 and of the conclusions I reached in *Staff of Oedipus*, I have recapitulated the book's concluding chapter here. I am very glad to have the opportunity to expand the investigation beyond physical disability in an attempt to gather clues about intellectual disability, elusive though it might be (cf. Kellenberger in this volume).[1]

Because disability was and is part of humanity, any ancient source has the potential to tell us something about its realities. Because the meanings and contexts of disability shift over time and from one culture to the next, one never knows where that reference might appear. Comedy and tragedy, for example, are very rich sources for the cultural perspective of disability and deformity (Garland 1995 and cf. Garland in this volume).

The speeches and court cases as a whole provide a composite view of the process of democracy as it developed over the 5th and 4th centuries. The surviving individual documents reveal everyday life behind this machinery of peer decision-making. We see petty and grand accusations, wounded pride, hurt feelings, explanations and justifications, and other very human products of living in a face-to-face community (Clark 1993; Rose 1997). One case, for instance, concerns a man accused of removing the stump of an olive tree from his land (olive trees were sacred, therefore collectively owned), to which he argues forcefully and eloquently that he could not have removed a stump that had never existed (Lysias 7, *Before the Areopagus: Defence in the Matter of the Olive-Stump*). Another case enumerates the woes of a man whose wealth and honour had been swindled (Lysias 8, *Accusations of Calumny Against Fellow-Members of a Society*).

Whether olive-stumps or honour, we never learn the whole story. The cases are one-sided, literally: either the accused's or the defendant's arguments are lost. We rarely know the outcome of any case, nor can we be sure that some cases were actually presented. The authorship and exact date, and the identity of the principal speaker in any given case, are sometimes unknown. The identities of the witnesses called are usually unknown, as well as the content of their testimony, and when laws are read out but not transcribed, unless the speaker recaps them, one can only guess. Some pieces in the collection of orations might be school exercises rather than actually scripted for a court of law. Nevertheless, and altogether, the writings of the orators offer an unparalleled view into Athenian boundaries of acceptable behaviour and lifestyle.

Lysias 24

Lysias 24, *On the Refusal of a Pension to the Invalid*, is likely a genuine speech both in authorship and in that it was meant for presentation before the Athenian Boule, the council that ran the affairs of state on behalf of the entire citizen body. The speech probably dates to the closing years of the 5th century.[2] Lysias composed this speech, in which the words of the defendant are in the first person, for the defendant to deliver before the Boule; whether or not it actually was presented, we do not know. The defendant, whose name we never learn, had been classed among 'the unable' (*tôn adunatôn*), and because of this, he had been receiving a state pension.

The defendant

The defendant, anonymous to us, is now accused of being 'able-bodied' (*sômati dunasthai*), thus ineligible for the pension. Specifically, the evidence that the defendant is able-bodied includes the charges that he mounts and rides horses, carries out a trade and associates with wealthy friends (4–5). Christopher Carey summarizes the speech and analyses the structure, concluding that because the defendant does not have a strong case, Lysias has him rely on 'verbal guerrilla tactics' instead (Carey 1990: 48–9).

The defendant has a physical handicap. This impairment affects his mobility. Well into the speech, he mentions casually the two sticks on which he relies to walk (12). He is, furthermore, unable to walk long distances at all. Indeed, although the defendant has a significant mobility impairment, which might have consisted of anything from weak and gnarled legs to no legs at all – we are never told – he cannot simply display himself to the council to prove that he is indeed 'unable' to earn a living. Many people had physical handicaps, but having a handicap did not put one in any special category (Rose 2003).

The case

If this defence was actually presented before the members of the Boule, they would know immediately that the defendant was physically impaired: he would have been standing before them on his two crutches. Furthermore, they'd likely have seen him around town: he's an old-timer, and he'd been receiving the pension for years. Yet being visibly and permanently physically handicapped – or disabled, as we would say today – does not automatically make him unable (or disabled) *(adunatos)*, and this is the crux of the case. When he refers to his bodily condition, he never uses the term 'unable' (*adunatos*). He refers vaguely to 'the afflictions of the body' and to the misfortune that makes it difficult for him to make long journeys, and he suggests sarcastically that it is he whose body is sound, and that his accuser ought to be voted the maimed one (13).

People with physical handicaps were not necessarily barred from playing any socio-economic role (Rose 2003). People could be significantly physically impaired yet capable of supporting themselves; this is, after all, the claim the accuser is making against the defendant, and the charge is serious enough to merit preparation for a hearing before the Boule. Lysias has the defendant argue that he should be categorized as 'unable' (*adunatos*), but not on grounds that he can barely walk. The defendant justly receives a pension, he argues, because he is categorized as unable for three reasons: a father who left him nothing, an aged mother whom he has had to support and the lack of children to support him when he reaches old age (5–6). Compounded with this, he adds, he is now growing older and weaker (7).

The defendant, in a calculated fit of frustrated sarcasm, says that if his pension is voted away, then he would be categorized as 'able', and therefore eligible to serve as archon, or chief magistrate. This indicates that people who received this pension were ineligible to serve as the archon (13). It is too easy, though, to leap to concluding that Athenian law prevented disabled people from holding key administrative positions, and, in fact, this is not the case. It is important to note that the speech does *not* suggest that men with physical impairments were ineligible to serve as archon. It only suggests that men – with or without physical impairments – who were unable to support themselves *and* were classified among the unable (*adunatoi*) were ineligible to serve as archon.

Blemished men may also have been restricted from holding religious office, but we do not know what constituted a blemish (a scarred face? the lack of testicles, Persian-style?), and the extent to which the restriction was practised is far from clear. After all, lack of wealth would be a far greater deterrent to holding a high office than the display of a limp. Veronique Dasen, in her work on dwarfs in ancient Egypt and Greece, suggests that there was an 'unwritten religious taboo' against people with physical disabilities holding office, and finds confirmation in the absence of reference to handicapped officials of sacred functions except for Medon, the legendary ruler of Athens, who, Pausanias (7.2.1) tells us, was given Athenian rule by the Delphic oracle after his brother tried to deny him the rule because Medon was lame in the foot (Dasen 1993: 212). No hard conclusions can be drawn from a single anecdote; Dasen may well be correct. Perhaps, though, there was no reason to point out that an office-holder had a physical handicap unless, as in this legendary case, it was relevant to his ascension (for Roman magistrates with disabilities see Baroin 2010).

Just as we must be careful to avoid drawing conclusions about political and religious restrictions of people with disabilities, we also have to avoid projecting back onto the ancient world the modern tendency to pity and vilify disabled people. This is not to say that people in the ancient world lacked pity (see Laes 2014: 291), only that pity was not linked automatically to a disabling appearance. Whatever our anonymous defendant's physical configuration or means of mobility, his physical impairment did not in itself evoke pity or admiration. Throughout the speech, the defendant never solicits pity for his impairment, even though an appeal to one's misfortunes was an acceptable courtroom tactic (Garland 1995: 37). There was no assumed pity or awe involved in the Greek concept of physical impairment because there were no categorical assumptions about what people with disabilities could or could not do, should or should not do, nor were disabilities associated with generalized character traits.

A physical impairment in itself did not constitute or even suggest impoverishment (Stiker 1979: 59). It is quite possible that, among beggars, some were impaired, but there is no indication that begging was the specialty of disabled people. It is also worthwhile to note that there are important differences between the modern and ancient notions of begging. There is a distinction in modern thought between 'legitimate' handicapped beggars and impostors who mimic a missing leg or a limp (Ré 1938: 21–2 discusses the 'impersonator'). Rosa Maria Perez Estevez (1976: 57–8) contrasts 'legitimate' beggars, on the one hand, and beggars disguised to look needy, on the other. This distinction rests on the assumption that a physical handicap in itself signifies helplessness and merits alms, a notion that was foreign to the Greeks (Hands 1968: 77–8). We see disguises of disability in Greek literature, but the disguises never induce pity and alms, nor are they meant to. Odysseus' disguise (Homer, *Odyssey* 17.202–4) gets him anything but pity; the despicable Aristogeiton's sham, in Plutarch's *Phocion* (10.1–2), only gets him out of military service. Indeed, far from impairment being linked with dispossession and begging, it was the other way around: if one is so helpless as to beg, one is disabled.

Lysias' speech demonstrates, furthermore, that one could be 'unable in body' yet not *adunatos* and therefore in need of a pension. Xenophon provides another example of physically disadvantaged people who did not need financial help when he suggests that the money for cavalry should come from, among other parties, wealthy men who are 'unable in body' (*Cavalry Commander* 9.5–6). In Lysias 24, the charge implies that the defendant is living a lifestyle so rich that he can afford horses rather than using the transportation for common people who were unable to walk: that ancient equivalent of the wheelchair, the donkey (Rose 2003: 24). The nature and significance of the defendant's physical impairment is not the issue in Lysias 24; the issue is his ability to make a living. Nor is the defendant feigning physical disability to gain state aid, as in the well-known scenario of insurance fraud in the United States today. The question in Lysias 24 is to what extent the defendant is able to function within the community. The accuser charged, apparently, that he functions very well indeed. In spite of his obvious physical handicap, the defendant may have been voted non-disabled. We do not know the results, if any, of the trial.

The pension

The pension in question is summarized in the Aristotelian Athenian Constitution. Each year, the Boule assesses the men who are classed as 'unable' (*adunatous*). People in this class, who have very little wealth or who are impaired so as to be unable to earn a living, receive a very small grant from the state. Plutarch (*Solon* 31) probably refers to the origins of this dole when he reports the Athenian law – that anyone maimed in war should be maintained by the state – as one that the 6th-century tyrant Peisistratus devised. Plutarch also tells us that the 4th-century BCE writer Heracleides of Pontus offers a conflicting report in which Peisistratus' law was not original, but based on Solon's support of one such man, Thersippus, who was maimed in war (Wehrli 1953: 110 discusses this statement of Heracleides of Pontus (frag. 149) as an example of trying to attribute all good things to Solon the Sage, the Solon of Herodotus). That Plutarch's account in *Solon* 31 of the origins of the dole, the dole described in Lysias 24 and the law described by the author of *The Athenian Constitution* (49.4) all describe the same law is basically agreed on (Hands 1968: 137–8; Garland 1995: 36; Rhodes 1981: 570). This pension has been taken to indicate the humanitarian nature of the Athenian community, but, while not ruling out compassion, Matthew Dillon makes the more astute suggestion that it was also a means to avoid aristocratic patronage, which leads to the tendency of the enfranchised poor to be in debt to aristocratic factions (Dillon 1995: 57 and Dillon in this volume).

The pension in question in Lysias 24 is not a 'pension for the handicapped', a prototype for or antecedent of any modern system of disability compensation. If it were, the case would have been about proving that the defendant is genuinely handicapped. That is not an issue. He is. The accuser charges that the defendant rides horses. This charge does not imply that the defendant is faking or exaggerating his handicap while he is actually well enough to mount and ride a horse (11). Carey (1990: 50) points out, correctly, that 'for riding in ancient Greece strong thighs were essential, yet our speaker is supposedly disabled in his legs'. Because the defendant could mount and ride a horse, though, does not preclude any number of physical handicaps involving the legs. For all we know, he had clubfeet, was missing one or both feet or lower legs, or was affected by multiple sclerosis, the symptoms of which are sporadic, varying with factors such as heat. He never mentions battle as a cause of whatever impairment caused him to rely on two crutches to get around, and it seems likely that he would have, if he had performed military service, since his 'verbal guerrilla tactics' included indignantly stating that he was a good citizen – and a better one than his accuser (3).

The vocabulary of ability and disability

In this chapter, I focus on a specific group of terms for ability and lack thereof – *dunamos* and *adunatos* – and especially on the way in which the terms are used by the orators. Many other terms refer to various types of physical disability (Garland 1995; Rose 2003; see also Samama in this volume).

Disability and ability

Lysias 2, *Funeral Oration for the Men who Supported the Corinthians*, gives us an example of the range of nuances of 'able' (*dunamenos*), showing that the possible meanings are flexible and relative to the situation. Writing early in the 4th century BCE, Lysias (if the author really is Lysias) recalls an event, a bit wistfully, from the middle of the 5th century, when alliances were such that Athens and Corinth were enemies. The regular Athenian troops were occupied in a two-front blockade of Aegina and Egypt. Taking advantage of the situation, the Corinthian enemy approached, and seized a position near Megara, which borders Athens. The men who had remained at Athens – those who were older and those who were too young to serve in the Athenian army – met the enemy outside Athens and defeated them; the defeat was even more glorious for the Athenians and shameful for the enemy because these were not men who would ordinarily fight.

> [T]he elderly and those below the age of service thought fit to take the risk upon themselves alone: the former had acquired their valor by experience, the latter by nature; those had proved their own worth on many a field, while these would know how to imitate them, and as the seniors knew how to command, so the juniors were able to carry out their orders. With Myronides as general they made a sally of their own into the land of Megara and conquered in battle the whole force of the enemy with troops whose strength was already failing or not yet capable (*tois êdê apeirêkosi kai tois oupô dunamenois*), of an enemy who had chosen to invade their country, but whom they had hastened to meet on alien soil. There they set up a trophy of an exploit most glorious for them, but most disgraceful for the foe. One part of them had ceased, and the other part had not begun, to be able-bodied (*hoi men ouketi tois sômasin, hoi d' oupô dunamenois*), but together they took strength from their spirit.
>
> *(Lysias 2.50–3)*

The older group was disabled by age in the same way as the younger group was disabled by youth, but neither group of men was composed of disabled men in the modern sense – or rather, if there were any men with physical impairments, the impairments were not worth mentioning.

Ability and inability

Isocrates, at 82 years of age, provides another example of the flexible meaning of ability according to context. Isocrates defends his character and career in a discourse titled *Antidosis*, the name of a charge that had been filed against him decades earlier. In this apologia, Isocrates names many of his students and associates, including the general Timotheus who 'lacks a robust physique' (*oute tên tou sômatos phusin*) (Isocrates, *Discourses* 15, *Antidosis* 115). Unlike generals who were elected superficially, on account of their bodies (*sômasi*) and their foreign military experience, Isocrates goes on to say, Timotheus met the criteria of being a good general by (among other qualities) being able to win battles and pay his soldiers even though he was handicapped (*periistamai dunamenon* – his ability was compromised by Athens' negligence in equipping him, 120).

In the same vein, possessing ability and disability (*dunasthai; adunatos*) can indicate a range of capacities: in Lysias 17, *On the Property of Eraton: Against the Treasury*, the petitioner opens his speech by dispelling the assumption that some among his audience might have formed, i.e. that he is an excellent speaker: he says that he is not even competent (*dunasthai*) to speak; he fears, even, that he will unable (*adunatos*) to speak sufficiently (1). The speaker does not have any sort of speech disability; this is a formulaic introduction to his argument. Isocrates in *Discourses* 21, *Against Euthynus* (1) opens more bluntly: Isocrates is presenting the plaintiff's plea because the plaintiff is his friend, is in need, has been dealt an injustice and lacks the ability to speak (*adunatos epein*). Nicias (the plaintiff) is not mute; he is untrained in speaking skilfully. There are no witnesses to support the claim that the plaintiff is indeed owed money from the treasury, so Isocrates argues that Nicias' accusation against Euthynus *must* be valid because he has gone to the trouble to bring suit when he does not have much to gain. Isocrates follows by using Nicias' lack of skill in speaking as a point in his legal favour, implying that ordinarily, wealthy men who cannot speak, such as Nicias, are taken advantage of by less wealthy, glib opportunists, such as Euthynus. In case his audience missed it the first time, Isocrates repeats that Nicias is bringing a charge against a glib, less wealthy man and, by this logic, it should be obvious that the charge is valid, for he would not waste his time otherwise (5). This line of argument, convoluted as it might seem, almost reaches the point of tedium when it is repeated, once again, not much later (9). For these purposes, the tedious point simply provides another example of the range of meanings behind an inability to speak.

Intellectual ability and disability

The works of the orators offer us an unequalled view into the fabric of community decision-making in the shifting meaning of 5th- and 4th-century Athenian democracy – and, during some years of the late 5th and early 4th centuries, after the Athenian empire collapsed so ignobly, of a very shaky and nervous democracy. The *Exordia,* a collection of over fifty introductions to legal speeches and attributed to Demosthenes, appears generic and formulaic, and perhaps it is: none of the prologues is very exciting on its own. Together, though, the collection serves as a sort of foundation for references to intellectual disability in the speeches.

How to be a good democrat

These preambles warn their audience against people who participate poorly in the democracy – and the audience, of course, were the participants. Significantly, it is not those men who speak foolishly who are poor participants, but the men who are not able to listen and deliberate. The responsible Athenian needs to listen to fools speaking frivolously, and he needs to listen all the way through, even if the speech is long, leaving it to the speaker to show his inability to make a point rather than pre-empting him (*Exordia* 5.2). The exhortation to listen to everything, avoiding any impulse to dismiss a speaker if he says something stupid, is the bedrock of democracy. 'For,' Demosthenes tells us, 'it often happens that the same person is wrong on one point and right on another' (*Exordia* 4).

On the other side of the coin, Athenians must beware of being misled by the cunning words of intelligent people who are so thoroughly in the wrong that they have nothing but the fantastic products of their intelligence to offer. Here (*Exordia* 24), Demosthenes goes so far as to warn the jury, no doubt at least gaining their attention, and possibly winning their confidence, that their simplicity (*euêthaseis* or guilelessness) has already been taken advantage of by such scoundrels (*Exordia* 24.2). This scenario of putting the jury on notice is repeated in *Exordia* 32.3, in which Demosthenes accuses the jurors, using the terminology of magic, of having succumbed to the spell of clever but false words. Here, Demosthenes says that it would be foolish of *him* to yield to fear and do anything other than speak his mind.

Mind/body

Physical and mental disability are not separated one from the other, although until recently they have been treated by historians, myself included, as separate phenomena. The mind/body split is so ingrained into the developed western world that most of us automatically think of seeing a physician (or another such professional trained in physical medicine) for somatic ills and a psychiatrist (or some professional trained in taming the mind) for psychological ills. But this is a modern (post-Locke) concept, and cannot be applied usefully to pre-modern societies (Goodey 2011; Goodey and Rose 2013, forthcoming).

Just as a variety of factors such as age and socio-economic station affects the meaning of one's overall ability in terms of community role, so too do factors such as mental state affect physical appearance and action. In the premodern world, before the functions of the mind and those of the body became compartmentalized to the point of segregation, one's state of mind, behaviour, and somatic characteristics were all of a system (Clark and Rose 2013; Goodey and Rose 2013, forthcoming). This system is of course reflected in the vocabulary, and we see it in the records of the orators. People display madness (*manian*) physically (Lysias 3, *Against Simon* 3.8) and act monstrously (Dinarchus, *Against Aristogiton* 10: in this case, Aristogiton is called a beast – *to thêrion*).

Reason (*gnômên*), when destroyed, has a physical manifestation of tasting good food as bad (Lysias 6, *Against Andocides: For Impiety* 1–2). In the same speech, Lysias uses an interesting turn of phrase when he wonders, rhetorically, if some god destroyed Andocides' reason (*gnômên diephtheiren*) (23). Isocrates, in his last oration, a tribute to Athens, juxtaposes his frail health and his writing. He is 94, he says, and his hair is grey (3). He goes on to reveal his fear that this discourse might be perceived as more feeble (*malaktêpôteros* – softer, weaker, of less substance) than his earlier ones, in which he used rhetorical flourish. And, truth be told, it is, a bit (*Discourses* 12 *Panathenaicus* 4).

For better or worse, the orators' writings do not provide an example of 'mental disability' comparable to the 'physically disabled' man of Lysias 24. Such an example might help us to understand how intellectual disability was perceived in classical Athens. Perhaps, though, it is just as well that there is no case of a man 'disabled in mind' to invite anachronistic interpretations.

Idiocy and other rhetorical expressions

Patricia Clark made an exhaustive study of the Greco-Roman vocabulary for mental disorders in *The Balance of the Mind: The Experience and Perception of Mental Illness in the Ancient*

World, and concluded that some disorders were thought to be recognizable and clearly marked. Other distinctions made today, though, such as between extreme emotional upset and depression, physical illness and fever, senility and psychoses, seem not to have been made among the general populace in Antiquity. The same vocabulary of madness served for all, and when different causes were recognized, the resultant states themselves were simply described by multifarious but unspecific terms (Clark 1993: 404).

The ancient/modern contrast is not absolute, Clark goes on to explain: the modern, educated public uses psychological terms with some sophistication and dexterity (if questionable accuracy), describing an individual for example as bulimic, or compulsive, or depressed, or senile – or simply neurotic or psychotic – but a large proportion of the populace does not attempt to differentiate between diagnoses, content to refer to people as 'crazy', or, perhaps, 'having a nervous breakdown'. Some people simply indicate, by a variety of suggestive but non-specific terms, that there is something wrong inside another person's head; more commonly, the indication is non-verbal. The ancient vocabulary of mental illness was rich in such non-specific terms, and we can reasonably speculate that the language of gesture also indicated mental impairment (Clark 1993: 404; Clark and Rose forthcoming).

The same framework – a large, non-specific and not necessarily codified vocabulary for psychiatric disability – can be assumed for intellectual disability. In many cases, we see cultural impressions and indications of awareness and experience rather than named cases of what we today call intellectual disability (cf. Gourevitch in this volume). In the oratory, the references to anomalous thought processes and weak cognitive abilities are oblique at best.

Lysias 10, *Against Theomnestus* 1 crafts an accusation based on the common understanding of terms (Theomnestus has claimed that he did not slander the speaker with patricide because he only said that he killed his father; he did not say that he murdered him) by saying that only fools would misunderstand the obvious meaning of similar words. Thus Theomnestus must be very stupid (*skaion* – literally, left-handed; see Humer 2006) to have thought that 'kill' and 'murder' do not mean the same thing (15), and the speaker makes a display of 'educating' him, in front of the jury, about obvious synonyms such as 'vow' meaning 'swear' and flee meaning running away (15–21). The speaker goes on, pointing out that if one is not a numbskull (*sidêrous* – iron-head), one will recognize common synonyms (20; see Goodey 2005). Only an idiot (*êlithon* – an idle fool) would insist on the literal meaning of 'wood' when everyone knows that 'wood' is a way of saying 'stocks' (16). In the *First Tetralogy* of Antiphon, the same supposition is used by the defendant: he claims with a flourish that his accusers must think him a simpleton (Antiphon, *Tetralogy* 1.1).

We see this formula again when the defendant in 'Olive-Stump' asks if he would have been so foolish (*môriôn*) as to clear out a lone, sacred olive-stump in clear view of the road (Lysias 7, *Before the Areopagus: Defence in the Matter of the Olive-Stump* 29.2). The flourish also appears in the *Panathenaicus* when Isocrates rhetorically ponders what he should do, discarding each possibility because he would be thought a simpleton (*môros*) (Isocrates, *Discourses* 12 *Panathenaicus* 22–3; we see *môros* again used in the same way, 270). Interestingly, he discards another possible action – convincing 'those of the lay public' (*idiôtôn*) – because, again, he would be charged with great folly. The choice of words here shows us that, although our 'idiot' has a Greek etymology, the Greek idiot was, in the context of democratic decision-making, the man who kept his thoughts private rather than participating among the public.

Definitions of incapacity, ancient and modern

We see reference to the conditions that render a man incapable of legal decision-making in *Apollodorus Against Stephanus* 2, an oration attributed to but probably not authored by

Demosthenes. The plaintiff Apollodorus has the clerk read out an inheritance law. This law allows any man without sons to will his property in any way he likes, 'unless his mind be impaired' (*paranoôn*) by lunacy (*maniôn*) or old age (*gêrôs*) or medication (*pharmakôn*) or illness (*nosou*), or by being under the influence of a woman, or under legal constraint (Demosthenes, *Orations 46 Apollodorus Against Stephanus, Charged with False Testimony* 2.14). Apollodorus repeats the conditions a few sentences later, emphasizing that a man must be of sound mind to make a valid will, 'but if he be impaired by disease or the effect of drugs, or be under the influence of a woman, or be the victim of old age or of madness, or be under constraint, the laws ordain that he be incompetent (*akuron* – having no power in terms of the law)' (15).

None of these references depicts an individual with an intellectual disability in the modern sense of the word, and even as a whole, the collection of terms reveals little about the realities of living with an intellectual or learning disability in Greece. Unless stunning evidence is unearthed, we will never be able to differentiate among fine distinctions in the style of modern diagnosis (see Figure 10.1), and to do so in the absence of testimony risks imposing anachronistic retrospective diagnosis (Goodey and Rose forthcoming).

Figure 10.1 breaks down disability into several types of disorders: the largest category is Physical and Other Disorders (40.6%); then clockwise, Intellectual Disorders (20%), Mood Disorders (17%), Schizophrenic and Psychotic Disorders (9%), Other Mental Disorders (4.2%), Organic Mental Disorders (4.2%) and Other Disorders (3%). The point of interest for our purposes is the display of measured and differentiated disabilities (even though the broad categories are somewhat crude) and the separation between physical and mental disorders.

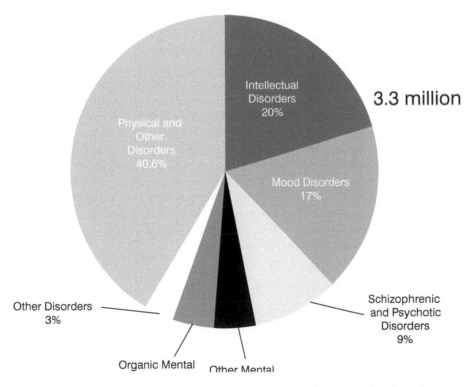

Figure 10.1 Chart of physical, intellectual, mental and other disorders. From the March 2012 Report to the Congress on Medicaid and CHIP, available from the Medicare and CHIP Payment and Access Communication website www.macpac.gov

Athenian citizenry

A few tentative conclusions can be drawn from the vocabulary of mental ability and disability in the orators' writings. It is safe to conclude that there was not much of a line between displaying characteristics of foolishness and being a chronic fool. The law restricting mentally impaired people from making legal decisions intimates that there was hardly a nosology of intellectual impairment: one's judgement could be clouded, temporarily or permanently, by various factors. Another safe conclusion is that the descriptions of fools and numbskulls and so on that the orators mention did not refer to standard categories of mental disability, but to loose sketches of men who did not express valuable opinions. Even the more definite restriction against men with clouded judgement making valid wills is not very specific. A pie chart equivalent to the one shown in Figure 10.1 showing the various types of impairments would have been inconceivable, not to mention useless. Incompetence due to drugs, incompetence due to old age, to mania, or to female influence were not standard, etiologically based diagnoses, but rather conditions significant enough to have been observed and codified, even if judgement about mental fitness or lack thereof was made on a case-by-case basis. The charge of incompetence itself – physical or mental or both – could have been made on an ad hoc basis as well. A person accused of an impaired mind would not be able to submit data to fight the charge, just as the accused in Lysias 26 cannot prove disability by displaying his disabled body,

Read optimistically, one might conclude from the speeches that, at least in the ideal, anyone's voice could and should be heard in Athenian democracy. One would not be banned from participating in the government a priori on the basis of an intellectual disability. We have to remember, though, that 'anyone' excluded females, children, slaves, foreigners and other people who were not Athenian citizens. But all Athenian citizens possessed the fully developed deliberative function that allowed them to participate – by speaking and by listening – in the democracy (Goodey 1999). In his tireless campaign against Philip of Macedon, Demosthenes (or more likely an imitator of Demosthenes), making a point about their lack of horror over Philip II's actions, scolds the Athenians, 'who are supposed to be superior to all men in understanding and culture (*sunesei kai paideia pantôn proexien dokounta*) and have also maintained here for the unfortunate (*atuxêsasin*) common refuge in all ages' (Demosthenes, *Letters* 3, *Concerning the Sons of Lycurgus: Demosthenes to the Council and the Assembly Sends Greeting* 11). Continuing his dismay over the lack of alarm among the Athenian citizenry, (pseudo-)Demosthenes (13) reminds his audience that Athenians and their allies form 'a culture which is thought capable of making stupid people tolerable' (*anaisthêtous* [literally, anaesthetized] *anektous poiein dokei dunasthai*). This may be a mere rhetorical flourish, or it may indicate an ideal similar to that expressed in Lysias' Funeral Oration, discussed above, where men who were not fully able to do so on their own were still able to band together to use their common strengths and abilities to defend Athens.

In summary: three methodological caveats

The dangers of reading the term *adunatos* as 'disabled' with all of the word's modern social and political connotations provide an opportunity to summarize three interrelated points about disability in the ancient world. It is human nature to find what we seek and to see what we expect to exist ... or to have existed (cf. Kellenberger in this volume for the tendency of modern scholars, especially regarding intellectual disability, to excavate nonexistent evidence). The skill of the historian to ask the right questions is perhaps nowhere more important than in disability studies.

Caveat one: the medical model

First, it is not possible to determine any one set of attitudes towards people with disabilities because the notion of physical or mental disability as classifications – and especially as discrete classifications – was foreign to the Greeks. There was no dichotomy of ability and disability; rather, there was a range of physical and mental conditions to which every human being was always susceptible. In contemporary disability studies, the medical model, although not as vilified as it was a decade ago, refers to the process by which people are deemed inherently able-bodied or disabled according to medical definition and categorization. By extension, the medical model also refers to the perception of disabilities as permanent illnesses, and of disabled people as in perpetual need of medical attention. Disability today in the developed world is an institutionalized phenomenon: in present-day thought, physical and mental disability has medical parameters. One is pronounced officially 'physically disabled', and to what degree, by a medical doctor. The Workers Compensation formula for calculating disability, with a range of points assigned to each body part's economic worth, is a reminder to United States citizens of the very real consequences behind this conceptualization (Figure 10.2).

An official medical entity also pronounces one psychiatrically, mentally, or intellectually disabled. This classificatory impulse was not part of the reality of ancient Greek disability.

Caveat two: the assumption of incompetence

Second, a set of expectations accompanies people with physical and mental disabilities in the modern world. A man who loses his arm in an industrial accident, say an assembly line, is not usually expected to heal up and get back to the same job, an assumption that seems both humane and practical, but the flip side is the assumption, based on the presence of a disability, of incompetence for certain tasks. Some assumptions are reasonable (no totally blind person can drive a bus competently); some are not (the latter situation is called discrimination).

In ancient Greece, we see very few instances in which people with disabilities were banned *a priori* from certain roles by collective expectation. Completely blind men could not serve in the front lines of the army; prelingually deaf people, because of the corollary misunderstanding of stupidity, would not have been eligible for a political career; a man with no legs would not train as a competitive runner.

These were not codified rules: only a modern perspective would see this collection of practical circumstances as a set of restrictions related to disability. From the modern perspective, some expectations about disability are codified to the extent that people with some physical disabilities are banned from certain roles: notoriously, in the Second World War, flat feet were enough to keep men from participating in active duty. It is useful to keep this difference between modern and ancient concepts of competence in mind in order to avoid making false assumptions.

Caveat three: pity and awe

The third implication of disability in the modern developed world that must not be assumed of ancient communities is that disability can evoke pity and the resulting condescension. Portraying children as 'the poster child with doom-dripped eyes' (Wade 1997 and see Rose 2011), the infamous Labor Day Telethon against Muscular Dystrophy, now thankfully retired, provides an example of intermingled pity and objectification (Longmore 1997).

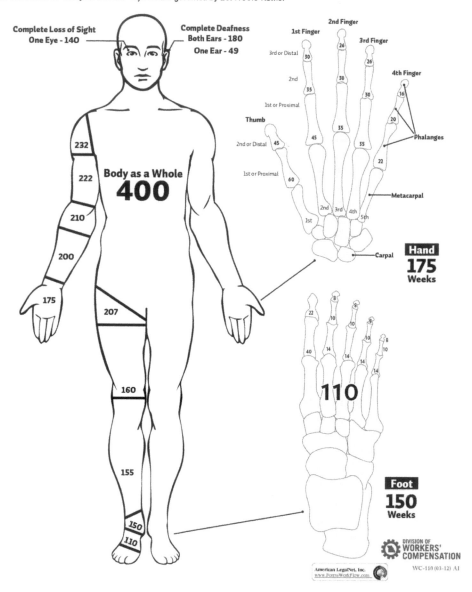

CHART NUMBER ❶ **PERMANENT PARTIAL DISABILITY**

Visual chart showing number of weeks of compensation payable for scheduled and non–scheduled permanent partial disabilities. Scheduled disabilities are governed by 287.190.1 RSMo.
Non–scheduled or "Body as a Whole" injuries are governed by 287.190.3 RSMo.

Figure 10.2 Chart of permanent physical disability showing number of weeks of compensation payable for scheduled and non-scheduled permanent partial disabilities. The human body is sectioned into portions and labelled according to weeks lost, e.g. the ear is worth 49; the body as a whole, 400. To the right is a diagram of the hand, labelling its 20 components, below that is a foot (totaling 150 weeks). Available on the Missouri Department of Labor site www.labor.mo.gov

Both physical and mental disability can also evoke the flip side of pity: awe. Misplaced awe moves some people to admire accomplishments all out of proportion and based solely on the disability. This is the 'Supercrip' phenomenon, seen in the media from time to time as a celebration of a person for having a mundane life – getting dressed, going to work, having a hobby – because the person has this or that disability (Shapiro 1993; Scully 2008).

In the ancient Greek world, people with a wide variety of disabilities participated in a wide variety of social, economic and military roles without fanfare. People with even the most significant disabilities participated in communities that accommodated all ranges of ability, not by some humanitarian design but out of practicality. Men who could not walk at all had military roles. Congenitally deaf people were considered impaired intellectually, but intellectual impairment was not the disaster that some surviving literature suggests (Rose 2003).

Finally, we must remember that attitudes towards and concepts of disability – in all its manifestations and parameters – changed over time (cf. contributions by Dillon, by Mitchell and by Metzler in this volume).

Conclusions

There is no indication in the works of the orators that being disabled in ancient Greece was horrible, categorically, nor that it was wonderful, nor do the Greek records on the whole suggest either extreme (Rose 2003). Blind people, for example, are as unfortunate as beggars, exiles and even the dismembered Orpheus (Isocrates, *Discourses* 11 *Busisris* 39). Being mad, or being foolish, is presented only as an undesirable trait in the orators' works – but then intelligence is also presented as a danger. Disabilities seem to have lacked mystique, and they had not combined and hardened into a phenomenon, let alone a tragic phenomenon. The criteria of ability and disability rested not on one's ability to function as an individual, but on one's functional ability within the community. And therein lies the problem for the investigator: we would see that people who we would label disabled, were we to go back in a time machine armed with diagnostic and testing manuals, were not hidden away at all, but carrying on in plain sight. This is the cloak of invisibility.

Moses Finley, a pioneer scholar of ancient social and economic history, pointed out that, because the elderly were not isolated from society, it is difficult to consider them separately (Finley 1981). This is the crux of the problem in looking at people with disabilities in ancient Greece. It is difficult to find and make sense of information about people with disabilities in Greek society because they were integral to the society and, as such, usually not remarkable.

There is no indication that people with physical or mental impairments in the ancient Greek world identified themselves or were identified as a distinct category. The inclusion – to the point of invisibility – of people with disabilities into the ancient Greek landscape was not an early form of humanitarian thought, legal accommodation or enlightened charity. Rather, disabled people did not have to be reintegrated: they had not been segregated.

Notes

1 Unless indicated otherwise, references to and translations of all Greek works are from the digital edition of the Loeb Classical Library from Harvard University Press, general editor Jeffry Henderson, available from: <loebclassics.com> (accessed Feb. 2015).

2 Carey 1990: 50, n. 3 argues that there is no basis for precise dating of this speech; Dover 1968: 189 concludes that, linguistically, there is no reason to think that Lysias 24, is not genuine. In addition, Carey 1990: 50 assumes that the speech was intended to be read before the Boule.

Bibliography

Baroin, Catherine, 'Integrité du corps, maladie, mutilation et exclusion chez les magistrats et les sénateurs romains', in F. Collard and E. Samama (eds), *Handicaps et sociétés dans l'histoire: L'estropié, l'aveugle et le paralytique de l'Antiquité aux temps modernes* (Paris, 2010), 49–68.

Bosman, Philip (ed.), *Mania: Madness in the Greco-Roman World* (Pretoria, 2009).

Carey, Christopher, 'Structure and Strategy in Lysias XXIV', *Greece and Rome* 37 (1990), 44–51.

Cilliers, Louise, and Retief, François P., 'Mental Illness in the Greco-Roman Era', in Ph. Bosman, *Mania: Madness in the Greco-Roman World* (Pretoria, 2009), 130–40.

Clark, Patricia A., 'The Balance of the Mind: The Experience and Perception of Mental Illness in Antiquity' (unpublished PhD, University of Washington, 1993) <www.historyoflearningdisability.co>.

Clark, Patricia A., and Rose, Martha Lynn, 'Psychiatric Disability and the Galenic Medical Matrix', in C. Laes *et al.* (eds), *Disabilities in Roman Antiquity* (Leiden, 2013), 45–72.

Clark, Patricia A. and Rose, Martha Lynn, 'Celsus and Somatic Misbehaviour' in M. McGlynn and B. Reynolds (eds), *Pre-Modern Madness Sacred and Profane* (forthcoming)

Dasen, Véronique, *Dwarfs in Ancient Egypt and Greece* (Oxford, 1993).

Dillon, Matthew, 'Payments to the Disabled at Athens: Social Justice or Fear of Aristocratic Patronage?', *Ancient Society* 26 (1995), 27–57.

Dover, Kenneth, *Lysias and the Corpus Lysiacum* (Berkeley, CA, 1968).

Edwards, Martha Lynn [= Rose, Martha Lynn], 'Constructions of Physical Disability in the Ancient Greek World: The Community Concept', in D. Mitchell and S. Snyder (eds), *The Body and Physical Difference: Discourses of Disability* (Ann Arbor, MI, 1997), 35–50.

Finley, Moses, 'The Elderly in Classical Antiquity', *Greece and Rome* 28 (1981), 156–71.

Garland, Robert, *The Eye of the Beholder: Deformity and Disability in the Graeco-Roman World* (Ithaca, NY, 1995).

Goodey, Chris F., 'Blockheads, Roundheads, Pointy Heads: Intellectual Disability and the Brain Before Modern Medicine', *Journal of the History of the Behavioral Sciences* 41/2 (2005), 165–83.

Goodey, Chris F., *A History of Intelligence and 'Intellectual Disability': The Shaping of Psychology in Early Modern Europe* (Farnham, 2011).

Goodey, Chris F., 'Politics, Nature, and Necessity: Were Aristotle's Slaves Feeble Minded?', *Political Theory* 27/2 (1999), 203–24.

Goodey, Chris F., and Rose, Martha Lynn, 'Mental States, Bodily Dispositions and Table Manners: A Guide to Reading "Intellectual Disability" from Homer to Late Antiquity', in C. Laes *et al.* (eds), *Disabilities in Roman Antiquity* (Leiden, 2013), 17–44.

Goodey, Chris F., and Rose, Martha Lynn, 'The Construct of Disability', in M. Rembis, K. Nielsen and C. Kudlick (eds), *Oxford Handbook of Disability History* (Oxford, forthcoming).

Hands, Arthur, *Charities and Social Aid in Greece and Rome* (London, 1968).

Harris, William V. (ed.), *Mental Disorders in the Classical World* (Leiden, 2013).

Hermsen, Lisa, *Manic Minds: Mania's Mad History and its Neuro-Future* (New Brunswick, NJ, 2011).

Horstmanshoff, Manfred, 'Klein gebrek geen bezwaar? Over de klompvoet in de oudheid', *Lampas* 46/2 (2013), 203–21.

Humer, Edith, *Linkshändigkeit im Altertum: Zur Wertigkeit von Links, der linken Hand und Linkshändern in der Antike* (Tönning, 2006).

Laes, Christian, *Beperkt? Gehandicapten in het Romeinse Rijk* (Leuven, 2014).

Laes, Christian, Goodey, Chris F., and Rose, Martha Lynn (eds), *Disabilities in Roman Antiquity: Disparate Bodies A Capite ad Calcem* (Leiden, 2013).

Laes, Christian, Goodey, Chris F., and Rose, Martha Lynn, 'Approaching Disabilities *a Capite ad Calcem*: Hidden Themes in Roman Antiquity', in C. Laes *et al.* (eds), *Disabilities in Roman Antiquity* (Leiden, 2013), 1–16.

Longmore, Paul, 'Conspicuous Contribution and the American Dilemma: The Telethon Ritual of Cleansing and Renewal', in D. Mitchell and S. Snyder (eds), *The Body and Physical Difference: Discourses of Disability* (Ann Arbor, MI, 1997), 134–58.

Perez Estevez, Rosa Maria, *El Problema de los Vagos en la España del Siglo XVIII* (Madrid, 1976).

Ré, Juan Alejandro, *El Problema de la Mendicidad en Buenos Aires* (Buenos Aires, 1938).

Rhodes, P. J., *A Commentary on the Aristotelian Athenaion Politeia* (Oxford, 1981).

Rose, Martha Lynn, *The Staff of Oedipus: Transforming Disability in Ancient Greece* (Ann Arbor, MI, 2003).

Rose, Martha Lynn, 'Gender, Generation, Aging, and Disability: The Case of Cheryl Marie Wade', in H. Ehlers, G. Linke, B. Rudolf and H. Trappe (eds), *Geschlecht-Generation-Alter(n)*: *Geistes- und sozialwissenschlaftliche Perspectiven* (Berlin, 2011), 167–89.

Scully, Jackie Leach, *Disability Bioethics*: *Moral Bodies, Moral Difference* (Lanham, MD, 2008).

Shapiro, Joseph P., *No Pity*: *People with Disabilities Forging a New Civil Rights Movement* (New York, 1993).

Stainton, Tim, and McDonagh, Patrick, 'Chasing Shadows: The Historical Construction of Developmental Disability', *Journal of Developmental Disabilities* 8 (2001), pp. ix–xvi.

Stainton, Tim, 'Reason and Value: The Thought of Plato and Aristotle and the Construction of Intellectual Disability', *Mental Retardation* 39/6 (2001), 452–60.

Stiker, Henri-Jacques, *Corps infirmes et sociétés* (Paris, 1979).

Wade, Cheryl Marie, 'Cripple Lullaby', in Lennard Davis (ed.), *The Disability Studies Reader* (New York, 1997), 409.

Wehrli, Fritz, *Der Schule des Aristoteles, VII. Herakleides Pontikos* (Basel, 1953).

Websites

MACPAC (Medicare and CHIP Payment and Access Communication) 2012, *Report to the Congress on Medicaid and CHIP*, Government of the United States. <www.macpac.gov> (accessed Feb. 2015).

Missouri Department of Labor 2011, *Chart No. 1, Permanent Partial Disability*, Government of the United States. <www.labor.mo.gov> (accessed Jan. 2015).

11

DISABILITIES IN TRAGEDY AND COMEDY

Robert Garland

Both Greek tragedy and comedy have provided us with some memorable characters afflicted with disability, notably those who are blind, lame, and temporarily insane. Deafness rarely features. The playwrights we shall be drawing upon are Sophocles, Euripides and Aristophanes. There are no disabled characters in either the surviving plays of Aeschylus or Menander. My principal focus will be the depiction of the disabled in drama and the evidence that drama provides for the treatment of the disabled. Though we have to proceed cautiously when seeking to draw inferences about social attitudes from drama, its evidence is hardly less trustworthy than that which derives from any other genre or indeed artistic medium.

Disability as tragi-comic

Is disability comic or tragic? It can be either, of course, depending on one's degree of sympathy for the afflicted individual. It can be a provocation to pity or a stimulus to derision. After all, life is a tragedy to those who think and a comedy to those who feel. Its tragi-comic aspect is brilliantly captured in the first appearance of a disabled person in western literature. Thersites, a commoner whom we encounter in book 2 of the *Iliad*, is not merely 'the ugliest man who came beneath Ilion', but a veritable monstrosity. He is balding, bandy-legged, crippled, round-shouldered, pigeon-chested and turricephalous (*Il.* 2.216–19). And yet Thersites alone of the Greeks has the effrontery and the courage to challenge Agamemnon in the assembly that Odysseus has called to deal with the crisis that has arisen as a result of Achilles' withdrawal from the fighting. Like Achilles in the opening scene of the poem, Thersites criticizes Agamemnon for his poor leadership, and he does so utterly fearless of the consequences.

Instead of receiving plaudits for his outspokenness, however, he is beaten so severely by Odysseus that he is reduced to tears and returns to his place thoroughly chastened. In response to the cripple's humiliation, his comrades 'laughed sweetly at him, for all that they were sorely vexed' (*Il.* 2.270). The poet does not tell us why they laugh sweetly nor why they were sorely vexed. Perhaps we are to suppose that they routinely derive enjoyment from the spectacle of others' sufferings, particularly when it involves someone like Thersites who cannot defend himself. Or perhaps they are relieved that Odysseus stepped in before Agamemnon vented his anger on the cripple. It is a complex moment in the poem, productive of several interpretations.

Their vexation may have something to do with the irritation that they are feeling at this moment towards Agamemnon, though it is not inconceivable as well that it is prompted in part by the violence of Odysseus' treatment of Thersites. If that is the case then their laughter, however sweet, may not have been totally sincere (see Garland 2010: 80–1; Laes *et al.* 2013: 7 for discussion of Thersites).

It may have occurred to some of Homer's audience that the cripple alone had the courage to declare in public what the rest of the army had only thought or muttered in private.

Pity and contempt

Just as in the *Iliad*, so in Greek tragedy the disabled are treated with a mixture of pity and contempt. In Sophocles' *Oedipus the King*, for instance, the blind seer Teiresias accuses Oedipus of having sought to 'shame him for his blindness'. It is as if the king in some way holds Teiresias responsible for his disability (ll. 372 and 412). The heated exchange that follows is suggestive of the barely concealed animosity that often existed between the blind and the sighted in Antiquity (see discussion of Neocleides below). Later in the play, when the Messenger reports how he found the infant Oedipus with pierced ankles in the wooded glades of Mount Cithaeron, Oedipus squirms at the allusion to what he calls 'that ancient evil' and confesses that his mutilation 'was a terrible mark of shame that I had from the time I was in swaddling bands' – an indication of the stigma that he has borne throughout his life (ll. 1033 and 1035). The suggestion that some at least of the whole-bodied looked with disdain upon the disabled and made them feel ashamed for their affliction is likely to have been drawn from life. It would surely have found an echoing chord among those in the audience who, because of similar experiences, had reason to sympathize with the likes of Oedipus and Teiresias. It is important to bear in mind that a sizeable proportion of the Athenian audience would have been physically challenged, given the very high incidence of disability in Antiquity.

Disdain and contempt were by no means universal responses to the disabled, however. When Oedipus asks the Theban Shepherd why he disobeyed Jocasta's order to kill him when she and her husband Laius learned from the oracle that he would commit incest and parricide, and why he handed the infant over to the Corinthian Messenger instead, the Shepherd disarmingly replies at the end of a barrage of questions and answers, 'Because I pitied it, master' (l. 1178). It is one of the most moving moments in the whole of Greek tragedy and it serves as a warning against the assumption that disabled infants were inevitably left to perish, even if they were commonly exposed, as required by law in Sparta and no doubt in other Greek communities (cf. Pudsey and Dillon and Lepicard in this volume).

Elsewhere in Sophocles, too, there is evidence of compassion for the disabled. We might expect that the Chorus of Sailors in his *Philoctetes*, comprising as it does men who are inured to hardship and the horrors of war, would be utterly indifferent to the plight of the lame archer Philoctetes, who is afflicted with a festering, putrid and incurable wound caused by a snakebite. A social outcast because of his repulsive and stinking sore, he has lived alone on the island of Lemnos for the entirety of the war. Instead, however, the Chorus speaks feelingly of his plight as they imagine his life:

> I pity him since he has no one to care for him and no one to be with, and he's wretched and alone, and he suffers from a terrible sickness and he is at a loss whenever a need arises (...) and he has no share in the amenities of life and he makes his bed beside beasts that are either dappled or furry.

> *(Sophocles, Philoct. 169–85)*

Later, too, the Chorus echoes Philoctetes' appeal to Neoptolemus to take pity on him (ll. 501, 507). The fact that Philoctetes describes himself in terms that anticipate the Chorus's description of him may well be intended to point up its sensitivity to his wretched plight (cf. ll. 225–8).

Conversely, Odysseus, who is on a mission to abduct the skilled archer because of a prophecy that the Greeks will need his help to win the Trojan War, expresses not the least iota of compassion towards him and is quite happy to deceive him in pursuit of his goal. Evidently, too, the Greeks were content to leave him to rot, quite literally, for ten whole years – the duration of the war – until they learned from the captured Trojan seer Calchas that he and his bow were vital to their success.

The isolation of the socially rejected

Pity extends only so far, and isolation and alienation would have been the condition of all those in the Greek world whose ailment was repellent to the whole-bodied. The pathetic lifestyle of the socially rejected is described in vivid detail in the *Philoctetes*. When scouring the island for the archer, Odysseus and his young companion Neoptolemus discover 'rags that are drying, reeking with the stench of a terrible sore' (ll. 38–9) – a pitiful image indeed. Later Philoctetes tells Neoptolemus how, whenever he shot a bird with his bow to acquire food, 'I would crawl along, alone and wretched, dragging my wretched foot' (l. 290–1). The Chorus, too, describes him as 'crawling like a child who does not have its loving nurse' (ll. 702–3). We might infer from this that the actor playing Philoctetes did so by crawling across the stage. However, this may not necessarily have been the case. Later Philoctetes states that he is falling to his knees before Neoptolemus, adopting the abject attitude of a suppliant, when pleading to be granted a place on board ship so that he can finally leave the island (l. 485). Elsewhere he declares, 'My affliction no longer permits me to stand upright' (l. 820).

The Chorus describes Philoctetes' wound as a 'fiery flux that oozes from the ulcers of his infested foot' (ll. 696–7, cf. 783–4, 824–5). Much more harrowing to the audience than mere description, however, is the scene in which the cripple experiences a sudden seizure that causes his whole body to be racked in torment. The actor would doubtless have used his vocal chords to the full to emit the several blood-curdling cries of pain that Sophocles wrote into the script, while at the same time providing a virtuoso display of bodily contortion (ll. 732, 739, 745, 754, 782 and 790).[1]

Sight and blindness

Blindness occupies a central place in Greek tragedy, principally for two reasons. First, it is an eloquent metaphor for humanity's ignorance about the future and limited understanding of the present and past, to which fatal weakness the root of tragedy can often be traced. We may even go so far as to state that blindness is an apt metaphor for the human condition *per se*, beset as that condition is by the ever-present possibility of imminent and unexpected catastrophe. In this regard mortals are starkly differentiated from the gods, who see everything and comprehend everything perfectly. Second, the antithesis between sight and blindness offers ample scope for the kind of dramatic irony that was so favoured by the tragedians, who never tired of pointing out that 20/20 vision does not guarantee any depth of self-awareness, whereas its antithesis, blindness, may actually be conducive of insight since it tends to prompt a deeper engagement with life's meaning and mystery. Hence the importance of the blind Theban seer Teiresias, who appears both in Sophocles' *Antigone* and *Oedipus the King*, and in Euripides' *Bacchae* and *Phoenician Women*.[2]

It is Sophocles who explores most richly the antithesis between those who have sight but are ignorant or deluded and those who are blind but endowed with insight or gifted with prophecy. His *Oedipus the King* features the cripple Oedipus, whose name may perhaps mean 'Swollen Foot' or 'Swell Foot'. Early in the play Oedipus summons Teiresias in the hope that he will provide information leading to the identification of the killer of Laius, the previous king of Thebes. Immediately prior to his entry, the Chorus of Theban Elders refers to him reverentially as 'the lord Teiresias who sees identically to the lord Apollo' (ll. 284–5) – high praise indeed – and in equally flattering terms Oedipus greets him on arrival as 'you who arrange all things, both those things that can be taught and those that are unspeakable, those that are in heaven and those that walk upon the earth' (ll. 300–1). Barely two minutes later, however, Teiresias' refusal to reveal any information to Oedipus prompts the king to accuse him of having conspired in the planning of the murder. He actually goes further and states rashly, 'Were it not for the fact that you are blind, I would accuse you of having undertaken the deed alone!' (ll. 348–9). This in turn provokes Teiresias, who has anger issues himself, to reveal what he had struggled to conceal – namely that Oedipus is guilty of both parricide and incest. Hearing this, Oedipus' anger knows no limits and he derides the seer for being 'blind in ears, mind, and eyes' (ll. 370–1) and for having 'only eyes when it comes to making a profit but being blind in the practice of your art' (ll. 388–9) – a similar charge to the one that is made by Creon to Teiresias in Sophocles' *Antigone* when the king suspects the seer of conspiring against his authority for personal gain (ll. 1033–47, 1055).

Teiresias is no less scornful in response and he turns the accusation of blindness back on his accuser. He taunts Oedipus with 'having sight but being blind to your evil situation' (l. 412), and he ends his own rant by predicting that Oedipus 'will go upon the earth, blind instead of sighted, poor instead of rich, leaning on a stick' (ll. 454–6) – a prophecy that will indeed come to fulfilment very soon. When Oedipus begins to realize that he may indeed be the killer of Laius even though he has no suspicion at this point that he is Laius' son, he retracts his former verdict and confesses, 'I am terribly afraid that the seer may have sight' (l. 747). Oedipus' belated acknowledgement that the blind man is not only honest but also insightful marks the beginning of his painful journey of self-discovery that will result in his being on a par with the seer. As Seale (1982: 224) points out: 'In the blind figure of Teiresias Oedipus is face to face with his own imminent destiny.'

There are other ways in which Greek tragedy explores the twin concepts of sight and blindness. The plot of every tragedy requires that the truth be brought to light. It thus follows that, prior to the final revelation, the dramatis personae including the Chorus are stumbling sightlessly. In addition, when the living contemplate death in Greek tragedy more often than not they talk about no longer seeing the light of the sun. Thus Polyxena, about to be dragged to death by Odysseus, renounces what she calls 'this unconstrained light that enters my eyes' in Euripides' *Hecuba* (ll. 367–8). Thus too Ajax greets for the last time 'the radiance of bright day' in Sophocles' *Ajax* (ll. 847–8). The ability to comprehend the sun's brightness is what best expresses the experience of being alive, whereas the inability epitomizes the condition of being dead. So when Oedipus wishes he were dead he apostrophizes the light in the hope that he may look upon it for the last time (Sophocles, *Oedipus the King* 1183).

Blinding as punishment

Blinding was a common method of punishment in the late Byzantine world, used against criminals and political rivals (cf. Beal, Kellenberger and Coloru and Efthymiadis in this volume). When Oedipus eventually realizes that he is guilty of both parricide and incest, he blinds himself with the golden pins that he takes from Jocasta's dress after she has hanged herself. He performs this horrific act of self-mutilation as the Messenger, who reports it, explains, 'so that his eyes should not see his terrible sufferings or his deeds, and so that in the future they should see in darkness those they ought not to have seen and those whom they ought not to have known' (ll. 1271–4). The eschatological conclusion to be drawn from this statement is that the disabled were believed to experience the same disabilities in the world below. If blind and crippled in life, they remain blind and crippled in Hades.

The entry of Oedipus immediately after this speech, groping his way helplessly across the stage, no doubt wearing a mask whose eye sockets are covered with blood and a robe that is bloodstained, would have shocked the audience. Shortly after, when the Chorus declares that he would have been better dead than alive in such a condition, Oedipus angrily retorts that he could not have gazed upon his parents and children when they eventually meet in Hades. He goes so far as to tell the Chorus that he would have rendered himself deaf as well, 'if there were a way to provide a barricade to the stream of hearing through the ears' (ll. 1386–7). And so it is, as Dawe (2006: 16) indicates, that 'Oedipus, who began life with two pierced feet, is to end it with two pierced eyeballs'.[3]

Blinding as an act of punishment occurs in Euripides' *Hecuba*. Hecuba takes revenge upon Polymestor, king of the Thracian Chersonese, who has treacherously murdered her son Polydorus in order to steal the gold that Polydorus had left in his safekeeping. Feigning ignorance of her son's murder and assisted by the Chorus of captive Trojan women, Hecuba lures Polymestor and his two sons offstage into a tent set up on the shore. As they blind Polymestor, the king emits a blood-curdling cry (l. 1035). The queen then proceeds to murder his children. Since Euripides chose not to interrupt the action with a messenger speech, the audience is left to imagine both the blinding and the killing from the horrific cries offstage. Immediately afterwards Hecuba emerges from the tent and addresses Polymestor exultantly: 'Never will you gain back your sight or see your sons, for I have killed them!' (ll. 1045–6). Soon afterwards Polymestor emerges as well, 'like a wild animal that hunts a pack of maddened hounds', as he later states (l. 1173), vainly seeking to track down Hecuba and the Chorus. 'O god of the sun!' he cries, 'Heal my bleeding eyes!' (1066–7).

Hecuba's atrocity is a measure of the intensity of her grief. The Greek commander-in-chief Agamemnon acknowledges as much when Polymestor calls him to witness her crimes and threatens to tear her limb from limb. An informal trial now takes place, over which Agamemnon presides as judge. Polymestor justifies his killing of Polydorus by claiming that it was motivated by his concern for the common good. He devotes most of his speech, however, to a description of the butchering of his sons and of his blinding at the hands of the captive Trojan women. 'They removed their brooches and stabbed the pupils of my wretched eyes so that they ran with blood,' he declares (ll. 1170–1). Hecuba dismisses his defence as pure sophistry and is entirely indifferent to his suffering, claiming that what she has done is fully justified.

It is unclear whether Euripides expected the audience to side with Polymestor or with Hecuba. Both are reprehensible. Some modern scholars have expressed repugnance at Hecuba's ability to gloat over her deed. Others see her as a helpless victim of events (ll. 1254–8; cf. Mossman 1995: 188–203). In the event Agamemnon finds Polymestor guilty of premeditated murder, especially heinous in light of the fact that the victim was his guest, and condemns him to solitary confinement on a deserted island. Before departing Polymestor prophesies that Hecuba will be transformed into a dog and drown at sea and that Agamemnon will be killed by his wife Clytemnestra when he returns home.

Though Polymestor's conversion from sight to foresight is hardly comparable in intensity to Oedipus' conversion from sight to insight in the *Oedipus the King*, there is some overlap between the two plays, not least in the fact that both involve a change from ignorance to recognition – Polymestor recognizes that Hecuba, whom he thought to be ignorant of his crime, was in fact fully informed – and both involve blinding with brooch pins. However, Polymestor's bloodcurdling offstage scream seems to be unique to Euripides' play. There is no evidence that Oedipus cries out from offstage when he pierces his eyeballs.

Distorted vision

Sight and blindness feature in Sophocles' *Ajax*, where human vision is seen to be limited and subject to interference from a god, and where, too, the inability of humans to discern the physical presence of a god serves as a useful dramatic device. In the Prologue the goddess Athena comes to Odysseus to explain that she has deluded the wits and the eyesight of his hated adversary Ajax. 'Voice of Athena, you who are dearest to me of the gods, how easily I hear your voice and grasp what you say, even though you are invisible to me,' Odysseus replies (ll. 14–16). We are perhaps to imagine Odysseus casting his eyes around the stage like a sightless man, trying to detect where her voice comes from. Athena then explains how she induced Ajax to slaughter cattle in the belief that he was murdering Agamemnon and Menelaus, loathsome and abhorrent to him because they awarded the prize of Achilles' arms to Odysseus instead of to him. She managed to do this, she tells him, 'by casting on his eyes evil fancies' (ll. 51–2).

Athena now declares that she will reveal Ajax's madness to Odysseus so that he can report it to the army. 'I shall prevent him from seeing you by diverting the rays of his eyes,' she says, seeking to reassure him (ll. 69–70). When Odysseus expresses his reluctance to see Ajax humiliated in this way, she becomes scornful:

Athena: Do you shrink from seeing a man who is obviously mad?
Odysseus: I would not have hesitated when he was sane.
Athena: But now he won't see you.
Odysseus: How can that be if he sees with the same eyes?
Athena: I will darken his eyes even though they see.
Odysseus: Everything can happen when a god purposes it.

(Sophocles, Ajax 81–6)

The goddess reveals herself to Ajax, who greets her with the words, 'You who have stood beside me loyally' (l. 92), in gratitude for the supposed help she rendered him in the slaughtering of his enemies. She proceeds to mock him in the same way that one might mock a blind man for his blindness. Odysseus, observing the scene, declares:

I pity him for his misery, even though he is my enemy, because he is yoked to evil. I think of my fate as much as of his; for I see that all of us are nothing but ghosts and empty shadows.

(Sophocles, Ajax 121–6)

A similar distortion of vision occurs in Euripides' *Heracles*. Hera, who hates Heracles on the grounds that he is the product of Zeus' extramarital affair with Alcmene, sends Iris and Lyssa (madness personified) to inflict the hero with temporary insanity. The onset of his insanity and the murder that he perpetrates under its influence are described by the Messenger, who begins his narrative as follows (ll. 931–4): 'He was no longer the same person. His face was distorted, his eyes rolled in their sockets, their veins filled with blood, and drool began to soak his bearded chin.' Heracles goes on a killing spree 'directing a wild gorgon gaze' at one of his sons in the deluded belief that he is the offspring of his sworn foe Eurystheus, king of Tiryns (l. 990). After slaughtering all his sons and his wife, he is on the point of killing his foster father Amphitryon when the goddess Athena intervenes and causes him to fall into a deep coma. Out of mercy it seems – albeit belatedly – Zeus has dispatched his daughter from Olympus to call a halt to the bloodbath.

Following a choral interlude, the doors of the palace open to reveal the still sleeping Heracles bound with ropes and surrounded by the bodies of his wife and children (on binding, cf. Gourevitch in this volume). Amphitryon urges the Chorus to let Heracles continue sleeping but he soon wakes up. The old man gently leads him to the realization of what he has done. Heracles' instinctive reaction is to commit suicide, but before he has a chance to act upon it, his close friend Theseus arrives. Heracles covers his head in shame, an act which epitomizes what Arrowsmith (1956: 278) memorably calls 'the dark night of his soul' (ll. 1140, 1159, 1104–5, 1198, 1216 and 1226–7).

Theseus eventually succeeds in persuading Heracles to unveil his head. He then offers him refuge in Athens where he will be able to undergo purification and find redemption. It is the unwavering friendship and support that Theseus extends to the broken and dependent hero that provides the play's uplifting resolution. At the end Heracles departs for Athens, 'being towed in Theseus' wake like a boat' (l. 1424), no longer capable of independent action. It is one of the most striking reversals in Greek tragedy. It is noteworthy that both Amphitryon and Theseus are more appalled by divine cruelty than they are by human brutality because they comprehend that the latter is a function of the former. As the Chorus says towards the end of the play, 'O Zeus, why do you hate your own son so vehemently? Why have you brought him to this sea of grief?' (ll. 1086–7).

In Euripides' *Bacchae*, the god Dionysus distorts the vision of Pentheus, king of Thebes, because he has insulted him by rejecting his claims to godhead. Pentheus is thus incapable of realizing that Dionysus is playing with him and sees double. At the same time the fact that the god can delude him so easily is an indication of the depths of his lack of self-awareness. Having been persuaded to dress up as a maenad so that he will be able to witness the Bacchic rites, he is lured up onto Mount Cithaeron. After a choral interlude, the Messenger enters to describe how Pentheus' mother Agave and his aunt Autonoe, accompanied by the maenads, mistook him for a wild beast. Possessed and driven temporarily mad by Dionysus, they proceed to tear Pentheus limb from limb. Lambert (2009: 19–35) compares the behaviour of the maenads in Euripides' play to that of Zulu women known as Amandiki in colonial records. As he notes, Euripides

> presents us with the two faces of Dionysiac madness: the one (…) which is destructive and an ominous threat to patriarchal values and their constructions of women; the other, the madness of those who have accepted Dionysus, which (…) embodies values (peace, prosperity, the feast, wine), which are perfectly acceptable to any patriarchy.
>
> *(Lambert 2009: 29)*

Agave, her vision still distorted, returns from the kill boasting of her hunting skills and clutching the head of Pentheus, which she believes to be that of a lion cub (ll. 1168–1210). Her father Cadmus, who greets her on return, gently leads Agave to the painful realization of what she has done in much the same way that Cadmus brought Heracles back to sanity and reality (ll. 1263–99). It is a uniquely human moment of shared misery and commiseration that demonstrates the gulf between humanity and divinity, since Dionysus demonstrates no compassion for the havoc he has brought down on the family, innocent and guilty alike. Agave, Autonoe and the maenads became maniacal murderers through no fault of their own, having piously committed themselves to the worship of Dionysus. We might legitimately wonder what will be the maenads' reaction to the atrocity when their sight is restored to them.

Exile, blindness and old age

Nowhere in tragedy is disability explored with greater understanding than in Sophocles' *Oedipus at Colonus*.[4] The play, which was written at the end of the poet's long life but not performed till several years after his death, opens with the same scene as the one that ends the *Oedipus the King*, which was written a generation earlier. The similarity is unlikely to have been lost on those in the audience, themselves now elderly, who had attended the performance of the earlier play, for we see the blind Oedipus being guided onstage by his daughters Antigone and Ismene just as they had led him offstage. They have been performing the function of his staff and eyes (ll. 848, 866–7). Oedipus introduces himself as a blind old man and makes repeated references to his blindness throughout the play (ll. 21, 33–4, 74, 138. 146–7, 1549). His condition is contrasted with that of the 'all-seeing Eumenides' (l. 42), into whose sacred grove he and his daughters have inadvertently strayed.

When a Stranger encounters them and orders the family to leave, Oedipus reveals that he has a great boon to give Athens. 'What help can come from one who has no sight?' the Stranger asks, perplexed and incredulous. 'In all that we speak there will be sight', Oedipus replies, ascribing insight not to himself but to the words themselves, as Jebb (1899: 24) aptly notes.

When the Chorus of Elderly Athenians enters, Oedipus declares, 'Here is the man you seek. In sound is my sight, as it is said [viz. of the blind]' (ll. 138–9). Though the Chorus is horrified to discover his identity, Antigone successfully urges compassion upon them. Theseus arrives soon afterwards and, learning of the benefit Oedipus promises to his city, agrees to give the exile sanctuary. After rejecting a highly emotional appeal from his son Polyneices to return to Thebes, Oedipus senses intuitively that he has reached the end of his life and is confirmed in his belief by a roll of thunder. 'My children, follow me', he urges, his sight seemingly restored to him. 'In a strange way I have become your guide, just as you were once your father's guide' (ll. 1542–3).

Following a choral interlude, a Messenger describes Oedipus's mysterious passing from life. Just as he had exited 'with no friend to lead him but guide to us all' (ll. 1588–9), so he again acted as a guide, somehow able to pick his way unaided through the features of the grove as if possessed of a highly detailed knowledge of the terrain. After washing and clothing himself in a white robe, the customary clothing of the dead, Oedipus bade farewell to his daughters by 'feeling for them with his blind hands' (l. 1639), as if his sight has miraculously abandoned him again or as if he is near-sighted . He then urged his daughters to quit the place. His mysterious departure from life is alone witnessed by Theseus. The Messenger tells us that Theseus observes his final moments on earth with his hand raised to his face, as if seeking to protect his eyes from a blinding light (ll. 1650–2).

Blindness in comedy

Disability features marginally in Greek comedy. The only disabled person who appears prominently in the works of Aristophanes' is Ploutos, the god of Wealth, the eponymous 'hero' of the play of that name. Following in the tradition of the sixth-century Ionian poet Hipponax (fr. 36), Aristophanes depicts Wealth as blind. The play opens with Chremylus, who is a modestly well off Athenian farmer, explaining to Cario, his slave, that Apollo ordered him to offer hospitality to the first man he encountered after leaving his shrine at Delphi. The person in question happens to be Wealth, who is later described as 'filthy, hunchbacked, wretched, wrinkled, mangy, and toothless' (l. 266).

When subjected to interrogation, the god is reluctant to reveal his identity because of his well-justified fear that he will be put under house arrest, though when threatened with violence he eventually yields. He explains to Chremylus that Zeus blinded him when he was a young man because he had promised to visit the homes of 'law-abiding, wise, and decent folk'. Zeus, he goes on to say, resents the human race, especially good people (ll. 87–92). No doubt Zeus' blinding of Wealth evoked in the audience the recollection of his blinding of the Thracian king Lycurgus for having persecuted the worshippers of Dionysus – a much more justifiable act of punishment, it would seem (Homer, *Iliad* 6.130–40; see Rose 2003: 81–2). When Chremylus offers to restore his eyesight, Wealth refuses, claiming that Zeus will exact further vengeance upon him if he goes about distributing wealth to the poor (ll. 112–19).

Eventually Chremylus persuades Wealth to undergo a cure at the sanctuary of the healing god Asclepius in the Piraeus. Chremylus and Cario accompany him to the sanctuary, where he spends the night, as was customary for those seeking a cure. The popular hope was that the god would visit the sick in a dream and indicate what procedure to adopt. Alternatively he would perform the healing himself. Following an interval of time perhaps marked by a lost choral interlude or entr'acte, Cario announces to the Chorus that the cure has been successful with the following quote from Sophocles' lost play the *Phineus* (fr. 710): 'Instead of being blind he now has perfect eyesight and his pupils are bright, thanks to Asclepius the kindly healer!'

Chremylus' wife emerges from the house and Cario provides her with a vivid and quite lengthy description of the night he spent in the sanctuary. The culminating moment in the cure is described as follows:

> The god seated himself beside Wealth and wiped his eyelids with a clean gauze. Panacea [Asclepius' daughter] then covered his head and all his face with a purple cloth. Next the god whistled and two exceptionally large snakes crawled out from inside the temple (…) They quietly slid beneath the purple cloth and began licking his eyelids. Before you could drink ten cups of wine, Wealth sprang up and could see.
>
> *(Aristophanes, Plut. 727–34)*

It is unclear whether we are to laugh at this or merely take it with a grain of salt. Either way the report does little to suggest much faith on Aristophanes' part in incubation and the miraculous cures ascribed to it.

Since Wealth is described as hunchbacked or stooped earlier in the play, it is not improbable that he now undergoes rejuvenation like other characters in Aristophanic comedy. As a result of the god's cure Chremylus becomes wealthy and the rest of the play is devoted to exploring the consequences for society of his restored sight.

Though it is possible that Wealth was a character in earlier comedies, there is nothing to indicate that the healing of Wealth as a blind god featured in any of them (Sommerstein 2001: 8). That said, Wealth's blindness amounts to little more than a convenient plot device. The audience is never invited to sympathize with the god because of his disability. The character makes no reference to his blindness other than in the brief explanation of how he came to be blinded, nor does he express any gratitude at having his sight restored to him. It is unclear, too, whether the actor who played him would have sought to render his blindness either by gesture or movement.

However, it is important to point out that Wealth is not mocked for his blindness, as he might well have been. On the contrary, he is treated like anyone else, despite his unprepossessing appearance. The opposite is the case in Euripides' satyric play the *Cyclops*, where the one-eyed giant Polyphemus, after he has been blinded by Odysseus, gropes his way pathetically around the stage in search of his assailant, to the evident amusement of the audience:

Cyclops: Where is he?
Chorus: Over here beside the rock. Are you grasping him?

Cyclops:	Bloody hell, I've given my head a terrible bang.
Chorus:	They're on the run.
Cyclops:	I thought you said they were over here.
Chorus:	Not over there but over here.
Cyclops:	Where?
Chorus:	Over here on your left.
Cyclops:	You're mocking me. You're ridiculing me when I'm in a wretched situation.

(Euripides, Cycl. 682–7)

There are a number of disparaging references in Aristophanes' plays to a well-known purblind Athenian called Neocleides. In the *Thesmophoriazousai* or Assemblywomen one of the women imagines the following scene taking place in the Assembly where a debate is taking place 'regarding the safety of the city':

Immediately Neocleides the Squinter groped his way forward to be the first speaker, whereupon the people shouted as loud as you can imagine, 'Isn't it dreadful that this fellow has the effrontery to address the Assembly about how to save ourselves when he can't even save his own eyelids?' At this he squints around and shouts back, 'What can I do about that?'

(Aristophanes, Thesm. 397–404)

It is not improbable that the passage alludes to a memorable incident that had recently taken place in the Assembly when the purblind man had indeed been shouted down. The scene is strangely reminiscent of the one in which Thersites addresses the Greek army and is abused for his pains, as we discussed at the beginning of this chapter. Neocleides also features in the *Ploutos*. He is described as 'having outshot the sighted in his thefts' (ll. 666–7) and is castigated for being a loudmouth and a busybody. When he goes to Asclepius' sanctuary in the Piraeus seeking a cure for his ophthalmic disease, the god seizes the opportunity to plaster up his eyes in order to prevent him from 'interrupting meetings of the Assembly with affidavits' (ll. 716–25). We, the audience, are evidently expected to take pure pleasure at the thought of the 'squinter' being punished in this way.

Whether the invective that is directed towards Neocleides reflects a general prejudice towards the blind or whether it is an ad hominem attack on a particularly unsavoury character is unclear. Though the latter is more likely, the suggestion that Neocleides only pretended to be blind in order to increase his chances of stealing may well have been a common charge that was levelled against those who claimed to be blind, particularly when they were making application for a disability allowance from the public exchequer (cf. contributions by Rose and Dillon in this volume).

Old age in tragedy and comedy

The helplessness of old age is occasionally foregrounded in tragedy. Geriatrics are typically characterized either by their irascibility, as in the case of Teiresias in Sophocles' *Antigone* and his *Oedipus the King*, and of both Oedipus and Creon in his *Oedipus at Colonus*, or by their feebleness, as in the case of the Chorus of Argive Elders in Aeschylus' *Agamemnon*, whose members complain that their strength is 'like that of a child' (ll. 74–5). Similarly the Chorus of Theban Elders in Euripides' *Heracles* speaks of old age as 'a weight that is heavier than Aetna's rocks, which hides in darkness the light of my eyes' (ll. 639–41). In addition, there are choruses of the elderly in five other surviving tragedies, namely Aeschylus' *Persians*, Sophocles' *Oedipus at Colonus*, and Euripides' *Alcestis, Children of Heracles*, and *Suppliants*.

The aged Hecuba, queen of Troy, who occupies centre stage in Euripides' *Hecuba* and *Trojan Women*, is a particularly haunting symbol of the utter degradation that was often the lot of the elderly, especially elderly women, in Greek society. Both strong and resourceful she is also possessed of a chilling capacity for administering a particularly grotesque form of vengeance, as we have seen. Another memorable image of old age is that of Teiresias and Cadmus in Euripides' *Bacchae*. We meet them, dressed incongruously as worshippers of Dionysus, just as they are about to depart to perform revels in his honour. As there are no stage directions, we cannot know whether the spectacle of two elderly men, one of them blind, about to indulge in revels, was intended to be primarily comic or pathetic. When the pair departs, Teiresias in a striking role reversal invites Cadmus to follow him 'doing service to Dionysus, the son of Zeus' and promises to support him if he stumbles (ll. 363–6). In the *Children of Heracles* the elderly Iolaus is transformed into an ephebe and wins military honours, even though the scene of his arming before the battle is invested with considerable pathos and humour (ll. 732–40, 843–60).

The mockery of old age is common to many early cultures.[5] In Aristophanes old age may well have been the subject of much visual humour of which we have no record. Of his eleven surviving plays, only the *Frogs* does not feature any geriatrics. Typically the elderly are portrayed as either pitiable and helpless or bellicose and cantankerous, and sometimes a combination of both. In the *Acharnians* the Chorus of elderly hoplites from the deme of Acharnae who fought against the Persians at the Battle of Marathon sixty-five years earlier personifies helpless but indomitable militancy. Painting a pathetic picture of itself as the victim of persecution by sharp-witted youngsters in the lawcourts, the Chorus tells of an old man, appropriately called Tithonus, who sucks on his toothless gums in a state of almost imbecilic bemusement (ll. 687–91). A specially memorable portrait of a geriatric is that of Philocleon in *Wasps*. Philocleon is a superannuated delinquent who looks back wistfully on his youth as a time when he was able to break the law with impunity. His sole remaining pleasure is to serve on the jury and pass waspish verdicts on those who break the law as a way of revenging himself on life for his physical decline. The drama ends with Philocleon's rejuvenation (ll. 1341–87). In the *Knights,* the 'bad-tempered, half-deaf, elderly' Demos undergoes a similar rejuvenation (ll. 42–3). When reminded of his former behaviour, he demands of the Sausage-seller, 'Was I so stupid and senile? (l. 1349). Presumably the actor who played Demos would have sought to make an extreme contrast between his first and second appearances on stage (ll. 727–1263, 1335–1408).

In his late plays Aristophanes repeatedly extracted cruel humour from the supposedly ludicrous spectacle of sex-starved old women chasing after young men less than half their age. The poet's point is that their desire to remain sexually active is the height of absurdity, given their repulsive appearance. Nothing in the comic theatre is in poorer taste than the ridicule that Aristophanes heaps upon those whose vitality is unimpaired. Further evidence of the way the elderly were portrayed in comedy is indicated by the fact that there was a large variety of masks depicting elderly women with unflattering and stereotypical characteristics. As the 2nd century CE grammarian Pollux (4.150) notes, they included the *graïdion ishnon* (little old shrivelled woman), the *graïdion lukainion* (little old she-wolf), the *graïdion oxu* (sharp-tongued or sharp-witted old woman) and the *graus pacheia* (obese old woman).[6]

Conclusions

Sophocles alone of the dramatists has provided us with some striking portraits of the physically disabled, notably in the figures of Oedipus, Philoctetes, and Teiresias. This, we may suspect, is due primarily to the myths upon which he chose to base his dramas, rather than to any specific interest in the plight of the disabled, though it may be that his exploration of blindness and old age in the *Oedipus at Colonus* was in part motivated by his own increasing infirmity. It is noteworthy, too, that Sophocles gives attention both to the psychological effects of disability on the disabled and to the social response towards the disabled, which is often a convincing blend of compassion and contempt. The gods' ability to distort the vision of those they seek to ruin is a prominent theme in tragedy. Euripides' depiction of temporary insanity and its terrifying effects is clinically observed. Memorable, too, is the depiction of the deranged Ajax in Sophocles' play of that name. Only one character is disabled in Aristophanes, namely Wealth, and his disability is treated cursorily and without any interest in either the psychological or physical consequences of his blindness.

Notes

1 See Edwards 2000: 55–69 for a discussion of Sophocles' play in its social context. She concludes (66), 'Because there was no military, social, or economic category of the wounded veteran, the plight of the individual wounded and disabled veteran could produce mixed feelings of pride and pity, admiration and repulsion.' Similar mixed feelings are directed towards Philoctetes. Wilson 1947: 272–95 compares Philoctetes to Oedipus, both of whom are outcasts.
2 On blindness in Greek tragedy, see Roig Lanzillotta 2014: 186–7. On blindness in the plays of Sophocles and myth, see Buxton 1980: 22–37. Trentin 2013: 89–114 discusses the causes of visual impairment, as well as the condition of the visually impaired, in the Roman world, though many of her observations pertain to the Greek world as well.
3 For Oedipus's self-blinding see Devereux 1973: 36–49 and Calame 1996: 17–48. Devereux 1973: 40–2 lists other instances in classical literature where sexual trespass is punished by blinding. As he (48) notes, Oedipus' act of self-blinding 'may well be a Sophoklean invention'.
4 For the imagery of blindness in Sophocles' play, see Shields 1961: 63–73. For a discussion of blindness in Greek society and in Greek tragedy with particular reference to the Oedipus at Colonus, see Bernidaki-Aldous 1990.
5 As Parkin 2003: 87 notes: 'On the Roman stage, particularly in the plays of Plautus ... every conceivable negative quality associated with old age is highlighted, with special emphasis on the old man's sexual, though impotent proclivities.' See also the famous description of the onset of old age in Ecclesiastes 12: 1–8.
6 Oeri 1948 provides a full investigation of old women in Greek comedy, including discussion of masks. See Parkin 2003: 351, n. 131, for extensive bibliography of the topic.

Bibliography

Arrowsmith, William, 'Introduction to Heracles', in D. Grene and R. Lattimore (eds), *Euripides II* (Chicago, IL, 1956), 44–59.

Bernidaki-Aldous, Eleftheria, *Blindness in a Culture of Light: Especially the Case of Oedipus at Colonus of Sophocles* (New York, 1990).

Brandt, Hartwin, *Wird auch silbern meine Haare: Eine Geschichte des Alters in der Antike* (Munich, 2002).

Buxton, Richard, 'Blindness and Limits: Sophocles and the Logic of Myth', *Journal of Hellenic Studies* 100 (1980), 22–37.

Calame, Claude, 'Vision, Blindness, and Mask: The Radicalization of the Emotions in Sophocles' Oedipus Rex', in M. Silk (ed.), *Tragedy and the Tragic: Greek Theater and Beyond* (Oxford, 1996), 17–48.

Dawe, R. D., *Sophocles: Oedipus Rex*. Rev. edn (Cambridge, 2006²).

Devereux, Georges, 'The Self-Blinding of Oedipous in Sophokles' Oedipous Tyrannos', *Journal of Hellenic Studies* 93 (1973), 36–49.

Edwards, Martha Lynn [= Rose, Martha Lynn], 'Philoctetes in Historical Context', in D. A. Gerber (ed.), *Disabled Veterans in History* (Ann Arbor, MI, 2000), 55–69.

Garland, Robert, *The Eye of the Beholder: Deformity and Disability in the Graeco-Roman World* (London, 2010²).

Goheen, Robert F., *The Imagery of Sophocles' Antigone* (Princeton, NJ, 1951).

Jebb, Richard C., *Sophocles: Oedipus Coloneus* (Cambridge, 1899).

Laes, Christian, Goodey, Chris F., and Rose, Martha Lynn (eds) *Disabilities in Roman Antiquity: Disparate Bodies* A Capite ad Calcem (Leiden, 2013).

Lambert, Michael, 'The Madness of Women: The Zulu Amandiki and Euripides' Bacchae', in P. Bosman (ed.), *Mania: Madness in the Greco-Roman World* (Pretoria, 2009), 19–35.

Mossman, Judith M., *Wild Justice: A Study of Euripides' Hecuba* (Oxford, 1995).

Oeri, Hans Georg, *Der Typ der komischen Alten in der griechischen Komödie* (Basel, 1948).

Parker, Robert, *Athenian Religion: A History* (Oxford, 1966).

Parkin, Tim, *Old Age in the Roman World: A Cultural and Social History* (Baltimore, MD, and London, 2003).

Roig Lanzillotta, Lautaro, 'Blindness', in Hanna M. Roisman (ed.), *Encyclopedia of Greek Tragedy* (Oxford and Malden, MA, 2014), I: 186–7.

Rose, Martha L., *The Staff of Oedipus: Transforming Disability in Ancient Greece* (Ann Arbor, MI, 2003).

Seale, David, *Vision and Stagecraft in Sophocles* (Chicago, IL, 1982).

Shields, M. G., 'Sight and Blindness Imagery in the Oedipus Coloneus', *Phoenix* 15 (1961), 63–73.

Sommerstein, Alan H., *Aristophanes: Wealth* (Warminster, 2001).

Trentin, Lisa, 'Exploring Visual Impairment in Ancient Rome', in C. Laes *et al.* (eds), *Disabilities in Roman Antiquity* (Leiden, 2013), 89–114.

Wilson, Edmund, 'Philoctetes: The Wound and the Bow', in E. Wilson (ed.), *The Wound and the Bow: Seven Studies in Literature* (Oxford, 1941), 272–95.

12

LEGAL (AND CUSTOMARY?) APPROACHES TO THE DISABLED IN ANCIENT GREECE

Matthew Dillon

Written law (*nomos*) as opposed to customary law hardly acknowledged the existence of the disabled and their physical disabilities in ancient Greece. As always, the exception was Athens, where one particular law of the 5th and 4th centuries BCE made provision for physically disabled citizens, who were incapable of work, to be paid a small daily allowance. Overall, it was customary, unwritten law which largely defined the status and treatment of the disabled in the ancient Greek world. Mentally disabled individuals were by custom kept inside, and Plato in his ideal state would have a law that these were definitely to be kept inside by their relatives, and not allowed to wander the streets. At Sparta, new-born babies who were deformed and had physical disabilities would be exposed in a pit-like place near Mount Taygetos, and this had the force of law, for all infants had to be inspected by the eldest of the fellow-tribesmen of its father; it was they not he who made their decision on whether an infant was to live or die. Once again, this was reflected by Plato, who formulated a law that physically disabled infants were to be quietly disposed of. Yet apart from Athens, laws did not deal with those who had disabilities, except in religion: decrees concerning the sale of priesthoods on Kos, in particular, do not specifically address those who were disabled or disfigured, but rather emphasized that those who were the ritual agents of the gods, as priests and priestesses, had to be physically 'whole'. Epigraphically, studies of the Greek disabled are extremely disappointing – the inscribed law codes tend not to focus on physical disabilities, but rather the emphasis is on legal standing with respect to the status of people, not on their appearance. But the Gortyn law code specifically allowed for the killing of children, without reference to whether they were disabled or not, and general Greek practice permitted exposure: it is apparent that to dispose of a disabled infant was not only possible, but not even socially reprehensible.

Greek legislation exposing disabled babies

In the *Theaitetos*, Plato compares the testing and scrutinizing of one of Theaitetos' ideas to an examination of a new-born infant, a woman's first child, and it being taken away from its mother after such an examination if found 'not worthy to be reared' (161a; all translations are the author's). As required by the proposed legislation of Plato's utopia in the *Republic* (*Politeia*), babies who were born disabled (*anapēron*) were to be disposed of secretly, so that their fate would be unknown to others. In this way, 'the purity (*katharos*) of the Guardians [who govern the state] will be preserved' (*Republic* 460c). Such a law was clearly modelled on Sparta's customs (see below), Plato's debt to which is clear throughout the *Republic* and the *Laws*, as well as, presumably, to the customary practice of Athens. No law at Athens protected the rights of the new-born infant and no child was legitimate until the father acknowledged this in the ceremony of the household ritual of the Amphidromia. He carried the infant around the household hearth, naming it, legitimizing it and transforming it into a proto-citizen (Laes 2014: 366–9, esp. 367; Dillon 2015). Killing a baby after this ceremony would presumably be punishable by law, as a case of child-murder.

Aristotle in the *Politics* is specific, and argues that in the ideal state there ought to be a specific law that, 'no deformed (*pepērōmenon*) child is to be raised' (Aristotle, *Pol.* 1335b20–1, cf. 1335b4–1336a3). This seems to indicate, not necessarily that Plato and Aristotle were reflecting such an actual law in any specific state, but rather that there was a deficiency of such laws in the Greek world, which these philosophers chose to rectify through these legislative promulgations, which presumably reflected customary practice. (For Plato and Aristotle on physical disabilities, and advocating laws for the exposure of deformed, disabled infants: Patterson 1985: 105–6; Rose 2003: 32; cf. 37, citing Diodorus Siculus 2.57.4–5 and 17.91.4–7.)

Sparta provides specific, historical evidence of the physical exposure of a 'defective' new-born baby (*paidarion*) (this evidence is not accepted by all: see Laes 2008: 92–3). As a state, Sparta did have law but much of it was oral – yet Delphi approved Sparta's constitution, laws and reforms, traditionally introduced by Lykourgos. Plutarch in his *Life of Lykourgos* provides a full biography of the Spartan law-giver, even though he admits that he has no real information to make use of, and even suspected that the man he is writing about was a myth (Plutarch, *Lyc.* 1.1). Nevertheless he gives details of many Spartan practices which had the force of law, and writes (in the past tense) about the exposure of deformed children at Sparta:

> A father of a newborn baby did not have the power to decide whether to rear it or not, but carried it to a certain place called a meeting-place, where the eldest of his fellow-tribesmen sat. They examined the infant, and if it were sturdy and robust, they told him to rear it … But if it was weak and deformed, they sent it off to the so-called Place of Exposure (*Apothetai*), a place like a pit by Mount Taygetos, considering it better for both the child itself and the city that what was not properly formed with a view to health and strength right from the very beginning should not live.
>
> *(Plutarch, Lyc. 16.1–2)*

Perhaps some caution is due here from a methodological point of view, for Plutarch writes a few centuries after the demise of classical Sparta, and Xenophon in his 4th-century BCE treatise *Spartan Constitution* makes no reference to compulsory infanticide for those who did not 'pass the test'. Xenophon refers to many Spartan social practices concerning the rearing of boys, most notably the *agoge*, the system of physical education for the boys from 7 years on. His admiration of Sparta, and his deliberate editing in his historical work, the *Hellenika*, suppressing Spartan activities which cast them in a poor historical light, might perhaps be responsible for his omission of this aspect of a Spartan infant's possible fate. He discusses the 'gestation' of children and various Spartan social customs with regard to this, including physical exercise for both male and female, with running competitions and contests of strength for both genders, and approves of these. He invites his reader's opinion: 'whether Lykourgos had success in peopling Sparta with a tribe of men large and strong, anyone wishing to do so can decide for themselves' (Xenophon, *Spartan Constitution* 1.10, with chapter 1 as a whole; cf. Aristotle, *Politics* 1338b9–19 for a negative view of this training). From there, without writing about the birth of Spartan babies meant to be procreated both by this process and the marriage customs he describes, he turns to when the boys are 7 years old, and the girls teenagers. He expects his reader to think that this size and strength related only to their physical training, but neglects and passes over the birth of the child itself. Presumably, he is embarrassed to write of the process at which Plutarch has no scruples relating. Plutarch is more realistic: the fitness of Spartan children resulted from an inspection of the newly born infant by elders whose only interest lay in preserving the strength of Sparta's citizens.

This inspection is echoed by the lakonophile Plato who incorporated a birth inspection for the ruling class. Moreover, Plato's workers in the *Republic*, the *cheironoi*, were not allowed to breed, and any babies they did have were to be killed instantly (Plato, *Republic* 460c). These *cheironoi* were the equivalent of Sparta's helots, whom they had to allow to breed to have workers, but whose numbers they kept down through a regular slaughter in which the five ephors of Sparta annually declared war on them (Plutarch, *Lyc.* 28.1–7; Arist. F538). Soranos of Ephesos, a medical practitioner of the 2nd century CE, specifies amongst various criteria in considering whether a new-born child should be reared or not, that it should be *teleion* (perfect) in its constituent parts, and generally healthy (Soranos, *Gyn.* 11).

Moreover, in the 4th-century BCE Gortyn law code, the exposure of in fact perfectly healthy children was permitted by law. If a free woman bore a child after divorce, she was required by law to take it, along with three witnesses, to her former husband. If he did not recognize the child as his legitimate offspring, she could rear (*trapen*, from *trephō*) the child if she chose – or she could expose it (*apothemen,* from *apotithēmi*). Similarly, when a serf mother bore a child after divorce, taking two witnesses in this case to her former husband, the former husband could recognize the child, or not, and the law once again permitted the serf woman to rear or expose the child. If this procedure was not followed, the free woman would be fined 50 staters, the serf woman 25 (*Gortyn Law-Code,* col. iii, ll. 44–55, col. iv, ll. 1–17; see Willetts 1967: 29). In the case of a manumitted woman from Delphi, Dioklea, her manumission agreement included the provision that any child she bore after her manumission was hers to raise or strangle, but not to sell (*SGDI* 2171, ll. 16–21). These few examples indicate that newly born infants were not recognized by law, custom or legal agreement to have any rights: their exposure or strangulation was permitted. Law at Sparta demanded the exposure and death of the disabled infant, social custom elsewhere countenanced this at the least and at the worst encouraged the practice. No law protected the disabled new-born: such law would have seemed ridiculous to the Greeks (for disabled children in Antiquity, cf. Schmidt 1983–4).

Religious legislation concerning 'wholeness of body'

In some ways, legislation against disability and the physically disabled was quite overt. In religious matters, discrimination against those who were physically disabled was particularly clear, and is important for providing information from outside Athens. Sacrificial victims presented to the gods had to be free from blemishes, perfect for the deities whom the worshippers wished to please. Various priests and priestesses on the island of Kos had to be free from any physical disability: just as the sacrifices were pure, so too the holders of priesthoods and priestesshoods. This provision which is laid down by law on Kos reflected what was the social and cultural norm throughout the Greek world. Plato in the *Laws* is presumably reflecting actual Athenian, or more generally Greek practice, when for his ideal state he proposes a law that priests (among various other requirements) be *holokleros*, which can be translated as 'wholeness of body', or less prosaically, 'physically whole' (Plato, *Laws* 759c). If the disabled speaker of Lysias 24 were declared not disabled, he argues that he could put his name in the lot to be elected as one of the Athenian nine archons (24.13; see further below). He is not simply referring to the political duties of these nine, but also, as the bouletai hearing the case would understand, to be elected as the *basileus archon*, who had various important religious roles to perform throughout the year of his term of office ([Arist.] *Ath. Pol.* 57). But as a physically disabled man with two crutches, he would not be socially acceptable to appear in public leading the city in its worship, nor would the gods be seen as pleased with this (see Rose in this volume for a different interpretation). A twelfth-century CE lexicographical entry, which might well reflect an actual procedure, indicates that at Athens the *archontes basileis* and the priests were subject to a *dokimasia* to see if they were 'unblemished and whole (*holokleros*)' (*Etymologicum Magnum s.v. apheles*). This *dokimasia* would be similar to the one which the disabled man of Lysias 24 was undergoing (see below) – a physical examination to ascertain that they were fit and healthy individuals to act as ritual agents for the worship of the gods.

This aversion towards those who were disabled and not physically 'sound' was matched at its extreme by a predilection not just to have healthy individuals as priests, but to require them to be 'good-looking' into the bargain. Hence it was specifically decreed by the state on Kos that the priestess of Aphrodite Pandemos was not only healthy and *holoklaros*, but also unblemished (*teleia*), for the goddess of love would not wish her public rites to be carried out by a ritual agent who did not reflect the unblemished beauty of the goddess (*ED* 178a(A), ll. 6–8, end of the 3rd century BCE; *holoklaros* [Doric dialectal form]: see Dillon 1999: 65 and 2016; Wilgaux 2009). At Aigion in Achaia, a boy priest for Zeus was chosen through a contest for the best-looking lad: when the chosen boy priest began to grow a beard, another would be chosen in his place. Similarly in Boiotia, a well-born lad, 'well-endowed with looks and physically strong', was chosen to be priest of Ismenian Apollo (Pausanias 7.24.4, 9.10.4; Garland 1984: 85). Priestesses could specifically be described as 'beautiful' (*Iliad* 6.298, 13.365–6). Needless to say, the many parthenoi on the east frieze of the Parthenon are all sound of limb and attractive.

Other examples in which decrees ruled that cult personnel were to be healthy and whole of body are known from Kos, which has a fulsome epigraphic legal record concerning its priesthoods and priestesshoods, owing largely to the number of these which were put up for sale on the island by the state, a process which required formal decrees to be passed. So from Kos there are numerous cults requiring priests and priestesses who were *holoklaros*: the priestess of Dionysos Thyllophoros (*ED* 216.7–8: end of the 3rd century BCE; *LSCG* 166.8–10: 2nd or 1st century BCE); the priest of Asklepios, Hygineia and Epiona (*ED* 2A.13–15); the priest of Herakles Kallinikon (*ED* 180.15–16); the priest of Zeus Alseios (*ED* 215.8–9, 1st century BCE; restored in *LSCG* 162.14, 3rd century BCE); and the priest of King Eumenes (*ED* 182.5–7, 2nd century BCE). Similarly, the priest of Asklepios at Chalcedon had to be *holoklaros* (*LSAM* 5.9–10 [*SIG*[3] 1009], c.200 BCE). At Rome, the same situation held. Metellus, possibly the consul for 119 BCE, overcame his stuttering disability so that he could fulfil the Roman condition that prayers and ritual formulae had to be recited exactly, and without interruption (Pliny, *Nat. Hist.* 28.3–4), when he had to speak at the dedication of the temple of the goddess Opifera (Pliny, *Nat. Hist.* 11.174; see Laes 2013b: 149 and 176 no. 10). Decrees of the state requiring not simply physical soundness but beauty as a whole reflect a deep-rooted societal preference for the handsome and beautiful, which was also seen as a mark of the gods' favour.

Paranoia ('derangement'), *mainomanos* ('mad-man') and Athenian law

Mental disability can be harder to detect than physical (cf. Rose in this volume). At Athens there was a strongly developed ideology of the preservation of the *oikos*. Prosecutors in law cases accused opponents of wasting their patrimony, of using up their inherited property in fast living, and such an attack resonated with the Athenian jurors (Aeschines, *Tim.* 42, 101, 105 and 194). At Athens, the *basileus archon* was in fact charged with dealing with several types of cases involving the usurpation of another's property, as in cases of guardians and orphans' property. Related to these was another type of case, that of *paranoia* (derangement): 'when someone accuses another of *paranoia* causing him to squander his property' ([Arist.] *Ath. Pol.* 57.6). There was a *nomos* (law) at Athens that one could leave one's property to whomever one liked, with the qualification that this was not the case when the bequeather was 'insane, old, or in the power of a woman'. When the Thirty Tyrants came to power in Athens in 405 BCE, they removed the quoted clause, so that there were no such impediments ([Arist.] *Ath. Pol.* 36.2). Plato in his ideal state had a similar law to the Athenian, which could have the madman who was wasting his property constrained by his son (*Laws* 929d–e). Those who were mentally ill so that they could not work may well have been excluded from receiving the allowance for *adunatoi*, for it was the responsibility of their family to care for them. So those who suffered from a mental illness, that is someone who was a *mainomenos*, suffering from mania ('madness', 'frenzy'), would need to be looked after in the home by relatives, or be homeless and wander the streets. Plato in the *Laws* (934c–d) ruled that a madman (*mainomenos*) was to be kept indoors by his relatives, with fines being levied by law against them if they failed to do so.

Payments to Athenian citizens maimed in battle

Greek warfare produced numbers of men disabled by wounds. According to Herakleides of Pontos, writing in the 4th century BCE at Athens, Solon passed a law (594 BCE) that a certain individual, Thersippos (known only from this passage) who had been maimed in a battle be supported at the expense of the state, and that Peisistratos, in promulgating a law that all those maimed in battle be maintained at public expense, was following Solon's example, in extending an individual grant to the entire body of the war-wounded incapable of work. This, the only notice of this payment, finds no echo in the Aristotelian *Athenaion Politeia*, which does deal with payments made to citizens incapable of working, the *adunatoi*. Perhaps it is to be imagined that the payment to the war-maimed was extended and that they were subsumed into this category of disability. But it is more likely that they were kept in a separate category due to how they incurred their disability, in fighting for the polis (Herakleides of Pontos F149 (Wehrli) [Plut. *Sol.* 31.2; schol. Aeschines 1.103]; pensions at Athens for war-disabled: Jacoby *FGrH* vol. 3b Suppl. 1: 562-64; Dillon 1995: 30).

Adunatoi as disabled citizens at Athens

Athens was the only Greek state, as far as the evidence indicates, which had specifically legislated for a financial payment to be made to those male citizens whom the state considered to be physically disabled: a disabled citizen, speaking in defence of his right to collect an allowance due to his disability, notes: 'the city voted us this allowance' (Lys. 24.22: by a *psephisma*, decree). This law, it might seem to go without saying, applied only to Athenian male citizens. For this allowance, the ancient sources are limited. A passage in the Aristotelian *Athenaion*

Politeia, in its discussion of the political workings of the Athenian constitution, is the main source. Lysias wrote a speech for an actual legal case (24), in which a disabled individual who had in the past received the allowance made to the disabled had lost his right to this (cf. Rose in this volume, with a different interpretation). Aeschines in his lawcourt speech prosecuting an Athenian citizen, Timarchos (delivered in 346 BCE), accused him (amongst other things) of being a male prostitute, and of not assisting his uncle, Arignotos, to retain his allowance as a disabled citizen. These two speeches both, in fact, deal with cases in which *adunatoi* lost their allowances, a theme to be further explored below. This allowance was a payment, a *misthos*, the same term as employed for the salaries given to political officials and jurors.[1]

At the turn of the 5th century, when the defendant of Lysias 24 delivered his speech (*Concerning Not Having the Money for the* Adunatoi *Paid to Him*), the allowance given to the physically disabled was 1 obol per day, and this is the amount this defendant had been receiving (26). In the Aristotelian *Athenaion Politeia*, probably written in the 320s BCE, the allowance was 2 obols and had obviously been increased, while Philochoros wrote that it was 9 drachmas a month: this is a rough, imprecise estimate. For 2 obols a day for thirty days makes 60 obols, or 10 drachmas (or the lexicographer could have accidentally written nine instead of ten (Dillon 1995: 46): Philochoros *FGrH* 328 F197a (Harpokration and Suida *s.v. adunatoi*; cf. Rhodes 1972: 175–6). These increases in the allowance reflect the increase in jury pay, which had originally been 1 obol per day of active duty for each juror, was then increased to 2, and eventually reached 3. This amount for the juror's allowance was designed to meet the living expenses of a juror while he was serving in the courts. Many of the jurors were old men, who would have been too old and infirm to work, and are satirized as such by Aristophanes in the *Wasps*. At least in the case of the old juror who is the main protagonist in the *Wasps*, he lives at home with his family, and his 3 obols will have been a welcome supplement to the family's income. One obol, eventually 3, for the *dikastai*, and 1 then later 2 for the *adunatoi*, would have met many incidental living expenses and been an important financial supplement for the poor and physically challenged. That the *adunatoi* received their allowance at a daily rate was an acknowledgement that the *adunatoi* had little or no capacity to work, and needed this money each day and, as in the case of the *adunatos* of Lysias 24, that they often had no family to support them (Lys. 24.6; cf. Grassl 1986; Fischer 2012). While it has been doubted that Lysias 24 was actually a speech delivered before the Boule (it has been suggested it is a rhetorical exercise), the sheer difficulties of the speaker in arguing his case and the complexities of his argument are strong proofs that this is an actual case heard before the Boule: for no legal case is straightforward and all rely on an element of deception on the speakers' part (Dillon 1995: 37–8, with references).

Scrutinizing the disabled: the *dokimasia* (examination) of the *adunatoi*

Athenian democracy was very much preoccupied with accounting for public monies spent. Officials underwent a *dokimasia* (examination) before they entered office, to ascertain they were fit to serve, and also rendered an official account, a *euthyna*, when they completed their term of office, including a record of all monies they had received and spent as part of their official duties. Athens' *adunatoi* also underwent a *dokimasia* at the beginning of each official year to confirm that they would continue receiving for another year the payment for being unable to work. It is unknown what happened to someone, such as a soldier, who became disabled as a result of battle at some stage before or after the annual *dokimasia*. Presumably, individual cases could be assessed throughout the year. *Dokimasiai* and *euthynai* of officials were conducted by the jury courts, the *dikasteria*, which were considered to be representative of the demos. For some reason, the *dokimasia* of the disabled was conducted by the Boule, rather than the courts.

A court such as was used in public cases, of 1,500 *dikastai*, could perhaps not provide a suitable environment in which to see if an individual citizen was disabled or not. Clearly the *dokimasia* of a disabled citizen involved him physically displaying the disability which rendered him unfit for work, and would need to take place within a venue and by a political body which could clearly see his infirmity, or in the case of infirmities such as blindness, could be carried out at close quarters. So the speaker of Lysias 24 enjoins the Boule to believe the evidence of its 'own eyes' as he speaks before them, rather than the mere words of the prosecutor (14).

Just as the Aristotelian *Athenaion Politeia* discusses other *dokimasiai*, it relates the one for the *adunatoi*:

> A *dokimasia* of the *adunatoi* is carried out by the boule: for there is a law (*nomos*) which prescribes that those who own less than 3 *mnai* worth of property and are disabled (*pepērōmenous*), with the consequence that they are unable to carry out any work, are to be scrutinized by the boule, which is to give them 2 obols a day for sustenance from public money. There is a treasurer for the *adunatoi*, being elected by lot.
>
> *(Arist. Ath. Pol. 49.4; cf. Grassl 1989: 54; Rhodes 1993: 570)*

Bodily incapacitation was the requirement to be classified as an *adunatos* by the Boule, as representative of the citizen body. While the *adunatos* in Lysias 24 (12) hobbles around on two sticks, Timarchos' uncle Arignotos was blind (Aeschines, *Tim.* 102). Both of these had received the payments for *adunatoi*, and are the only two references to the nature of the actual disabilities which would receive payments. Presumably those who were deaf would not have been eligible, with the disability needing to be one which actually made one incapable of doing any work.

In assessing the *adunatoi*, the Boule clearly had more than one responsibility (see Rhodes 1972: 175–6 for the Boule and its scrutiny of the disabled). It would have needed to ascertain that each applicant had less than 3 *mnai* of property. This is a relatively small amount, of 300 drachmas, with the daily wage of an unskilled labourer being about 1 drachma a day. So an *adunatos* was allowed to have 300 drachmai worth of property. It was not required by the state that the disabled person sell or use up this property and live on it until he was penniless, but rather it recognized that a disabled person would have property, such as clothes, cooking utensils and the like. What is interesting is that this maximum amount of wealth disqualified the disabled home-owner from receiving the allowance. What this seems to mean is that a disabled person who lived in their own home would be the responsibility of the *oikos* of which that home was the main constituent part. This too might be why Arignotos, another *adunatos*, was left off the list of *adunatoi* at a *dokimasia*, although in previous years he had been on it. For he had in the past been wealthy, quite wealthy in fact, and might not have been able to persuade the particular Boule of the year that he was in possession of no more than 300 drachmas. Aischines refers to his case:

> And finally, and most horribly, when the old man's name [Arignotos] had been left off at the *dokimasia* of the *adunatoi*, and he brought a supplication (*hiketēria*) for the allowance (*misthos*) to the boule, [Timarchos, his nephew] although a *bouleutes* and one of the presiding officers (*proedroi*) for the day, did not condescend to speak on his behalf, but stood by and let him be deprived of his monthly allowance (*misthos*).
>
> *(Aischines, Tim. 104; cf. Suida s.v. Timarchos [Adler T495])*

Those who had been *adunatoi* in previous years had to submit to an annual *dokimasia*. Yet their disabilities presumably did not change or go away (be healed). This is a reflection of the Athenian scrupulousness that state financial issues be revisited annually. A previous council may have made decisions about who was to receive about 360 obols a year, but this then needed to be corroborated each year by a new Boule, of 500 new members. In addition, the Boule was to ensure that other provisions of the *nomos* were met – not just that the *adunatos* was still disabled, but also that they still possessed no more than 3 *mnai*, i.e. 300 drachmas.

Payments for the disabled 'incapable of performing any work'

Defending his right to the allowance, which he has received for many years but which had been disallowed in the latest *dokimasia*, the speaker of Lysias 24 stresses that he has no property:

> My father bequeathed me nothing, and I only stopped looking after my mother when she died two years ago, and at this stage I have no children to care for me. I carry out a trade (*technē*) which gives me but little help, and it's a difficult one for me to work at, and I'm not able yet to find someone who could take over the work of it for me. I have nothing to live on bar this payment: if you take it away from me, I would be in grave danger of being in the most dreadful circumstances.
>
> *(Lysias 24.6)*

He is aiming to show that he has no money – 'My father left me nothing'. Yet his statement is in some ways a strange one. His father has left him nothing; he mentions no siblings, and perhaps he was an only child. He has been supporting his aged mother until two years ago, and presumably his 1 obol a day was going towards this, as well as some little money which he can earn himself, as becomes apparent later in the speech (24.6, 19–20, 26). At this stage he has no children 'to care for' him. Does this mean that he expects the Boule to believe that at some stage he will marry, and support not only a wife but also children, until such a stage as the children are adults and can support him? Now this could not be done on 300 drachmas worth of property, the maximum amount an *adunatos* could possess and draw the allowance, and 1 obol a day. There is in the *nomos*, as reported by the *Athenaion Politeia* (49.4), no provision made for a disabled person who can undertake some work: those classified as *adunatoi* by the Boule were to be 'unable to carry out any work'. If this passage is taken as a literal reflection of the actual law, the disabled person who can perform some work would not receive any allowance. This is a point which is clearly at dispute in the case of which Lysias 24.

Technically, if the Aristotelian *Athenaion Politeia* is correct, an *adunatos* had to be incapable of work. This is clearly a point the accuser in the speech has raised, arguing that the defendant is 'able with respect to his body' and not one of the *adunatoi* (24.4–5). For the prosecution, the case rested largely on this charge of able-bodiedness, and his working at a trade. In any case in which a citizen who applied for the disabled allowance for the first time, or for its continuance, the disability would need to be proved by the applicant. If he was missing an arm or leg, or any combination of such, or was clearly physically afflicted in some way (such as being a hunchback), proving status as an *adunatos* and being able to benefit from the law concerning *adunatoi* would seem easy enough to ascertain. But there will have been borderline cases, as always with disabilities.

In Lysias 24, the prosecutor has set out to prove that the *adunatos* is not disabled: he has pointed out to the Boule that the *adunatos* is 'able-bodied' (4), 'strong of body' (5), so this is obviously a point that according to the law would disqualify a citizen from *adunatos* status. This strength of body is shown, the prosecutor alleges, because the defendant rides horses.

(Riding a horse can indeed require a degree of bodily strength, particularly in the thighs, but many trained horses can be ridden for distances without requiring that the rider be physically strong – it is simply a matter, of course, of sitting on the beast, especially if the travel is to be at a walking pace, rather than a gallop.) Meeting this equine point, the *adunatos* argues that he rides horses which he borrows from friends (10–11). It is precisely because he is disabled that he rides a horse, particularly for the longer trips which he has to make. Mounting and riding a horse, he argues, is not a sign of his wholeness of body, but of the reverse. He employs the horses as an aid to mobility, to ameliorate his crippledness, as is the manner of all those, he argues, who suffer from some misfortune (*dystychēma*: 10). His riding borrowed horses is the strongest proof (*megiston tekmērion*) of his disability; moreover, a little later he stresses the infrequency of this mode of transport: he is 'compelled every once and a while to borrow other men's horses' (12). This argument will have had a resonance with a jury, for borrowing in kind (as opposed to money) was very much a part of Athenian and Greek culture generally (Theophrastos, *Characters* 10.13; Millett 1991: 38; at Sparta, horses and dogs were borrowed when not in use by their owners: Xenophon, *Spartan Constitution* 6.3).

Yet clearly the prosecutor has linked this borrowing with the alleged prosperity of the *adunatos*, for the defendant moves on from borrowing the horses to arguing that if he were indeed a 'man of substance' (11), he would ride upon a saddled mule, and would not borrow other men's horses. (A saddled mule would be more comfortable for a cripple than an unsaddled one, more comfortable than a horse, and be easier to mount and dismount.) By this, he presumably means that he would hire the mule as occasion required – and if his prosecutor saw him on a saddled mule he would say nothing, for what would be more natural for a crippled man (12)? Yet, he asks rhetorically, given that he uses two sticks to walk – others use one – his prosecutor should argue that this shows that he is in fact 'able-bodied' for he employs the horses and his two sticks for the self-same purpose, for transportation (12). These sticks are clearly proof of his disability, a way of showing to the Boule that he is indeed handicapped (cf. Plutarch, *Mor.* 922b: the lame (*khōloi*) cannot walk without a stick). Yet, of the many weak points in Lysias 24, that he does not even mention his trade (tempered perhaps by his assertion that all the *bouleutai* know of it, 5) is the least strong. He is very vague on the amount of wealth which he has: his father left him nothing (6), and he asserts that his trade (*technē*) gives him *little* financial assistance (6). For despite his poverty, he did associate with many who, as his prosecutor notes, are men of means and own horses (4–5).

Disabled citizens and political office at Athens

This leads the speaker on to a point which has been explored above – state decrees concerning religious positions. At Kos and other places, laws discriminated against the disabled, not by naming disabilities which made people ineligible for religious roles, but by ruling that priests and priestesses had to be 'whole of body'. Appealing to the religious sensitivities of the *bouleutai*, the *adunatos* facing disqualification in Lysias 24 advances a very persuasive argument when he puts this proposition to the *bouleutai*: if the prosecutor convinces them that he is not disabled, he can exercise his citizen rights to their fullest possible extent:

> If he should convince you that I am sound of body, boule, what is to stop me from drawing the lot to hold office as one of the nine archons, and you from divesting me of the one obol, as being of sound health (*hygiainontos*), and all of you voting to award the obol to this man as being a cripple (*anapēros*)? For actually, if you took away this allowance from me because I am sound of limb (*dynamenos*), the

thesmothetai could not disqualify me from seeking election by lot to this position because I am disabled (*adunatos*)?

(Lysias 24.13)

Here, the argument is that, if the Boule judges him to be healthy of body, they might as well judge his prosecutor to be a cripple, so absurd would this be. If he can be one of the nine archons, he could well be the *basileus* (king) archon, charged with various religious rites and acting as the ritual agent of Dionysos on behalf of the city (Demosthenes 59; ([Arist.] *Ath. Pol.* 57.1; Garland 1984: 112). He could in fact be any of the three most important of the nine archons – so as well as the *basileus*, he could hold office as the eponymous archon (and so give his name to the year) or the *polemarchos* (war-archon), and both of these also had specific religious duties ([Arist.] *Ath. Pol.* 3.3, 56 and 58.1; Garland 1984: 112); the other six archons were the thesmothetai, a 'law-officer' type of position. One can readily imagine the defendant *adunatos* making his two sticks prominent as he made this point. He must also be referring to the political duties that were in the competence of these offices. A question here is whether there was a custom that *adunatoi* could not put their name forward for selection to these archonships, or was there actually a *nomos* that prevented them from doing so? Was it simply socially expected that disabled citizens would not apply for and fulfil these roles?

Athens had several hundred political posts, and the defendant is clearly using the archonships as the most prominent and graphic example of these positions – and he is using them to convince the Boule. As the Aristotelian *Athenaion Politeia* notes, the Athenian state maintained many of its citizens by paying them for their public offices (in the heyday of the 5th-century empire, up to 20,000 citizens could serve the polis for pay: *Ath. Pol.* 24.1–3, cf. 62.2). Payments to the *adunatoi* were a realization of the fact that *adunatoi*, unlike other citizens, could not draw pay (*misthos*) for political office, and in particularly could not draw the most common payment which 6,000 citizens did, chosen each year to be *dikastai* jurors.

Poverty and disability

Yet it is his poverty that he needs to prove as well. Having argued that his crippled nature leads him to borrow horses, and that if he actually did have some money he would hire a saddled mule, he now must prove that he is penniless, as his father left him. So he mockingly challenges his accuser to an *antidosis*, a formal, legal procedure. If a man found himself nominated for a public liturgy, he could nominate another to take his place, maintaining that the other citizen was wealthier and more able to meet the financial obligations of this position. If the other man refused, he could challenge him to an *antidosis*, to 'swap' properties (Harrison 1971: 236–8). So the *adunatos* argues:

> The greatness of my impoverishment can, it seems to me, be demonstrated more clearly by the prosecutor than by any other man. For if I were compelled to undertake the liturgy of the costs for a chorus for a tragedy, and I were to challenge him to an exchange of property (*antidosis*), he would rather pay for the expenses of the chorus ten times than to exchange property with me just once.

(Lysias 24.9)

Athenian jurors took liturgies and their performance very seriously, and it is likely that the members of the Boule did as well. Another neat way in which he secures his impoverished state is to mock the prosecutor: he is carrying on as if he were prosecuting a case about an heiress and her estate (14). How could he the defendant be hybristic and savage, as described by the prosecutor: 'for it is not probable that hybris would be shown by those who are stricken with extreme poverty, but rather by men who are in possession of much greater than the mere necessities of life' (16, cf. 15).

His prosecutor has accused him of having a *technē*: and this presents a problem for the *adunatos*. He does not name this, but simply indicates that the Boule will be aware of it (5). Many wretched men (*ponēroi*) meet up at his shop, argues the prosecutor, who have wasted their own means and plan to deprive others of theirs (so has he been accused of running a den of thieves? 19). Yet this, counters the *adunatos*, can happen at any establishment – the perfumery, a barber's or a shoemaker's (19–20), all of which the *bouleutai* frequent. But why does he not name his own establishment – it is not a perfumery, barber's or shoemaker – so what was it? He has a *technē*, the prosecutor asserts, that would enable him to do without his obol a day, a *technē* that provides, 'an abundance of means that permits me to fraternize with men who have the funds to spend up big' (5). Something is a little odd here, as Lamb noted: the Boule is hearing about 'the humble way of life of a small, struggling tradesman, who has to conceal his uneasy sense of being able to do a certain amount of work under the brave air of a crippled man who is making a hard fight for existence' (Lamb 1930: 517).

After hearing this case, the Boule for this year needed to make a decision on the basis that the *nomos* specifically states that an *adunatos* is someone incapable of work, who can receive 1 obol a day (the level of the allowance at the time of his speech). Yet this *adunatos* admits that he has a *technē*, as the prosecutor accuses. Why then does he want this 1 obol a day, for which he would need to be quite financially desperate? To answer this objection, he argues: 'my trade can render me but little assistance', and he practises it with difficulty (alluding of course to his disabled state; 24.6).

Part of the law concerning *adunatoi*, presumably part of the original decree, was to establish a treasurer for the Boule, who paid their allowance to them: 'There is a treasurer (*tamias*) for the *adunatoi*, being elected by lot' ([Arist.] *Ath. Pol.* 49.4). Aeschines refers to the *adunatos* Arignotos receiving his monthly allowance (Aesch. 1.104), so the *nomos* for the disabled must have stipulated that they would receive their obol per day (or two) once a month. This was only humane – for the *adunatoi* to collect their allowance on a daily basis would have been inconvenient to them, making their way to the collection point and then waiting, each day, to receive it. Moreover, a monthly payment was administratively easier than a daily pay-out, with the *tamias* handing out the allowance just once a month. This *tamias* will have been elected for one year, as were other Athenian officials. It would not have been one of the *adunatoi* themselves as the disabled did not hold political office, and moreover, that would not be seen as physically qualified to do so. This *tamias*, like all other officials, would have been required to undergo a *dokimasia* to ascertain his fitness for office, and then a *euthyna* before the courts at the completion of his office, involving a written account of all the sums he had received and disbursed for the payments.

Reconstructing the Athenian law (*nomos*) for payments to the disabled

Probably at some stage in the 5th century BCE the original law was passed by the *ekklesia*, and can be partially reconstructed as follows from the Aristotelian *Athenaion Politeia* 49.4, Lysias 24, and Aeschines 1.103–4:

- the Boule each year would conduct a *dokimasia* of those male citizens who claimed to be *adunatoi*;

- the Boule would decide if an individual was an *adunatos* to the extent that they could not carry out any work whatsoever for a living;
- the *Boule* would assess the property which such an *adunatos* owned; if it were less than 3 *mnai*, the citizen was paid the allowance; if his property was more than this, the Boule was not to grant him the *misthos*;
- it was solely the decision of the Boule as to who was classified as an *adunatos* and who was not;
- (those wounded in war were dealt with separately under the provisions of Solon and Peisistratos);
- the allowance was to be for 1 obol per day (increased by subsequent decree to 2 obols);
- any citizen could challenge, before the Boule, the claim of another citizen to be an *adunatos*, and the *adunatos* could answer in turn;
- the *adunatos* could supplicate the Boule to be reinstated on the list of *adunatoi* receiving the allowance;
- others could speak in favour of the *adunatos*, including members of the Boule;
- there was to be a *tamias* (treasurer), elected each year by lot from amongst the citizen body, from the requisite property classes (treasurers were drawn from the top two, the *pentakosiomedimnoi* and the *hippeis*), who would pay the amount of the allowance to the *adunatoi* once a month;
- like others, this law would have been inscribed on stone.

Athenian pity for the disabled citizen

This *nomos*, as far as the evidence allows, was unique in the ancient Greek world. Apparently only Athens, with its preoccupation with democratic ideology and a concern for the poor, had such a law. At a politically pragmatic level, it prevented the poor disabled citizen from falling into the patronage of aristocrats (Dillon 1995). But humanitarian feelings for fellow male citizens were obviously to the forefront: when Aeschines attacks Timarchos for not assisting his blind and impoverished uncle to be enlisted again as an *adunatos* (1.104), even though Timarchos was actually not only on the Boule but present at the hearing of his case, in fact was one of the presiding officers (*proedroi*) for that day, the jurors were obviously meant to feel outraged at this. Timarchos both failed to assist a relative, and one whom he had impoverished (Aeschines claims), and abandoned a blind man when he could give him assistance at the *dokimasia*. Such behaviour was clearly meant to arouse anger, that Timarchos could not pity even his blind uncle.

As Aeschines does with the *dikastai*, so too does the speaker make a strong appeal to the humanitarian feelings of the *bouleutai*. He claims that he has no money except this obol (6), and there is a strong element of piteous appeal in his argument (for which see esp. Carey 1990: 47; cf. Dillon 1995: 53–4): 'If someone envies those whom others feel pity for, from what type of evil would such a man not shrink from?' (2). If the Boule deprives him of this allowance, he argues:

> I would be in danger of falling into the most dreadful circumstances. So don't, boule, when it is in your power to succour me justly, unjustly destroy me. And don't snatch away from me what you gave to me when I was younger, now that I'm older and weaker. Moreover, given your former renown for displaying an extreme of pity towards those men who are actually not in trouble, don't be persuaded by this man to treat harshly those who are piteous even to their enemies. Nor should you have the hardness of heart to treat me unjustly, and make all the other (*adunatoi*) in my position feel wretched … When my difficulty was but slight, I was then seen taking

this money, but now, when I am assaulted by old age, sicknesses, and the problems that are go hand in hand with these, I have it taken away from me.

(Aeschines, Tim. 7)

Old age, disease, infirmity, poverty and what will otherwise be his grievous plight: these are mentioned precisely because they will raise pity amongst the *bouleutai*, which along with appearing before it with two sticks, will make him an object of pity. Interestingly, the *adunatos* refers to the community of the *adunatoi* – it is not his individual plight alone, but that of all the physically disabled citizens who are disabled and receiving this allowance. If his is cancelled, it will send a ripple effect through this group. For it is to be imagined that many did indeed supplement the obol in some way, possibly even by begging, or through some small trade or even commerce in public places. There was a sense, too, amongst the Athenians, that it was certainly not the disabled's fault that he was so, for it was fate that apportioned the condition of an *adunatos*, and so the city decreed that the payment be made, 'considering the chances of evils and of good things to be the same for all in common' (22). (For pity of the poor in ancient Greece, see Hands 1968: 77–86; Laes 2008: 114 and 2013a: 137 on blame and sin.)

This official payment was not so much a charity, but rather a form of social assistance to those in need: it was specifically for those who through no fault of their own were physically impaired to the extent that they could not generate their own income. Related to this was the Greek aversion to beggars, who were seen as capable of earning their own livelihood, but as being too lazy to do so (cf. Hands 1968: 64–5). There was no charity as such towards the poverty-stricken: the Athenians were of the view that 'the actual disgrace of poverty is not so much in not recognizing it, but in doing nothing to extricate oneself from it' (Thuc. 2.40.1). Athens expected the poor to work, but considered that social aid was just for those who could not do so.

Aeschines' speech prosecuting Timarchos dates to 345 BCE, and the Aristotelian *Athenaion Politeia*, which gives the details of the law, was written in the early 320s BCE. This is the last reference to the law. It is probable that it became redundant when democracy was overthrown in 322 BCE, and possibly not reintroduced when it was reinstated, for nothing more is ever heard of it. Athenian *adunatoi* without 3 *mnai* of property will have no longer received the allowance, and the ancient world's first system to provide financial support for those who could not work because of their physical disability came to an end.

Conclusion

Spartan infants who were born disabled were left to die in a pit, either by written or unwritten law; Plato would legislate that physically disabled babies be killed at birth. Athens cared for physically disabled citizens by a law granting them a specific daily allowance, paid monthly. But it was scrupulous about the award of this single obol, or later two, and the physically disabled had to prove their disability and their lack of property. That the cripple with two sticks in Lysias 24 can earn some money ought to have disqualified him, for the law specifically stated that the allowance was for those who were 'unable to carry out any work' ([Arist.] *Ath. Pol.* 49.4). However, the Athenians with their usual pragmatism do not seem to have, until the date of this speech, adhered to the letter of this law, though if this Boule accepted the case of the prosecution, this cripple would be forced back onto his *technē* (and his associates) alone. Aeschines and this crippled speaker evoked pity and appealed to the Boule's sense of it; such pity provided much of the original motivation for this *nomos* and its allowance, and indicate that the ancient Athenians did have a sense of pity for the plight of others who could not work – not for those, necessarily, who lived in poverty, but to those who could not escape it through hard work. Athens was also conscious that the poor might become dependent on wealthy patrons, and sought through the allowance to ensure an independent citizenry not dependent on the rich for its livelihood. As such, through this legislation, Athens was perhaps unique in the Greek world in providing monetary assistance to those citizens who suffered from physical disabilities.

Abbreviations

ED   Mario Segre, *Iscrizioni di Cos*. 2 vols (Rome, 1993).

LSAM   Franciszek Sokolowski, *Lois sacrées de l'Asie mineure* (Paris, 1955).

LSCG   Franciszek Sokolowski, *Lois sacrées des cités grecques* (Paris, 1969).

SGDI   Hermann Collitz, Friedrich Bechtel, *et al.* (eds), *Sammlung der Griechischen Dialekt-Inschriften*. 4 vols (Göttingen, 1884–1915).

SIG³   Wilhelm Dittenberger, *Sylloge Inscriptionum Graecarum*. 4 vols (Leipzig, 1915–1924³).

Note

1   The terms used are: *misthos* (pay): Aeschines, *Against Timarchos* 1.103; *trophē* (sustenance): [Arist.] *Ath. Pol.* 49.4; *to argurion* (the silver): Lys. 24.8. For the *adunatoi* and their allowance, the main ancient sources are [Arist.] *Ath. Pol.* 49.4; Philochoros *FGrH* 328 F197a (Harpokration and Suida *s.v.. adunatoi*); Lysias 24; Aeschines, *Against Timarchos* 1.103–4. See Rhodes 1993: 570 (on [Arist.] *Ath. Pol.* 49.4); Dillon 1995 (with previous bibliography); Garland 1995: 35-38; brief comments: Hands 1968: 10, 173 n. 165; Edwards 1997: 37–8; Stiker 1999: 45–6. See also Rose 2003: 95–8, and in this volume.

Bibliography

Carey, Christopher, 'Structure and Strategy in Lysias XXIV', *Greece and Rome* 37 (1990), 44–51.
Dillon, Matthew P. J., 'Payments to the Disabled at Athens: Social Justice or Fear of Aristocratic Patronage?', *Ancient Society* 26 (1995), 27–57.
Dillon, Matthew P. J., 'Post-Nuptial Sacrifices on Kos (Segre, *ED* 178) and Ancient Greek Marriage Rites', *Zeitschrift für Papyrologie und Epigraphik* 124 (1999), 63–80.
Dillon, Matthew P. J., 'Home and Hearth. The Classical Greek Experience of Domestic Religion', in E. Eidinow and J. Kindt (eds), *The Oxford Handbook of Religion in the Ancient World* (Oxford, 2015), 241–55.
Dillon, Matthew P. J., '"Chrysis the Hiereia Having Placed a Lighted Torch Near the Garlands Then Fell Asleep (Thucydides iv.133.3)": Priestesses Serving the Gods and Goddesses in Classical Greece', in S. Budin (ed.), *Women in Antiquity: Real Women from across the Ancient World* (Oxford and New York, 2016), 683–702.
Edwards, Martha L. [= Rose, Martha L.], 'Constructions of Physical Disability in the Ancient Greek World: The Community Concept', in D. T. Mitchell and S. L. Snyder (eds), *The Body and Physical Difference: Discourses of Disability* (Ann Arbor, MI, 1997), 35–50.
Fischer, Josef, 'Behinderung und Gesellschaft im klassischen Athen: Bemerkungen zur 24. Rede des Lysias', in R. Breitwieser (ed.), *Behinderungen und Beeinträchtungen/Disability and Impairment in Antiquity* (Oxford, 2012), 41–5.
Garland, Robert, 'Religious Authority in Archaic and Classical Athens', *Annual British School at Athens* 79 (1984), 75–123.
Garland, Robert, *The Eye of the Beholder: Deformity and Disability in the Graeco-Roman World* (Ithaca, NY, 1995).
Grassl, Herbert, 'Behinderung und Arbeit', *Eirene* 26 (1989), 49–57.

Grassl, Herbert, 'Behinderte in der Antike', *Tyche* 1 (1986), 118–26.

Hands, Arthur Robinson, *Charities and Social Aid in Greece and Rome* (London, 1968).

Harrison, Alick R. W., *The Law of Athens*, II. *Procedure* (Oxford, 1971).

Laes, Christian, 'Learning from Silence: Disabled Children in Roman Antiquity', *Arctos* 42 (2008), 85–122.

Laes, Christian, 'Raising a Disabled Child', in J. Evans Grubbs and T. Parkin (eds), *The Oxford Handbook of Childhood and Education in the Classical World* (Oxford, 2013a), 125–44.

Laes, Christian, 'Silent History? Speech Impairment in Roman Antiquity', in C. Laes, C. F. Goodey and M. L. Rose (eds), *Disabilities in Roman Antiquity: Disparate Bodies* A Capite ad Calcem (Leiden, 2013b), 145–80.

Laes, Christian, 'Infants between Biological and Social Birth in Antiquity: A Phenomenon of the *Longue Durée*', *Historia* 63 (2014), 364–83.

Lamb, Walter R. M., *Lysias: With an English Translation* (London, 1930).

Millett, Paul, *Lending and Borrowing in Ancient Athens* (Cambridge, 1991).

Patterson, Cynthia, '"Not Worth the Rearing"': The Causes of Infant Exposure in Ancient Greece', *Transactions and Proceedings of the American Philological Association* 115 (1985), 103–23.

Rhodes, Peter John, *The Athenian Boule* (Oxford, 1972).

Rhodes, Peter John, *A Commentary on the Aristotelian Athenaion Politeia* (Oxford, 1993²).

Rose, Martha L., *The Staff of Oedipus: Transforming Disability in Ancient Greece* (Ann Arbor, MI, 2003).

Schmidt, Martin, 'Hephaistos lebt: Untersuchungen zur Frage der Behandlung behinderter Kinder in der Antike', *Hephaistos: Kritische Zeitschrift zur Theorie und Praxis der Archäologie und angrenzender Wissenschaften* 5–6 (1983–4), 133–61.

Stiker, Henri-Jean, *A History of Disability,* tr. W. Sayers (Ann Arbor, MI, 1999).

Wilgaux, Jérôme, 'Ὑγιὴς καὶ ὁλόκλαρος: Le corps du prêtre en Grèce ancien', in P. Brulé (ed.), *La norme en matière religieuse en Grèce ancienne* (Liège, 2009), 231-42.

Willetts, Ronald F., *The Law Code of Gortyn* (Berlin, 1967).

13

THE HELLENISTIC TURN IN BODILY REPRESENTATIONS

Venting anxiety in terracotta figurines

Alexandre Mitchell

In the archaic age (600–480 BCE), Greek sculptors began to represent the human body in the round, their limbs finally losing their matchstick appearance. According to the 5th-century BCE sophist Protagoras (Plato, *Theaetetus* 152a–f), man was 'the measure of all things'. It is as if that Greek artists took this motto to heart and from the archaic age until the dawn of the Roman Empire in the late 1st century BCE, focusing their entire powers of observation and creativity on the human body. The representations underwent many changes, struggling between two poles, realism (*mimesis*) and idealism, either trying to show mimetically the human body as accurately as they could or, alternatively, showing it as well as they could according to certain notions of beauty. Disability did not earn a rightful place in representations until late in the Hellenistic age (322–31 BCE), and mainly in a cheap and mass-produced art form, terracotta figurines. After a quick review of the various artistic movements that preceded the Hellenistic age, we will consider a selection of physical deformities represented in terracotta figurines and what the function of some of these objects may have been.

Preliminary thoughts

Art often expresses a society's deepest joys and fears, its limitations and taboos. There is something pervasive in Greek art, a latent form of anxiety that may have originated in their appalling view of the afterlife. They had no vision of paradise but instead one of ever growing numbers of ghosts in the land of shadows, the Underworld – Hades (also called 'Plouton' which meant the 'rich one' in Greek). This awful view of death and its aftermath may explain their obsession with youth, with living life to the full, and their fear of inexorable decrepitude and old age. The greatest gift the gods could bestow on humans was to pluck them in the flower of youth (Herodotus 1.31). Their anxiety may also have come from constant warring between similar people, with often no end in sight, or possibly something even deeper, a sense of divine injustice. One could come to terms with losing limbs from a sudden disease or combat, treachery or pillage, but how did men reconcile their faith in the gods' almighty powers, wisdom and just retribution when children were not all born physically or mentally able? To avoid feeling powerless, Greek artists made sure the mimetic, experimental approach of their art was reined in by idealism which sought to show what one could be or should be rather than what one actually was. As a society, the Greeks sought to control their surroundings by reaching for order and balance. And their idealized art served this *kosmos*, this worldview. The Greek word *kosmos* contained the notions of 'order', 'arrangement' and 'beauty' all in one. Thus, there was very little space in such an ordered universe, where the order itself was beauty, for images of disability. From about 600 to the 330s, idealized representations tend to take over most other representations. They were best embodied in the aristocratic young Greek male, well-proportioned, white and athletic.

Greek artists' stock-in-trade for hundreds of years consisted mainly in idealized types, reproducing famous marble or bronze sculpture. A statuette originally found in Smyrna (Figure 13.1), measuring 0.29 m and dating to the 1st century BCE, is a small-scaled clay imitation of the famous *Diadoumenos* of Polykleitos, a youth tying a fillet around his head after a victory in an athletic context, in c.430 BCE. The life-size *Diadoumenos*,[1] is 1.86 m in height.

The Diadoumenos was evidently still favoured by customers as it was being reproduced in terracotta series, i.e. in large numbers, four hundred years later. Numerous terracotta copies of famous sculptures by Polykleitos and later Lysippos, were found throughout the Mediterranean. These images were archetypes of what men sought to be, images of winning athletes, living among the *aristoi*. The sculptor Polykleitos attempted to capture the ideal proportions of the human (mostly male) figure and wrote a treatise called *Kanon*, which exemplified his aesthetic principles, or mathematic proportions, called *symmetria* in Greek. To this day, we commonly use the term canon as 'rule'.

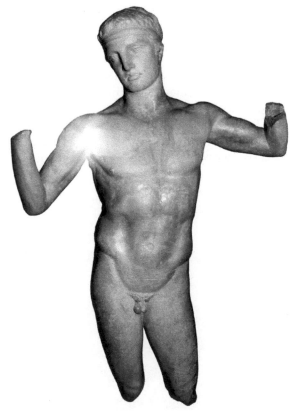

Figure. 13.1 The Diadumenos.Terracotta figurine, Paris, Musée du Louvre, on loan from New York, The Metropolitan Museum of Art, 32.11.2. Photograph © Alexandre G. Mitchell.

Images of disability in the Greek iconographic landscape are extremely rare prior to the Hellenistic age, whether in marble statuary, clay terracotta figurines or painted vases in the black- or red-figure techniques.[2] The 'others' consist in representations of women, old age, foreigners, figures from the Dionysian world and dwarves, none of which count as disabled human beings. Of course, even though dwarfism is not a disability, dwarves in Greek art offer a stark visual contrast with the *Kanon* or male athlete. However, if the affected individuals also suffered from related debilitating physical ailments like a front-to-back curvature of the spine, a pronounced sway of the lower back (lordosis) and bowed legs, then they would be considered disabled – from our point of view, as the status of disabled individuals in Antiquity was more complex than today. *Achondroplasia* was the most common type of short-limbed dwarfism, which often included *macrophally*. Dwarfs played a similar role as the other representatives of the 'otherness' category (ethnic jokes are rooted in the fear of the 'other' and his perceived difference): they lent their distinctive traits to the genre of caricature, to amuse the greater public and reaffirm the *kanon*, almost pay homage to the ruling imagery.

Caricature was a well-known genre since the archaic age. The word itself comes from the Italian *caricare* ('to load': first used in descriptions of some of Annibale Carracci's works). It consists in the grotesque or ludicrous representation of persons or things by exaggerating their most characteristic and striking features. In Greek caricature, African facial traits were often used in conjunction with dwarfism to emphasize the contrast with normally proportioned Greek men and women with Caucasian facial traits.

On one side (Figure 13.2) of a small *askos* (wine drinking vessel), a bald, deformed man leans on a staff; the other side shows a roaring lion. The man's body is absurdly small compared to his enormous head, larger than the whole body. He is leaning, his cloak folded under his left arm and hanging off the staff. He is strikingly caricatured. When examining unusual imagery, as we shall in this chapter, one should always keep in mind the visual representation of usual or 'common' imagery. The contrast ensures we do not overlook any potentially abnormal or grotesque representations. The figure's attitude is that of many nonchalant strollers or bystanders at the palaestra or the agora, seen in thousands of Greek vase-paintings. With such a huge head and pensive attitude, this figure could be a caricature of a sophist; not one in particular but what the common artisan in the Potters quarter thought of sophists, who spent their time thinking or chatting at the palaestra (for a physiognomic study and interpretation, see Zinserling 1967).

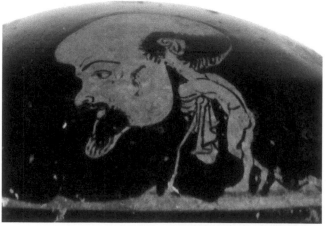

Figure 13.2 Caricatured bystander. Attic red-figure askos, Paris, Musée du Louvre, G610, 460–440 BCE. Photograph © Alexandre G Mitchell.

With the sudden changes in the geopolitics of ancient Greece, the loss of democracy, becoming part of Alexander's new empire, then refragmented at his death into smaller kingdoms, and eventually being beaten into shape by the Roman Empire, there was a simultaneous, distinct and almost paradigmatic shift in artistic experimentation. The need to show humans as they are, mimesis, was a need almost as strong as that of showing an idealized view and it was contained for a long time. The Greek anxiety which had previously turned to balance and idealism in the archaic and classical periods had a new way of venting its distress: *pathos*. For the first time, one could see faces contorted in pain or extreme pleasure. One could identify the fear of the unknown in the deep-set eye sockets of works by the famed Hellenistic sculptor Scopas. Idealism had not disappeared; it was just subdued in favour of mimesis. The Greek world had become much larger within a few decades: it extended all the way to India. One can scarcely imagine the conflicting artistic influences that infused and merged at the time. Still, there was no space in expensive materials and art forms, like marble sculpture or metal works, for images of disability. One must look in an entirely different art form: cheap market-produced, easily copied and moulded, clay terracotta figurines.

Grotesque terracotta figurines

With a few exceptions, it is only in this material and art form that we find thousands of representations of so-called 'grotesques', a wide-ranging umbrella term that refers to figurines displaying various forms of physical deformities. They were first studied in depth by Jean-Martin Charcot's team at the Salpêtriere in Paris in the 19th century (Régnault 1900, 1909a, b and c). These medical doctors with a passion for archaeology offer fascinating insights into previously unidentified objects. Despite their good intentions, we now understand that iconodiagnosis is fraught with dangers, chiefly overinterpretation of artistic objects as medical objects whilst disregarding their intended use or function. But the potential results are worth the risk. When D. Gourevitch teamed up with the medical doctor M. Grmek (Grmek and Gourevitch 1998), they produced excellent results, models of the fine balance required in the study of 'pathological grotesques'.

Indeed, as I have discussed elsewhere (Mitchell 2013) these figurines do not all show pathologies and need to be differentiated. Some of the caricatured, grotesquely deformed faces and bodies are in fact standardized caricatures, typical theatrical types, small versions of stage comedy actors, probably reproduced in terracotta as mementos of plays that people had seen performed or knew of. Other grotesques were in fact visual parodies of specific, well-known 'serious' models. The aim of these was to be humorous, to attract the eye and be purchased by prospective buyers at the market. There was nothing pathological about them. The close inspection of some of these parodies reveals a clever and bitter sense of humour, parodying boxers or famous types, like the *spinario*, a bronze sculpture which shows a young idealized boy pulling out a thorn from the sole of his foot. Others still were representative of what one might call a social realistic vein. They produced terracotta figurines in a veristic style with, apparently, no other interest than to show a failing body in old age or similar subjects. Pathological grotesques followed a mimetic approach that was very close to that of portraiture, but just as portraiture always included at least a small dose of idealism, pathological grotesques might have been true to their model in the observation of individual parts of the body, yet, as we shall see, still more often than not presented 'idealistic' *reconstructed* bodies and types.

A great many grotesques are in fact caricatures. There is a clear distinction between a pathological grotesque and a caricature: a caricature consists in the *intentional exaggeration* of someone's most characteristic features to produce a comic effect, whereas a pathological grotesque is an *intentional realism* towards the actual representation of a phenomenon: in other words, a portrait. Of course, artists did not follow our distinctions and principles, so a number of caricatured aspects coexist with realistic mimetic pathologies. Here, we will only discuss pathological representations, pathologies that would have been so debilitating that they would probably have been considered to be a *disability.*

Our first terracotta figurine (Figure 13.3), from Smyrna in Asia Minor was produced towards the end of the Hellenistic period. It shows a hunchback suffering from *acromegaly*, an uncommon chronic metabolic disorder in which there is too much growth hormone and the body tissues gradually enlarge in addition to other deformities. This male figurine in the Louvre[3] is unusual as it shows a number of deformities in one same body and exemplifies the problem suggested above: at first glance we have a hunchback dwarf with his head dug in between the shoulders. His ribs are pushed forward, and his hips deformed. These would definitely categorize this individual as being disabled. He is also bald, his nose large and hooked, his head anatomically placed where his neck should be, at the level of the clavicle, the insertion of the neck's trapezius muscle.

The age of the individual, which can be surmised from observing his face, seems far older than the muscular upper body. A man with such deformed hips and weak legs, could not have carried the weight of the upper body and still reached a ripe old age. Even if we imagine that his lips are swollen because of an allergic reaction, why would they be missing the line joining them? This figurine is a mixture of closely observed pathologies and unrealistic aspects.

The next figurine, also from Smyrna (Figure 13.4),[4] shows a crowned dwarf with a hump on his back, a gaping mouth and a prominent ribcage. This deformity may be caused by Pott's disease (Grmek and Gourevitch 1998: 217–19). A few details make this 'pathological' grotesque something more than a medical showcase: his enormous phallus, the suspension hole in his back and traces of red paint.

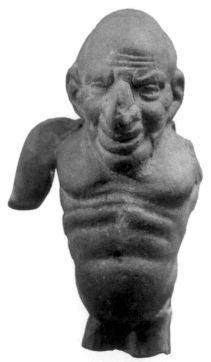

Figure 13.3 Hunchback suffering from acromegaly. Terracotta figurine, height 8 cm, Paris, Musée du Louvre, MNC266 (Myr 705) 100 BCE–100 CE. Photograph © Alexandre G Mitchell.

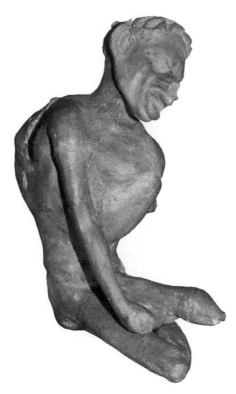

Figure 13.4 Dwarf with Pott's disease. Terracotta figurine, from Smyrna, height 7.5 cm, Paris, Musée du Louvre, CA5190. 2nd century BCE. Photograph © Alexandre G. Mitchell.

Traces of red paint have been found on many pathological grotesques and is the apotropaic colour *par excellence* throughout antiquity and to this day in many parts of the world. As far as the large phallus is concerned, it was 'talismanic in itself' (Stevenson 1975: 47). And, to quote Gourevitch (Gourevich and Grmek 1998: 214), 'the frequency of hunchbacks in ancient art is not as much caused by the real frequency of this pathological state than the magical meaning that is attributed to them … to reinforce this apotropaic effect, hunchbacks in good-luck artefacts were often given a huge phallus'. A suspension hole implies that the figurine was designed to be hung from a hook on a wall for example, like an amulet. The dwarf was crowned with ivy, which needs to be explained. The figure is not an athlete, evidently, but could be participating in a banquet as a comic entertainer, which is in itself a good reminder that being disabled did not mean that one could not work or earn a living in antiquity or at least earn one's keep. E.-J. Graham (2013) in a seminal study discusses this very problem from the point of view of palaeopathology, showing from the close examination of bones of 'disabled' individuals that they were also afflicted with certain bone or cartilage ailments linked to repetitive gestures, all typical of manual labour.

The crown could be a Dionysian sign. Smith (1991: 136) writing about unusual representations, genre and peasant imagery, states 'part of the Dionysian countryside is an impressive series of old labourers, derelict women and peasant boys. Many carry explicit badges of Dionysian membership, like ivy wreaths and most should be seen as part of his realm.' He might also serve as an apotropaic figurine, with the talismanic power of a priapic god and the focal power for envy and physical disability all in one. D. Gourevitch (Gourevich and Grmek 1998: 329) suggests that this figurine and other similar ones may have been inspired from truly observed clinical patients, especially with certain developmental diseases linked to a dysfunctional hormonal activity.

Whether the figurine was apotropaic or medical in nature, both these aspects are 'means of control' to counteract human powerlessness in the face of nature's random choices. Medicine is a rationalization, an attempt at naming, identifying and possibly curing what must have seemed a divine whim; producing 'anti-disease' figurines was a magical attempt to avert from what was perceived as being evil. Medical classification and magical amulets to control human fears and anxiety.

An uncommon facial acromegaly is shown in a small terracotta head in Brussels (Figure 13.5). This endocrine disorder is astonishingly rendered, with excess growth hormone production, characterized by gigantism and facial features with frontal bossing, a thick and hard nose, deepening of creases on the forehead and nasolabial folds, enlargement of the lower lip, nose and auricles (Volteranni 2002). The individual is also bald and his eyes closed which may indicate he is asleep or dead. Acromegaly takes a number of forms. It is an unusual affection, not genetically inherited, linked to growth hormone hypersecretion.

The most common cause for this affliction is a tumour of the hypophysis but as D. Gourevitch notes (Gourevich and Grmek1998: 199) these internal aspects are not artistically represented; only the external effects that manifest themselves with large hands and feet, prominent maxillaries, are shown in the figurines.

The next head (Figure 13.6), was described by F. Régnault (1907: 26–7) as one of a number of representations of leprosy. S. Mollard-Besques (1972: 234) felt that the nasal deviation was due to a clumsy gesture during the production. This is quite unlikely as these figurines are very precisely detailed and the artist would have simply rectified his mistake. D. Gourevich (Gourevich and Grmek 1998: 250) noted that the curious nasal deformity resembled the outward effects of a different and very specific infectious disease called rhinoscleroma. This is a chronic granulomatous condition of the nose and other structures of the upper respiratory tract.

Rhinoscleroma was not lethal in itself, but left untreated could lead to sepsis, bleeding or other chronic conditions that could be fatal. It is a disease which is however more often identified in tropical climates, in Africa and South America than the Eastern Mediterranean where this figurine was found. Interestingly, the outward signs of leprosy, certain facial deformities, were sometimes called *leontiasis* in antiquity but *leontiasis ossea* is in fact an entirely different condition.

Cases of leontiasis were known in classical antiquity but also in ancient Egypt, as reported by various authors with different interpretations and descriptions (Ashrafian 2005). *Leontiasis ossea* describes a number of conditions where a patient's face resembles that of a lion. The

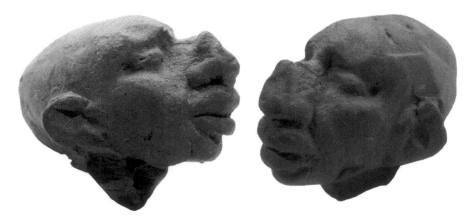

Figure 13.5 Facial acromegaly. Terracotta head, Brussels, Musées Royaux d'Art et d'Histoire M398, height. 3.2 cm. Photograph © Alexandre G. Mitchell.

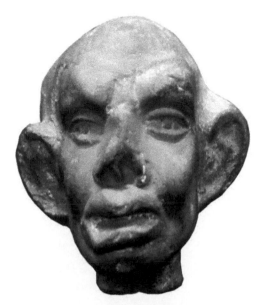

Figure 13.6 Leper (?). Terracotta head, from Smyrna, Paris, Musée du Louvre, E144. 1st century BCE
Photograph © Alexandre G. Mitchell.

main mechanism of true leontiasis ossea is a defect in differentiation and maturation with the replacement of normal bone with immature woven bone (craniofacial fibrous dysplasia). Many conditions may mimic a leontiasis face: endocrinopathy (gigantism or acromegaly, Cushing syndrome, secondary hyperparathyroidism after uraemia), neurology (neurofibromatosis), infection (syphilitic osteoperiostitis after the 15th century in Europe, Pott's disease by tuberculosis), tumour (paranasal sinus) that create an alteration of the cranial structures with cranial asymmetry, facial deformity, nasal stuffiness, bulging eyes (proptosis) and visual impairment or unilateral blindness (Mitchell and Lorusso 2014: 21–2). Another small terracotta head from Smyrna (Figure 13.7), shows some of the distinctive signs of leontiasis ('lion face') with hypertrophied maxillaries which give the impression of a lion's nose. The figure's grotesque facial features, are emphasized by the lack of facial hair, the baldness, a huge forehead and the fact that the ears are left unfinished. A human skull in Bologna (Figure 13.8), shows all the previously described outward signs of leontiasis ossea, the overgrowth of bone in the facial and cranial bones and just like in Figure 13.7, the maxilla must have progressively grown, eventually affecting the eye orbits, mouth, nose and sinuses. From a visual point of view, the lion face is clearly distinguishable, with a frightening prognathism because of the protruding lower maxilla.

In some cases, it is particularly unfortunate that the artwork should be fragmentary. For instance, a terracotta head in the Louvre (Ht. 6cm) is labelled 'monkey head' ('tête de singe hellénistique'). Yet, this very same head could well be a representation of a classic case of leontiasis ossea (Mitchell and Lorusso 2014: 28). The cranium of Figure 13.9 is different from the maxillofacial area. In a human the maxillofacial area, composed of the mouth, jaw, face, is smaller than the cranium. But in an ape (Figure 13.10), the two zones are almost identical in size. We have here a human face, slightly elongated into that of an ape's. But this head cannot be an ape's head. This is a mixture of various potential pathologies and unrealistic deformities. His hair is combed and parted in the middle, he has some facial hair, a rather trim beard that runs around the face but not over the upper lip. However, the pronounced facial features might be explained by a condition of leontiasis ossea.

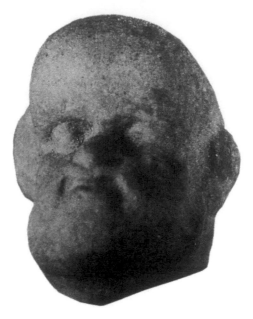

Figure 13.7 Leontiasis ('lion face'). Terracotta head, from Smyrna, Paris, Musée du Louvre, E/D 1747. 1st century BCE. (After Gourevitch 1998: fig. 179, pp. 233–4.)

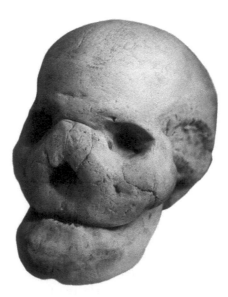

Figure 13.8 Human skull with leontiasis. Bologna, Luigi Cattaneo Museum, Institute of Human Anatomy. Photograph © Scott D. Haddow.

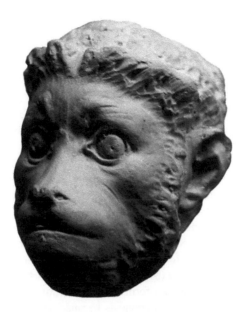

Figure 13.9 Leontiasis ('lion face'). Terracotta head, Paris, Musée du Louvre, CA3006, height 6 cm. 1st century BCE. Photograph © Alexandre G. Mitchell.

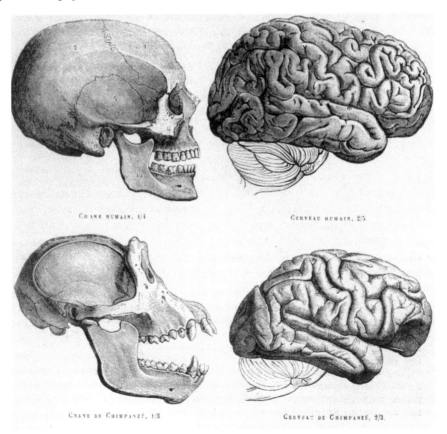

Figure 13.10 Comparison of ape and human skulls. Plate after Gervais 1854–5: 15

Conclusion

It is clear from the various representations that there was a wide range of representations in the Hellenistic period which differed greatly from those produced previously and, among the so-called grotesques, an almost equally vast number of different types, both male and female. What seems to be most interesting here, is that on close examination, while some of the representations display disabled individuals, the objects themselves are not straightforward medical wax figures. Even if some, if not many of these objects were produced based on the detailed observation of real clinical cases, the multiplicity or the improbable or impossible combination of certain diseases makes the interpretation of the objects all the more complex. None of the images described in this chapter were found in healing sanctuaries. If so, one might have been tempted to interpret them as ex-votos. We have numerous examples of ex-votos from healing sanctuaries dedicated to Asclepius, including hands, feet, eyes, noses, ears, breasts, brains and so on. Yet, none of these were injured or deformed. The ex-votos are perfect specimens (Stevenson 1975: 100, *contra* Roebuck 1951: pl. 40, no. 63).

The most plausible explanation for many of these objects remains an apotropaic one, i.e. good luck charms against the evil eye (Mitchell 2013). Some scholars imagined that a certain type found in numerous materials and art forms (clay terracotta figurines, clay lamps, mosaics, copper alloy figurines) suffered from tuberculosis because of the figure's distinctive choking gesture with both hands around its throat. Others thought it was the sign that the ingestion of a foreign object had blocked its breathing, others still that we were witnessing a form of autoerotic asphyxiation, as it is a known fact that strangulation increases the sense of pleasure and possibly explains the enlarged penis which is often found in this type. Yet, the penis is far too large to be in proportion with the rest of the body, and it is not in erection in these figures, whereas asphyxiation by hanging provokes the so-called 'death erection'. This type is found in large quantities, and often has a suspension hole in the back and sometimes visible traces of red paint. Thanks to an inscription in a mosaic in a Roman villa on the island of Cephalonia, this type was identified as a personification of Envy (*Phthonos*), suffocating with jealousy. The notion of the evil eye is based on envy (Greek: 'phthonos', Latin: 'invidia'), as envying consists in coveting by looking. The figurines probably hung near house thresholds as apotropaic symbols (Slane and Dickie 1993; Mitchell 2013). Most scholars agree on the talismanic properties of the phallus, of fertility and prosperity and a protection against the evil eye and evil spirits. Phallic amulets were ubiquitous in the Greek and Roman world, from good luck charms, to the numerous tiny (4-6 cm) bronze phallic amulets tied around the necks of babies and infants.

The need for these images was rooted in the precarious nature of human life in Antiquity, far more so than today, and the accompanying feeling of powerlessness when faced with a short life expectancy. Some of the images may have been produced to titillate the darker side of the human psyche, just like the preserved remains in the Hunterian museum in London, that reveal a morbid desire to be satisfied, or a way for viewers to reassure themselves they were still alive. These objects were a far cry from the visible pathos in the facial expression of *The Laocoon* for instance, but all the same they were produced in an effort to name and control an ever present fear, not to visually and faithfully present different physical disabilities to medical students. I chose the term anxiety because of its semantic weight. Anxiety is when anxious feelings are ongoing and do not subside. For those experiencing anxiety, these feelings cannot be easily controlled. Whether it was the terror of Apollo's priest, Laocoon, being torn apart by a divine snake come from the sea, whilst witnessing the murder of his own sons, or the fearful look in the eye of a Potts' disease sufferer with horrific physical deformities, these images were all produced in the same day and age. The difference between these images was their visual impact. Indeed, marble statues were costly and took time to be designed and produced for a patron, whether it was a private client, a corporation or a city. There are obvious limitations in this opulent and often propagandist form of art which are absent from cheaper materials like clay. Terracotta figurines were often moulded and produced in large series, for the marketplace. This means that they had to follow the laws of the market, i.e. follow or lead the fashion to be purchased. We find these grotesque terracotta figurines all around the Mediterranean and in great numbers. Their impact must have been relatively important as they continued to be produced for hundreds of years. As mentioned earlier, it is important to keep in mind that mainstream images were produced in far greater numbers than grotesque images. Small, easily transportable, terracotta versions of famous sculpted types were ubiquitous, because that was what most people could afford. But even if the grotesque figurines were but a fraction of the 'common' ones, they were still found in great numbers.

In a recent publication, Christian Laes (2014: 197–201) referred to the work of evolutionary psychologists who describe the various reactions of people throughout the ages when confronted to 'strangeness'. These attitudes, i.e. *shame, mockery, fascination, pity* and *fear*, were almost interlocked in the ancient Greek world. The feeling of shame may have occurred when confronted with disability in one's own family, tribe, close social structure, but only versus the outside world, the greater social circle or the foreigner. Indeed, one is only as strong as one's weakest link, and in a 'shame-culture', i.e. based on honour, shaming the other was as important as ensuring one's physical and intellectual integrity. Mockery was inherent to shame-cultures and very well explained by the philosopher Bergson in his study of social laughter. The guiding principle is social cohesion and according to Bergson, when we mock someone we do so because they are different or act differently from the rest of the main group. They are poked fun at to ensure they return to the fold and protect the integrity of the group. Yet other principles have their limitations. Bergson's other principle of comical deformity, a deformity that a normally built person could successfully imitate (1921: 23), is less pertinent: the philosopher was probably not aware of our pathological terracotta figurines when he wrote this. In societies where hubris was punished 'by the gods', where one tried to keep one's head down, pity may have come from the feeling that one's able-bodiedness or mental prowess could be diminished at any given time. Did they imagine that disabled individuals were punished by the gods, for personal or ancestral reasons? After all, Greek mythology has often been understood as generational curses or described ironically as 'une affaire de famille' (Giraudoux 1937), where individuals are punished generations later because of an ancestral evil deed. Fear was a natural reaction when confronted, like pity, with something one could have been afflicted with, or the fear of divine retribution or simply the fear of the unknown. The most interesting concept is 'fascination', a wonderfully multi-faceted notion explored by P. Quignard (1994) and which we have alluded to here in the morbid attraction viewers might have had to grotesque visual re-enactments of spectacular deformities and pathologies.

These five attitudes are useful to understand individuals' reactions to disabled individuals, but can they help us understand the large-scale clay production of pathological representations? And what does this say of the Greek visual conception of disability? Artists chose to show disabilities only in a popular kind of object that was ultimately found in funerary and domestic contexts and not in healing sanctuaries. The figurines were often syncretic, mixing clinically observed disabilities with other incongruous details that seriously complicate their interpretation. Some of the figurines even present incompatible diseases. It is as if physical disabilities were part of the building blocks of an art form that showed 'constructed' types, whatever their intended use, rather than realistic medical representations.

Notes

1 See Stewart 1993 173, figs. 383–5.
2 With a few exceptions, like the turned feet of Hephaestus on a number of vase-paintings, e.g. a Laconian cup from Rhodes (Mus. Arch. 10711, 550 BCE) or a Caeretan hydria (Vienna, Kunsthistorisches Mus., 3577 (M218), 550 BCE).
3 See also Mollard-Besques 1972: D1176, pl. 235.e.
4 See Mollard-Besques 1972: D1183, pl. 236.a.

Bibliography

Ashrafian, Hossein, 'The Medical Riddle of the Great Sphinx of Giza', *Journal of Endocrinological Investigation* 28 (2005), 866.

Ballet, Pascale, and Jeammet, Violaine, 'Petite plastique, grands maux : Les «grotesques» en Méditerranée aux époques hellénistique et romaine', in *Corps outragés, corps ravagés de l'antiquité au moyen âge* (Turnhout, 2011), 39–82.

Bergson, Henri, *Laughter: An Essay on the Meaning of the Comic* (London, 1921).

Boutantin, Céline, 'Une figurine caricaturale du Musée du Caire', *Chronique d'Egypte* 74 (1999), 161–70.

Bruneau, Philippe, 'Ganymède et l'aigle: Images, caricatures et parodies animales du rapt', *Bulletin de Correspondance Hellénique* 86/1 (1962), 193–228.

Burr, Dorothy, *Terra-cottas from Myrina in the Museum of Fine Arts, Boston* (Vienna, 1934).

Charlier, Philippe, 'Etude médicale d'ex-voto anatomiques d'Europe occidentale et méditerranéenne', in C. Bobas and C. E. Evangelides (eds), *Croyances populaires: Rites et représentations en Méditerranée orientale: Actes du colloque de Lille (2–4 décembre 2004), 2e colloque interuniversitaire des Universités Capodistrias d'Athènes et Charles-de-Gaulle-Lille* (Athens, 2008), 271–96.

Clarke, John. R., *Looking at Laughter: Humor, Power, and Transgression in Roman Visual Culture, 100 B.C.–A.D. 250* (Berkeley, CA, 2007).

Daehner, Jens, and Lapatin, Kenneth (eds), *Power and Pathos: Bronze Sculpture of the Hellenistic World* (Exhibition from March 14 to June 21, 2015) (Los Angeles, CA, 2015).

Dasen, Véronique, *Dwarfs in Ancient Egypt and Greece* (Oxford, 1993).

Dasen, Véronique, 'Amulettes d'enfants dans le monde grec et romain', *Latomus* 62 (2003), 275–89.

Dasen, Véronique, 'D'un monde à l'autre: La chasse des Pygmées dans l'iconographie impériale', in J. Trinquier and C. Vendries (eds), *Chasses antiques: Pratiques et représentations dans le monde gréco-romain (IIIe siècle av.–IVe siècle apr. J.-C.)* (Rennes, 2009), 215–33.

De Francesco, Maurizio, 'Di alcune terracotte figurate caricaturali da Agrigento', *Sicilia Archeologica* 17 (1984), 69–71.

Devoize, Jean-Louis, 'Hemifacial Spasm in Antique Sculpture: Interest in the "Other Babinski Sign"', *Journal of Neurological Neurosurgical Psychiatry* 82 (2011), 26.

Dunbabin, Katherine M. D., and Dickie, Matthew W., 'Invida rumpantur pectora: The Iconography of Phthonos-Invidia in Graeco-Roman Art', *Jahrbuch für Antike und Christentum* 26 (1983), 7–37.

Dundee, Alan, *The Evil Eye: A Folklore Casebook* (New York, 1981).

Ewigleben, Cornelia, *Götter, Gräber und Grotesken: Tonfiguren aus dem Alltagsleben im römischen Ägypten* (Hamburg, 1991).

Gervais, Paul, *Histoire naturelle des mammifères: Avec l'indication de leurs moeurs et de leurs rapports avec les arts, le commerce et l'agriculture* (Paris, 1854–5).

Giraudoux, Jean, *Electre* (Paris, 1937).

Gourevitch, Danielle, and Grmek, Mirko, 'L'obésité et ses représentations figurées dans l'antiquité', *Archéologie et médecine : Rencontres internationales d'archéologie et d'histoire d'Antibes 7, 1986* (Juan-les-Pins, 1987), 355–67.

Gourevitch, Danielle, and Grmek, Mirko, *Les maladies dans l'art antique* (Paris, 1998).

Graham, Emma-Jayne, 'Disparate Lives or Disparate Deaths? Post-Mortem Treatment of the Body and the Articulation of Difference', in C. Laes *et al.* (eds), *Disabilities in Roman Antiquity* (Leiden, 2013), 249–74.

Himmelmann, Nikolaus, *Alexandria und der Realismus in der griechischen Kunst* (Tübingen, 1983).

Huysecom-Haxhi, Stéphanie, 'Terres cuites animales dans les Nécropoles grecques archaïques et classiques du bassin méditerranéen', *Anthropozoologica* 38 (2003), 91–103.

Jeammet, Violaine (ed.), *Tanagras: Figurines for Life and Eternity. The Musée du Louvre's Collection of Greek Figurines* (Chicago, IL, 2010).

Kassab, Domique, 'Recherches sur quelques ateliers de coroplathie de Myrina à l'epoque hellénistique: Étude archéologique et analyses de laboratoire' (unpublished PhD dissertation Paris IV-Sorbonne, 1982).

Kassab, Dominique, 'Myrina, petite cité grecque de la côte occidentale de l'Asie Mineure', in E. Frézouls (ed.), *Sociétés urbaines, sociétés rurales dans l'Asie Mineure et la Syrie hellénistiques et romaines : Actes du colloque organisé à Strasbourg (novembre 1985) par l'Institut et le Groupe de Recherche d'histoire romaine et le Centre de Recherche sur le Proche-Orient et la Grèce antiques, Université des sciences humaines de Strasbourg. Contributions et travaux de l'Institut d'Histoire Romaine* 4 (Strasbourg, 1987), 173–89.

Kassab, Dominique, *Statuettes en terre cuite de Myrina: Corpus des signatures, monogrammes, lettres et signes* (Istanbul, 1988).

Khodza, Yelena, 'On the Problem of Greek Comedy as Reflected in Terracotta Figurines', *Travaux du Musée de l'Ermitage* 24 (1984), 6–71 (Russian with English summary).

Khodza, Yelena, 'The Grotesque in the Hellenistic Coroplastics', *Vestnik drevnei istorii* 3 (2006), 156–82 (Russian with English summary).

Laes, Christian, 'Ik zie er niet uit! Gehandicapten, invaliden en mismaakten in de Romeinse oudheid', *Hermeneus* 83/1 (2011), 19–25.

Laes, Christian, *Beperkt? Gehandicapten in het Romeinse Rijk* (Leuven, 2014).

Laes, Christian, Goodey, Chris F., and Rose Martha Lynn (eds), *Disabilities in Roman Antiquity: Disparate Bodies A Capite ad Calcem* (Leiden, 2013).

Laugier, Ludovic, 'Les grotesques de Smyrne, types pathologiques et caricatures', in J.-L. Martinez *et al. D'Izmir à Smyrne: Découverte d'une cité antique* (Paris, 2009) 170–3.

Laumonier, Alfred, 'Terres cuites d'Asie Mineure', *Bulletin de Correspondance Hellénique* 70 (1946), 312–18.

Laumonier, Alfred, *Les figurines de terre cuite.* 2 vols. *Exploration Archéologique de Délos* 23 (1956).

Leyenaar-Plaisier, Paula G., *Les terres cuites grecques et romaines: Catalogue de la collection du Musée national des antiquités à Leiden.* 3 vols (Leiden, 1979).

Lorusso, Lorenzo, 'Neurological Caricatures since the 15th Century', *Journal of the History of the Neurosciences* 17 (2008), 314–34.

Maloney, Clarence (ed.), *The Evil Eye* (New York, 1976).

Martinez, Jean-Luc, Laugier, Ludovic, and Rous, Isabelle Hasselin (eds), *D'Izmir à Smyrne: Découverte d'une cité antique* (Paris, 2009).

Mitchell, Alexandre G., 'Humour in Greek Vase Painting', *Revue Archéologique* (2004/2), 3–32.

Mitchell, Alexandre G., *Greek Vase Painting and the Origins of Visual Humour* (New York and Cambridge, 2009).

Mitchell, Alexandre G., 'Disparate Bodies in Ancient Artefacts: The Function of Caricature and Pathological Grotesques among Roman Terracotta Figurines', in C. Laes *et al.* (eds), *Disabilities in Roman Antiquity* (Leiden, 2013), 275–97.

Mitchell, Alexandre G., and Lorusso, Lorenzo, 'La caricatura nell' antichità', in *Il sorriso della mente: La caricatura nella storia delle neuroscienze* (Pavia, 2014), 13–31.

Mollard-Besques, Simone, *Musée National du Louvre: Catalogue raisonné des figurines et reliefs en terre-cuite grecs, étrusques et romains*, II. *Myrina. Figurines et reliefs : Musée du Louvre et collections des Universités de France* (Paris, 1963).

Mollard-Besques, Simone, *Musée National du Louvre: Catalogue raisonné des figurines et reliefs en terre-cuite grecs, étrusques et romains*, III. *Epoques hellénistique et romaine Grèce et Asie Mineure* (Paris, 1972).

Potter, Timothy, W., 'A Republican Healing-Sanctuary at Ponte di Nona near Rome and the Classical Tradition of Votive Medicine', *Journal of the British Archaeological Association* 138 (1985), 23–40.

Quignard, Pascal, *Le sexe et l'effroi* (Paris, 1994).

Régnault, Félix, 'Les terres cuites grecques de Smyrne', *Bulletins et Mémoires de la société d'anthropologie de Paris* 1 (1900), 467–77.

Régnault, Félix, 'Les figurines antiques devant l'art et la médecine', *Medicina* 4 (1907), 1–15; 21–28.

Régnault, Félix, 'Rhinologie et otologie devant l'iconographie antique (terres cuites grecques et smyrniotes)', *Archives internationales de laryngologie, d'otologie et de rhinologie* 28 (1909a), 195–201.

Régnault, Félix, 'Terres cuites pathologiques de Smyrne', *Bulletins et Mémoires de la société d'anthropologie de Paris* 10 (1909b), 633–5.

Régnault, Félix, 'La syphilis est-elle représentée sur les terres cuites grecques de Smyrne', *Bulletin de la Société d'Anthropologie de Lyon* 18 (1909c), 33–9.

Roebuck, Carl, *The Asklepieion and Lerna, Corinth XIV* (1951).

Rous, Isabelle Hasselin, 'Les ateliers de figurines en terre cuite de Smyrne', in J. L. Martinez *et al.* (eds), *D'Izmir à Smyrne* (Paris, 2009), 100–3.

Rous, Isabelle Hasselin, 'Les types idéaux', in J. L. Martinez *et al.* (eds), *D'Izmir à Smyrne* (Paris, 2009), 126–9.

Rous, Isabelle Hasselin, 'Les sujets de genre, les types ethniques et les types réalistes', in J. L. Martinez *et al.* (eds), *D'Izmir à Smyrne* (Paris, 2009), 156–7.

Rous, Isabelle, H., 'Autour de Smyrne, les autres ateliers de figurines en terre cuite de la région', in J. L. Martinez *et al.* (eds), *D'Izmir à Smyrne* (Paris, 2009), 200–3.

Rumscheid, Frank, *Die figurlichen Terrakotten von Priene: Fundkontexte, Ikonographie und Funktion in Wohnhausern und Heiligtumern im Licht antiker Parallelbefunde* (Wiesbaden, 2006).

Slane, Katherine W., and Dickie, Matthew W., 'A Knidian Phallic Vase from Corinth', *Hesperia* 62/4 (1993), 483–505.

Smith, Bert, *Hellenistic Sculpture* (London, 1991).

Stevenson, William, 'The Representation of the Pathological Grotesque in Greek and Roman Art' (unpublished PhD., University of Pennsylvania, 1975).

Stewart, Andrew, *Greek Sculpture: An Exploration* (New Haven, CT, 1993).

Turfa, Jean M., 'Anatomical Votive Terracottas from Etruscan and Italic Sanctuaries', in J. Swaddling (ed.), *Italian Iron Age Artefacts in the British Museum* (London, 1986), 205–13.

Turfa, Jean, M., 'Anatomical Votives and Italian Medical Traditions', in R. D. De Puma and J. P. Small (eds), *Murlo and the Etruscans: Art and Society in Ancient Etruria* (Madison, WI, 1994), 224–40.

Uhlenbrock, Jaimee P., *The Coroplast's Art: Greek Terracottas of the Hellenistic World* (New York, 1990).

Verbanck-Piérard, Annie (ed.), *Au temps d'Hippocrate: Médecine et société en Grèce antique. Catalogue d'exposition* (Mariemont, 1998).

Volteranni. Elena, *La medicina greco-medicina: Scienza e tecnologia nel mondo greco-romano* (Pisa, 1992).

Zinserling, Verena, 'Physiognomische Studien in der Spatarchaischen und Klassichen Vasenmalerei', *WZRostock* 16 (1967), 571–5.

14

PLUTARCH'S 'PHILOSOPHY' OF DISABILITY

Human after all

Michiel Meeusen

Introduction: discovering disability in Plutarch, and related problems

As the renowned American intellectual and essayist R. W. Emerson once wrote, 'Plutarch will be perpetually rediscovered from time to time as long as books last' (Emerson 1968: 322). The contribution at hand can only confirm this. Our aim is to document the multi-faceted notion of disability and its particular manifestations in the *corpus Plutarcheum* and to analyse its function and value in the various discourses of Plutarch's *Moralia* and *Vitae parallelae*. To interpret the work of the famous historian and philosopher of Chaeronea (c.45–120) in light of the relatively young discipline of disability studies is not an easy undertaking, though, for at least two reasons.

First of all, disability features only as a minor topic throughout the Chaeronean's writings, in that it is never 'thematized' in the form of a treatise or a dialogue (as collected in the so-called *Moralia*). Neither does the Lamprias catalogue (an ancient list of Plutarch's writings, where several of his works are listed that are now lost) give us any leads. Surely, Plutarch must have lived among people with sight or hearing problems, or who had limited mobility, or suffered chronic illnesses of various sorts – we read, for instance, about the 'monster-market' in Rome, where handicapped slaves were put on display (*De curiositate* 520c), or about the fact that doctors diagnose their patients with mental illness if they cannot find another explanation (*De cupiditate divitiarum* 524d–e) – but his treatment of such disabilities does not add up to a coherent or systematic approach to the topic. It remains to be seen, therefore, whether or not we can really speak of a 'philosophy' of disability in Plutarch. Most of the time, the topic of disability contributes to the central argument or narrative of Plutarch's writings only in a digressive way, so that it fulfils an inferior discursive role. For instance, in the imagery Plutarch uses regarding religious matters, atheism is compared with blindness (*De superstitione* 167a–b) and superstition with an eye disease that needs to be cured (*Non posse suaviter vivi secundum Epicurum* 1101c). This does not imply, however, that the *corpus Plutarcheum* is lacking in passages that are of interest to the history of disability more generally. In the case of Plutarch's biographies of famous Greek and Roman statesmen (the *Vitae*), we actually learn about the lives and achievements of renowned handicapped persons (we, for instance, read about Demosthenes' speech disorder and Agesilaus's limp). However: 'Plutarch cared more about portraying the internal characteristics of great Greek and Roman men than about portraying their historical contexts. His commentaries demonstrate the Roman penchant for equating appearance with character and for interpreting nature as providing physical "deformities" as warnings' (Albrecht 2006: 65; on monstrous births, see *Coniugalia praecepta* 145d–e, *Septem sapientium convivium* 149c–e, *Quaestiones convivales* 8.9, 731f–732a, *Pericles* 6.2–4). It will be of specific interest for our study to determine how the topic of disability functions in Plutarch's biographical narratives and to examine how it contributes to the global character sketch of Plutarch's heroes. If this means that the topic of disability needs to be gleaned from the margins of the Chaeronean's texts, then let that be the purpose of this contribution.

As is well known, secondly, disability is a socially and culturally determined phenomenon, meaning that its concrete conceptualization and assessment is relative to the very context in which it occurs. Our general take on the matter rests on the idea that Plutarch, as an exponent of Middle Platonism, has a fundamentally philosophical view on the human body, its mortal nature and inherent imperfection. In line with Platonic orthodoxy, Plutarch accepts that the human soul is anchored in the material realm of the natural world by being incarnated in the human body. The human soul is akin to the world-soul, from which the Demiurge made it, but only the rational part of it (as opposed to the spirited and appetitive parts) can transgress the cycle of reincarnation.[1] By consequence, Plutarch is especially interested in the (ethical-intellectual) abilities and disabilities of the soul, while those pertaining to the physical body are of inferior interest. In a passage in *De sollertia animalium*, for instance, Plutarch mentions several types of disabilities, but his main focus is on mental disorders. In an attempt to prove that animals have rational abilities, Plutarch there notes that some of them can lose their reason and become mad (as is the case e.g. in dogs). The topic of bodily disabilities is introduced only for the sake of the argument (corroborating animal rationality) and is, therefore, of secondary importance:

> It is my opinion that each part and faculty has its own particular weakness or defect or ailment which appears in nothing else, as blindness (τυφλότητα) in the eye, lameness (χωλότητα) in the leg, stuttering (ψελλότητα) in the tongue. There can be no blindness in an organ which was not created to see, or lameness in a part which was not designed for walking; nor would you ever describe an animal without a tongue as stuttering, or one voiceless by nature as inarticulate (τραυλόν). And in the same way you would not call delirious or witless or mad (παραπαῖον ἢ παραφρονοῦν ἢ μαινόμενον) anything that was not endowed by Nature with reason or intelligence or understanding; for it is impossible to ail where you have no faculty of which the ailment is a deficiency or loss or some other kind of impairment (κάκωσις).
>
> *(Plutarch, De sollertia animalium 963c–d)[2]*

Notably, Plutarch considers the diseases of the soul to be worse than those of the body. In *Animine an corporis affectiones sint peiores* 501e, he writes that 'it is worse to be sick (νοσεῖν) in soul than in body; for men afflicted in body only suffer, but those afflicted in soul both suffer and do ill'. These diseases are to be understood primarily in terms of vice and ethical corruption. It is especially these types of human weakness Plutarch tries to remedy by providing moral philosophical recommendations to his readers. We should bear this typically ethical penchant in mind on interpreting the passages about physical disability in Plutarch. In doing so, and confronted with the immensity of the material, we will restrict ourselves to a selection of seminal passages that will be of interest to the reader of this volume. It goes without saying, therefore, that this study cannot make any claims towards exhaustiveness.

The reality of disability and grief: Plutarch as a scholar, philosopher and human being

Throughout his writings, Plutarch sporadically refers to the everyday realities of his own life. As such, his texts give us a nice picture of the social, cultural and political situation of the wealthy Greek(-speaking) elite under the Roman Empire. This picture is often quite lively. Plutarch had a large circle of friends and acquaintances who lived all over the Mediterranean region and with whom he regularly corresponded via letters or conversed at symposia and dinner-parties. However, it's not all roses. At the symposia described in *Quaestiones convivales* Plutarch and his fellow symposiasts discuss a number of problems (προβλήματα) regarding all kinds of physical-medical issues (such problems are also treated separately in Plutarch's *Quaestiones naturales*). There is sporadic interest in bodily afflictions and mental disorders. We read, for instance, about alcoholism (*Quaestiones convivales* 1.6, 623d–625a: on Alexander's excessive drinking; 1.7, 625a–c: old men are very fond of strong wine; 3.3, 650a-e: as opposed to women, old men are more liable to drunkenness; *Quaestiones naturales* 31, 919c: heavy drinkers are bald), eating disorders (*Quaestiones convivales* 6.8, 693e–695e: on the cause of bulimia, 'ox-hunger' – not to be confused with the modern disorder (!); *Quaestiones naturales* 3, 912d: on weak and undernourished people; 26, 918d pregnant women eat stones and dirt; *Quaestiones naturales* 6, 913f: obese women soak up dew on their clothes in order to dissolve their excess fat), and, connected with it, infertility (*Quaestiones naturales* 30, 919c, *Quaestiones convivales* 2.6, 640f–641a, and 8.4, 724e: no generative residue is produced if the entire nourishment is used up in the body), mental disorders (*Quaestiones convivales* 6.7, 693a–b: hellebore cures insanity), etc. We can only assume that these topics hint at a genuine reality of suffering and distress, but for Plutarch and his peers they rather provide *gefundenes Fressen* to fuel scholarly debate among intellectuals. Scholarly pedantry was, in fact, highly valued in Plutarch's milieu. Notably, some of these issues had become recurrent topics for rhetorical deliberation, as is the case with the problem of 'Which was Philip's lame leg?' (*Quaestiones convivales* 9.4, 739b; see Samama 2013: 244 – we will come back later to the war-wounds of Philip II of Macedon). Clearly, the symposiasts are not interested in the actual reality of disability (not much is said on how these disorders could be remedied). Their main attention goes to the physical etiology, i.e. the material causes, of these problematic 'phenomena' (this type of research is informed by Aristotelian natural-medical problem literature: see Meeusen 2016; for instance, problems on wine drinking and drunkenness are treated in the third book of Pseudo-Aristotle's *Problemata physica*).

On other occasions the situation is very different, though. In one of his letters, we find Plutarch painfully confronted with the frailties of human existence: the death of his 2-year-old daughter, Timoxena. As a father trying to cope with his loss, Plutarch consoles his mourning wife (also named Timoxena). Some of his 'arguments' may seem rather outlandish if not untactful today, but this can be explained in view of Plutarch's Platonic convictions about life and especially the afterlife. This is the case, for instance, with the idea that the earlier one dies the better (*Consolatio ad uxorem* 611c–612b). Plutarch even gives some hygienic advice for grieving people (*Consolatio ad uxorem* 610a: after all, 'in its own suffering the soul should be helped by a vigorous condition of the body'). In an attempt to convince his wife to maintain her moderated attitude in mourning their beloved child, Plutarch intertwines some of his insights in the fields of moral philosophy and psychology. The soul is immortal and survives after death. Therefore, that the child 'has passed to a state where there is no pain (ἄλυπον) need not be painful to us' (*Consolatio ad uxorem* 611c). There is not a word about the cause of death or about the physical condition of their deceased child (this would only pour salt into the fresh wound). Nevertheless, one may wonder if the younger Timoxena perhaps had a disorder of some kind or suffered an acute or chronic disease. Or was her death caused by a fatal accident? There is no need to mention that child mortality was probably a far more 'common' phenomenon in Antiquity than it is nowadays, statistically speaking at least. In consoling his wife, Plutarch (*Consolatio ad uxorem* 609d) actually reminds her of the previous death of their eldest child and also of 'fair Charon'. This means that only two of their five children survived childhood. (Plutarch and his wife had four sons – Soclarus, Autobulus, Plutarchus, Charon – and one daughter, Timoxena: cf. *Consolatio ad uxorem* 608c.) But even so, and even if Plutarch's consolation is clearly informed by a rational Platonic subtext (De Lacy and Einarson 1959: 577), we see in him not just a man of philosophy but also a caring husband and father, who was not born 'from oak or rock', after all (*Consolatio ad uxorem* 608c, cf. Homer, *Iliad* 22.126; *Odyssey* 19.163). Plutarch actually wrote a treatise *On affection for offspring* (*De amore prolis*).

Disability in the early years: the παιδεία of physical impairment

There is one contrasting passage in Plutarch's writings where we find a far less caring (read: simply cruel) attitude towards the frailties of early human life than in the *Consolatio ad uxorem*. Plutarch there tells us about the Spartan selection procedure of new-born babies in the time of Lycurgus. We read that flawed and deformed babies were condemned to death in Sparta.

> Offspring was not reared at the will of the father, but was taken and carried by him to a place called Lesche, where the elders of the tribes officially examined the infant, and if it was well-built and sturdy, they ordered the father to rear it, and assigned it one of the nine thousand lots of land; but if it was ill-born and deformed (ἀγεννὲς καὶ ἄμορφον), they sent it to the so-called Apothetae, a chasm-like place at the foot of Mount Taÿgetus, in the conviction that the life of that which nature had not well equipped at the very beginning for health and strength, was of no advantage either to itself or the state. On the same principle, the women used to bathe their new-born babes not with water, but with wine, thus making a sort of test of their constitutions. For it is said that epileptic and sickly infants (τὰ ἐπιληπτικὰ καὶ νοσώδη) are thrown into convulsions by the strong wine and lose their senses, while the healthy ones are rather tempered by it, like steel, and given a firm habit of body.
>
> *(Plutarch, Lycurgus 16.1–3)*

In his biography of Lycurgus (where this passage is found), Plutarch describes the life and political achievements of the legendary Spartan law-giver, notorious for the far-reaching reformation of the Spartan state in the 9th century BCE. He does this against the background of the Spartan society of that bygone time, with its laws and customs. Plutarch is clear in the prologue that the history of these times is very obscure, by which he marks the nearly 'legendary' status Lycurgus (and his Spartan state) had obtained in later times. He notes that, 'although the history of these times is such a maze, I shall try, in presenting my narrative, to follow those authors who are least contradicted, or who have the most notable witnesses for what they have written about the man' (*Lycurgus* 1.3). But even so, his discourse clearly contains a high degree of historical idealization, so that one can cast considerable doubt on the historical accuracy of the passage about the new-born babies. Whether we actually find 'legendary' elements in the passage at hand is difficult to say, though (there is, for instance, no archaeological proof or disproof). This does not, however, seem to have bothered Plutarch as much as it does modern historians. In fact, Plutarch seems to have had good reasons to include this account in his biographical narrative, since it serves as a nice illustration of the austerity of Sparta's society, as institutionalized by Lycurgus. A little earlier on, Plutarch stated that 'Lycurgus did not regard sons as the peculiar property of their fathers, but rather as the common property of the state' (*Lycurgus* 15.8). It is in view of Plutarch's 'totalitarian' outlook on childhood and education (παιδεία) – a key concept in Plutarch's time – that the passage about the new-born babies should be interpreted. As such, this passage directly contributes to the development of Plutarch's biographical narrative, since it further illustrates the strict Spartan regime, a severe, communal παιδεία being the very fundament of the Spartan 'utopic state'. Throughout the *Lycurgus*, Sparta is represented as a polis that will not tolerate any form of weakness in its citizens, be it physical or ethical. In the passage about the new-born babies, the emphasis is clearly on the physical condition and physiological purity of the human body, but this is framed in the larger context of the education of the ideal citizen. With regard to the education of female youths, Plutarch notes that Lycurgus 'made them exercise their bodies in running, wrestling, casting the discus, and hurling the javelin, in order that the fruit of their wombs might have vigorous root in vigorous bodies and come to better maturity, and that they themselves might endure the times of pregnancy with vigour, and struggle successfully and easily with the pangs of child-birth' (*Lycurgus* 14.2). Plutarch, thus, implies that a 'healthy' state cannot welcome 'unhealthy' citizens. Such an austere selection procedure of new-borns is necessary, then, at the time of birth, since this moment is the absolute beginning of an individual's education and is, thus, critical for the welfare and stability of the Spartan state. As such, the digression about new-born babies was 'real enough' for Plutarch to incorporate it in his narrative (cf. Dillon in this volume for a different interpretation).[3]

The fact that the ancient Spartan society was probably not as severe towards handicapped individuals as the *Lycurgus* passage would suggest can be illustrated from Plutarch's description of the bodily impairments of the Spartan king Agesilaus II (see Luther 2000). In describing Agesilaus's youthful years among the so-called 'boys-bands' (ἀγέλαι), Plutarch gives some valuable information about the man's physique and character. We read that Agesilaus was deformed in the legs and was crippled (χωλός, lit.: lame), in addition to being markedly small in stature. (As scholars point out, Plutarch's use of χωλός is undefined. He uses it to describe both Agesilaus's limp and the lameness of Artemon, the engineer who, due to his handicap, had to be carried around on a stretcher (*Pericles* 27.3–4). See Rose 2003: 13; Laes 2014: 168.) Plutarch suggests that Agesilaus's bodily impairments did not, however, influence his character in a negative way – in fact, Agesilaus was the first to scorn his own handicap, and it revealed his enduring character and his ambition all the more clearly.

> As for his disabling (πήρωσιν) in the legs, the beauty of his person in its youthful prime covered this from sight, while the ease and gaiety with which he bore such a misfortune, being first to jest and joke about himself, went far towards rectifying it. Indeed, his lameness (χωλότητα) brought his ambition (φιλοτιμίαν) into clearer light, since it led him to decline no hardship and no enterprise whatever. We have no likeness of him (for he himself would not consent to one, and even when he lay dying forbade the making of 'either statue or picture' of his person), but he is said to have been a little man (μικρός) of unimposing presence.
>
> *(Plutarch, Agesilaus 2.2)*

As this passage shows, physical deformity and disability was not a valid criterion to exclude an individual from Spartan society, let alone to administer him a marginal socio-political position – to the contrary, Agesilaus eventually made it to the rank of king. He did not, however, mount the throne unhindered, and his handicap was, indeed, to blame. Resistance came in the figure of Diopeithes, the diviner, who declared that it is 'contrary to the will of Heaven that a lame man should be king of Sparta' (*Agesilaus* 3.4; Diopeithes' divination recurs in *Agesilaus* 30.1 in the context of the imminent war between Sparta and Thebes – if only the Spartan populace had obeyed the diviner's words!). Apparently, this was not so evident after all, but one may wonder how radical the Spartan aversion towards handicapped persons really is, seeing that this is framed in a very political context. Leotychides, an adoptive son of king Agis, also made a claim to the throne, but his 'handicap' is of a more ethical (and therefore much worse) kind, since he was born out of Alcibiades's *illicit* intercourse with Timaea, Agis's wife. Agesilaus, by contrast, enjoyed the favour of the Spartan populace, and received the same public training (the so-called ἀγωγή), in spite of his royal descent (he was a son of king Archidamus and Agis's half-brother) and especially his physical impairments (see *Agesilaus* 1).

Clearly, then, the topic of Agesilaus's disability is very central to the development of Plutarch's biography, since it had a major impact on his hero's education, career and character, but even so it is not of interest *per se* to Plutarch. A parallel passage is found in a different context in *De profectibus in virtute*. The topic of disability there serves as a rhetorical *exemplum* underscoring Plutarch's argument about how one can recognize one's progress in virtue (the central theme of the essay).

> But just so long as a man (...) by passing some jest about himself for being dwarfed or humpbacked (μικρὸν ἢ κυρτόν), imagines that he is thus showing a spirit of youthful bravado, while, at the same time, the inward ugliness of his soul, the despicable acts of his life, his displays of pettiness or love of pleasure or malice or envy, he covers up and conceals as though they were ulcerous sores (ἕλκη), and allows nobody to touch them or even see them because of his fear of being reprehended for them – such a man's part in progress is little, or rather none at all.
>
> *(Plutarch, De profectibus in virtute 82b)*

Plutarch here compares moral vice with deformity of the body, more precisely with dwarfism and kyphosis ('humpback': for the literary value of this image, see Fuhrmann 1964: 152 and 272). He implies that treating one's moral depravity lightly is not the right procedure in making moral progress. The parallelism with the *Agesilaus* passage is striking, but the context is obviously different (Agesilaus takes his handicap lightly, thus revealing his ambitious character, rather than concealing his vice). As such, the connection between a person's bodily impairments and his ethical disposition is a recurrent topic in Plutarch's writings, but its concrete application largely depends on the literary contexts where it occurs. As we will see in the next sections, a similar moralizing dynamic lies at the basis of several other passages where the topic of disability is at issue.

Vir bonus dicendi peritus? Demosthenes' disabled rhetoric

According to ancient physiognomic theories it is possible to interpret a person's mental constitution on the basis of his external, physiological characteristics. In line with such theories, Plutarch believes that education exerts influence on the formation of the body (Soares 2014: 380). In *Demosthenes* 4.4, we read that the famous rhetorician had a weak and fragile body (ἀσθένειαν καὶ θρύψιν) when he was a youth and that this was one of the reasons why he could not pursue the studies that suited a free-born boy – the main reason being that his guardians had squandered his inheritance that would have financed such studies. Moreover, Demosthenes's mother did not allow him to train his body in the palaestra, so he had 'a lean and sickly physique (κάτισχνος καὶ νοσώδης) from the beginning' (*Demosthenes* 4.5). Demosthenes's physical weakness does, indeed, provide a key element in the orator's rhetorical *Werdegang*, and it plays a crucial role in the further development of Plutarch's narrative.

At a later age, when Demosthenes started to declaim in public, he was not very successful at first, since his physical feebleness had a negative impact on the delivery of his speech. Plutarch writes that he had 'a certain weakness of voice (φωνῆς ἀσθένεια) and indistinctness of speech (γλώττης ἀσάφεια) and shortness of breath (πνεύματος κολοβότης) which disturbed the sense of what he said by disjoining his sentences' (*Demosthenes* 6.4). It is unclear from this passage whether Demosthenes stuttered or had another speech impairment (did he clutter, mumble or lisp, perhaps? On the indefinability of Demosthenes' speech disorder, see Rose 2003: 50. In *Demosthenes* 11.1 we read that Demosthenes had a lisp (τραυλότης). Perrin 1919: 27, n. 1, notes that this is '[s]trictly, an inability to pronounce the letter "r," giving instead the sound of "l."' Cf. Pseudo-Aristotle, *Problemata physica* 11.30, 902b22–3). What is probably more important, though, is the implicit allusion Plutarch is making here to ancient theories about voice and breathing. The ability to control one's breathing in order to modulate one's voice and speech (in terms of a correct pronunciation, syntax, rhythm, etc.) was considered essential for the success of a rhetorical performance in Antiquity. (On the risks connected with unnecessary straining of the voice, see, however, *De tuenda sanitate praecepta* 130f–131a and Renehan 2000.) To this end, a rhetorician should actually train and prepare his body for the *actio*, a point Plutarch emphasizes in the passage where he portrays Demosthenes' frustration for having failed as a public orator.

> And finally, when he had forsaken the assembly and was wandering about dejectedly in the Piraeus, Eunomus the Thriasian, who was already a very old man, caught sight of him and upbraided him because, although he had a style of speaking which was most like that of Pericles, he was throwing himself away out of weakness and lack of courage, neither facing the multitude with boldness, nor preparing his body for these forensic contests, but suffering it to wither away in slothful neglect.[4]
>
> (*Plutarch, Demosthenes 6.5–7.2*)

In explaining Demosthenes' public failure as a rhetorician, Plutarch thus connects the man's physical weakness with his lack of courage and boldness, an important aspect of his character and an important element in Plutarch's biography. In what follows, the topic of Demosthenes' cowardice in rhetorical matters is foregrounded even more *vis-à-vis* his sporadic demonstration of courage (notably, Demosthenes only exceptionally had the courage to extemporize on a given topic). Clearly, Demosthenes was not naturally talented to take the role of a rhetorician. As Plutarch notes, therefore, 'it was thought that Demosthenes was not a man of good natural parts (εὐφυής), but that his ability and power were the product of toil' (*Demosthenes* 8.3). Indeed, the *Demosthenes* can be read as a coming-of-age story, in which the protagonist conquers his natural weakness and disability by heavy training and exercise. The methods Demosthenes used to work his voice were rather unconventional. He built a subterranean study where he trained his gestures and cultivated his voice (*Demosthenes* 7.6). To this end, he also discoursed while running up steep places, and recited speeches or verses at a single breath. In order to correct the indistinctness and lisping in his speech he held pebbles in his mouth while reciting (*Demosthenes* 11.1).

Notably, other famous Greeks had similar speech disorders. Plutarch reports that Alcibiades also had a lisp, but in his case it is seen as a positive feature contributing to his remarkable physical beauty (*Alcibiades* 1.6). (The whole dossier on speech impairment has been treated extensively in Laes 2013: see esp. 172 on Alcibiades; 173–4 on Demosthenes.) In Plutarch's description of Demosthenes's lisp, by contrast, the aspect of rhetorical training and education is central. Obviously, the spoken word and one's ability to master it plays a central role in the rhetorical culture of Greco-Roman Antiquity – this had not changed in Plutarch's times. The fact that Demosthenes had the character to fight his own weak nature and to overcome his bodily feebleness by intensive training and schooling is, for Plutarch, what eventually made him one of the greatest rhetoricians of Greek history.

Disability in military service: the ethics and aesthetics of honourable wounds

As the *Demosthenes* has shown, Plutarch in describing the character of his heroes pays specific attention to their physiological disposition. This is the case also in his other biographies. When dealing, for instance, with Aratus' military achievements, Plutarch mentions the physiological manifestations of the general's alleged fear in the presence of seeming peril: viz. his heart palpitations, change in the colour of his skin and looseness of the bowels. Plutarch doubts that this is accurate, but he notes that the general's fear is, nevertheless, a popular topic of discussion in the philosophers' schools and explains that the symptoms are generally accounted for in a twofold manner, viz. by reference to the general's cowardice or to some defective disposition and coldness in his body (*Aratus* 29.6; see Meeusen 2016: 127–8). In ancient biological-medical literature, a connection is often drawn between a person's physiological and ethical disposition. Parallels are found, for instance, in book 27 of Pseudo-Aristotle's *Problemata physica*, which deals with the physiological manifestation of fear and courage in the human body more generally (see Castelli 2011; Meeusen 2016: 67). As opposed to cowardice, which is associated with a cold disposition of the body, bravery is associated with the presence of physiological heat.

Of course, the actual proof of someone's bravery in battle is most clearly demonstrated by his military actions and their effects. In some cases, these effects can be read from the body itself and from a person's physical appearance (εἶδος). Considering the long list of wars and battles in Greco-Roman times, disability through military service must have been relatively common in ancient society (see Salazar 2000: with 209–27 for a useful epilogue on literary motives related to war-wounds). No wonder, therefore, that the theme of wounded generals and soldiers is a recurrent motif in several Plutarchan writings. Plutarch sporadically reflects on the topic of war-wounds in light of his heroes' characters. This is mostly phrased in terms of pride and shame: pride for having 'gained' such disfigurements by bravery in battle (in an ethical sense), and shame for the bodily disfigurement such wounds and scars cause (in an aesthetic sense).

At the beginning of his *Cato Maior*, Plutarch describes Cato's military repute and bravery in battle. We read that Cato had participated in the campaign against Hannibal at the age of 17 (217 BCE), and that 'while he was yet a mere stripling, he had his breast covered with wounds (τραυμάτων)' (*Cato Maior* 1.7). The fact that Cato had these wounds on the front of his body (ἐναντίων, lit.: opposed) and *not* on his back implies that he obtained them while facing danger, not while fleeing from it.[5] It is unclear from the text whether these scars filled Cato with pride or shame, but in light of the well-known Roman reverence of the heroic veteran body, the former seems more likely.[6] In any case, these wounds put Cato's cardinal virtue of bravery on show – some kind of a family trait, since 'Cato himself extols his father, Marcus, as a brave man and good soldier. He also says that his grandfather, Cato, often won prizes for soldierly valour, and received from the state treasury, because of his bravery, the price of five horses which had been killed under him in battle' (*Cato Maior* 1.1). Clearly, military courage and bravery was in Cato's blood, and his bodily disfigurements were there to prove it. The topic of war-wounds thus provides a suitable occasion for Plutarch not just to describe the physical appearance of his hero, but also to concretize his character and nature.

The topic of war-wounds recurs in the *Life of Agesilaus* (*Agesilaus* 36.2), where Plutarch deals with Agesilaus's decision to start a new military expedition in his eighties with a body covered with wounds (τραυμάτων). The topic is again mentioned here in light of Agesilaus's ambitious character (φιλοτιμίαν, cf. the passage above), but Plutarch criticizes this decision as indecorous – after all, Agesilaus was way past the proper age to start a new military campaign, and, as his scars revealed, his body was tired of fighting. Agesilaus agreed to take a command under Tachos the Egyptian in his war against the Persian king. Plutarch sees this not as a decision of a reputable commander but of an old mercenary greedy for money: after all, 'honourable action has its fitting time and season'. Notably, Xenophon's account of this event in his *Agesilaus* is very different from Plutarch's. This can be explained by the different historiographical projects both authors had in mind. Whereas Xenophon's account of Agesilaus's decision (to 'again set free the Greeks in Asia, and chastise the Persian for his former hostility': Xenophon, *Agesilaus* 2.29) is part of the author's encomium of the Spartan king (with whom he was personally and politically affiliated), Plutarch rather focuses on Agesilaus's personal failure to find a proper balance in his actions. Clearly, the main intention of Plutarch's biographical narrative is more 'introvert', in that it displays an overtly moralizing interest and dynamic (as is flagged in the passage at issue with such concepts as καλόν and μέτριον).[7] As such, the aspect of Agesilaus's disability is entirely subordinated to the moralizing teleology of Plutarch's narrative. The fact that Agesilaus's body is old and covered with wounds (τραύματα) indicates that he had arrived at a certain point in his life where it is beyond socio-ethical decorum to still be actively involved in (military) politics – a topic Plutarch treats separately and more at length in *An seni respublica gerenda sit* (esp. 790c, where Agesilaus is named among several other kings and politicians who remained in office up to an advanced age).

Some war-wounds do not just result in scars, however, but cause genuine handicaps. Plutarch mentions Sertorius's loss of an eye resulting from bravery in battle. Nevertheless, the general still prided himself on this disfigurement (just as was the case with Cato's scars), since it proved his courage:

> Others, he said, could not always carry about with them the evidences of their brave deeds, but must lay aside their necklaces, spears, and wreaths; in his own case, on the contrary, the marks of his bravery remained with him, and when men saw what he had lost, they saw at the same time a proof of his valour.
>
> *(Plutarch, Sertorius 4.3–4)*

Notably, at the beginning of the biography, Sertorius is named as an example of the coincidence that many generals had lost one of their eyes in battle. Plutarch writes that 'the most warlike of generals, and those who achieved most by a mixture of craft and ability, have been one-eyed men (ἑτερόφθαλμοι)' (*Sertorius* 1.8). Among these generals, Plutarch also mentions Antigonus, Hannibal and Philip II of Macedon, father of Alexander the Great (Lycurgus can be added: he was blinded in one of his eyes during an uprising of the Spartan aristocracy; see *Lycurgus* 11). From other sources we know that the Macedonian king had lost his right eye and was deeply ashamed of his disfigurement – he even forbade the use of the words 'eye' or 'Cyclops' in his vicinity.[8] Elsewhere, Plutarch deals with yet another handicap Philip suffered as a consequence of his bravery on the battlefield. The Macedonian king walked with a limp, due to a spear wound in his thigh. We read that he was ashamed also of this handicap.

> When the thigh of his father Philip had been pierced by a spear in battle with the Triballians, and Philip, although he escaped with his life, was vexed with his lameness (χωλότητι), Alexander said, 'Be of good cheer, father, and go on your way

rejoicing, that at each step you may recall your valour.' Are not these the words of
a truly philosophic spirit (φιλοσόφου) which, because of its rapture for noble things
(καλοῖς), already revolts against mere physical encumbrances? How, then, think you,
did he glory in his own wounds (τραύμασι), remembering by each part of his body
affected a nation overcome, a victory won, the capture of cities, the surrender of
kings? He did not cover over nor hide his scars (οὐλάς), but bore them with him
openly as symbolic representations, graven on his body, of virtue and manly courage.

(Plutarch, De Alexandri Magni fortuna aut virtute 331b–c)

Scholars have read this passage as a tipping point in the conceptualization of war-
wounds, where the (Greek) aesthetic tradition of physical beauty and the (Roman) tradition
of glorification of the heroic veteran body are unified. They even speak of a paradigm shift,
where the figure of Philip functions as a pivotal point between the two traditions (see Laes
2014: 166; this remains hypothetical, of course: see Salazar 2000: 218; Samama 2013 links it
to the shift from classical Greek to Hellenistic aesthetics, rather than explaining it in terms of
Greek *vis-à-vis* Roman identity). Whereas Philip is ashamed about his handicap and sees it as
a physical stain on his body and its integrity, Alexander rather sees it as a mark of his father's
virtue (ἀρετή). This is why Alexander is not at all ashamed to display his own war-wounds,
as if they are the 'bas-reliefs de son grand courage' (Fuhrmann 1964: 107). The same motive
returns elsewhere in Plutarch (e.g. in *Lacaenarum apophthegmata* 241e–f: Spartan soldiers
return from the battlefield ashamed of their wounds and handicaps, but their mothers are proud
of their sons' bravery in battle; cf. also *Pompeius* 64.4: Sextus Teidius was jeered at, since he
was very old and lame in one leg, but Pompey welcomes him heartily since he chose his side
and came to face danger with him; see Rose 2003: 44).

The combination of these two motives – viz. the classical Greek custom of hiding external
ailments and the later tradition of proudly displaying such deficiencies – was already common by
Plutarch's time. A similar anecdote that intertwines the motives of shame and courage is found
e.g. in Cicero, *De oratore* 2.249 (Spurius Carvilius was ashamed of his lameness, caused by a
wound he obtained during military service, but his mother says that every step he takes should
remind him of his courage). In Plutarch's case, however, this is tilted on a higher philosophical
level, where Alexander the Great is represented as having great philosophical (i.e. Platonic)
insight – clearly Plutarch's projection at work here! – since he, far from idolizing the body,
despises its material inferiority by his 'enthusiasm for more noble things (καλοῖς)'. Plutarch's
main interest is not so much in the topic of disability as such, but rather in Alexander's reaction to
his father's sorrow and what it can tell us about his philosophical character. This was previously
marked in *De Alexandri Magni fortuna aut virtute* 330e: 'let us examine his sayings too, since it
is by their utterances that the souls of other kings and potentates also best reveal their characters
(ἤθη)'. (The same idea is expressed in *Regum et imperatorum apophthegmata* 172d.)

Conclusion: Plutarch's 'philosophy' of disability?

As this contribution has tried to show, there are a number of interesting *loci* in the *corpus
Plutarcheum* that can give us some insight – even if it's only a glimpse – into the impact a
handicap could have on an individual's character, life and career in Antiquity. The aspect of
idealization is never far away in these passages, though, since they mostly concern renowned
figures from the ancient past. In some cases the concept of disability actually functions as
a literary motive with a tradition of its own (as is especially the case with the topic of war-
wounds). As such, we are *en pleine littérature* here, and we should keep up our guard not to

interpret Plutarch's biographies as merely historical records (a *caveat* he makes himself in *Alexander* 1.2; see n. 6). Nevertheless, the fact that Plutarch's biographical project includes the lives of renowned handicapped figures (that mostly belonged to the top layer of Greco-Roman society from the time of the mythological founding fathers up until the end of the Republic) can only lead one to suspect that disability was omnipresent in ancient society, even in the highest strata of political life – and perhaps therefore it did not *need* a separate treatment.

Disability is a minor topic that is treated only marginally in Plutarch's writings. The Chaeronean does not seem to have been specifically interested in this topic, or he did not at least ascribe any other relevance to it than purely narrative or digressive. The theme of handicaps and bodily deformities is foregrounded in some of his writings (esp. in the *Vitae*), where it mostly contributes to his description of the character and ethical profile of his heroes. On other occasions (especially in the *Moralia*), it provides the typical content for scholarly discussions or for literary comparisons and rhetorical *exempla* that provide only little information about the author's personal outlook on handicaps or handicapped individuals. Moreover, when Plutarch speaks about the deviating status of handicapped individuals in society, the image is mostly blurred (e.g. in Sparta, deformed babies could either be eliminated or make it to kings, as proven by Agesilaus).

Those passages that do provide the reader with some insight into how the Chaeronean looked at physical ailments, deformities, handicaps – in short, human frailty – are generally set in a Middle Platonic framework that displays a typical 'enthusiasm for more noble things' (cf. *De Alexandri Magni fortuna aut virtute* 331c), to which the materiality of the body is totally subjected. The topic is not treated systematically, let alone separately (such a systematic approach is, in fact, absent in ancient literature), but it is rather incorporated in a broader philosophical construct that has an obvious ethical teleology. If we raise the question of how 'philosophical' Plutarch's 'philosophy' of disability really is, then (if we are to label it 'philosophical' to begin with), let us be reminded that for the Chaeronean, philosophy is primarily an 'art of life' (*Quaestiones convivales* 1.1, 613b: τέχνην περὶ βίον) and should have a concrete application in human relations. Nevertheless, human weakness (in an *ethical* sense) is pardonable, insofar as it is essentially human. As such, Plutarch's moral philosophy is a relatively flexible system that allows for slips and mistakes, at least if one is prepared to learn from them. Morality is omnipresent in the Chaeronean's writings, but it is always balanced by a deeply rooted humanity (φιλανθρωπία) and a degree of sympathy for human fragility (on Plutarch's humanity, see the contributions in Ferreira *et al.* 2009).

Arguably, Plutarch's personal view on human disability and bodily deformities is also based on his φιλανθρωπία. This is the case most notably in his account of the Roman nomenclature in *Coriolanus* 11.4, where he discusses the Roman custom of giving three names to one person (see Laes 2014: 28; the same topic recurs in *Cicero* 1.3–6). Plutarch praises the Roman usage of *cognomina*, even if they often indicate a negative bodily feature or physical abnormality.

> From bodily features they not only bestow such surnames as Sulla, Niger, and Rufus, but also such as Caecus and Claudius. And they do well thus to accustom men to regard neither blindness (τυφλότητα) nor any other bodily misfortune (ἀτυχίαν) as a reproach or a disgrace, but to answer to such names as though their own.
> *(Plutarch, Coriolanus 11.4)*

Is this the philosopher speaking, reluctant to attach any intrinsic value to material things, or the man not born 'from oak or rock' – or is it both? I would say that if we want to speak of Plutarch's 'philosophy' of disability, we should probably do this in view of his deeply rooted humanity. In any case, as R. W. Emerson already knew: 'The reason of Plutarch's vast popularity is his humanity' (Emerson 1968: 298).

Notes

1 For the relation, more generally, between the world soul and the human soul in Plutarch, see Opsomer 1994. According to Plutarch's conception of the world soul, its irrational part explains the existence of evil, imperfection and deformity in the context of creation.
2 All translations are borrowed from the LCL with sporadic adaptations.
3 Notably, authors like Plato or Xenophon, who were well-disposed towards the Spartan regime, did not mention the selection procedure of new-born babies. Nevertheless, Plato's description of the 'ideal state' may still function as a general subtext for Plutarch's *Lycurgus*. Cf. Plato, *Respublica* 415c, 460c (selection procedure), *Timaeus* 19a (children of bad parents are to be brought to other cities). Cf. also Plato, *Theaetetus* 161a (Socrates discredits an argument by comparing it with a child that should be left to death) and Aristotle, *Politica* 7, 1335b19–26 (a law which forbids to raise deformed babies). See Laes 2008: 93; Laes 2014: 37. See also Rose 2003: 29–49 more generally. On abortion in Sparta, cf. *Lacaenarum apophthegmata* 242c. On children and childhood more generally in Plutarch, see Pelling 1990; Soares 2014 (esp. 378, n. 7, for further literature on the passage about the new-born babies).
4 On Pericles' 'sublime' style of speech, see *Pericles* 5.1; 8.1–2 and Meeusen 2016: 51–2.
5 Cf. *Amatorius* 761c and *Pelopidas* 18.3 (a soldier who had fallen in battle on his face asks his enemy to wait a moment and strike him in the chest so that his lover will not see him wounded from behind). See Salazar 2000: 217.
6 See Samama 2013. In *Coriolanus* 14.1, Plutarch reports that it was a Roman custom for candidates for the consulship to go to the forum in their toga, without a tunic under it. 'This was either because they wished the greater humility of their garb to favour their solicitations, or because they wished to display the tokens of their bravery, in case they bore wounds.'
7 In line with the Chaeronean's overarching biographical project, this passage is clearly embedded in a broader moralizing-philosophical framework that is primarily concerned with ethical paraenesis (towards the reader), rather than with historical accuracy (on the author's side). In *Alexander* 1.2, Plutarch famously notes that 'it is not Histories that I am writing, but Lives' (οὔτε γὰρ ἱστορίας γράφομεν, ἀλλὰ βίους). His biographical narratives provide very moralizing portrayals of the heroic protagonists and contain an obvious ethical *appel*. As such, they give very concrete (descriptive, rather than normative) moral guidance to the reader. See Duff 1999: 13–98.
8 See Pseudo-Demetrius, *De elocutione* 293 (Samama 2013: 237–8). Cf. also *Alexander* 3.1 (an oracle predicts Philip's eye loss). The fear of soldiers of becoming disfigured in the face recurs in *Caesar* 45.2–4 and *Pompeius* 69.5–6 (Caesar instructs his troops to aim at the face and eyes of the enemy). See Salazar 2000: 35; Soares 2014: 380; Laes 2014: 195.

Bibliography

Albrecht, Gary L. (ed.), *Encyclopedia of disability*, 5 vols (Thousand Oaks, CA, 2006).
Castelli, Laura Maria, 'Manifestazioni somatiche e fisiologia delle "affezioni dell'anima" nei *Problemata aristotelici*', in B. Centrone (ed.), 'Studi sui *Problemata Physica* aristotelici', *Elenchos* 58 (2011), 239–74.
De Lacy, Phillip H., Einarson Benedict, *Plutarch's Moralia in fifteen volumes*, VII (Cambridge, MA, and London, 1959).
Duff, Timothy E., *Plutarch's Lives: Exploring Virtue and Vice* (Oxford, 1999).
Emerson, Ralph Waldo, *The Complete Works of Ralph Waldo Emerson: Lectures and Biographical Sketches*, X (New York, 1968).
Ferreira, José Ribeiro, Leão, Delfim, Tröster, Manual, and Barata, Dias Paula (eds), *Symposium and Philantropia in Plutarch* (Coimbra, 2009).
Fuhrmann, François, *Les images de Plutarque* (Paris, 1964).
Laes, Christian, 'Learning from Silence: Disabled Children in Roman Antiquity', *Arctos* 42 (2008), 85–122.
Laes, Christian, *Beperkt? Gehandicapten in het Romeinse Rijk* (Leuven, 2014).
Laes, Christian, 'Silent History? Speech Impairment in Roman Antiquity', in C. Laes, C. F. Goodey and M. L. Rose (eds), *Disabilities in Roman Antiquity Disparate Bodies* A Capite ad Calcem (Leiden, 2013), 145–80.
Luther, Andreas, 'Die χωλὴ βασίλεια des Agesilaos', *AHB* 14 (2000), 120–9.

Meeusen, Michiel, *Plutarch's Science of Natural Problems: A Study with Commentary on* Quaestiones Naturales (Leuven, 2016).

Opsomer, Jan, 'L'âme du monde et l'âme de l'homme chez Plutarque', in M. G. Valdés (ed.), *Estudios sobre Plutarco: Ideas religiosas* (Madrid, 1994), 33–49.

Pelling, Christopher, 'Childhood and Personality in Greek Biography', in C. Pelling (ed.), *Characterization and Individuality in Greek Literature* (Oxford, 1990), 213–44.

Perrin, Bernadotte, *Plutarch's* Lives *in Eleven Volumes*, VII (Cambridge, MA, and London, 1919).

Renehan, Robert, 'A Rare Surgical Procedure in Plutarch', *Classical Quarterly* 50/1 (2000), 223–9.

Rose, Martha L., *The Staff of Oedipus: Transforming Disability in Ancient Greece* (Michigan, 2003).

Salazar, Christine, *The Treatment of War Wounds in Graeco-Roman Antiquity* (Leiden, 2000).

Samama, Evelyne, 'A King Walking with Pain? On the Textual and Iconographical Images of Philip II and Other Wounded Kings', in C. Laes, C. F. Goodey and M. L. Rose (eds), *Disabilities in Roman Antiquity: Disparate Bodies* A Capite ad Calcem (Leiden and Boston, MA, 2013), 231–48.

Soares, Carmen, 'Childhood and Youth', in M. Beck (ed.), *A Companion to Plutarch* (Chichester, 2014), 373–90.

III

The Roman world

15

PERFECT ROMAN BODIES

The Stoic view

Bert Gevaert

Introduction

In several European languages the word 'stoic' is used to describe or call someone who accepts his misfortune (whether it be mental or physical) without complaining or showing emotion. Though the modern use of the word 'stoic' is only a very superficial and extremely narrow interpretation of the complexity of 'one of the most important philosophical schools of ancient Greece and Rome' (Strange and Zupko 2014: p. iii), which shows many similarities with ancient Christianity (Thorsteinsson 2010: 1–5), being 'impassible' to (or undisturbed by) misfortune is indeed one of the main characteristics of Stoic philosophy. Impassibility (or *apatheia*) is the ultimate goal for each Stoic philosopher and he who can completely control his emotions (which could be disturbed by misfortune) is called *vir sapiens* ('sage') (Sellars 2006: 36). Bearing of misfortune (*constantia*) is an important aspect of moral strength (*fortitudo*) and when the gods decide against our expectations, we should not be unhappy with their decisions (Setailoli 2014: 297–8). Misfortune usually happens in the area of the so-called *indifferentia* (indifferent things), which are neither good nor bad and have no actual value in the eyes of Stoic philosophers: one's own life, reputation, health, poverty, social status, etc. (Sellars 2006: 110).

According to many Greek and Roman Stoics, the perfect *vir sapiens* and role model for all moral philosophers after him, is – without any doubt – the Athenian philosopher Socrates (469–399 BCE) (Graver 2007: 208). When condemned to die by drinking hemlock, Socrates remained calm and didn't complain, in contrast to his friends, who were crying over his death (Xenophon, *Apologia Socratis* 28–34).

If Stoic philosophers don't consider their own death or that of their friends worthy of shedding any tears, what are their thoughts about being affected with a mental or physical impairment? It seems logical that impairments are also seen as *indifferentia*, but how can we explain that the famous Stoic philosopher Seneca Minor (4 BCE–65 CE) mocks the disabilities of emperor Claudius (41–54) in his infamous *Apocolocyntosis*?

Thus, in this contribution I will focus on the Stoic take on the mind–body distinction. In addition I will explore the compatibility of this distinction with the fact that such an important Stoic philosopher as Seneca Minor explicitly ridicules bodily impairment.

Moral excellence as ultimate goal

Instead of worrying or complaining about misfortune – such as slavery, torture, death, disease or mental and physical disability – Stoic philosophers only care about virtue (*virtus*) (Lagrée 2010: 150): 'excellence in the activity of rational agency' (Becker 2010: 272).[1] These misfortunes, which can happen to the body, are not evil and when we inspect them later, we will see that they are not as serious as we first thought (Lagrée 2010: 157). According to this vision, the body is less important than moral virtue, as Seneca Minor writes several times in his *Epistulae Morales ad Lucilium*:

> I am too big and I am born for bigger things than to be a slave of my body. I can only see my own body as a sort of chain by which my freedom is bound. Thus, I offer this body to Fortune, where she can obstruct me, but I do not allow any wound to hurt me through that body. Whatever in me can suffer an injury, that is my body. In this feeble house a free spirit lives. (…) Despising your own body is sure freedom.
>
> *(Seneca, Epistulae Morales 65.21–2)[2]*

Similar ideas can be found in other places in the same work (*Epistulae Morales* 71.18 and 79.16) and also in other texts from Seneca (*De Constantia* 10.4) and other Stoic philosophers such as Epictetus (50–130) (*Dissertationes* 3.1; 3.22.21 and 40; *Enchiridion* 9). To illustrate the futility of the body, Seneca writes:

> Out of a small cabin, a great man can come and out of a deformed and humble little body a beautiful and great soul can come. It seems to me that nature generates such people in such shape to show that virtue can be born in any body. If nature would be able to produce naked, independent bodies, she would have done this already, but now she does something more: she produces several people who are bodily impaired, but nevertheless these people break all boundaries (…). Thus we can know that the soul is not made ugly by the deformity of the body, but the body becomes beautiful by the pulchritude of the soul.
>
> *(Seneca, Epistulae Morales 66.3–4)[3]*

The Stoic emphasis on virtue and by consequence the lower appreciation of a physically healthy or perfect body (Seneca, *Epistulae Morales* 92.19) doesn't imply that embodiment is entirely distinct from mental well-being and that a Stoic philosopher can neglect the care of his own body. Sometimes bodily disease is even compared to weakness of the soul, an old idea that can be found as early as in Plato's work (Inwood 1985: 127). Illness of the body is dangerous, because it is often accompanied by mental lowness or confusion (Graver 2007: 18). Mental lowness or even mental disability does not even belong to the concept of ethics; it is an illness of the soul caused by humoral imbalances, leading to actions not voluntarily chosen (Graver 2007: 110). Thus, suffering from a mental disability makes it almost impossible for an individual to achieve virtue.

According to Epictetus, a Stoic philosopher (and a Cynic philosopher) needs a good and healthy body for other reasons as well. People won't have much confidence in a skinny philosopher, for he has to prove the benefits of his (philosophical) way of life with his body. His body must show that his simple life under the open sky doesn't harm his physical wellbeing. When people feel pity for a philosopher, it is because he is similar to a beggar, who elicits only contempt (*Dissertationes* 3.22.86–9).

Impassibility towards bodily injuries

It seems logical that a healthy body is generally preferred by a Stoic philosopher, but what happens when the same philosopher is suddenly afflicted by a specific physical impairment? Seneca's commentary is very detailed about this:

> When a disease or enemy takes off his hand, when an accident makes him lose an eye or both of his eyes, then what is left will suffice for him and in spite of his weakened and mutilated body, he will be as happy as if his body was unharmed. But he doesn't long for what he is missing and he doesn't prefer that these are missing.
>
> *(Seneca, Epistulae Morales 9.4)*[4]

Of course the point is here again that everything is useful for the sage 'but nothing, including his or her own body is needful' (Graver 2007: 183). Musonius Rufus, another Stoic philosopher (1st century CE), even says that one should forgive evildoers, as happened to Lycurgus (9th century BCE), the legendary Spartan leader who lost an eye in an attack by a fellow citizen. When Lycurgus kept this young man as a prisoner and had the opportunity to take revenge upon him, he treated him well and trained him to be a good man. In the end he even returned this young man to the Spartans with these words:

> This man I received from you is an insolent and violent creature; I return him to you a reasonable man and good citizen.
>
> *(Epictetus, Fragmenta 5; tr. W. Oldfather)*

This anecdote about the life of Lycurgus also illustrates another Stoic idea about bodily harm: this apparent harm was not really done to him and the Sage must forgive those who do him evil (Musonius Rufus, *Fragmenta* 39; see Harris 2001: 116).

The most incredible story, however, about being impassible towards bodily injuries is about Epictetus, who was probably the only philosopher in Antiquity whom we actually know suffered from a disability, in his case being crippled (Moser 2012). When Epictetus was still a slave, his master tortured him and deliberately broke his leg. When the torturer wrenched his leg, Epictetus smiled and warned him that he would break the leg. When his leg broke, Epictetus commented that he had foreseen that this would happen (Origen, *Contra Celsum* 7.53). Thus Epictetus became a cripple and considered himself 'an old crippled man' (*Dissertationes* 1.16.20). This was the role he played in his life (*Enchiridion* 17), and as such, he did not complain.

In the end, it is probably better to laugh at misfortunes because this benefits human beings more than crying about them (Seneca, *De animi tranquillitate* 15.2–3). People should behave as the Stoic emperor Marcus Aurelius says:

> To be like the rock that the waves keep crashing over. It stands unmoved and the raging of the sea falls still around it. It is unfortunate that this has happened. No. It is fortunate that this has happened and I have remained unharmed by it – not shattered by the present or frightened by the future. It could have happened to anyone. But not everyone could have remained unharmed by it.
>
> *(Marcus Aurelius, Meditationes 4.49, tr. G. Hays)*

At the same time, it is still normal for people to prefer health to illness (Inwood 1985: 201). The famous Roman politician, philosopher, orator and publicist Cicero states that people by nature prefer those things which they think to be good, and avoid their opposites (Cicero,

Tusculanae Disputationes 4.12). This living *secundum naturam* ('according to nature') can only be achieved when we are free from earthly goods and emotions which can only cause misfortune (Sellars 2006: 125).

Being ill or suffering from impairment is against nature, but above all it is important to remain calm because this state of mind is considered as living according to nature (Seneca, *Epistulae Morales* 66.38). The sage is not unaware of his misfortune, but remains impassible in that his virtue stays untouched (Lagrée 2010: 151).

Besides this, being healthy doesn't make people happier (Seneca, *Epistulae Morales* 92.94) and being healthy is sometimes even a bad thing when a dictator wants to take advantage of you. In this case, is much better to be ill and because of this neither reason, nor health, nor possessions are at all beneficial, and neither are their opposites harmful (Graver 2007: 49). Every human being must know that, in the end, beauty and power have less effect than (the destructive power) of old age (Seneca, *Epistulae Morales* 31.10). In this way, not one person is ever exempt from being disabled or losing his bodily strength and power.

Condemnation of deriding disabled people

Though Marcus Tullius Cicero encourages mocking physical flaws as a strategy in juridical speeches (Cicero, *De oratore* 2.239, 245, 246 and 249), philosophers generally tend not to laugh at (disabled) people (Halliwell 2008: 266, 305–55 and Laes 2014: 199–200). Since virtue is the highest good, a true Stoic philosopher never mocks disabled people; he only mocks others who don't share his vision on life. This mocking or laughing has to happen without anyone noticing it, without an accompanying feeling of superiority or the need to make a point (Halliwell 2008: 306).

According to Seneca Minor life is about avoiding hatred, envy or contempt and the only purpose is achieving – as mentioned earlier – virtue (*Epistulae Morales* 14.10). Never mock another person; because people must treat their fellow human beings as they themselves want to be treated (Seneca Minor, *Epistulae Morales* 47.11). Besides the moral condemnation that results from mocking others, people must also be aware of the risk that the derided person may take his revenge when he can (Morgan 2007: 99), a common knowledge that can also be found in ancient fables (Phaedrus, *Fabulae* 1.28). To illustrate his point, Seneca tells the story of Cassius Chaerea, whom emperor Caligula constantly mocked because of his feeble voice. Chaerea could not stand these insults any more, and was in essence forced to use his sword against the emperor (*De Constantia* 18.3–5).

It is also important not to be upset when you are insulted (Seneca, *Epistulae Morales* 74.20): you must remain calm and try to understand why you were insulted (Epictetus, *Enchiridion* 42). Musonius Rufus even claims that the only person suffering damage from an insult is the insulter, not the insulted (*Dissertationes* 10). Epictetus advises ignoring the opinions of other people (*Enchiridion* 42 and 50), while Seneca considers it a good idea to laugh with people when they laugh at you, following Socrates, who didn't have any problem with the jokes people made about him (*De Constantia* 19.1).

The best way to deal with people making fun of you can also be read in Seneca:

> What to think when we are insulted, when someone imitates our language, our way of walking, when someone imitates any impairment of your body or of your language? As if these would become better known when someone imitates them instead of when we are showing them. Some people don't like to hear about old age, grey hair and other things that (other) people wish to achieve (…). Thus the subject is taken away

from impudent people and people who try to be funny by insulting you, when you take this subject away before them. Nobody provides laughter when he finds the laughter in his own person.

(Seneca, De Constantia 17.2)[5]

For people suffering from a disability, self-deprecation is the best solution to cope with derision (De Libero 2002: 91). To illustrate his point, Seneca provides the example of the famous enemy of Cicero, Publius Vatinius, who, though not known as a Stoic philosopher, used self-deprecation as a way of self-preservation (Corbeil 1996: 46–56; Laes 2014: 195–196). This Vatinius 'was born to be derided and hated' (Seneca, *De constantia* 17.3: *hominem natum et ad risum et ad odium*) and suffered not only from gout, but also from *strumae*, cushion-like swellings in his face and neck. This deformity is described in ancient medical texts (Celsus, *De medicina* 5.28) and today we know that these swellings are the symptom of a malfunction of the thyroid gland, caused by a lack of iodine (Breitwieser 2005: 542). A funny anecdote about the hatred of the people towards this Vatinius can be found in Macrobius (5th century CE):

Because people had thrown stones at Vatinius, when he was the organizer of gladiatorial games, he obtained the decree of the *aediles* that not one person could throw anything towards the arena, except an apple. During those days someone asked Cascellius casually whether a conifer cone is an apple, to which the latter replied: 'If you plan to throw it at Vatinius, it is an apple.'

(Macrobius, Saturnalia 2.6.1)[6]

According to Plutarch Vatinius suffered from swellings in his neck and on several occasions Cicero made fun of this deformity (*Vita Ciceronis* 9 and 26). Another author, Velleius Paterculus even draws a parallel between the evil character of Vatinius and his bodily deformity:

in him, the deformity of his body was in competition with the ugliness of his character, thus his soul seemed to have been enclosed in the most suitable dwelling.

(Velleius Paterculus, Historia Romana 2.69.3)[7]

In the eyes of Seneca (*De constantia* 17.3–4), Vatinius is a fine example of teaching us how to deal with derision by others:

If he could do this thanks to the harshness of his speaking – his continuous insulting had made him forget to feel shame – why would this not be possible for someone who made some progress because of his study in the free arts and cultivation of wisdom? Here, one must add that it is a sort of vengeance to ruin the pleasure of someone who has insulted you. The insulter might say, of his intended victim, 'Oh woe is me! I think that he didn't understand it!' The success of an insult rests on the indignation of the person harmed by it.

(Seneca, De constantia 17.3–4)[8]

Approval of deriding disabled people

Only one question remains: how is it possible that Seneca, one of the most famous and most productive Stoic philosophers, who undoubtedly sees virtue as the highest good and who openly condemns the mocking of people with disabilities, was able to write a work titled

Apocolocyntosis divi Claudii (the gourdification of the divine Claudius)? In this political satire, Emperor Claudius is represented as a human *monstrum,* displaying his bodily disabilities:

> Word comes to Jupiter that a stranger has arrived, a man of fair height and hair well sprinkled with grey; he seemed to be threatening something, for he wagged his head ceaselessly; he dragged the right foot. They asked him what nation he was of; he answered something in a confused mumbling voice: his language they did not understand. He was no Greek and no Roman, nor of any known race. On this Jupiter bids Hercules to go and find out what country he comes from; you see Hercules had travelled over the whole world, and might be expected to know all the nations in it. But Hercules, at the first glimpse he got, was really much taken aback, although not all the monsters in the world could frighten him; when he saw this kind of object, with its extraordinary gait, and the voice of no terrestrial beast, but such as you might hear in the leviathans of the deep, hoarse and inarticulate, he thought his thirteenth labour had come upon him. When he looked closer, the thing seemed to be a kind of man.
>
> *(Seneca, Apocolocyntosis divi Claudii 5, tr. W. H. D. Rouse)*

In this passage it is very clear that Seneca is mocking the physical disabilities of Emperor Claudius, which are also described in the works of other authors (Suetonius, *Claudius* 30) and are probably symptoms of cerebral palsy (Leon 1948; Emberger 2012) or Little's disease also known as dystonia (Laes 2013: 164), although the difficult issue of retrospective diagnosis comes up again. Is this the same Seneca who previously praised Vatinius and condemned mocking people with disabilities? Seneca is certainly the author of this text and not one scholar doubts the authorship of Seneca, who seems to contradict Stoic philosophies by mocking the disabilities of emperor Claudius. We must understand Seneca's portrait of Claudius in the *Apocolocyntosis* in a different way: in a context, different from his philosophical writings, Seneca clearly wants to present us the image of an ideal emperor by showing us the opposite: an emperor who is unable to speak, who is a non-human animal or even a *monstrum* ('and the voice of no terrestrial beast') (Laes 2013: 166).

But Seneca doesn't only mock emperor Claudius. Elsewhere he mocks the baldness of women:

> The greatest amongst the physicians and the founder of this science said that the hair of women never falls out and that they never suffer from gout. But they also lose their hair and they also become ill in their feet. The nature of women has not changed, but it is defeated. Because they are now equal in the excessive behaviour of men, they are also equal in the bodily incommodities of men. They stay equally awake all night, they equally drink as men, and they challenge men in sporting and in drinking activities. They remove food from their reluctant intestines through their mouth and then they measure all kinds of wine again, while they are vomiting. They equally consume snow, as a remedy for their burning stomach. In lust they don't have to cede for men (…). So why do we have to be amazed when the greatest of all physicians, who knows most about nature, can be caught in a lie when there are so many women who suffer from gout and who are bald? They have lost the beauty of their gender because of their vices and because they have cast off their female nature, they are condemned to male diseases. (…) We now pay the interest for our exaggerated and boundless pleasures. You don't have to wonder about the amount of diseases. Count the cooks.
>
> *(Seneca, Epistulae Morales ad Lucilium 95.20, 21 and 23)*[9]

The reason why baldness and gout are criticized by Seneca is obvious: these deformities of the body are the results of a deviant way of life: both are clear signs of drunkenness (alcoholism?) and debauchery, so they don't deserve our pity (Laes 2014: 198–200).

Aristotle (384–322 BCE), who was highly esteemed by Stoic philosophers, explains why it is permitted to criticize and make fun of certain disabilities and to blame people for having them:

> But not only are the vices of the soul voluntary, but those of the body also for some men, whom we accordingly blame; while no one blames those who are ugly by nature, we blame those who are so owing to want of exercise and care. So it is, too, with respect to weakness and infirmity; no one would reproach a man blind from birth or by disease or from a blow, but rather pity him, while every one would blame a man who was blind from drunkenness or some other form of self-indulgence. Of vices of the body, then, those in our own power are blamed, those not in our power are not. And if this be so, in the other cases also the vices that are blamed must be in our own power.
>
> *(Aristotle, Ethica Nicomachea 1114a, tr. W. D. Ross)*

It is clear that men and women who lose their hair or suffer from gout can be blamed for their own misfortunes, so they deserve to be mocked. But what moral mistake did emperor Claudius make to deserve the same fate? Seneca gives an explanation in the *Apocolocyntosis*: Claudius is stupid and morally repugnant (*Apocolocyntosis divi Claudii* 8.10 and 11), so the ugliness of his character has an influence on his physical appearance. Claudius also lacks self-control (Seneca, *Apocolocyntosis divi Claudii* 10), another important Stoic virtue (Laes 2013: 166–7). All these aspects, and the portrait of Claudius as the opposite of the ideal, rhetorically gifted emperor, explain Seneca's derision of the physical disabilities of emperor Claudius: the emperor is the human monster, not only physically but also morally (Laes 2013: 166–7). If Claudius had been a good and wise emperor, his body would have appeared normal, and if he were suffering from disabilities, Seneca would either ignore them or praise Claudius in the same way he praised Vatinius. Now, the deformities of Claudius are an indisputable proof of the bad character of the emperor. Thus, the Stoic ideas about the origin of some disabilities amongst certain bad people can be put in line with the tradition of ancient physiognomy. In this pseudoscience, Greek and Roman physiognomists try to investigate the character of people by studying their physical traits, with special attention to the face (Corbeil 1996: 31–5; Barton 1994: 95–131). According to this pseudoscience – in a narrow sense – people having physical similarities with certain animals bear the characteristics of these animals, e.g. a person with ears as long as a donkey's is also as stupid as a donkey. In the broader sense, an ugly or deformed body denotes a deformed character (Weiler 2002), so when an ugly or deformed person is being mocked, he deserves this scorn by his fellow human beings because his ugliness betrays his evilness. Thus, it is very surprising that Seneca, in another work, praises Vatinius about whom Velleius Paterculus wrote that 'his soul seemed to have been enclosed in the most suitable dwelling' (cf. *Historia Romana* 2.69.3). For ancient believers in physiognomy, beauty was clearly in the eyes of the beholder (Garland 2010). In this way, the 'science' of ancient physiognomy was stronger than the important distinction Stoic philosophers made between body and mind.

Conclusion

No philosophy in Antiquity has challenged the ancient – and even present-day – ideal of having a beautiful body as much as the philosophy of Stoicism, replacing it with the ideal of virtue as the highest good. Is having a beautiful, healthy body important when your character is deformed and unhealthy? The philosopher Epictetus provides a clear example of how a disabled person can be a great philosopher, helping other people on the path to wisdom. And wasn't Socrates known as an ugly man who had the appearance of a satyr? This Stoic morality explains why Stoic philosophers won't laugh at deformed people or people suffering from disabilities. There is, however, one exception to the rule of not mocking other human beings: deformed, disabled and ugly people deserve to be loathed and scorned if they themselves are responsible for their own misfortune. This is made clear by the examples of women suffering from baldness and gout and, notably, by the stupidity and evil of emperor Claudius.

Did Stoic philosophers have any influence on larger segments of Roman society? Probably not, since these philosophers more or less concentrated on an elite, well-educated minority. But Shadi Bartsch and other historians have tried to render it plausible that the Roman Stoa introduced a new attitude towards the body and ushered in a culture in which people regarded and defined themselves as bodies susceptible to pain and suffering. Was this accompanied by a different attitude towards disabilities and people with disabilities, at least amongst a small part of the population (Bartsch 2006; Bartsch and Wray 2009; Laes 2014: 202)?

For a true Stoic philosopher the famous Roman saying *mens sana in corpore sano* ('a healthy mind in a healthy body') can easily be shortened to *sola mens sana* (only a healthy mind). All other things are *indifferentia* – and not worthy of consideration.

Notes

1 This vision can also be found in the works of the famous French philosopher René Descartes (1596–1650) and because of his influence in present-day philosophy, the Stoic vision is called a 'Cartesian' vision: Descartes saw a human being only as *res agens*, but trapped in a physical body. Today this Cartesian vision is seen as outdated: people not only have a body, but they also are a body and it is hard – nearly impossible – to make a distinction between body and mind.

2 *Maior sum et ad maiora genitus quam ut mancipium sim mei corporis, quod equidem non aliter aspicio quam vinclum aliquod libertati meae circumdatum; hoc itaque oppono Fortunae, in quo resistat, nec per illud ad me ullum transire vulnus sino. Quidquid in me potest iniuriam pati hoc est in hoc obnoxio domicilio animus liber habitat. ... Contemptus corporis sui certa libertas est.*

3 *Potest ex casa vir magnus exire, potest et ex deformi humilique corpusculo formosus animus ac magnus. Quosdam itaque mihi videtur in hoc tales natura generare, ut approbet virtutem omni loco nasci. Si posset per se nudos edere animos, fecisset; nunc quod amplius est facit: quosdam enim edit corporibus impeditos, sed nihilominus perrumpentis obstantia. ... ut scire possemus non deformitate corporis foedari animum, sed pulchritudine animi corpus ornari.*

4 *Si illi manum aut morbus aut hostis exciderit, si quis oculum vel oculos casus excusserit, reliquiae illi suae satisfacient et erit imminuto corpore et amputato tam laetus quam [in] integro fuit; sed <si> quae sibi desunt non desiderat, non deesse mavult.*

5 *Quid quod offendimur, si quis sermonem nostrum imitatur, si quis incessum, si quis vitium aliquod corporis aut linguae exprimit? Quasi notiora illa fiant alio imitante quam nobis facientibus! Senectutem quidam inviti audiunt et canos et alia ad quae voto peruenitur; ... itaque materia petulantibus et per contumeliam urbanis detrahitur, si ultro illam et prior occupes; nemo risum praebuit qui ex se cepit.*

6 *Lapidatus a populo Vatinius cum gladiatorium munus ederet obtinuerat ut aediles edicerent, nequis in harenam nisi pomum misisse vellet. Forte his diebus Cascellius consultus a quodam an nux pinea pomum esset respondit: 'Si in Vatinium missurus es, pomum est'.*

7 *... in quo deformitas corporis cum turpitudine certabat ingenii, adeo ut animus eius dignissimo domicilio inclusus videretur.*

8 *Si hoc potuit ille duritia oris qui adsiduis conuiciis pudere dedidicerat, cur is non possit qui studiis liberalibus et sapientiae cultu ad aliquem profectum peruenerit? Adice quod genus ultionis est eripere ei qui fecit factae contumeliae uoluptatem; solent dicere 'o miserum me! puto, non intellexit': adeo fructus contumeliae in sensu et indignatione patientis est.*

9 *Maximus ille medicorum et huius scientiae conditor feminis nec capillos defluere dixit nec pedes laborare: atqui et capillis destituuntur et pedibus aegrae sunt. Non mutata feminarum natura sed victa est; nam cum virorum licentiam aequaverint, corporum quoque virilium incommoda aequarunt. Non minus pervigilant, non minus potant, et oleo et mero viros provocant; aeque invitis ingesta visceribus per os reddunt et vinum omne vomitu remetiuntur; aeque nivem rodunt, solacium stomachi aestuantis. Libidine vero ne maribus quidem cedunt ... Quid ergo mirandum est maximum medicorum ac naturae peritissimum in mendacio prendi, cum tot feminae podagricae calvaeque sint? Beneficium sexus sui vitiis perdiderunt et, quia feminam exuerant, damnatae sunt morbis virilibus. ... Has usuras voluptatium pendimus ultra modum fasque concupitarum. Innumerabiles esse morbos non miraberis: cocos numera.*

Bibliography

Barton, Tamsyn S., *Power and Knowledge: Astrology, Physiognomics, and Medicine under the Roman Empire* (Ann Arbor, MI, 1994).

Bartsch, Shadi, *The Mirror of the Self: Sexuality, Self-Knowledge, and the Gaze in the Early Roman Empire* (Chicago, IL, 2006).

Bartsch, Shadi, and Wray, David (eds) *Seneca and the Self* (Cambridge, 2009).

Becker, Lawrence J., 'Stoic Emotion', in S. K. Strange and J. Zupko (eds), *Stoicism: Traditions and Transformations* (Cambridge, 2010), 250–75.

Breitwieser, Rupert, 'Kropf', in K. H. Leven (ed.), *Antike Medizin: Ein Lexicon* (Munich, 2005), c. 542.

Corbeil, Anthony, *Controlling Laughter: Political Humour in the Late Roman Republic* (Princeton, NJ, 1996).

Damschen, Gregor, and Heil, Andreas (eds), *Brill's Companion to Seneca, Philosopher and Dramatist* (Leiden, 2014).

De Libero, Loretana, 'Dem Schicksal trotzen. Behinderte Aristokraten in Rom', *Ancient History Bulletin* 16 (2002), 75–93.

Emberger, Peter, 'Kaiser Claudius und der Umgang mit Behinderten', *Journal of Early Medicine* 4 (2012), 75–81.

Garland, Robert, *The Eye of the Beholder: Deformity and Disability in the Graeco-Roman World* (London, 2010²).

Graver, Margaret R., *Stoicism and Emotion* (London and Chicago, IL, 2007).

Halliwell, Stephen, *Greek Laughter: A Study of Cultural Psychology from Homer to Early Christianity* (Cambridge, 2008).

Harris, William V., *Restraining Rage: The Ideology of Anger Control in Classical Antiquity.* (Cambridge and London, 2001).

Inwood, Brad, *Ethics and Human Action in Early Stoicism* (Oxford, 1985).

Laes, Christian, 'Silent History? Speech Impairment in Roman Antiquity', in C. Laes, C. F. Goodey and M. L. Rose (eds), *Disabilities in Roman Antiquity: Disparate Bodies A Capite ad Calcem* (Leiden, 2013), 145–80.

Laes, Christian, *Beperkt? Gehandicapten in het Romeinse Rijk* (Leuven, 2014).

Lagrée, Jacqueline, 'Constance and Coherence', in S. K. Strange and J. Zupko (eds), *Stoicism: Traditions and Transformations* (Cambridge, 2010), 148–76.

Leon, Ernestine F., 'The Imbecillitas of the Emperor Claudius', *Transactions and Proceedings of the American Philological Association* 79 (1948), 79–86.

Morgan, Teresa, *Popular Morality in the Early Roman Empire* (Cambridge, 2007).

Moser, Peter Daniel, 'Epikt – ein Porträt des Philosophen als behinderter Mensch', *Journal of Early Medicine* 4 (2012), 65–74.

Sellars, John, *Stoicism* (New York, 2006).

Setailoli, Aldo, 'Epistulae Morales', in G. Damschen and A. Heil (eds), *Brill's Companion to Seneca, Philosopher and Dramatist* (Leiden, 2014), 191–200.

Strange, Steven K., and Zupko, Jack (eds), *Stoicism: Traditions and Transformations* (Cambridge, 2010).

Thorsteinsson, Runar M., *Roman Christianity and Roman Stoicism: A Comparative Study of Ancient Morality* (Oxford, 2010).

Weiler, Ingomar, 'Inverted kalokagathia', *Slavery and Abolition: A Journal of Slave and Post-Slave Studies* 23 (2002), 9–28.

16

FOUL AND FAIR BODIES, MINDS, AND POETRY IN ROMAN SATIRE

Sarah E. Bond and T. H. M. Gellar-Goad

In Petronius' *Satyricon,* Encolpius, the narrator of the work, at first insists that Eumolpus cover Giton and himself with ink so that they might pass as Ethiopian slaves. All this in an elaborate attempt to sneak off a ship they had boarded without being noticed by two passengers from their past they wished to avoid. Giton rejects the idea, saying it was as ludicrous as circumcising yourself to look like a Jew, piercing your ears to look Arabian or rubbing chalk all over your face to look like a Gaul (102). To truly pass as an Ethiopian slave, dying yourself with ink would not be enough. Giton notes that it would also require fuller lips, curled hair, bowed legs, turned ankles, beards, and – above all – carving *cicatrices* (scars) into their foreheads. After all, tattoos and, less frequently, branding were common penance for slaves recaptured after running away (Jones 1987). Thus when Martial (8.75) mentions four *inscripti* who were carrying a body to be thrown on a mass pyre, the audience would have easily understood that the reference was to servile funeral workers. Rather than endure such intense body modification, however, the clever Eumolpus suggests instead that they put fake scars on their foreheads and shave all their hair off (103.1) so as only to appear to be slaves. However, when Lichas, the archenemy of the duo, finds out about the on-board haircuts, he orders them to be flogged. Even if the scars on their foreheads were fake, the wounds on their backs would leave permanent, visual and real reminders of their foiled ruse.

Describing the distinguishing marks, tattoos, scars or blemishes on another's skin sent translatable signals to the readers of Roman satire. Satirists used them to provide a character map that could indicate the ethnicity, status, experiences, morality and dignity of the individual in question, drawing a mental picture for the reader. In Antiquity, satirists were people who could 'read past' the corporeal in order to view the inner health, morality or nature of one's soul (Barchiesi and Cucchiarelli 2005: 207). However, the satiric body goes beyond simply making the internal manifest. These bodies demonstrate pragmatic and vocational aspects of ancient society as well. In a world without driver's licences, social security databases or passport photos, the body was an important indicator of identity (Cernuschi 2010). In the midst of their punishing lashes, Giton's cries reveal himself to his former mistress, whereas it is the naked genitals of Encolpius that communicate his true identity to Lichas. Encolpius' travels were meant as a satiric echo of Odysseus' journey in Homer's *Odyssey*, and likewise, this scene alludes specifically to Eurycleia, Odysseus' nurse in the *Odyssey*, who recognizes him from his scar (19.467). Similarly, we are told by Suetonius (*Vita Augusti* 65) that Augustus examined all of the freedmen and slaves that attended upon his daughter Julia in her banishment and recorded their age, stature, complexion and scars. Papyri and inscriptions indicate a similar focus on scars and distinguishing features for all members of society, both free and enslaved. A papyrus recording members of a voluntary association from Roman Tebtynis (*P.Mich.* 5.247) noted any scars on the bodies of its members, a loan receipt listed the scars of the participants involved (*P.Oslo* 1046), and runaway slave notices frequently referred to scars, warts or any other differentiating mark that might singularize the escapee (*P.Lond.* 7.1950). Although satire may have enhanced bodily dysfunction and used it for various purposes, Greco-Roman society as a whole appears to have been much more focused on such marks than we are today.

Encolpius and Giton are just two examples of the ways in which satirists manipulate the body. As this chapter explores, a host of vulnerable, foul, abnormal, ill and even deceased bodies populate the genre. Because ridicule and over-exaggeration of the human form had the ability to draw laughter, satirists often heighten age, ugliness, deformity, mental disability and even odour for comedic effect. In many ways, elegy is like the language one uses to convince a friend to go on a blind date, whereas satire is the language one uses to describe that date to a friend after the fact. Although he recognized there were limits to this form of mocking comedy, it was Cicero who stated that laughter often stemmed from the 'hideousness and blemishes of the body' (*De oratore* 2.239). Despite Cicero's claim, in Roman verse satire, at least, humour based on physical appearance or physical disability does not appear frequently. Yet the body is an important interpretive locus for the study of *satura* (Labate 1992; Braund and Gold 1998; Miller 1998, Walters 1998; on bodies in Horace specifically, see Oliensis 1991; in Persius, see Dessen 1996, Bramble 1974, Migliorini 1990, Reckford 1998; in Juvenal, Gold 1998). The satiric body is and was a distended, hyperbolic canvas that spoke to the literary masses, but it also a canvas that illuminates many elite pretensions. While not a direct reflection of social reality, the foul bodies depicted in Roman satire are still valuable for their instructional purposes, pointing us to elite Roman attitudes, phobias and perceptions. In this chapter we argue that dirty, disabled, putrid and otherwise deficient bodies play an important role in doing satire's work of distancing the satirist and his audience from the dangerous Others that populate his literary landscape; that these bodies reflect back on the satirists themselves and on their literary worldviews; and that the discourse of healthy mind and healthy body in Roman verse satire holds moralizing, metapoetic valence.

Abused and inviolable bodies

The antics of Encolpius and Giton aboard the ship point to the fact that control over one's body was a sign of dignity and social position in the Roman Republic and early imperial period. Whereas citizens and those with *dignitas* retained many corporeal rights, the disreputable body – a prostitute, an actor, a gladiator, a slave, a criminal – was more vulnerable to sexual penetration, whips, cudgels and any number of corporal punishments (Bond 2014: 16–22). Thus in Apuleius' tale of Cupid and Psyche in *Metamorphoses*, the goddess Venus has the ability to turn the mortal Psyche into an *ancilla* (house slave) for breaking the rule barring her from staring at Cupid. At the whim of her new *domina,* the servile Psyche is then repeatedly whipped, insulted and put to hard labour by Venus' other slaves: Habit, Anxiety and Depression (*Metamorphoses* 6.9–10). By the end of her labours for Venus, she resembles but a *dormiens cadaver* (sleeping corpse), but is revivified by Cupid, whose wound had finally healed into a scar (6.21). Unlike the fortunate, mythical Psyche, many real slaves must have been more physically altered while in servitude. In the *Satyricon,* Trimalchio, himself a former slave, is constantly threatening or inflicting corporal punishment on his *servi*: a slave gets his ears boxed (34), servile gladiators are flogged for a poor performance (45), a slave is stripped down for a beating (49) and another threatened with death (52). Although battle scars could certainly distinguish a soldier or king (Samama 2013) and a mangled gladiator could still be found sexually attractive (Juvenal 6.104–10), the marks gained during enslavement were not generally viewed as a badge of honour. In Horace's *Epodes* (4.1–6), the speaker differentiates himself from an antagonist by focusing on the physical marks of the latter's former enslavement (whip- and fetter-scars). This former slave bears his possibly criminal past on his body, having been *sectus flagellis hic triumviralibus* ('lashed by the triumviral whips'), and is deemed a disgrace to the post of military tribune (4.11, 20). We can compare this military tribune with Fonteius Capito, suffect consul of 33 BCE, whom Horace described as a polished gentleman with 'no flaw on him anywhere' (*Sermones* 1.5.32–3). The depiction of the abused, threatened, and vulnerable body is common in Roman satire. It communicated the relative status of an individual to the reader, just as the pristine body advertised privilege.

Satire transmits a rich vocabulary of violence to the reader, but not all corporal abuse was inflicted by others. The disgust that Trimalchio represented to readers stemmed in part from his gluttonous appetite and his partaking in unheard of luxury. Satirists like Petronius, Horace and Persius used the excessive consumption of food and drink – the abuse of one's body through *luxuria* – as a means of communicating immoral and often un-Roman behaviour. Medical writers such as Celsus, who encouraged balanced, moderate meals, similarly decried living to excess and taught that vomiting for the sake of luxury was ill advised (*De medicina* 1.3). Horace notes the self-abuse of the body by eating luxurious foods, and cites the abandonment of Roman ideals (*Sermones* 2.2), whereas Persius (*Satirae* 2.41–3) notes physical disability caused by poor diet. According to Persius, although you may pray for strength in old age, grand dishes and the pursuit of wealth keep the fortune bestowed by the gods away. Juvenal (1.140–4) notes the distended belly of someone who recently dined on peacock and emphasizes the gastrointestinal distress and even death that came from too much or too luxurious food (cf. Juvenal 3.232–4). Just as bodily marks could advertise a lack of personal liberty, the self-abuse of the body through obesity, gout and vomiting could function to separate the conservative, elite Roman from the upstart, nouveau riche, or foreigner. The juxtaposition of the pristine master beating the wounded slave, or the muscular rustic attending the dinner party of an obese freedman, spoke to Roman ideas of hierarchy and traditional values through the prism of the body (See Laes 2016 on obese bodies and the history of disability).

Dirty and clean bodies

In the first book of Apuleius' *Metamorphoses,* Aristomenes tells the harrowing tale of his meeting with a witch and *scortum scorteum* – a leathery whore –by the name of Meroe (1.8). After ostensibly killing her former lover, Socrates, while Aristomenes watched in horror, Meroe and her female companion then urinated on the dumbfounded Aristomenes (1.13) as a kind of final injustice. The *spurcus* (foul) stench from this urine did not dissipate later, but clung to Aristomenes while he spoke to the miraculously revived Socrates, who was repulsed and mystified by his friend's stench (1.17). Just like severe beatings sustained by slaves and those of lower status, the defiling of a body by urine was degrading, though to a lesser extent than physical harm. Whereas water and the bathing of the body represented civility for Romans (as when Aristomenes drags Socrates to the baths to strigil the filth off of him, see *Metamorphoses* 1.7), being urinated upon was shameful. For instance, Horace notes a number of painful bodily punishments received by adulterers enamoured with deriving pleasure from other people's spouses: leaping from a roof, flogging, falling in with a gang of thieves, extortion, castration and being urinated on (*Sermones,* 1.2.40–4). Not coincidentally, *meio, mingo* and its compounds could denote urination or ejaculation, and the verb used here by Horace (1.2.44) is *permingo* (Richlin 1992: 251, n. 8). Consequently, there may be an additional assertion of sexual dominance. While all of these punishments existed within an articulated hierarchy of shame, they were each actions that served to distance an individual corporally from the rest of the populace as a physical repercussion for a transgressive action that marked off the dirty from the clean.

How should we define the dirt that sullied the satiric body? The anthropologist Mary Douglas famously proposed that the definition of dirt was simply 'matter out of place' (1966: 2). Dirt is disorder. However, it is important to keep in mind that this notion of dirt is also dependent on the space within which it exists. As Anne Carson notes, 'The poached egg on your plate at breakfast is not dirt; the poached egg on the floor of the Reading Room of the British Museum is' (2002: 87). The 'dirt' that was attached to or flowing outward from the bodies in Roman satire was all the more humorous because of the spatial taboos they often punctured. The crossing of these boundaries also made for good metaphor. In Persius' *Satires* (1.112–14) the sacred land upon which a tomb was built was used as an allegory for the boundaries of poetry, and the poet mimics the public signs that warned off visitors from defecating or urinating on a tomb (*CIL* 6.2357; imitated in *CIL* 4.8899). The poet essentially remarked that satire can be used irreverently to urinate upon the genre of epic. Dirt was a fact of life in ancient Rome, but Persius exemplifies the fact that the substance occupied a set place within society (on Roman sanitation, see Scobie 1986; Koloski-Ostrow 2015). A soldier, who pees in a circle in the *Satyricon* before becoming a werewolf, is in a cemetery (62) rather than a latrine or a street-side amphora. Latrines, chamber pots or the workshops of tanners and fullers were the proper spaces for urine. Thus Petronius is commenting on the wealthy freedman's inappropriate use of space when he notes that Trimalchio signalled to a eunuch with a chamber pot to place it underneath him while playing a ballgame at the baths (*Satyricon,* 27). Satire often closely linked sewers, faeces and insults, but could also sully whole neighbourhoods with such excremental language (Koloski-Ostrow 2015: 110–11). Thus the Subura of Rome, known for its mix of taverns, impoverished workers and foreigners, became a depraved borough personified by the sewer that seethed beneath it – at least to Juvenal (5.105–6).

Romans did not reject filth completely; they simply wished to organize it. It was the elite that had the luxury of distance from this filth. As Mark Bradley has deftly shown, conservative elites used the human body as a locus for articulating alterity within Roman society and used the senses to separate those on the fringe from traditional Romans (2015: 133). Satire tested this spatial organization and often tied things that smelled, tasted, felt, sounded, or looked disgusting to morality. A prime example of the satiric use of spatial and bodily filth as commentary comes within the works of Horace. In his *Sermones* (1.8), he focuses in on Priapus, the lowly scarecrow god in charge of guarding the new garden of Maecenas on the Esquiline. The garden was built overtop the old cemeteries and trash middens of the earlier Republic. In the poem, the garden represents a 'transitional space', and both the bodies and magical actions of the witches indicate that the area's previous status lies under a thin veneer (Pagán 2006: 51). Canidia wears a black robe with bare feet and unkempt hair, while loudly yelling with Sagana. Horace remarks that their pale faces made them a frightening sight to behold (1.8.25–6). Using two proxies for their love curse victims – an *effigies* made of wax and another of wool – the two witches clawed the earth, ripped apart animals and sprinkled blood. It is only when the Priapus lets go a startling fart that the two unsightly bodies scurry away back to the urban centre, leaving their fake teeth and hair behind. Just like the space itself, the two witches (and the love they promise for their patrons) are but a facade. Their spatial tie to cemeteries manifests in their corpse-like appearance, demonstrating that the body and the location could work in tandem within satire.

It is with some irony, perhaps, that we should note that, when Horace died, he was buried near Maecenas on his lavish estate there on the Esquiline hill.

Corpses and living bodies

It was not simply the body but also the space inhabited by that satiric body that served to either marginalize or legitimize an individual. This is particularly true when considering the roles of the corpse, the cemetery and the funeral in Roman satire. A number of taboos surrounded corpses and the subsequent treatment of the body after death; these cultural attitudes are often commented upon, toyed with and frequently inverted in satiric works. Rome was a matrix of boundary zones both tangible and imagined. The *urbs Roma* (city of Rome) itself was surrounded by a kind of invisible boundary called the *pomerium*. This boundary separated the city from the *agri* (fields) with a conceptual, religious and juridical boundary. Dead bodies, soldiers with weapons and foreign cults were supposed to stay outside of this boundary, though there were a few exceptions over the years. The *pomerium* then made certain binary oppositions clear: there were the living versus the dead, the civilian versus the soldier and the Roman versus the foreigner. Such stark binary pairs can also be seen in Roman satire. Even if ambiguity and grey area existed in reality, the literary genre of satire projected films shot almost exclusively in black and white – at least at first viewing.

As far back as the Twelve Tables, corpses were legally kept from burial within the city (Cicero, *De legibus* 2.23, 58). The dead were themselves polluting agents that could defile both individuals and objects, and render those that came into contact with them disreputable both legally and socially within Roman society (Bodel 2000: 144). Hence we can see why the narrator and the other dinner guests in Petronius were moved to the level of extreme *nausea* (sickness) when Trimalchio began to recast the feast at Trimalchio's house as a funeral for himself (*Satyricon* 78). Talk of death, corpses and funeral pyres had no place at the dinner couch, and certainly the guests must have been stunned to see the flood of musicians and performers pour in for the mock-procession. Petronius has tongue in cheek when he notes that the *servus libitinarii* (slave of the undertaker) was the most *honestissimus* (honourable person) at the soirée. After all, in the world of Roman satire, spaces perceived as defiling or disreputable – cemeteries, bars, brothels – tended to seethe with disreputable bodies polluted by both vice and other agents, like death pollution. Take a scene from Juvenal's *Saturae* (8.171–6), which reiterates the old adage that you are the company you keep: 'Send to Ostia, Caesar, send, but look for the *legatus* in the big bar, and you will find him lying with some murderer, hanging out with sailors, thieves, and runaway slaves, among hangmen, bier-makers and the idle tambourines of a *gallus*, laid out from drunkenness.' Juvenal is using this scene in order to cast the *legatus* as immoral and perhaps even an *infamis* (infamous) person. Moreover, the bar is a place for criminals, theatrical persons and funereal workers to intermingle in the city of Ostia, and perhaps within other Italian cities as well. Marginal persons sullied by crime, the stage and death are here heaped together in one amoral pile within the bar. The *legatus* had walked into a den of iniquity.

The constant tension that existed between the living and the dead is also seen in the satiric portrayal of magic. In Horace's *Epodes,* we again have the character of the wild-haired, gnarly-toothed witch Canidia, who, along with Sagana, Folia and Veia, wishes to make a love potion from the *aridum iecur* (dried-up liver) of a boy they have kidnapped (5.37) and are now sucking the life out of. The young boy is literally being transformed into a corpse for the purposes of these ugly and nefarious women. In addition to producing corpses from actual murder or death, satire also used the corpse metaphorically and as invective. The invective poems within Horace's *Epodes* and *Satires* were modelled after the invective of Hipponax and Archilochus, in which slander was often heavily centred on the body. For instance, the narrator of *Epode* 8 blames the fact that he is impotent on the decrepit, black-toothed, wrinkled, spongy-stomached, flabby-chested, scrawny-thighed corpse of a whore that he is sleeping with. Although an old woman, she subverts the stereotype by being both sexually hungry and aggressive to the point of being masculine (Cokayne 2003: 140–1). For those in old age, being called a corpse appears a common insult. An old woman, who tended a robbers' cave in Apuleius' *Metamorphoses,* provides a prime example. Upon entering the cave, the returning robbers called to the woman: *Etiamne tu, busti cadaver extremum et vitae dedecus primum et Orci fastidium solum ...* (What's up, you last corpse on the funeral pyre, number one disgrace of life, and the only reject of Orcus ...). The language of death and the disgust conjured from such language is what satirists banked on and on which invective was predicated.

The discourse of sanity in Roman verse satire: mind, body, morality and metapoetics

One of Juvenal's most famous verses comes near the end of his tenth satire, a treatise on the Vanity of Human Wishes (as Samuel Johnson's imitation of it is titled). After deflating and mocking the foolish hopes and false poetry of those who pay for wealth, power, long life and so forth, the Juvenalian speaker, in a rare moment of positive recommendation, tells the addressee what to pray for: *orandum est ut sit mens sana in corpore sano* ('pray to have a healthy mind in a healthy body', *Saturae,* 10.356, cf. Seneca *Epistulae Morales* 10.4 and Weiler 1996: 159, who sees 'ein kausaler Konnex' between a healthy mind and body). The mind–body linkage encapsulated in this motto appears earlier in Roman satire, when the Horace *ego* compares his well-bred character with a few flaws to a nice body with a few moles:

> And yet if my nature/character is flawed by middling vices, but otherwise upstanding, just like if you'd criticize moles sprinkled on an otherwise outstanding body, [I owe it to how my father raised me].
>
> *(Horace, Sermones 1.6.65–7)*[1]

The 'middling vices' (*vitia mediocria*) appear earlier in Horace, at *Sermones* 1.4.130–1 and 139–40. This passage contrasts the satiric topos of infatuated lovers who apply terms of endearment to the physical and social defects of their beloveds (Lucilius fr. 17.2C = 540–546M = 567–573W = 541–547K; Lucretius, *De rerum natura* 4.1160–70; Horace, *Sermones* 1.2.80–105, 1.3.38–75; Juvenal 8.32–8).

The Roman satirists, each in his own way, hold up the image of the healthy mind in a healthy-enough body as the *aurea mediocritas* that they want their audience and their targets to strive for – and at the same time, they use this image metapoetically, as a metaphor for their own satiric aesthetics. A principal vector for this image, we argue, is a particular kind of disability, namely mental illness, and the discourse of sanity and insanity in Roman verse satire is one key to accessing the genre's poetic concerns. The discourse (which runs parallel in some ways to the voyeuristic, perverted 'libidinal rhetoric of satire' examined by Gunderson 2005) plays out in the simple usage of 'insane' as an insult (not too distant from ableist language in modern western societies), in moralizing diagnoses of insanity, in the moral shading of the mind–body connection and in metapoetic undertones of satiric mental illness.

The tactic of insulting someone by calling him or her insane has a long pedigree in Latin poetry. An early example is Plautus' *Menaechmi*, wherein one of the title characters, misrecognized as his identical twin by a certain Cylindrus, makes a joke about purificatory ritual:

M. responde mihi,
adulescens: quibus hic pretieis porci ueneunt
sacres sinceri? **C.** nummeis. **M.** nummum a me accipe:
iube té piari de mea pecunia.
nam équidem | insanum esse te certo scio,
qui mihi molestu's homini ignoto quisquis es.

Menaechmus:	Tell me, boy: what's the price for a whole sacrificial pig 'round here?
Cylindrus:	A *nummus*.
Menaechmus:	Well then, here, take a nummus, and have yourself cleansed at my expense. 'Cause I damn sure know you're insane, botherin' me, a guy you don't even know, whoever you are.

(Plautus, Menaechmi 288–93, cf. 314–15, 517)

Because he is bothering Menaechmus Sosicles, Cylindrus must be mentally ill. The adjective *insanus* functions similarly as a general-purpose insult at Horace, *Sermones* 2.6.29. So also in Juvenal insanity can be a standard-issue comparand for negative qualities: at 2.71, insanity is less disgusting/shameful (*turpis*) than wearing see-through clothes in public, and at 6.28, Postumus' erstwhile sanity (*certe sanus eras*) is questioned because he has decided to get married. Insanity as a token comparison point – as a stock basis for satire's negative value judgements – even finds a mythological *exemplum* in Orestes (Horace, *Sermones* 2.3.133–7; Persius 3.118, where the target of satiric critique is accused of doing things even Orestes would avoid; Ajax, too, at Horace, *Sermones* 2.3.187–213).

Satire's play with Stoic philosophy contributes two points to the satiric discourse on mental health (cf. Gevaert in this volume). First, both Horace, *Sermones* 2.3 and Persius' poem 3 build their critiques upon the Stoic precept that 'everyone except for the philosopher is insane' (so e.g. Fuchs 1977: 28, n. 1, 31, n. 8). Avoidance of philosophy, or embrace of worldly concerns and foibles, is labelled 'insane'. In Horace, for example, the interlocutor Damasippus, who dominates the conversation, describes how he was cured of the 'disease' (*morbus*, 2.3.27) of commercial employment. He then calls the Horace *ego* 'mad' and everyone 'fools' (*insanis et tu stultique prope omnes*, 32), just as he claims his Stoic instructor Stertinius had previously called him. The rest of the poem, which is replete with terms for mental disability (*insanire, stultitia, furor, desipere, excors, mentis morbus*, etc.), features Damasippus' interrogation of this 'madness', a category including ambition, luxury, superstition and greed (77–83). The treatment for this 'madness' is described in Persius: learn the underlying logic of the universe (*causas cognoscite rerum*, 3.66), namely what is right and proper and moderate (67–72).

The second Stoic component of the satiric discourse of sanity, stemming from the first, is the moral interpretation of psychological and psychosomatic maladies, especially the claim that ailments of the mind (i.e. character or behavioural flaws) are expressed by the body (so e.g. Reckford 1998: 339). As Barchiesi and Cucchiarelli put it, '[t]he satirist's eye, like that of a physician or expert in physiognomy, is keen at detecting indications of sickness or health, vice or virtue' (2005: 207, citing Lucilius fr. 26.65C = 638M = 678W = 662K: 'when someone is sick in mind we see an indication on the body', *animo qui aegrotat, videmus corpore hunc signum dare* – cf. Gevaert in this volume for the links between Stoicism and physiognomics). Indeed the satirists frequently diagnose their targets as insane on the ground of immoral activity. Prominent symptoms (or perhaps causes) of insanity in satire include vengeance (e.g. Juvenal 13.190–1), greed (e.g. Juvenal 1.92–3) and mercantile entrepreneurship (a product of greed: Juvenal 14.284–91, cf. Persius 5.52–61). Some people are so unbalanced by greed, the speaker of Juvenal's thirteenth satire alleges, that they would prefer physical disabilities such as blindness or gout to losing money (13.92–8). In Persius, the lust of tyrants (for power, wealth, sex) causes a derangement of their character (*ingenium*) that in turn produces both a loss of excellence and crippling anxiety- or fear-induced hallucinations (3.35–43).

And these mental-moral debilities are often inscribed upon the body – a causal pattern that Galsterer suggests is already implicit in the Juvenalian *mens sana in corpore sano* (1983: 35). Thus, as in the Lucilius fragment cited above, Juvenal's speaker claims that 'you can discover the mind's maladies hiding in a sick body, and pleasures too, as the face draws each disposition from these' (*deprendas animi tormenta latentis in aegro / corpore, deprendas et gaudia; sumit utrumque / inde habitum facies*, 9.18–20), and thus the turgid poetic spirit of one Furius makes his body itself distended (Horace *Sermones* 2.5.40–1, cf. Barchiesi and Cucchiarelli 2005: 209, n. 4). Gunderson's claim about the sexual physiognomy of satiric bodies – '[t]he narrator requires us to accept the (rhetorical) proposition that "bodily style is the man"' (2005: 228)– applies equally well to the satiric discourse on mental state. Psychological disability in satire (as in some strands of ancient medical thought) carries physical manifestations, such as the overabundance of blood that the Juvenal *ego* enjoins to be drained by doctors (*o, medici, nimiam pertundite venam*, 6.46, cf. 14.56–8 with e.g. Braund 2004: 238, n. 9, 463, n. 10). Again, this mind–body connection is often moralizing in tone, so that the madness causing (or caused by) greed, ambition, gluttony and other human faults is borne out by physical symptoms, the most extreme of which is death, as with the recurrent motif of fools given over to excess who die in their baths (Juvenal 1.140–4, 3.232–4; cf. Horace, *Sermones* 2.2, Persius 2.41–3, 5.52–61).

Moral turpitude, death, excess and the discourse of insanity all coalesce into a causal relationship in Juvenal's fifteenth satire, on cannibalism in Egypt, his last wholly surviving poem. In the first two lines, the speaker rhetorically asks, 'who doesn't know what sorts of monsters crazy Egypt worships?' (*quis nescit ... qualia demens / Aegyptos portenta colat?*, 15.1–2). Amid a catalogue of exotic and pedestrian animals supposedly deified by Egyptians, the speaker suggests that Egyptian religious practices are morally suspect because they omit reverence to gods more ordinary to Roman minds ('entire towns venerate a dog – but nobody Diana', *oppida tota canem uenerantur, nemo Dianam*, 15.8). This impious piety in turn generates an everlasting blood-feud between the denizens of two neighbouring Egyptian towns (33–8) – a rivalry metaphorically described as a chronic injury (*numquam sanabile uulnus*, 34). The intercity strife that arises from the controversy is a mental illness, an 'epidemic madness' (*inde furor uolgo*, 36). The product of this madness is a violence that extends not only to slaughter but even to gratuitous cannibalism (77–92), which is termed insanity (*rabies*, 126) and is contrasted (at 93–109) with the necessity-driven, understandable and excusable cannibalism of the besieged Vascones suffering from the 'madness of an empty belly' (*uacui uentris furor*, 100).

So for the satiric speaker in Juvenal 15, 'insane' religious belief leads to immoral impiety, from there to violent 'madness', and from there to the 'insanity' of cannibalism, a psychological disease physically expressed. Furthermore, Juvenal's Egyptians are throughout this poem presented as deficient humans, as lacking some aspect of human psychosocial capacity. The poem is filled with terms of wildness, barbarism and beastliness, as well as comparisons to beasts (e.g. *saevus*, 17, 115, 164; *feritas*, 32; *horridus*, 44; *barbarus*, 46; *saeuire*, 54, 126; *truces*, 125). The Egyptians' behaviour is contextualized within the decline of humankind from the mythic age to the time of Homer to now (69–70). The speaker digresses to explain that what separates humans from animals is our capacity for empathy (143–7) – and, by implication, that the Egyptian perpetrators of cannibalism in this satire are bestial and inhumane. He even says outright that animals are morally better than his satiric targets, since animals at least do not murder and consume their own species (159–64; at 163, a tigress is 'crazed', *rabida*, but still gets along with another tigress, unlike these humans). The capacity for and practice of cannibalism is thus figured not only as insanity but also as a psychic disability that reclassifies the cannibals as less than human.

Juvenal's fifteenth satire is also thoroughly metapoetic (as the speaker himself indicates by calling his story 'more serious than all the tragedies put together', *cunctis grauiora coturnis*, 29) and the poem's self-referentiality in this regard offers an entry point into the metapoetics of insanity in Roman satiric verse. Ehrhardt (2014) shows how this satire uses cannibalism as a metaphor for the poet's intertextual relationship to his literary predecessors, especially Ovid: the earlier poet(ry) becomes subject matter consumed by, digested within and absorbed into Juvenal's poetic *corpus* (cf. the potentially gruesome metaphor of poetry as a dismembered body in Horace, *Sermones* 1.4.53–61 and *Ars Poetica*). We argue that the mental illness of which the cannibalism is an expression is itself another metapoetic device. The rage directed at intercity rivals in Juvenal 15 answers the rage at poetic rivals or pretenders in Juvenal poem 1 (cf. Horace *Sermones* 1.4, 1.10, 2.1; Persius 1) and the resultant insanity/*rabies* of metapoetic cannibalism in 15, a madness that poisons the body by way of a poisoned mind, reflects the role of these rivals as the very sustenance of satiric production. Without something to mock, satire cannot be.

The metapoetic work performed by disability and especially psychological disability appears across the satiric corpus, not only at the end of Juvenal's opus. Barchiesi and Cucchiarelli claim that 'it is actually *through his own body* that the satirist finds a complete and economical means for expressing his poetic consciousness' (2005: 209–10; italics theirs) – and we would add 'through his own mind' as well as body, *mens in corpore*. In the opening of Horace's second book of *Sermones*, for instance, the reader learns that the Horace *ego* suffers from insomnia (*nequeo dormire*, 2.1.7) and at the same time lacks the strength, be it mental or physical, to write epic (*cupidum ... uires / deficiunt*, 'my strength fails me even though I want [to write poetry in praise of Augustus' deeds]', 12–13). Given Roman satirists' consistent endorsement of a mind–body connection in matters of psychology, we suggest that the topos of pinkeye (*lippitudo*), which Horace's and Persius' speakers use for their metapoetic *recusationes* of epic and of political affairs (Horace, *Sermones* 1.3.25–7, 1.5.30–1; Persius 1.79; so also Cucchiarelli 2001: 66–70, Barchiesi and Cucchiarelli 2005: 218), is in satire not merely a physical ailment but rather a psychosomatic condition. The ocular malady is linked with an intellectual disability, with the inability to tackle more serious subject matter and higher forms of poetry. Thus when the interlocutor of Persius' third satire reminisces about faking pinkeye to avoid studying declamations (3.44–5), he is suggesting that a poet's conjunctivitis is a failure not of the eyes but of the mind.

To return to the *mens sana in corpore sano* of Juvenal: that this is the sum of all prayers recommended by the satirist-speaker means metapoetically that he wishes simply for the ability to compose verse within healthy bounds of moderation and at a level befitting the genre and contents of that verse. We read poetic 'sanity' and 'health', both psychological and physiological, as equivalent to the *aurea mediocritas* glorified in the programmatic slogan *est modus in rebus* of Horace's *Sermones* ('there is moderation in / a limit to all things', 1.1.106). The Horace of *Sermones* book 1 advocates moderation even to the point of being content with 'middling flaws' (*uitia mediocria*, discussed above), so long as the person remains good on the whole. Meanwhile, the Horace of *Sermones* book 2, who yields much of his poetic real estate and dominant voice to a series of interlocutors, responds to a poem-length lecture from Davus with mere threats of violence – threats that Davus characterizes as 'insanity or poetry in the making' (*aut insanit homo aut uersus facit*). Whereas the satirist himself links his poetic production with good mental health, the more sceptical Davus equates Horatian satire instead with poor mental health and, in doing so, suggests that satire is itself a violent act (cf. Keane 2010: 52 ad loc.).

This moment aside, Roman satire's connection of the healthy-mind-in-a-healthy-body trope to its own poetics carries an evaluative element, as well. Since, as we have shown, physical ailments are outward symptoms of mental illness, and since mental illness is a product of (or coexistent with) immorality, good poetry is thus for the satirists *morally* good as well. Each satirist at some point or another portrays himself as physically or intellectually or artistically debilitated – or, on the other end, as using satire to vent the psychosomatically overfull, often-bilious contents of his spleen, liver or *praecordia* (Horace, *Epodes* 3.5, 11.15; *Sermones* 1.4.89, 1.9.66; Persius 1.117, 3.8–9, 5.22, 5.144; Juvenal 1.45). Yet ultimately his positive prescription for moral, medicinal and metapoetic mantra is moderation.

Conclusions on reading the satiric body

This chapter has argued that Roman satire represented and explored issues of unfreedom, status, poetry, luxury, death and mental-moral debilities through the inscribed, sensual body. Roman satirists carefully craft and articulate the look of the body in order to influence the perceptions of the reader, but the textual description of the smell, sound, touch and even taste of that body also serves to communicate the otherness of the individual. We are neither the first nor the last to recognize the symbolic significance of the body; Mary Douglas and later Michel Foucault had similar ideas about its regulation and use as an 'inscribed surface' through which we can view historical transformations. More recently, Judith Butler (1989) and Mark Bradley (2015) have extended and critiqued their ideas.

These satiric bodies do not exist within a vacuum. Their ancient creators were influenced in their techniques of invective or humor by literary predecessors. Roman satirists take advantage of pervasive social norms that deprecated and disempowered those with bodily differences – norms of healthy and unhealthy, sane and insane, whole and unwhole, strong and weak – in order to pursue their own poetic and moralistic agendas. Dirty, disabled, putrid and otherwise deficient bodies function to distance the satirist and his audience from the dangerous Others that populated his literary landscape, to paraphrase the theory of satire of Bogel (2001). This imagined landscape must also be defined and understood along with the satiric body. The satiric body and the topography it inhabits together reflect back on the satirists themselves and map their literary worldview.

Note

1 *atqui si vitiis mediocribus ac mea paucis / mendosa est natura, alioqui recta, uelut si / egregio inspersos reprendas corpore naeuos …*

Bibliography

Barchiesi, Alessandro, Cucchiarelli Andrea, 'Satire and the Poet: the Body as Self-Referential Symbol', in K. Freudenburg (ed.), *The Cambridge Companion to Roman Satire* (Cambridge, New York 2005), 207–223.

Bodel, John, 'Dealing with the Dead: Undertakers, Executioners and Potter's Fields in Ancient Rome', in V. M. Hope and E. Marshall (eds), *Death and Disease in the Ancient City* (London, 2000), 128–51.

Bogel, Fredric V., *The Difference Satire Makes: Rhetoric and Reading from Jonson to Byron* (Ithaca, NY, 2001).

Bond, Sarah, 'Altering Infamy: Status, Violence, and Civic Exclusion in Late Antiquity', *Classical Antiquity* 33/1 (2014), 1–33.

Bradley, Mark, 'Foul Bodies in Ancient Rome', in M. Bradley (ed.), *Smell and the Ancient Senses* (London, 2015), 133–45.

Bramble, J. C., *Persius and the Programmatic Satire* (Cambridge, 1974).

Braund, Susanna H. Morton (ed.), *Juvenal and Persius*. Loeb Classical Library 91 (Cambridge, 2004).

Braund, Susanna H., and Gold, Barbara K., 'Introduction', *Arethusa* 31/3 (1998), 247–56.

Butler, Judith, 'Foucault and the Paradox of Bodily Inscriptions', *Journal of Philosophy* 86/11 (1989), 601–7.

Carson, Anne, 'Putting her in her Place: Woman, Dirt, and Desire', in D. M. Halperin, J. J. Winkler and F. I. Zeitlin (eds), *Before Sexuality: The Construction of Erotic Experience in the Ancient Greek World* (Princeton, 1990), 135–69.

Cernuschi, Giuseppina, *Nuovi contributi per lo studio dei connotati personali nei documenti dell' Egitto greco-romano* (Padua, 2010).

Cokayne, Karen, *Experiencing Old Age in Ancient Rome* (London, New York, 2003).

Cucchiarelli, Andrea, *La satira e il poeta: Orazio tra epodi e sermones* (Pisa, 2001).

Dessen, Cynthia S., *The Satires of Persius:* Iunctura Callidus Acri (Champaign, IL, 1996²).

Douglas, Mary, *Purity and Danger* (London and New York 1966).

Ehrhardt, Kristen, 'Cannibalizing Ovid: Allusion, Storytelling, and Deception in Juvenal 15', *Classical Journal* 109/4 (2014), 481–99.

Fuchs, Jacob, *Horace's Satires and Epistles* (Toronto, 1997).

Galsterer, Henry. '*Mens sana in corpore sano*. Der Mensch und sein Körper in römischer Zeit', in A. E. Imhof (ed.), *Der Mensch und sein Körper: Von der Antike bis heute* (Munich, 1983), 31–45.

Gold, Barbara, '"The House I Live in is Not my Own": Women's Bodies in Juvenal's *Satires*', *Arethusa* 31 (1998), 369–86.

Gunderson, Erik, 'The Libidinal Rhetoric of Satire', in K. Freudenburg (ed.), *The Cambridge Companion to Roman Satire* (Cambridge and New York, 2005), 224–40.

Jones, C. P., 'Stigma: Tattooing and Branding in Graeco-Roman Antiquity', *Journal of Roman Studies* 77 (1987), 139–55.

Keane, Catherine, *A Roman Verse Satire Reader: Selections from Lucilius, Horace, Persius, and Juvenal* (Mundelein, IL, 2010).

Koloski-Ostrow, Ann Olga, *The Archaeology of Sanitation in Roman Italy: Toilets, Sewers, and Water Systems* (Chapel Hill, NC, 2015).

Labate, Mario, 'Le necessita' del poeta satirico. Fisiopatologia di una scelta letteraria', in I. Mazzini (ed.), *Civiltà materiale e letteratura nel mondo antico* (Macerata, 1992), 55–66.

Laes, Christian, 'Writing the Socio-Cultural History of Fatness and Thinness in Graeco-Roman Antiquity', *Medicina nei Secoli* 28, 2 (2016) 585–660.

Migliorini, Paola, *La terminologia medica come strumento espressivo della satira di Persio* (Pistoia, 1990).

Miller, Paul A. 'The Bodily Grotesque in Roman Satire: Images of Sterility', *Arethusa* 31/3 (1998), 257–83.

Oliensis, Ellen, 'Canidia, Canicula, and the *Decorum* of Horace's *Epodes*', *Arethusa* 24 (1991), 107–38.

Pagán, Victoria Emma, *Rome and the Literature of Gardens* (London and New York, 2006).

Reckford, Kenneth J., 'Reading the Sick Body: Decomposition and Morality in Persius' Third Satire', *Arethusa* 31/3 (1998), 337–54.

Reckford, Kenneth J., 'Only a Wet Dream? Hope and Skepticism in Horace, *Satire* 1.5', *American Journal of Philology* 120 (1999), 525–54.

Richlin, Amy, *The Garden of Priapus: Sexuality and Aggression in Roman Humor* (Oxford, 1992²).

Samama, Evelyne, 'A King Walking with Pain? On the Textual and Iconographical Images of Philip II and Other Wounded Kings', in C. Laes, C. F. Goodey and M. L. Rose (eds), *Disabilities in Roman Antiquity: Disparate Bodies* A Capite ad Calcem (Leiden, 2013), 231–49.

Scobie, Alex, 'Slums, Sanitation and Mortality', *Klio* 68 (1986), 399–433

Steenblock, Maike, *Sexualmoral und politische Stabilität: Zum Vorstellungszusammenhang in der römischen Literatur von Lucilius bis Ovid* (Berlin and Boston, MA, 2013).

Walters, Jonathan, 'Making a Spectacle: Deviant Men, Invective, and Pleasure', *Arethusa* 31/3 (1998), 355–67.

Weiler, Ingomar, 'Physiognomische Überlegungen zu *Mens sana in corpore sano*', in C. Klodt (ed.), *Satura lanx: Festschrift für Werner A. Krenkel zum 70. Geburtstag* (Hildesheim, 1996), 153–68.

17

THE 'OTHER' ROMANS

Deformed bodies in the visual arts of Rome

Lisa Trentin

There are conspicuously few representations of disability, and none of the severely disabled, in the entire repertoire of Roman art. Even the god Hephaestus/Vulcan, famously characterized in the literary tradition as lame (the earliest reference comes from the *Iliad*, where he is described as 'crook-footed', or with 'feet turned backwards': 18.371 and 1.607) is never portrayed as overtly disabled in the visual tradition; his lameness, when represented, is always discreet (e.g. a slight twist of the foot, see, for example, the Albani Puteal, c.2nd century CE, now in the Capitoline Museums, Rome) and his body is otherwise youthful and physically robust (on the iconography of Vulcan in Roman art, see the *LIMC* VIII (1997), 283–97; on the earlier iconographic tradition of Hephaestus in Greek art, see the *LIMC* IV (1988), 628–54; on lameness in Antiquity more generally, see Pestilli 2005). Vulcan's representation underscores a tension in the (literary and) visual record and in our examination here of disability: if one of the most famous characters in Antiquity is rarely depicted as physically impaired, then perhaps we should wonder whether disability, as understood today, works at all as an ancient category of identification?

While images of the disabled body are very few indeed, images of the deformed body are to be found with greater frequency (but not with great frequency) in Roman art. Originating in the Hellenistic visual tradition (see Mitchell 2013 and his chapter in this volume), rife with anomalous bodies of, to list just a few: black Africans and pygmies, dwarfs, hermaphrodites, emaciated men and grossly obese women, Hellenistic, and thereafter Roman, artists pushed the boundaries of artistic convention so as to challenge viewers to find beauty in bodies of *all* types. These Others, characterized by their unusual physical features – black skin, disproportionately small or exaggeratedly thin bodies, corporeal deformities, etc. – nevertheless, form a comparatively small assemblage in the corpus of (Greco-)Roman art.

The Romans preferred to represent near-perfect bodies: though in the Republic verism was favoured in facial portraiture, this was oftentimes juxtaposed with a youthful, idealized (classical, Greek-style) body (see e.g. the Tivoli General, c.70 BCE); in the Empire, the ever-youthful face of Augustus matched his ever-youthful and physically flawless body (see e.g. the Augustus of PrimaPorta, c.20 BCE). Even representations of the emperor Claudius, who, according to literary sources, suffered from a speech and mobility impairment (he somehow stuttered and was lame: Suetonius, *Claudius* 30), never show any hint of this; rather, his portraits show a handsome emperor with a healthy body (see the sculpture from Aphrodisias of Claudius conquering Britannia, c.1st century CE).

But the representation of beautiful and able Roman bodies was, in fact, quite 'abnormal': recent anthropological evidence has revealed patterns of general poor health and nutrition and high levels of trauma and infection, suggesting that the majority of ancient viewers inhabited bodies far removed from the artistic ideal (see Graham 2013: 254, and Pudsey in this volume). Even the Hellenistic tradition, with its heightened artistic interest in diverse body types, doesn't bring us any closer to a 'realistic' representation of the body; here too the evidence is skewed towards the exaggeratedly ugly and abnormal or deformed. How, then, would ancient viewers have responded to these extremes of representation, the perfectly healthy and able-bodied versus the horribly diseased and deformed body?

This present chapter aims to uncover the ways in which Roman audiences engaged with, and ascribed meaning to, bodies of difference. I shall focus on artefacts that survive from across the Roman Empire, spanning a period of four hundred years, from the 2nd century BCE to the 2nd century CE, during which time we find an abundance of relevant visual material. I examine a wide range of deformed Others (dwarfs, pygmies, hunchbacks, etc.), all connected by their *atopia*, or unbecoming physical appearance, as represented in different media (mosaic pavements, wall paintings, large- and small-scale sculpture), so as to showcase the breadth of representation. Inevitably, however, the analysis that follows will be limited to a selection of examples, albeit ones that best reflect the corpus of Roman Others.

What follows then, is a careful rereading of (some) familiar images in an attempt to bring new meaning to our understanding of difference (see Laes *et al.* 2013: 5–6). We approach these artefacts as viewers, aiming to reconstruct how they would have been encountered in the ancient world: we examine their size, shape and medium; the context(s) in which they were displayed (when known); then delve deeper into the wider socio-cultural environment in which they were made, displayed, and viewed.

Different bodies, different meanings

There exists a universal fascination with confronting the body of the Other, but the meaning and significance attributed to these bodies varies from culture to culture, through time and space. How are we to interpret the bodies of deformed Others as represented in the visual arts of the Romans?

Only a handful of scholars have studied the corpus of Others in Roman art with rigour, fewer still the deformed and disabled Other. In his ground-breaking work, *The Eye of the Beholder: Deformity and Disability in the Graeco-Roman World* (first published in 1995, second edition published in 2010), Garland provides the earliest comprehensive analysis of 'Images of the Deformed', highlighting the different types of deformities and physical disabilities represented in the ancient (Greco-Roman) visual record, along with the problems inherent in the interpretation of their iconography. Images of the deformed appear most frequently in the so-called 'minor arts', e.g. miniature statuettes; Garland asserts that these were designed primarily to 'shock or amuse', with exceptions created by artists 'whose foremost concern was to render the plight of their subject with unsparing realism and attentive, if not always accurate, observation' (Garland 2010: 121). In Grmek and Gourevitch's foundational monograph, *Les maladies dans l'art antique* (1998) this 'realism and attentive observation' is contextualized within the medical tradition; Grmek and Gourevitch survey a multitude of deformed Others, attempting to diagnose the pathologies represented, hoping, in turn, to shed light on the existence and frequency of diseases and their social and psychological impact. Building on the work of earlier tradition (the study of the pathological grotesque is explored earlier, in Stevenson's 1975 doctoral thesis, 'The Pathological Grotesque Representations in Greek and Roman Art'), this study is important for understanding the representation of diseases in ancient art, and their diagnosis and treatment; nevertheless, it fails to address the broader social contexts in which these images were displayed, and viewed.

In studying individual types, scholars have attempted to nuance our understanding of the deformed Other, proposing a wider array of theories for their function, some better received, and indeed more convincing, than others: models (teaching aids?) of individuals suffering from various pathologies (medical context); votives to Asclepius and other (healing) divinities (religious context); prophylactic charms, charms to protect against the evil eye, charms to enhance sexual potency (social context); and representations of mimic actors, sympotic entertainers or imperial court jesters (artistic context).[1] In many ways, these interpretations echo the assertion of Garland: the power of the Other lies in its ability to shock and amuse.

As recent work on Hellenistic (Masséglia 2015) and Roman art (Trentin 2015) has demonstrated, however, these images resonated with viewers in more profound ways that went far beyond their initial shock or amusement. As objects made for display, representations of the deformed Other have been found decorating both public and private spaces, including tombs, bathhouses, and villas, throughout the Roman world. A large number also exhibit extraordinary artistic sophistication and exceptional workmanship. The diverse display contexts and fine quality of these images suggests that the body of the Other was invested with both symbolic and ideological capital. These images demand that a viewer do more than just gawk and laugh: they implore a viewer to look at these bodies and to engage (sometimes in very physical ways) with their otherness, forcing a viewer to consider their own corporeal relationship to the body of the Other, and their own privileged status as 'normal'-bodied (affirmed through race, gender, social status *and* ability) or, perhaps, more interestingly, their own distance from the norm. Reviewing the visual evidence will thus expose the content and context of these representations; I shall examine the scholarly framework within which these representations have been traditionally studied, namely their function as apotropaia, and then, highlight directions for future research, asking new questions about the relationship between viewer and image, pushing the limits of contemporary scholarship. In so doing, it shall become clear that the distance and difference traditionally associated with the body of the Other in the Roman world was neither fixed nor static; artists relished in blurring the boundaries between the beautiful and ugly, normal and abnormal, able-bodied and dis-abled body, to tease out the tension between *all types* of bodies and their associated meanings.

The other as apotropaion

The most widely recognized interpretation for the function of the Other is their use as apotropaia, charms to ward off the evil eye of envy. Indeed, the apotropaic power of the Other has been well established based on two conspicuous elements in their representation: emphasis on the hyperphallicism of the Other, that is, the presence of a disproportionately large and/or erect phallus, and the *atopia*, or unbecoming appearance, of the Other, specifically, the disproportion of the body, the caricature of facial features, and the presence of visible physical defects; all of which contributed to positioning the body of the Other on the outermost margins of Roman standards of normality, thereby eliciting laughter ('shock and amuse') and dispelling evil.

In as much these images served an apotropaic function, they could also, as shall be demonstrated below, take on additional meanings. Classifying these images as straightforwardly or singularly apotropaic negates other, often overlooked, modes of viewing. When we consider the gesture and posture of these Others, as well as the addition of other attributes, then we are forced, as the ancient Romans must have been, to re-evaluate the role of the Other in the construction of the Self. To demonstrate this, we shall examine a handful of artefacts which clearly served an apotropaic function, but, upon closer analysis, also served to highlight tensions in the valuation of one's own body.

Dwarfs in Roman art

The most systematic study of dwarfs in the Roman world is Garmaise's 1996 doctoral thesis ('Studies in the Representation of Dwarfs in Hellenistic and Roman Art'), though also important is Dasen's early work on dwarfs in the Egyptian and Greek worlds (1993), and her more recent work on the representation of Hellenistic and, to a lesser extent, Roman dwarfs (Dasen 2006, 2013). Representations of dwarfs depict women and men characterized by their full-sized heads and trunks but with short, bowed legs and arms, and disproportionately small toes and fingers. Appearing in a wide variety of media, particularly popular in miniature statuettes, or as tintinnabula (bells or chimes), and wall paintings (the blurring in iconography between dwarfs and pygmies is most clear here, see below, p. 241) and mosaic pavements, dwarfs are engaged in a variety of activities, from the civilized to the uncouth; most popularly performing as entertainers, playing instruments or engaged in ecstatic dancing, or both.

One of the most oft cited examples of the dwarf clearly serving as an apotropaion is the mosaic pavement that once decorated the main vestibule to the peristyle court in the so-called House of the Evil Eye, a Roman villa in Jekmejeh, south-west of Antioch, dating to the 2nd century CE (Figure 17.1) (see Levi 1941, 1947; Trentin 2015: 54–9). This mosaic, measuring 1.74 m high by 1.47 m wide, features a large eye (an evil eye) being viciously attacked by various animals and weapons, including a trident and sword, snake and scorpion, dog and panther, and a raven and centipede.

To the left of the eye is a naked dwarf who appears to be walking away from the eye. He carries rhythm sticks, which indicate he is dancing. The dwarf is endowed with a large phallus

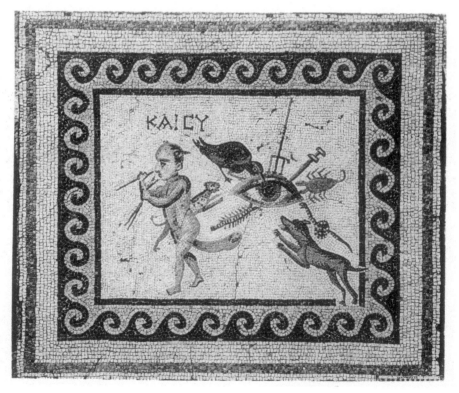

Figure 17.1 Mosaic pavement depicting an ithyphallic dwarf and the evil eye, c.2nd century CE. From the 'House of the Evil Eye' in Jekmejeh near Antioch, now Hatay Archaeology Museum, Antakya, 1024. [Photo after Stillwell 1941: pl. 56, no. 121]

that projects backwards from below his buttocks, stretching towards the eye, as if to attack it too (the 'tuck-for-luck' pose, as coined by Masséglia 2015: 289). Above the dwarf, the phrase καὶ σύ appears, in red tesserae. This cursory phrase has strong apotropaic associations: it likely served as a prophylactic curse, perhaps translated as 'may you also suffer ill' and understood as spoken by the dwarf and directed at the eye (and the viewer?).

Below this mosaic were discovered two smaller mosaic pavements, used as decoration at an earlier date, the apotropaic function of which is also clear and directly connected to the dwarf mosaic. The first mosaic (Figure 17.2), measuring 0.84 m high by 0.83 m wide, features a lone, dwarfed hunchback, depicted wearing a short, grey and white loincloth that does little to conceal his erect phallus. The dwarfed hunchback strides toward the left, looking back over his right shoulder, thus directing a viewer's gaze to his prominent hump. He carries in each hand a rhythm stick, similar to those carried by the dwarf. Above the hunchback the phrase καὶ σύ also appears, here in black tesserae.

The second mosaic (Figure 17.3), measuring 0.87 m high by 0.85 m wide, laid a few feet above, features Herakles as a baby strangling the snakes sent by Hera to kill him. Herakles' body is plump and infantile but his head, with dark brown-grey hair and full eyebrows, looks like that of an adult; this contrasts with the hunchback, who, even as an adult, is represented with a child's dwarfed body. Herakles is depicted kneeling on his left knee and wears a light-brown cloak with yellow highlights, thrown over his shoulder. He holds the head of one snake in his left hand close to his left thigh and the other in his right hand, without looking at either of them; rather, he gazes outside of the mosaic's frame towards the left in the opposite direction to the hunchback.

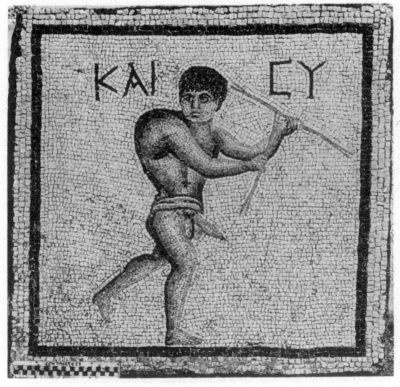

Figure 17.2 Mosaic pavement depicting an ithyphallic hunchback, c.2nd century CE. From the 'House of the Evil Eye' in Jekmejeh near Antioch, now Hatay Archaeology Museum, Antakya, 1026/a. [Photo after Stillwell 1941: pl. 56, no. 120 Panel A]

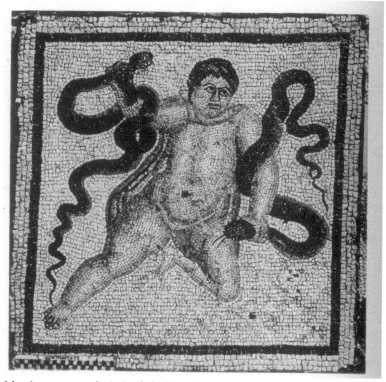

Figure 17.3 Mosaic pavement depicting baby Herakles strangling snakes, c.2nd century CE. From the 'House of the Evil Eye' in Jekmejeh near Antioch, now Hatay Archaeology Museum, Antakya, 1026/b. [Photo after Stillwell 1941: pl. 56, no. 120 Panel B]

In analysing all three of these mosaics, scholars have focused on their use as apotropaia, arguing that it was a viewer's laughter at the sight of the figures represented that would have dispelled the evil feared by a viewer (Levi 1941: 225; Clarke 2007a: 160). Although laughter may have been the anticipated response, and perhaps even the most common response, I have argued elsewhere (2015) that it was certainly not the only response. These mosaics engaged a viewer in active viewing. The sheer size of the mosaics and their placement in an entranceway suggests that a viewer might have had to be careful when passing through the vestibule to the peristyle court so as to not step on the hunchback or baby Herakles, although perhaps stomping on the eye in the dwarf mosaic would have been an added protective measure. The high quality of the mosaics, evidenced in their decoration and detailing, would have demanded that a viewer lean in or crouch down to get the best view of the fine figures depicted. Upon close inspection, a viewer might be compelled to question the meaning ascribed to the bodies of these figures: the pairing of the dwarfed hunchback with the baby Herakles is especially significant in that it places two extremes of appearance, one depiction of physical deformity, the other of physical strength, on the same plane so as to be viewed one against the other. The implication of the phrase καὶ σύ in both mosaics could perhaps be read outside of its cursory context: translated simply 'and you' it demands that a viewer weigh him/herself against these bodily extremes, prompting a viewer to consider his/her own (ab/normal) position along a sliding scale of divine and debased, normal-bodied and abnormal-bodied. This seems to have been the case with another example of an Other, a hyperphallic hunchback.

Hunchbacks in Roman art

Of all deformed Others, the corpus of hunchbacks is less copious, and has consequently received the least consideration, until recently, with my own work (2009, 2011, 2015) and that of Masséglia (2015). Representations of hunchbacks have survived in a variety of different media, from small-scale statuettes in terracotta, bronze and ivory, to hanging vases, a vase painting, a wall painting, a mosaic pavement, a bronze mirror, and one large-scale marble sculpture. Studied in connection with other Others (especially dwarfs), representations of the hunchback have often been attributed an apotropaic function; indeed, many examples explicitly served such a function, but other, complementary functions, equally important, are likewise key to understanding the hunchback's complex iconography.

Perhaps the most famous example of a hunchback is the sole surviving large-scale sculpture, dating to the 2nd century CE, now in the Villa Albani-Torlonia in Rome (Figure 17.4) (see Trentin 2009; Trentin 2015: 40–4).

Only the upper torso of this fine-grained Luna marble statue survives, measuring 56 cm high. The statue is remarkable not only because of its size (it is the only extant large-scale representation of a deformed Other), but also because of its context: it was found in the Baths of Caracalla in Rome (and is the only representation of a visibly deformed body to have decorated a monumental, public space.).

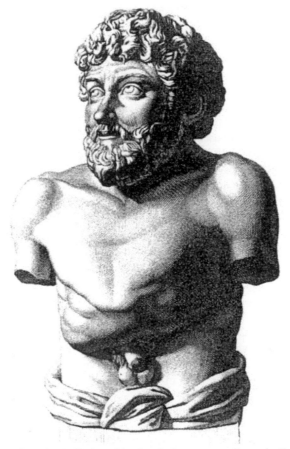

Figure 17.4 Engraving of an ithyphallic hunchback, c.2nd century CE. From the Baths of Caracalla, now in the Villa Albani-Torlonia, Rome, 964. [Engraving after Visconti 1811: II, pl. 12]

This hunchback juxtaposes disparate corporeal features: a handsome head paired with an unnaturally proportioned and physically deformed body. The hunchback has a full head of short, thick, curly hair, and wears a full, trimmed beard accompanied by a trimmed lip moustache. He has oval eyes, the irises of which have been drilled, a strong aquiline nose and thin lips. His head is angled to the right and he gazes upward with slightly furrowed brows, revealing a calm expression of quiet contemplation and reflection. His body is altogether different. He has a stunted torso and protruding chest box, which give the impression of a dwarf-like physical appearance; also noteworthy is the disproportion of parts: the hunchback's head is 27 cm long while the entire upper torso measures only 29 cm. He also has a prominent hump on his back, now significantly worn away on account of having been rubbed (for good luck?), and was originally endowed with a semi-erect penis, now covered by a fig-leaf. The fact that this hunchback is represented as (ithy)phallic would suggest that he likely served as an apotropaion. However, this attribution is complicated by the fact that he is represented with a remarkably handsome face.

The original display setting of this hunchback in the Baths of Caracalla remains unknown; however, as I have argued elsewhere (2009), based on the decorative programme of the Baths, the sculpture was likely displayed in one of the Baths' outdoor garden areas, seated upon a (rocky) base, set at ground level so as to be at an equal, or lower, height to passers-by. Viewing this sculpture fully in the round would have elicited a wide range of responses from a viewer; indeed this seems to have been the function of the hunchback, and many other sculptures in the Baths of Caracalla: the sculptures manoeuvre a spectator's viewing experience through their treatment of front and back, making the viewer the dupe of their programmatic character, shocking and surprising viewers in unexpected ways (on the sculptural programme of the Baths and viewer engagement, see Marvin 1983; Trentin 2009: 145–51). From whichever angle this sculpture is approached, a viewer would be unexpectedly confronted with a figure whose head is at odds with his body, thus causing the viewer to ponder the oddity of this disjunction. This hunchback, in its display of such disparate features (handsome face, deformed body and erect penis) was surely intended to confound a viewer's expectations (compare veristic portrait heads paired with physically robust bodies, as discussed above).

A hunchback is perhaps not the ideal piece of statuary to find in a bath complex – indeed, it is unusual in its public display setting – but perhaps this was the point of his display. This hunchback's deformity was not minimized or hidden away; rather it was placed in a grand, public setting for everyone to see and, more importantly, judge. The facial expression of the hunchback, of contemplation and reflection, perhaps encouraged a similar response from a viewer, who, after having examined this figure fully in the round, might have looked at this hunchback anew and thereafter reflect upon his own body and mind and to (re)consider what quality defined him. This thought-provoking introspection is likewise evidenced in the representation of other Others.

Pygmies in Roman art

Representations of pygmies, or 'very small negroid people' (Versluys 2002: 275), otherized by their dark skin colour, short stature, and hypersexual nature, become a popular type of representation of the black African in the Roman world by the middle of the 1st century CE (Clarke 2007b:160; for a full description of the physical features that characterize the pygmy, see Versluys 2002: 275–7; for the black African more generally, see the work of Snowden, esp. 1970: 5–11, but also 1976, 1978, 1983, 1996, 2001). Pygmies are most often represented engaged in unusual (and usually sexually explicit) exploits in Nilotic landscape scenes, depicted on wall paintings and mosaic pavements, in both a domestic and funerary context, especially in Italy, where the greatest number of Nilotic scenes have been found. The role of pygmies in such scenes has been systematically studied by Clarke (1998, 2007a), Dasen (1993, 1994), Meyboom and Versluys (2005), and Versluys (2002); all of whom agree that their representation is to be attributed an apotropaic function, in both life and in death (see especially Clarke 2007a). For a Roman viewer, images of the hyperphallic (foreign) Other engaged in sexual acts were meant to amuse and titillate; indeed, this bespoke their apotropaic power. As Clarke notes 'By having them [pygmies] carry out sexual acts in open nature, artists created a comic foil to the elegant couples on beds who represented 'bourgeois' lovemaking. The viewer could identify him- or herself with the refined representations, but the expected response to the crude pygmies' acts would be laughter' (Clarke 1998: 43–4). According to Versluys, however, these images also had additional, erotic power. Versluys has suggested that scenes of sexual intercourse associated with the Nile flood referred to the importance of the Nile in Egyptian religion (namely the divine union between Isis and Osiris) and emphasized the pygmies' symbolism with fertility and abundance; rather than depicting comic parodies of lovemaking scenes, these were genuine imitations of foreign sexual-religious rituals (Meyboom and Versluys 2005: 182–202). Of course, the very foreignness of these individuals and their rituals could have been amusing to a Roman audience, but the point seems to be that laughter was not the only response that these overtly sexual images could elicit.

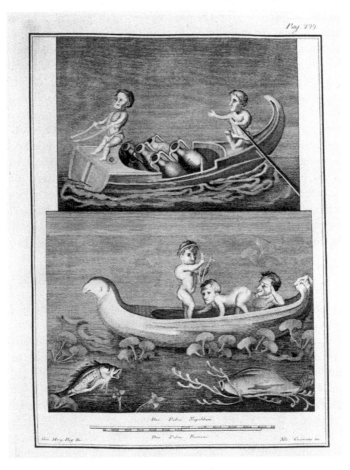

Figure 17.5 Wall painting depicting pygmies in a boat floating along the Nile, c.1st century BCE. From Pompeii, painting now lost. [Drawing after Carelli 1755–1831: VII: 297–9]

One example of the pygmy's dual nature, as apotropaion and erotic stimulus, comes from a 1st century BCE wall painting discovered in Pompeii (Figure 17.5) (see Trentin 2015: 65–7). The scene depicts three male pygmies on a boat. The pygmy on the left is a hunchback, depicted standing and facing the two other dwarfed pygmies.

This hunchbacked pygmy is nude and ithyphallic, although his erection has been expurgated from the 18th-century drawing. Next to him is another nude pygmy, bent on all fours with his buttocks in the air – he is in the coitus *a tergo* position – and looks as though he will soon be engaged in fellatio. Both he and the hunchback pygmy stare outside of the painting, as if looking directly at the external viewer. The third pygmy reclines, head propped by his left arm, directly behind (literally, behind the buttocks of) the second pygmy; he smirks, and his gaze tells us why: it is directed straight ahead, at the buttocks of the pygmy, rather than turned towards the viewer. The scene is one of misbehaving pygmies, an orgiastic threesome on a boat sailing along the exotic, fertile Nile, fecund with fish and river flora. In the repertoire of Nilotic paintings, scenes of pygmies involved in sexual acts were particularly popular as decorations in the garden areas of Pompeian houses; the *a tergo* position was exclusive to scenes of lovemaking on boats, and is usually, though not exclusively, reserved for male–male encounters (see Versluys 2002: 282 and Meyboom and Versluys 2005: 183).

But in this particular wall painting something more is going on. None of the pygmies are actually engaged in sexual activity, *yet*. The painting presents a moment at which time the action stops and all three pygmies debate what to do next: the external viewer is thus implicated in this debate – confirmed by the two pygmies who stare directly at the external viewer – and is permitted to play out a range of possible outcomes. As a homoerotic scene, this underscores a male viewer's own erotic desirability, both to other men and women. Given the importance placed on the role of active and passive sexual partners in the ancient world, this scene creates a tension by blurring the boundaries between soon-to-be-active pygmies, and passive, but perhaps also soon-to-be-active, viewer. The context in which this wall painting was displayed (the triclinium? the peristyle portico? Unfortunately, we don't know the recorded provenance of the painting) and the events surrounding its viewing (e.g. a banquet or drinking party, perhaps with lavish entertainment, performed by deformed slaves?) would certainly have affected a viewer's response to the scene. The 'crude' sexual acts of the misbehaving pygmies were thus a deliberate statement (or perhaps warning) about in/appropriate sexual conduct. The viewer remains at a safe distance to the orgy about to take place, thus maintaining the role of an outsider looking in and affirming the difference between 'normal' viewer and 'abnormal' Other, in body and action.

Disabled bodies in Roman art

It is much more difficult to recover the bodies of what we conventionally deem 'disabled' Others in the visual record of ancient (Greece and) Rome. No depictions survive of the severely disabled, and other (minor) disabilities are also difficult to identify in the visual record outside the sphere of the famously disabled: the lame god Vulcan, or the blind bard Homer, for example.

One remarkable, and indeed, anomalous, example in which we can positively identify a deformed and disabled Other comes from an Etruscan mirror from the necropoli at Tarquinia, dating to the 1st century BCE (Figure 17.6) (see Trentin 2015: 61–4). The decoration of the mirror consists of a garland of a continuous ivyleaf wreath pattern, with large, heart-shaped leaves with stems, surrounding the main medallion design without interruption.

The medallion features a naked, dwarfed hunchback with a protruding chest box. Notably, the dwarfed hunchback is represented with stumped feet, indicating that he is lame. He is

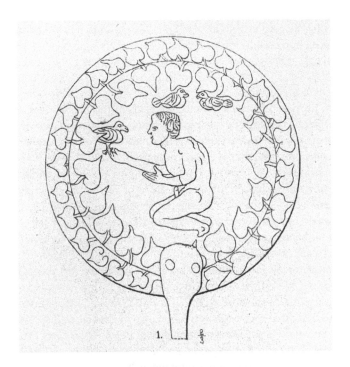

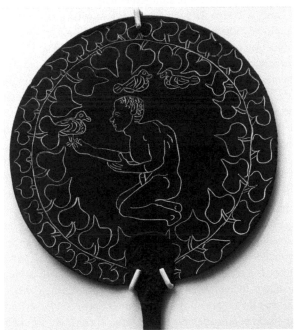

Figure 17.6 Bronze mirror depicting a lame hunchback, seated, and surrounded by birds, c.1st century BCE. From Etruria, now National Archaeological Museum, Tarquinia, RC 5776. [Drawing after Gerhard 1884–97: 186, pl. 141.1; photo by author ©2015]

depicted kneeling on the ground with his erect phallus pointing upward between his legs. His right arm is extended horizontally with a bird perched on his right hand. Two additional birds (flying or resting) appear above the lame hunchback's head facing one another.

Although most Etruscan mirrors with known provenance have been found in tombs, they were certainly not made specifically for the grave, but their secondary setting as a grave good suggests that they provided apotropaic protection both in life *and* in death. Used during the lifetime of the deceased as an object of adornment, mirrors not only served a utilitarian function, but also had symbolic and magical connotations. The user of the mirror was involved in rituals of (narcissistic) beautification, and thus was especially prone to eliciting the evil eye of envy from spectators. The mirror itself, which was a highly valued item of considerable craftsmanship, in metalsmithing, and creative skill, in the incised detail of the figural decoration, thus signified a level of status and wealth, adding yet another layer of potential envy. The user thus took the precaution of ornamenting this mirror with an apotropaic image – a lame, ithyphallic hunchback – to avert evil. As the hunchback does not appear as a stock image for Etruscan mirrors – indeed, no other image of a hunchback has been identified in the corpus of Etruscan mirrors – we can suppose that the owner of this mirror had a specific, personal reason for choosing the hunchback.

As an apotropaion, the mirror was equally important to its owner beyond their lifetime into their death, since it also functioned as a grave good. Based on analyses of other mirrors found at Tarquinia and other apotropaic tomb imagery found across Italy, we can make some inferences about the mirror's use as an apotropaion in death. Clarke has convincingly argued that representations of dwarfs and pygmies in Nilotic scenes on wall paintings decorating tombs in Italy had an apotropaic function, simultaneously providing protection from evil spirits to the guests of the tomb, and also frightening the evil spirits of death who looked upon these images. As we have already attributed an apotropaic function to the mirror in life, it follows that this apotropaic function continued in death, helping to deflect any harm that might come to the deceased. However, a curious feature of the mirrors found in situ at the tombs in Tarquinia is that they were oriented so that the figural scenes were hidden, meaning that the obverse, the reflecting mirror side, was visible. As an apotropaic device, we might expect that the figured representation of the hunchback would be face up (in fact, it may well have been) to avert evil forces and demons. But Carpino (2008: 24–5) and de Grummond (1991: 22) suggest that the 'reflection-death' superstition was more potent: because the obverse both projects and reflects the image of its user it was thus considered a receptacle for the soul of the deceased, helping the soul journey to the afterlife without harm. Thus, a mirror's use to both reflect and deflect images, in life and in death, demonstrates that it was well suited as an apotropaic device. The image of the hunchback as apotropaion on this specific mirror, however, would seem to have been more potent against the living than the dead.

But like the other deformed Others examined thus far, the significance of the dwarfed and lame hunchback depicted on this mirror goes beyond its apotropaic function. The fact that this hunchback is represented in an idyllic, outdoor landscape, but is depicted on an indoor object of adornment, and is then brought to the grave, highlights the Other's domestication. His domestication thus allows for a more intimate encounter between viewer and object. Holding the mirror in one's hand – held at arm's length much of the upper body would be in view – enabled the primary beholder to admire his/her own reflection. It also allowed secondary viewers to observe the hunchback on the reverse. For the secondary viewer, a curious play of visual imagery ensued: the image of the hunchback replaces the image of the primary beholder, or coexists in the same field of view. A viewer is thus presented with two extremes of appearance, the beauty of the beholder and the unsightly deformed hunchback. A viewer might thereupon situate him/herself somewhere along this sliding scale, or, read differently, having the ugly hunchback in direct opposition to the beauty of the beholder would make any homely viewer feel handsome or pretty in comparison. Thus, part of the appeal of this mirror and its figural decoration arises from the viewer's recognition of the ease with which beauty and ugliness could slide unsteadily into one another; indeed, it serves as a reminder that beauty eventually fades. This mirror thus explicitly draws out tensions in looking, much in the same way as the dwarf in the Antioch mosaic, with his cursory inscription, the hunchback now in the Villa Albani-Torlonia, with his handsome face and deformed body, and the pygmies in the wall painting from Pompeii, with their mischievous behaviour: these representations force a viewer to reconsider the meaning of the body of the Other and the function of his representation in relation to the Self.

Conclusions: viewing these 'other' Roman bodies

We see in representations of the deformed Other a fascination with that which is different – black skin colour, a dwarfed body, a humped back – and an emphasis on displaying these different bodies so as to highlight normative values associated with physical appearance and social status. These non-normative bodies were titillating to look at and indicate that there was a certain fascination with confronting the abnormal, whether that be to point at it or applaud it.

In all of the examples here presented, the deformed Other functions, on one level, as an apotropaion, and a particularly efficacious one at that; but as I have shown, the importance of these bodies goes far beyond this. The body of the Other was designed to generate strong responses, both negative and positive; it acts as an inverse symbol of the viewer's status, affirming his privileged health, wealth and social standing: everything that the *Other is not* serves as a stark and explicit validation of everything that the *viewer is*, or at least teases out the distance in between. On the whole, then, a viewer's encounter with these representations was a resonant, and in some ways, a reciprocal one: recognizing the otherness of the Other necessitated a recognition of the Self in relation to that Otherness, whether in opposition *or* alignment, revealing much about the place of the deformed body, and all bodies, including a viewer's own, in Roman society.

Acknowledgements

Sections of this chapter have been printed elsewhere (Trentin 2015). I am grateful to the editors of Bloomsbury Academic, an imprint of Bloomsbury Publishing Plc., for permission to reprint here.

Note

1 For the various traditional (though perhaps now dated) interpretations, see: Wace 1903–4 who asserted that they were used as apotropaic charms to ward off the evil Eye of envy; Perdrizet 1911: 58 who suggests that some grotesques were votives to Asclepius; Richter 1913 who argues they represent mimic actors; Binsfeld 1956: 43–4 who suggests that they were considered comical as well as apotropaic; Shapiro 1984: 391–2 who argues that the attribution of a large or erect phallus is an indication of sexual potency; Giuliani 1987: 701–21 who argues that they served as sympotic entertainment; Wrede 1988: 97–114 who suggests that they had Dionysian associations; Barton 1993 who suggest that they were court pets, as well as mimers and talismans; Fischer, Zachman 1994: 70–3 who suggests that they were cultic, but also served as talismans. For a more recent survey of function and meaning, see Mitchell 2013, Masséglia 2015 and Trentin 2015.

Lisa Trentin

Bibliography

Barton, Carlin, *The Sorrows of the Ancient Romans: The Gladiator and the Monster* (Princeton, NJ, 1993).

Binsfeld, Wolfgang, *Grylloi: Ein Beitrag zur Geschichte der antiken Karikatur* (unpublished PhD thesis, University of Cologne, 1956).

Bol, Robert, 'Porträt eines Buckligen (sog. Aesop)', in P. C. Bol (ed.), *Forschungen zur Villa Albani. Katalog der antiken Bildwerke,* I (Berlin, 1989), 207–31.

Bradley, Mark, 'Obesity, Corpulence and Emaciation in Roman Art', *Papers of the British School at Rome* 79 (2011), 1–41.

Braund, Susanna, and Gold, Barbara K. (eds), 'Vile Bodies', *Arethusa* 31/3 (Baltimore, MD, 1998).

Carelli, Francesco, *Le antichita di Ercolano esposte* (Naples, 1755–1831).

Carpino, Ann, 'Reflections from the Tomb: Mirrors as Grave Goods in Late Classical and Hellenistic Tarquinia', *Journal of the Etruscan Foundation* 11 (2008), 1–33.

Clarke, John, 'Hypersexual Black Men in Augustan Baths: Ideal Somatotypes and Apotropaic Magic', in N. Kampen (ed.), *Sexuality in Ancient Art* (Cambridge, 1996), 184–98.

Clarke, John, *Looking at Lovemaking: Constructions of Sexuality in Roman Art, 100 B.C.–A.D. 250* (Berkeley, CA, 1998).

Clarke, John, 'Look Who's Laughing at Sex', in D. Fredrick (ed.), *The Roman Gaze: Vision, Power, and the Body* (Baltimore, MD, 2002), 149–81.

Clarke, John, *Art in the Lives of Ordinary Romans* (Berkeley, CA, 2003).

Clarke, John, 'Three Uses of the Pygmy and the Aethiops at Pompeii', in L. Bricault, M. J. Versluys, and P. Meyboom (eds), *Nile into Tiber: Egypt in the Roman World* (Leiden, 2007a), 155–69.

Clarke, John, *Looking at Laughter: Humor, Power and Transgression in Roman Visual Culture, 100 B.C.–A.D. 250* (Berkeley, CA, 2007b).

Dasen, Véronique, *Dwarfs in Ancient Egypt and Greece* (Oxford, 1993).

Dasen, Véronique, 'Pygmaioi', *Lexicon Iconographicum Mythologiae Classicae* 7/1 (1994), 594–601.

Dasen, Véronique. 'L'enfant qui ne grandit pas', *Medicina nei secoli* 18/2 (2006), 1–13.

Dasen, Véronique, 'Des musiciens différents? Nains danseurs et musiciens dans le monde hellénistique et romain', in S. Emerit (ed.), *Le statut du musicien dans la Méditerranée ancienne: Égypte, Mésopotamie, Grèce et Rome* (Cairo, 2013), 259–77.

de Grummond, Nancy, 'The Usage of Etruscan Mirrors', in N. T. de Grummond (ed.), *A Guide to Etruscan Mirrors* (Tallahassee, FL, 1982), 166–7.

de Grummond, Nancy, 'Etruscan Twins and Mirror Images: The Dioskouroi at the Door', *Yale Bulletin* 10 (1991), 10–31.

Dunbabin, Katherine, '*Sic Erimus Cuncti.* The Skeleton in Graeco-Roman Art', *Jahrbuch des Deutschen Archäologischen Instituts* 101 (1986), 185–255.

Dunbabin, Katherine, '*Baiarum Grata Voluptas*: Pleasures and Dangers of the Baths', *Papers of the British School at Rome* 57 (1989), 6–49.

Dunbabin, Katherine, and Dickie, Matthew W., '*Invida Rumpantur Pectora:* The Iconography of *phthonos/invidia* in Graeco-Roman Art', *Jahrbuch für Antike und Christentum* 26 (1983), 7–37.

Fischer, Jutta, and Zachmann, Thomas, *Griechisch-römische Terrakotten aus Ägypten: die Sammlungen Sieglin und Schreiber: Dresden, Leipzig, Stuttgart, Tübingen* (Tübingen, 1994).

Garland, Robert, *The Eye of the Beholder: Deformity and Disability in the Graeco-Roman World* (London, 2010²).

Garmaise, Michael, 'Studies in the Representation of Dwarfs in Hellenistic and Roman Art' (unpublished PhD Thesis, McMaster University, 1996).

Giuliani, Luca, 'Die seligen Krüppel. Zur Deutung von Mißgestalten in der hellenistischen Kleinkunst', *Archäologischer Anzeiger* 102 (1987), 701–21.

Graham, Emma-Jayne, 'Disparate Lives or Disparate Deaths? Post-Mortem Treatment of the Body and the Articulation of Difference', in C. Laes *et al.* (eds), *Disabilities in Roman Antiquity* (Leiden, 2013), 249–74.

Grmek, Mirko and Gourevitch, Danielle, *Les maladies dans l'art antique* (Paris 1998).

Laes, Christian, Goodey, Chris F., and Rose, Martha Lynn (eds), *Disabilities in Roman Antiquity: Disparate Bodies A Capite ad Calcem* (Leiden, 2013).

Levi, Doro, 'The Evil Eye and the Lucky Hunchback', in R. Stillwell (ed.), *Antioch-on-the-Orontes,* III (Princeton, 1941).

Levi, Doro, 'House of the Evil Eye – Lower Level', in D. Levi, *Antioch Mosaic Pavements* (Princeton, NJ, 1947), 32–4.

Marvin, Miranda, 'Free-Standing Sculptures in the Baths of Caracalla', *American Journal of Archaeology* 87 (1983), 347–84.

Masséglia, Jane, *Body Language in Hellenistic Art and Society* (Oxford, 2015).

Meyboom, Paul, and Versluys, Miguel J., 'The Meaning of Dwarfs in Nilotic Scenes', in L. Bricault, M. J. Versluys, and P. Meyboom (eds), *Nile into Tiber: Egypt in the Roman World* (Leiden, 2005), 170–208.

Mitchell, Alexandre, 'Disparate Bodies in Ancient Artefacts: The Function of Caricature and Pathological Grotesques among Roman Terracotta Figurines', in C. Laes *et al.* (eds), *Disabilities in Roman Antiquity* (Leiden, 2013), 275–97.

Montserat, Dominic, *Changing Bodies, Changing Meanings: Studies on the Human Body in Antiquity* (London, 1998).

Perdrizet, Paul, *Bronzes Grecs d'Égypte de la Collection Fouquet* (Paris, 1911).

Pestilli, Livio, 'Disabled Bodies: The (Mis)representation of the Lame in Antiquity and their Reappearance in Early Christian and Medieval Art', in A. Hopkins and M. Wyke (eds), *Roman Bodies: Antiquity to the Eighteenth Century* (London, 2005), 85–97.

Richter, Gisela, 'Grotesques and the Mime', *American Journal of Archaeology* 17 (1913), 149–56.

Rose, Martha Lynn, *The Staff of Oedipus: Transforming Disability in Ancient Greece* (Ann Arbor, MI, 2003).

Shapiro, Alan, 'Notes on Greek Dwarfs', *American Journal of Archaeology* 88 (1984), 391.

Slane, Kathleen, and Dickie Matthew, 'A Knidian Phallic Vase from Corinth', *Hesperia* 62/4 (1993), 483–505.

Snowden, Frank Jr, *Blacks in Antiquity: Ethiopians in the Greco-Roman Experience* (Cambridge, MA, 1970).

Snowden, Frank Jr, 'Iconographical Evidence on the Black Populations in Greco-Roman Antiquity', in J. Vercoutter and J. Devisse (eds), *The Image of the Black in Western Art*, I (Cambridge, MA, 1976), 229–32.

Snowden, Frank Jr, 'Blacks in Antiquity through the Eyes of Greek and Roman Artists (Summary)', *Afrique Noire et Monde Méditerranéen dans l'Antiquité* (Dakar, 1978).

Snowden, Frank Jr, *Before Color Prejudice: The Ancient View of Blacks* (Cambridge, MA, 1983).

Snowden, Frank Jr, 'Bernal's "Blacks" and the Afrocentrists', in M. R. Lefkowitz and G. MacLean Rogers (eds), *Black Athena Revisited* (London, 1996), 112–27.

Snowden, Frank Jr, 'Attitudes toward Blacks in the Greek and Roman World: Misinterpretations of the Evidence', in E. M. Yamauchi (ed.), *Africa and Africans in Antiquity* (East Lancing, MI, 2001), 246–76.

Stevenson, William, 'The Pathological Grotesque Representations in Greek and Roman Art' (unpublished PhD. Thesis, University of Pennsylvania, 1975).

Stillwell, Richard, *Antioch on-the-Orontes*, III. *The Excavations 1937–1939* (Princeton, NJ, 1941).

Thompson, Lloyd, *Romans and Blacks* (London, 1989).

Tougher, Shaun, 'In or Out? Origins of Court Eunuchs', in S. Tougher (ed.), *Eunuchs in Antiquity and Beyond* (London, 2002), 143–59.

Trentin, Lisa, 'What's in a Hump? Re-examining the Hunchback in the Villa Albani-Torlonia', *Cambridge Classical Journal* 55 (2009), 130–56.

Trentin, Lisa, 'Deformity in the Roman Imperial Court', *Greece and Rome* 58/2 (2011), 195–208.

Trentin, Lisa, *The Hunchback in Hellenistic and Roman Art* (London, 2015)

Versluys, Miguel, *Aegyptiaca Romana: Nilotic Scenes and the Roman Views of Egypt* (Leiden, 2002).

Visconti, Ennio Quirino, *Iconographie grecque,* vol. I (Paris, 1811).

Vlahogiannis, Nicholas, 'Disabling Bodies', in D. Montserrat (ed.), *Changing Bodies, Changing Meanings: Studies in the Human Body in Antiquity* (London, 1998), 13–36.

Wace, Alan, 'Grotesques and the Evil Eye', *Annual of the British School at Athens* 10 (1903–4), 103–14.

Wrede, Henning, 'Die tanzenden Musikanten von Mahdia und der alexandrinische Götter- und Herrscherkult', *Rheinisches Museum* 95 (1988), 97–114.

18

MOBILITY IMPAIRMENT IN THE SANCTUARIES OF EARLY ROMAN ITALY

Emma-Jayne Graham

Introduction

> Nicanor, a lame man. While he was sitting wide-awake [in the sanctuary], a boy snatched his crutch from him and ran away. But Nicanor got up, pursued him, and so became well.
>
> *(IG 4.1.121–2: Stele 1.16; Edelstein and Edelstein 1945: 233)*

According to some of the first studies of ancient disability, physical impairments were viewed by the communities of Antiquity as a metaphor for divine punishment (Garland 1995; Vlahogiannis 1998). Hence, 'Every god could punish, and specific punishments were not restricted to specific deities. Disabilities – destruction of limbs through paralysis or injury, loss of the use of senses, personal appearance, sanity, impotence – became intertwined with punishment for violations of divine and moral order' (Vlahogiannis 1998: 29). However, attempting to interpret past attitudes towards impairment with reference to 'the anger of the gods' (Garland 1995: 59) overlooks the key fact that every god could also heal, and as the example of Nicanor and his crutch reveals, people of the ancient Mediterranean might look to the divine world for assistance with their impaired bodies as much as they feared punishment for moral wrongdoings. Inscribed on one of four stele erected at the Asclepieion at Epidaurus in the 4th century BCE the 'miracle tale' (*iama*) of Nicanor advertised the willingness of one of the great healing gods of the ancient world to intervene positively in the bodies of the diseased, injured and impaired. Regardless of whether this tale was founded on real events or embellished by the temple priests and officials in order to advertise the efficacy of Asclepius' curative powers, its presence alongside nearly seventy similar stories of pilgrims who had received divine healing for pain, illness, injury, infertility and a variety of chronic physical conditions demonstrates the existence of powerful ideas concerning the ability of the divine to remove or minimize potentially disabling impairments (LiDonnici 1992; Dillon 1994; Rynearson 2003).[1]

Examples such as that of Nicanor and his Epidauran contemporaries provide a glimpse of the physical impairments which drove people to seek divine healing. Other *iamata* from

Epidaurus refer repeatedly to instances of blindness, lameness and paralysis, malignant sores and tumours, oedema, abscesses, headaches, injuries and other conditions. Some of these produced symptoms which limited or otherwise affected a person's physical mobility, the subject of this chapter. The cures received at Epidaurus and the context in which these took place belong nevertheless to the religious world of the great sanctuary complexes of the Eastern Mediterranean. Moreover, they adhere to distinctive Asclepian forms of healing that were not necessarily experienced elsewhere, often entailing an overnight stay in the abaton of the sanctuary in anticipation of a meeting with the god or the receiving of a cure in the form of a dream (Rynearson 2003; Renberg 2006–7). Similar stories were inscribed at other Asclepieia as well as during later periods (for Roman Pergamum see Petsalis-Diomidis 2005; 2010), but it is difficult to be certain how common the ideas underpinning this behaviour were, or indeed how typical were the impairments recorded. There are, for example, several cases of 'paralysis' amongst the Epidauran *iamata* but whether these represent a generally high incidence of paralysing conditions within Greek communities, a tendency to visit the sanctuary only in the most extreme cases of mobility impairment or an emphasis placed by the official record-keepers of the sanctuary on the public display of the most dramatic instances of recovery is difficult to determine.[2]

For early Roman Italy comprehensive epigraphic attestation of divine healing and the bodily conditions for which it was sought is largely absent. Instead, many sanctuary sites of the Republic/Hellenistic period are abundant in clay and bronze models, often in the shape of human body parts, which were dedicated to the divine during a relatively restricted period of time (primarily the 4th to 1st century BCE). These 'anatomical votives' are interpreted most commonly as thank offerings connected with requests for divine healing similar to those expressed in the Greek inscriptions or with appeals for other forms of divine intervention to secure the wellbeing and safety of the dedicant. These objects were intended most probably to commemorate the occasion on which a request was granted and the suppliant's vow to provide an offering in return (*ex-voto*) was completed. By referencing the relevant part of the body anatomical votives remained a permanent reminder of the power of the deity and the presence of the suppliant's body in the sanctuary (for significant overviews of the subject see: Rouse 1902; Fenelli 1975; Comella 1981; van Straten 1981; Forsén 1996; Turfa 2004; Glinister 2006; Recke 2013; Draycott and Graham forthcoming; Hughes forthcoming). Despite sparking the curiosity of scholars and public alike, these votive objects remain a largely untapped source of information about the bodies and bodily understandings prevalent amongst members of Italic and early Roman communities (although see Turfa 1994; Hughes 2008, 2010, forthcoming; Draycott and Graham forthcoming). Even more significantly, unlike so many other visual representations of the ancient body (i.e. sculpture) anatomical votives appear to reference living bodies and body parts that were diseased, injured, impaired or otherwise malfunctioning, even if they do not depict discrete pathologies. This is something which, until now, has been largely overlooked in studies of Roman disabilities.[3] Equally remarkable is the fact that the terms 'disability' or 'impairment' feature only rarely in parallel scholarship on anatomical votives, even when the focus is primarily medical or pathological in tone (e.g. Oberhelman 2014; for a rare juxtaposition of anatomical votives with questions about disability see Adams forthcoming).

Importantly, however, these objects attest to particular types of bodies (impaired ones) in particular types of place (religious contexts), and it is the relationship between these impaired bodies and religious places as well as the consequent implications for experiences of mobility impairment which form the focus of this chapter. Rather than treating votive objects from the highly problematic perspective of retrospective diagnosis – which attempts to use them to identify specific conditions – this chapter adopts a new approach to anatomical votives and disability.

It is argued here that anatomical votives presents mobility impaired individuals and groups as religious performers within the context of ancient sanctuaries and that these material dedications to the divine therefore offer a route into exploring the significance of differential forms of mobility within religious settings. It is demonstrated that the presence and experience of mobility impaired bodies at sanctuaries produced discrete forms of religious knowledge and understandings of place.

Ancient mobility impairment and modern interactional theory

It is difficult to identify universal attitudes towards physical impairment in the ancient world, as existing scholarship has shown (Vlahogiannis 1998, 2005; Deris 2013; Kelley 2007; Bruce 2010; Trentin 2011; Graham 2013; Samama 2013; Southwell-Wright 2013, 2014). Perhaps, then, it is time to stop looking for them. Current approaches to this topic frequently take as their starting point either identifiable divine, mythological or mortal individuals whose particular impairments are signalled in written or visual sources (Hephaestus/Vulcan, Oedipus, Philip of Macedon, Caesar, Claudius), or fragments of evidence from different periods and places which represent, in broad terms, conditions which are recognized as potentially disabling in the modern world (sight or hearing impairment, dwarfism, kyphosis and so forth). Questions about 'disability' are then addressed to the predictably narrow or composite pictures of Antiquity produced by these respective approaches. If studies of ancient impairment and disability are to progress beyond descriptive 'top-down' accounts of generalized social attitudes or particular medical conditions, these methodologies must be refined.

One alternative is to seek to reconstruct and analyse the *experiences* of people with impairments (as far as our uneven and dispersed sources allow) in relation to specific contexts for which activities, behaviours and bodily performances can be determined. Given the sliding scale of corporeal disparity that existed for the bodies of the Roman world, physical impairment might be one aspect of personal and social identity for many people, but not necessarily always the most important (Graham 2013). Nonetheless, discrete embodied experiences and cultural practices almost certainly brought impairment into greater focus at particular moments in a person's life. Pursuing the lived experiences of impaired bodies in these situations, rather than merely attitudes towards them, makes it possible to shift our focus away from 'the bigger picture' towards an assessment of the role of impairment(s) in determining how people understood themselves, their actions and the world in which these took place. Early Roman healing cult offers one such context in which personal bodily experiences, and indeed disparate bodies themselves, inevitably took centre stage. Attested in material form by anatomical votives and readily defined in terms of space (the sanctuary) and time (4th to 1st century BCE), as well as in association with discrete types of behaviour (pilgrimage, religious performance and dedications), healing cult therefore provides a well-defined context in which the significance of experiences of impairment might be sought.

A contextualized approach to ancient impairment also makes it possible to address questions concerning both the physical and social dimensions of mobility impairment emphasized by recent studies of modern disability (Shakespeare 2006; Riddle 2013a, 2013b; see also the Introduction to this volume). Interactional approaches in particular seek to understand *experiences of impairment*, especially those arising as a consequence of a complex interweaving of both the underlying physical impairment (medical) and the world in which a person lives (social). By acknowledging that 'impairment has both physical and social dimensions' (Riddle 2013a: 32) interactional theory consequently compels the researcher to think about what it means (or, for ancient contexts, what it meant) to actually experience, as well as to be seen experiencing, a physical impairment in discrete settings and to explore the extent to which this might be significant for determining both personal identities and social attitudes. The case studies that interactional approaches can address may by necessity be narrow in scope, with generalizations about topics such as 'Roman mobility impairment' becoming more difficult to assert, but they promote a more thorough assessment of the significance of lived experiences of impairment against the backdrop of a much bigger kaleidoscope of past bodily identities. In this way, ancient disabilities studies become aligned more closely with early 21st-century applications of 'body theory' within classical studies and cognate historical disciplines (e.g. Hopkins and Wyke 2005; Garrison 2010; Rebay-Salisbury *et al.* 2010; Osborne 2011; Robb and Harris 2013). Ancient body studies have, for example, focused on embodied experiences of landscapes, cities and the bodily activities performed there, as well as sensory perception and the awareness of one's own physical movement in space, known as kinaesthesia or proprioception (examples include Favro 1994; Yegül 1994; Ingold 2004; Favro and Johanson 2010; Laurence and Newsome 2011; Betts 2011, forthcoming; Jenkyns 2013; Leary 2014a). Studies have also addressed the significance of walking and of being seen to move in specific ways in particular places for the construction and negotiation of identity. Hence, Timothy O'Sullivan has observed that:

> [Roman] viewers see someone walking ... and are immediately able to appreciate something about that individual's identity – whether because he is walking alongside others like him; or because he walks at the centre of a group of acolytes; or because he walks in a certain place, at a certain time, or on a certain occasions; or because he sits in a litter, and lets his slaves do the walking. *Or even because he moves his body in a certain way.* Roman walking, in other words, was not only a way of moving through space but also *a performance of identity*.
>
> *(O'Sullivan 2011: 7; emphasis added)*

O'Sullivan (2011: 14) goes on to suggest that Roman onlookers might see 'identity in motion' in the way in which bodies moved through space. Similar ideas have already begun to be explored for religious contexts, with Alexia Petsalis-Diomidis (2005: 205) arguing that at the Asclepieion at Pergamon 'the experience of the pilgrims was constructed on the one hand by the physical space of the sanctuary and on the other by the rules which governed their paths through that space', or in other words their bodily behaviours and movements. These are themes which the remainder of this chapter seeks to extend by adopting an interactional approach to Roman mobility impairment which addresses the consequences, for the negotiation of identities (the social), of bodily experiences in religious contexts (the physical). Rather than attempting to define 'mobility impairment' it draws upon evidence from settings in which a range of potential mobility impairments were experienced as a lens through which to explore the significance of those lived experiences. In order to do this the extent to which mobility impaired individuals were present in the ancient sanctuaries of Italy must first be determined before their encounters with these distinctive settings can be evaluated.

Identifying mobility impairment in ancient Italy

As noted above, concepts of movement and experiences of moving feature prominently in recent work on ancient space and place, including religious settings, but the possibility of impaired movement within, across, around and to or from these places is markedly absent. This is curious given that palaeoanthropological and palaeopathological examination of skeletal data has demonstrated the extent to which the bodies of ancient Roman urban and rural communities were far from perfect (Catalano *et al.* 2001, 2006; Cucina *et al.* 2006; Belcastro *et al.* 2007; Paine *et al.* 2009). Bodies might be damaged or modified by a range of factors including poor diet and living conditions, laborious physical activities, infectious diseases and injuries and the many other perils of living in a pre-industrial, pre-germ theory world (Scheidel 2010; Graham 2013). In some instances modifications to the upper parts of the human skeleton caused by prolonged use of crutches demonstrate the use of mobility aids by members of these communities (Belcastro and Mariotti 2000). Nevertheless, Richard Jenkyns recently offered the following summation of how Romans moved:

> How did their feet carry them through their town? The human body has two main sorts of forward locomotion: we can walk and we can run. … Human beings can also hop, skip, jump, and crawl … We can walk fast or slowly, and we can adjust the pace of a run.
>
> *(Jenkyns 2013: 143)*

Implicit in this description of movement is the assumption that these actions could be performed by all Romans; that everyone's body was capable not only of walking but of varying its speed at will in order to run, jog or skip. But osteoarchaeological evidence strongly suggests that in order to move 'through their town' some Romans would also have hobbled, limped, shuffled, used crutches or other mobility aids and prostheses, dragged or propelled themselves using their upper body or relied upon physical support from other people. Moreover, it was not just impairment which could be a factor. According to cultural theorist Kim Sawchuk:

> People are never simple abstract entities-in-movement. We learn and cultivate unique movement-repertoires comprised of distinct gestures and practices that change through any number of processes: age, exercise, illness, accident or injury. (…) We are 'differentially mobile.'
>
> *(Sawchuk 2013: 409)*

Non-normative bodies remain absent, however, when Jenkyns (2013: 143) asks further questions about how Romans moved and 'how did it feel to them?' Once again he seeks to identify a clear divide between the pace of walking and that of running but even basic pedestrian locomotion might be subtly nuanced by the nature and capabilities of individual bodies.[4]

To answer questions about the significance of how movement 'felt' for those who experienced physical impairment we must first locate and identify the mobility impaired of Roman Italy. Livio Pestilli (2005: 86) asserted that 'there are no Roman artefacts that attest to a presence of lame mortals in the visual tradition', but anatomical votives provide a significant corpus of material culture, which although not demonstrating discrete pathologies associated with recognizable impairments, appears to confirm the presence of 'lame mortals' at sanctuaries. Many thousands of terracotta representations of divine and human figures, heads, half-heads, eyes, ears, hands, open torsos, internal organs, wombs, hair and more rarely teeth and tongues were dedicated at sacred sites. Amongst these there were also large quantities of foot, knee, leg and lower torso models. In the majority of instances these probably signal requests for divine intervention concerning these parts of the body and therefore provide evidence for people with conditions and impairments which may have impacted upon mobility.

These types of anatomical votive are far from standardized in terms of size and detail, often varying from site to site, with examples made from both terracotta and bronze. Individual or paired feet might be life-sized, under life-sized or miniaturized, shown bare or sandaled, representing the right and/or left foot (Figure 18.1). Similarly, models of legs might include the foot or stop at the ankle and could extend from the sole of the foot to the knee or as far as the hip, including the genitals and buttocks, again appearing in pairs or as single limbs (Figure 18.2).

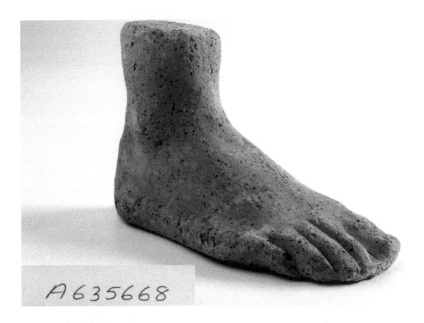

A635668

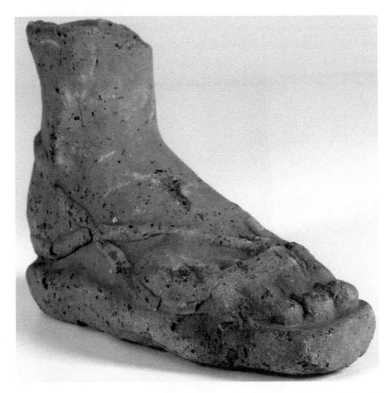

Figure 18.1 Votive feet of unknown provenance, one of which is shown bare and the other wearing a sandal (Science Museum inv. A635668 and inv. A635615). Source: Wellcome Images.

In 1975 Maria Fenelli collated information concerning the anatomical votives known from 150 individual assemblages from ninety-six locations across Italy with significant concentrations in areas associated with the territories of ancient Etruria and Latium. Of the individual sites and collections that Fenelli surveyed, forty-five (i.e. 30 per cent) featured at least one example of a lower torso, leg, thigh or knee and eighty-one (54 per cent) returned at least one example of a foot (with or without a sandal).[5] These figures, which already reflect the vagaries of excavation and publication, have undoubtedly been revised upwards in recent decades as a consequence of the publication of newly discovered and previously unpublished assemblages. Annamaria Comella (1981) included a further fourteen sites with 'lower limbs' in her own catalogue but, as in other publications, it is not clear whether this refers only to legs or to individual models of legs and of feet. The distribution of types can therefore be difficult to quantify in the absence of more recent surveys, with estimates of the total number of sites with anatomical votives now ranging up to around 300 (Glinister 2006: 13, n.11). Fenelli's figures do, however, offer an impressionistic view of how widespread and popular these types of votive offering were.

Excavation reports and publications supply more detail concerning the quantities of feet, legs and associated offerings dedicated to the divine at individual sites. At the monumental Ara della Regina temple at Tarquinia (Etruria), for instance, twenty-six legs (3 per cent of the assemblage) and 225 feet (30 per cent) were recorded within a deposit of 759 anatomical votives (excluding statuettes and swaddled babies; Comella 1982). Here, the number of feet was exceeded marginally by one other type: models of wombs (233 examples = 31 per cent). At the coastal site of Pyrgi (the international port of Caere also in Etruria) the total number of complete and fragmentary anatomical votives recovered was 734, with 458 (62 per cent) of those representing models of feet and/or legs (Bartoloni 1970). Further south, in Latium, 719 anatomical votives

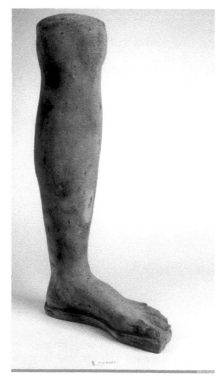

Figure 18.2 Terracotta model of a leg of unknown provenance (Science Museum inv. A129321). Source: Wellcome Images

recovered from the Tiber at Rome have been catalogued, including sixteen legs (2 per cent) and 402 feet (56 per cent) (Pensabene *et al.* 1980). Well-preserved life-size lower male torsos have been found at Cales (Campania) where at least nine examples (4 per cent) are catalogued within an assemblage of 247 anatomical votives (excluding heads) held by the Museo Nazionale di Napoli (Ciaghi 1993). These take the form of pairs of free-standing, stocky, well-muscled legs cut off at the waist and shown standing on a slab. At Cales, once again, feet represent the most frequent type of offering with 155 (63 per cent) in the catalogued collection, to which can be added 52 additional foot fragments and 21 fragments of legs (Ciaghi 1993). Feet certainly outnumber legs at this selection of sites from across the central Italian regions of ancient Etruria, Latium and Campania but in each case the ratios appear to be very similar.

Moreover, feet and legs were dedicated at both 'urban' and 'rural' sanctuaries (for discussion of what constituted ancient sanctuaries of different types see Glinister 1997). At Ponte di Nona, a road-side rural sanctuary 9 Roman miles (approx. 13.3 km) east of Rome, large numbers of feet and lower limbs were found in a votive deposit of more than 8,000 items (Potter and Wells 1985; Potter 1989). Here 'almost one terracotta in three consisted of part of a foot', leading the excavators to suggest that the sanctuary specialized in curing foot injuries and was associated with a dense local agricultural population for whom such injuries might be particularly critical (Potter and Wells 1985: 30, 39). Similarly, however, high numbers of legs (685), legs with genitals (8) and feet (1,654) were recovered from the sanctuary connected with the urban centre of Fregellae, about 100 km south-east of Rome, where together they make up more than half of the entire assemblage of over 4,000 offerings (Ferrea and Pinna 1986). This suggests that mobility impairments might be equally as critical for urban dwellers as for those of more dispersed agricultural communities. Together, Ponte di Nona and Fregellae caution against making assumptions about causes of injury and disease as well as the mobility risks facing the communities who frequented urban and rural sanctuaries. This is reinforced by skeletal evidence recovered from (imperial period) cemeteries associated with areas of intense industrial activity, which demonstrates the extent to which heavy labour took its toll on urban bodies in the form of significant physical impairment (Musco *et al.* 2008).

The sites identified above represent either those with particularly large (and well-published) deposits of anatomical votives which lend themselves to meaningful observations concerning the relative quantities of different types, or those at which feet/legs are especially predominant. It must be observed, however, that these votive objects appear in much smaller quantities at other sites and are entirely absent from some deposits. Many of the most well-known and highly monumentalized sanctuaries of Italy, including those at Veii (Latium) and Caere, Graviscae and the Porta Nord sanctuary at Vulci (Etruria), lack the large numbers of feet and legs described above. At these sites other types are more common (e.g. wombs at Graviscae) raising questions about specialization, local custom and the extent to which excavated assemblages represent all offerings made at a site over the course of its active life. Nor should all sites at which anatomical votives appear be categorized necessarily as 'healing sanctuaries' since all ancient gods had the capacity to heal as well as to bestow other forms of divine favour: sanctuaries were visited for a multitude of reasons (Glinister 2006: 13). These discrepancies are nevertheless potentially significant. Without wishing to argue that deities or sanctuaries specialized in treating particular conditions, these variations suggest that the living bodies which collectively visited and animated ancient sanctuaries might be appreciably different from location to location, creating different types of bodily community.

The exact quantities and densities of foot/leg offerings made across the whole of Italy between the 4th and 1st century BCE and the extent to which this varied over time are yet to be determined. Nonetheless, the representative examples described above indicate that many of the sanctuaries of Italy were places that might be frequented by quite considerable numbers of individuals who chose to commemorate that visit or to acknowledge their relationship with the divine in the form of the material citation of the feet, legs or lower torso. Even if we acknowledge that these offerings might have had a range of more abstract meanings, healing is ordinarily considered to have been the primary reason for the dedication of anatomical votives (Glinister 2006: 11–13; Recke 2013; Hughes forthcoming).[6] Even so, Jean Turfa (2006) has argued that there was little space for medical treatment or overnight accommodation in most Italian sanctuaries and that this, along with the inaccessible location of some isolated rural shrines, suggests that people suffering from illness, injury or debilitating impairments did not visit them. These people would, according to Turfa, visit a sanctuary in order to deposit their offering only once they had been cured, completing a vow that had been made elsewhere. The journey to some sacred sites was undoubtedly arduous and difficult even for people without mobility impairments, but the sacrifice and physical effort required in order to reach a sacred place might also be part of the gift given to the god (Leary 2014b: 13). What is more, vows were considered more efficacious if they took place in the presence of the deity being petitioned so it is to be expected that the majority were made on the occasion of a visit to the sanctuary (Petsalis-Diomidis 2006: 205). Particularly isolated sites may not have been regular places of pilgrimage for large numbers of worshippers with restricted mobility but the distribution of foot, leg and lower torso anatomical votives at sites across central Italy indicates unquestionably that they were well-represented at many.[7] It is possible, then, to infer that during the Republic/ Hellenistic period Italian sanctuaries were frequented by individuals seeking divine assistance with foot and leg conditions which might be associated with mobility impairments.

To what extent can these mobility impairments be reconstructed? Retrospective diagnosis is highly problematic and modern studies of anatomical votives avoid associating specific conditions or injuries with individual objects. The vast majority of anatomical votives do not, in fact, display any evidence for pathologies which might indicate a precise motive for dedication. A terracotta foot in the Science Museum, London (inv. A634921) has been described as possibly evidencing signs of the congenital condition *talipes equinovarus* (clubfoot) because of a slight turn at the ankle (Science Museum, n.d.) but this is difficult to verify and may be the consequence of the use of an old mould or another production error (Figure 18.3). Similarly, although votive models of feet frequently show the big toe separated from the second this can be understood as a consequence of the long-term wearing of sandals in the ancient world (Potter and Wells 1985: 30). Under normal circumstances this modification to the structure of the foot does not cause pain or bring about any limited or reduced mobility (Ingold 2004: 334). Traces of paint survive on anatomical votives of all types, indicating that many were perhaps painted in order to emphasize points of detail (Turfa 2004: 361–2). Injuries, infections, lesions and other potential impairments were possibly depicted on leg and foot models in this way but the absence of definitive examples makes it impossible to reconstruct what these might have represented.

Despite these *caveats* concerning detailed diagnoses it is possible to speculate about the more general range of requests that might have been associated with these objects and to consider the consequences for the presence of mobility impaired individuals within the sanctuary. Some may have been connected with petitions to a deity for recovery from acute foot or leg injuries such as sprains, fractures and broken bones, dislocations, pulled ligaments, ruptures of the Achilles tendon, torn anterior cruciate ligaments, punctures and other wounds, including those caused by crushing. Extremely rare examples of apparently 'bandaged legs' reported for a votive deposit at Lucus Feroniae (Etruria) may also fall into this category, indicating injuries or perhaps skin conditions such as psoriasis (Baggieri 1996: figs 15–16; Turfa 2004: 362). Overuse or repetitive strain injuries, many of which become particularly painful and debilitating during physical activity, might also be represented in this way, including metatarsalgia, plantar fasciitis and

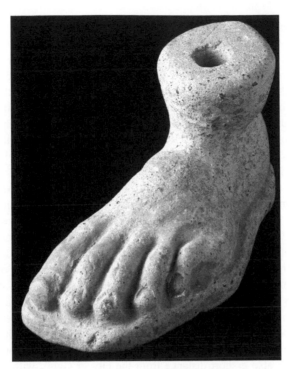

Figure 18.3 Terracotta votive foot of unknown provenance (Science Museum, inv. A634921). Source: Wellcome Images.

retrocalcaneal bursitis. Others might have been connected with longer lasting chronic conditions such as fallen arches, clubfoot, ingrown toenails, valgus ankles or pigeon toes (Potter and Wells 1985: 41–2) or with other walking difficulties caused by conditions such as osteoarthritis or gout. Models of the lower torso may have been emblematic of recovery from pain caused by sciatica or osteoarthritis in the hip or more substantial mobility impairments brought about as a consequence of injuries to the spinal cord, cerebral palsy, multiple sclerosis or muscular dystrophy/atrophy. Although it cannot be stated with any degree of certainty that these were indeed the conditions with which anatomical votive objects of feet, knees and legs were associated, collectively this range of possibilities suggests that the bodies of visitors to a sanctuary might demonstrate a range of mobility impairments. Moreover, these range from acute, temporarily debilitating ailments and injuries to chronic congenital anomalies or the result of more serious illness or accident. Together these objects commemorate the presence and actions of a host of differentially mobile people who engaged, in significant numbers, with religious activities within the ancient sanctuary.

Differentially mobile bodies at the sanctuary of Ponte di Nona: a case study

Religion does not exist autonomously, it is produced, negotiated, created and modified through bodily experiences of worship and sensory interactions with material culture and place, including movement (Boivin 2009; Howes 2011; Graham forthcoming). As David Chidester (2005: 56–7) has observed, 'For the study of religion, kinaesthesia calls attention to embodied movements – kneeling, standing, prostrating, walking, climbing, dancing, and so on – not only as types of ritual performance but also as instruments of knowledge.' If experiences of bodily performance produce religious knowledge and understanding then what happened at an ancient sanctuary, how it happened and how it was experienced through the body *was* ancient religion. Roman cult performances were highly kinaesthetic in nature as worshippers moved around the sanctuary, negotiated its terrain and engaged with its architectural topography, supplicated the divine, made offerings, encountered past offerings and participated in other ritual activities (see Petsalis-Diomidis 2005, 2010). As David Morgan (2010: p. xiv) notes, religion is produced by exactly these sorts of sensory experiences, or as he refers to them: 'the patterns of feelings and sensations bound up with performances, objects, and spaces'. Juxtaposing these conclusions with the observations above concerning the relationship between Roman walking, movement and identity compels us to explore how movement in the course of ancient religious acts produced distinctive religious identities and understandings of religious space. But, as the evidence of anatomical votives reminds us, in the context of the ancient sanctuary these movements were not always as uncomplicated as scholars tend to assume, with a range of mobility impairments being shared by the disparate bodies which animated these places. To borrow the question asked by Jenkyns above, what did it 'feel like' for these people to engage in healing cult and in what ways was that significant for the production of religious knowledge and identities?

To investigate this we can examine in more detail the sanctuary at Ponte di Nona, where especially large quantities of votive feet were dedicated. The site is usually described as a 'rural' sanctuary although it was in fact located close to the Via Praenestina, a major thoroughfare (Figure 18.4). The name of the sanctuary and the small road-station constructed on a ridge of high ground overlooking the crossing of a river valley is derived from its location at a place known as Ad Nonum, a name which acknowledged its distance from Rome (Potter and Wells 1985: 23–5).[8] It was also a short distance from the city of Gabii, with its own monumental

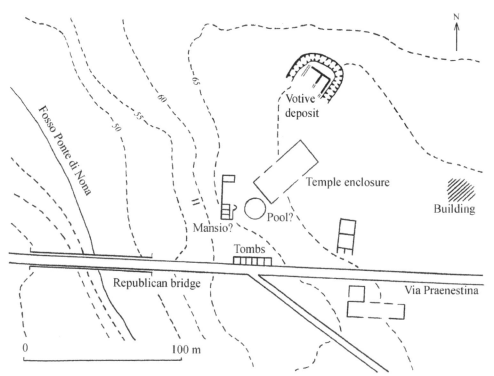

Figure 18.4 Sketch plan of the site at Ponte di Nona. Redrawn by the author (after Potter and Wells 1985: 26, fig. 2)

temple dedicated to Juno. Destroyed by quarrying in the 1960s, the site once comprised a large enclosure interpreted as the *temenos* (although no temple remains were discovered) as well as two irregular cavities containing many of the terracotta *ex-votos* described above (Potter and Wells 1985: 24). The area of high ground also included a structure interpreted as a *mansio* (but perhaps accommodation for pilgrims), a circular feature which was possibly a pool (fed by the nearby magnesium-bearing spring?) and buildings and tombs belonging to later periods. Excavations in the 1970s revealed further terracotta votives but no evidence for the identity of the presiding deity (Potter and Wells 1985: 34).

Although little is known about the nature of the buildings associated with this sanctuary it is possible to use it as a case study through which to consider how the sacred landscape and the religious activities which took place at Ponte di Nona were experienced by pilgrims with mobility impairments (their presence attested by anatomical votives). The ridge was not particularly high or steep and was relatively accessible by virtue of its location adjacent to the road but anyone visiting the sanctuary (certainly from the direction of Rome) would be compelled to walk up a slight rise in order to reach it. For those for whom walking was challenging or physically demanding this would have entailed a strenuous effort at the end of an already potentially arduous journey.[9] Pilgrims with mobility impairments may also have required mobility aids or support from other people; some were perhaps carried on stretchers or litters by relatives, friends or slaves who, in turn, would have experienced the strain of this through their own bodily movements. It is unlikely that hordes of people could be witnessed hobbling, limping or being carried up to the sanctuary at any one time but other users of the road may have noticed that it was here that some of their fellow travellers, including those who moved in a range of non-normative ways, turned off the main road and headed up to the sacred site on the ridge.

The distance from road to sanctuary at Ponte di Nona was not considerable (perhaps 50 m at most) and for many visitors was probably negligible. However, experiences of that short walk will have been very different for those visiting the sanctuary in order to seek healing or a cure for mobility impairments which affected their legs or feet, especially when these conditions caused pain. Indeed, studies of experiences of pain have emphasized its impact on understandings of space and bodily movement. When researching chronic pain conditions in modern Finland, for instance, Marja-Liisa Honkasalo (1998: 37–8) noted that 'space and time are the main constituents of sufferers' stories', to the extent that people 'often define their pain in terms of spatiality. Some spaces are associated with pain or memories of pain, and, on a more abstract and metaphorical level, in symptom experience space is seen as a dimension of self.' She went on to observe that, 'In pain narratives the experience of one's own body becomes present in a way it never normally does. The relationship between space and body becomes weird, pointing both to the lack of space and the overwhelming presence of the body. Everything in the living space is the painful body' (Honkasalo 1998: 43). Pain which restricts or otherwise impacts upon a person's mobility or mobility impairments which cause pain can therefore shape understandings of space and place in highly personal ways. Pain causes distances to become warped and space to take on new meanings as a person's spatial world is defined with direct reference to the painful body at its heart. Observations such as this which emphasize the complex connection between experiences of pain, movement (physical) and perceptions of places and the activities which people perform there (social) are especially relevant to an interactional assessment of mobility impaired encounters with ancient sacred space. Evaluated from this perspective the comparatively short walk from the main road towards the sanctuary at Ponte di Nona had the potential to produce a world shaped not only by religious expectations and the emotional prospect of healing, pain relief or improved mobility but by the limitations of the specific body in motion in that place and at that moment. Pain, discomfort, muscle strains in other parts of the body caused by the use of prostheses, mobility aids or non-normative bodily articulation as well as physical sensations of fatigue, anticipation, anxiety or even fear will consequently have combined to bring the meaning of that sacred place – and the presence of *that* body, moving in *that* way, in *that* place – into sharp focus. This warping of painfully embodied space into one which had particular meaning in the experience and memory of the supplicant would have continued during the performance of the cult activities which took place as part of the subsequent supplication of the deity, especially as the pilgrim moved around the topography of the sanctuary in order to participate in the ritual activities required of them. To revise Honkasalo's observation, under these circumstances for the individual pilgrim everything in that religious space was the impaired body and, simultaneously, the impaired body was that religious space. Religious knowledge was therefore produced in embodied terms.

But these bodies were not alone. Petsalis-Diomidis (2005: 204–5) has written of the 'imagined communities' of pilgrims at the Asclepieion of Pergamon. These were produced by the viewing of past votives which attested to shared healing experiences (and undoubtedly shared pre-healing experiences of impairment), as well as by communal acts of worship such as processions (involving movement once again) and the wearing of ritual clothing. At a sanctuary such as Ponte di Nona encounters with large quantities of anatomical offerings which testified to the presence of others with comparable levels of bodily impairment must have encouraged similar connections to be made between the disparate bodies of past and present communities of religious practitioners. Personal encounters with the divine and embodied experiences of the sacred topography may have varied in accordance with the differentially mobile bodies that experienced it, but these remained united by the fact that they shared a relationship with the deity and with the sanctuary landscape which was produced via mobility impaired and potentially painful bodies.[10]

Any collective identity produced in this way may also have been significant for defining the nature of the sanctuary as a certain type of 'religious place'. O'Sullivan's (2011: 7) comments concerning the importance of a Roman being seen 'walking alongside others like him' have already been noted, and as Kirk Woolford and Stuart Dunn (2014: 116) have also pointed out, 'the quality of moving bodies contributes to the qualities of the spaces in which these bodies move'. Work in cultural studies has also stressed the ways in which 'walking bodies communicate meaning through rhythms and gestures, constituting racial, ethnic, class and subcultural allegiances which are "signalled, formed and negotiated through bodily movement"' (Edensor 2000: 82, citing Desmond 1994: 34). In other words, a community *seen by others* to be moving in non-normative ways can define and give meaning to the spaces in which these movements take place. This, too, aligns with Riddle's (2013a) comments concerning the application of interactional theory within disability studies and the importance of exploring the connection between experiences of impairment and social attitudes. It can therefore be suggested that some (but not all) ancient sanctuaries were commonly understood as places where non-normative mobility was to be expected, the latter thereby effectively being transformed into 'normative' behaviour for those contexts. Certain types of ancient religious space, including sanctuaries visited for healing purposes, may therefore have been defined not only by their association with the powers of a specific deity but by the potentially erratic and certainly non-normative, cumulative movements and experiences of the mortal people who used them as well as by the material attestation of the presence of differentially mobile bodies that they left behind in the form of anatomical votive offerings. In these settings differential types of movement were on display both bodily, in the case of living worshippers, and artefactually in the form of votive dedications. Together these marked that place out from a range of other social, cultural, political and religious places and helped to define it as a place in which specific types of embodied religious knowledge were produced.

Conclusions

This chapter has argued that lived experiences of mobility impairment were highly significant in the context of healing cult in ancient Italy. Movement has the potential to define collective identities not only as a consequence of acute personal experience but from the perspective of an external audience witnessing bodies in motion. In ancient Italy it also produced specific forms of religious knowledge concerning the nature and experience of healing cult and contributed towards the production of understandings of sanctuaries such as that at Ponte di Nona as particular types of religious place. More importantly, however, these conclusions are predicated on an assessment of the role of *differential* mobility in religious contexts. The bodies which engaged with religious practices in these settings were highly disparate, many perhaps evidencing mobility impairments of varied types. Incorporating these differential bodies and mobility experiences into discussions of the role played by the phenomenology of sacred places and material culture in the production of religious knowledge represents not only a new way of thinking about past religious experiences but also about the significance of physical impairments. The discussion of mobility impaired bodies presented here suggests that there was no single 'experience' of ancient sanctuaries and consequently no single all-encompassing 'understanding' of religious space. Movement, mobility and kinaesthetic experience combined as instruments of religious knowledge textured by the differentially mobile bodies which animated the disparate topographies of each sacred site.

Of course, mobility impairment was not the only reason for visiting a sanctuary or dedicating an offering. Many other types of votive objects attest to other physical impairments affecting sight, hearing, upper limbs and hands, heads and internal conditions which might cause pain and other symptoms which could manifest themselves in terms of physically limiting conditions. It should not be forgotten, then, that there were people present at these sanctuaries whose experiences of religious performances and votive cult were mediated through other forms of bodily impairment: sight or hearing impairments, upper body conditions, incapacitating migraines and headaches, cognitive impairment, heart conditions, cancers and so forth. Indeed, the possibility that models of heads and the distinctive half-heads found at many sites were associated with cognitive impairment has yet to be explored. Moreover, it is far from clear that each of these individual offerings was associated directly with a request for healing and many might be associated with more abstract concerns about wellbeing, fertility, social status, life-course events, economic prosperity, personal safety, long journeys or even conflict. There were, after all, many people without impairments present within the sanctuary too. It is not my intention to argue that mobility impairment was the most important or even the most common reason for a votive offering which referenced the feet, legs or lower torso. Instead, these types of anatomical votive have been spotlighted as a means of contextualizing bodies which might demonstrate differential mobilities in order to ask more searching questions about experiences of ancient impairment. Questions now need to be asked about how these experiences compared, conflicted or interacted with others and what the implications might be beyond the sacred confines of the sanctuary. The impaired body in the sanctuary represents one of the pieces of the jigsaw puzzle that is Roman disability but one that compels us to place discrete experiences of impairment at the heart of our ongoing investigations.

Notes

1 This behaviour is not restricted to the ancient world. People experiencing bodily impairments and debilitating illnesses continue to turn to the divine or supernatural for cures or additional support, as the dedication of anatomical offerings and related items at modern Catholic, Orthodox, Hindu and Islamic sacred sites and shrines confirms.

2 Instances include the healing of 'Hermodices of Lampsacus, paralysed in body' (*IG* 4.1.121–2: Stele 1.15; Edelstein and Edelstein 1945: 232–3), an unknown man from Epidaurus who was 'lame' and carried on a stretcher (*IG* 4.1.121–2: Stele 2.35; Edelstein and Edelstein 1945: 236) and Cleimenes of Cirrha 'paralysed in his knees' (*IG* 4.1.121–2: Stele 2.38; Edelstein and Edelstein 1945: 237). Others recount serious toe conditions and foot injuries, with one also recording 'A man whose fingers, with the exception of one, were paralysed' (*IG* 4.1.121–2: Stele 1.3; Edelstein and Edelstein 1945: 230).

3 See e.g. Pestilli (2005: 85) who observes that, 'Images of the disabled that have survived from classical Roman art are limited primarily to representations of the smith-god, Vulcan, whose distinctive trait was the infirmity of his feet. *This paucity of archaeological evidence* is certainly at odds with what must have been the historical reality of communities where congenital deformities, illnesses, disease and war indelibly altered human bodies' (emphasis added). It is sometimes noted that anatomical votives point towards large numbers of diseased or 'disabled' people within ancient communities, but analysis does not extend far beyond this observation.

4 It is disingenuous to single out Jenkyns's otherwise excellent book for criticism without observing that the same is true of other recent works devoted to the study of 'walking', 'movement' and 'mobility. None of the chapters in the methodologically wide-ranging volume edited by Laurence and Newsome (2011) indicate that mobility impairments might have consequences for the type of movements under discussion, and O'Sullivan's (2011) examination of Roman walking as seen through the lens of elite literature also overlooks the non-normative moving body. Beyond the classical world, contributions to Leary (2014a) omit discussion of those who found mobility painful, difficult or impossible.

5 Pelvis models ('bacino') have been excluded because it is not always clear whether these were intended to reference the locomotive function of the hips and pelvis or to make specific reference to the genitals. All percentages have been rounded to the nearest per cent.

6 Amongst these more 'abstract' meanings are acknowledgements of pilgrimage or dangerous journeys (Dunbabin 1990), movement across life-course stages, strength, athletic prowess or the well-being of male youths (in the instance of well-muscled lower torso models). They may even have had economic connotations associated with businesses in which the feet were especially important, including fulling and tanning. The relationship between votive offerings and ideas of movement more generally will be explored in another paper.

7 In the strictest sense, as *ex-votos*, these objects represent the bodies of those who had received healing or divine assistance, being dedicated as a thank offering rather than in anticipation of a cure. However, little is known about the formal processes involved in the making of votive dedications and even if these artefacts were in fact dedicated subsequent to healing, or even upon the occasion of a return visit to the sanctuary once health had been restored, they still attest to the earlier presence in that place of mobility impaired individuals seeking divine healing.

8 The bridge existed from at least the early 2nd century BCE but archaeological evidence indicates that the area was probably first occupied in the 4th century BCE (Potter and Wells 1985).

9 The precise origin of the worshippers who left dedications at Ponte di Nona is unknown. Some may have come from the nearby city of Gabii, others perhaps from Rome or villages close to the via Praenestina. If Potter and Wells (1985) are correct in their assessment of this site as one which served local agricultural communities, pilgrims may well have come from anywhere within the surrounding region, making their way to the sanctuary across country and along tracks and other routes not as well maintained as the via Praenestina.

10 It is possible that the so-called *mansio* at Ponte di Nona actually provided accommodation for pilgrims as much as it served the needs of more general travellers. Although it may not have served the same religious function as the *abaton* of an Asclepieion, it may have offered a place in which people experiencing considerable impairment could congregate and share their experiences, thus strengthening this sense of community.

Bibliography

Adams, Ellen, 'Fragmentation and the Body's Boundaries: Reassessing the Body in Parts', in J. L. Draycott and E.-J. Graham (eds), *Bodies of Evidence: Ancient Anatomical Votives Past, Present and Future* (Abingdon, forthcoming).

Baggieri, Gaspare (ed.), *L'antica anatomia nell'arte dei donaria* [Ancient anatomy in the art of votive offerings] (Rome, 1996).

Bartoloni, Gilda, 'Le terrecotte votive', in *Pyrgi: Scavi del Santuario Etrusco (1959–1967)*. Notizie degli Scavi di Antichità 8/24, suppl. 2 (1970), 552–78.

Belcastro, Maria Giovanna, and Mariotti, Valentina, 'Morphological and Biomechanical Analysis of a Skeleton from Roman Imperial Necropolis of Casalecchio di Reno (Bologna, Italy, II–III c. A.D.): A Possible Case of Crutch Use', *Collegium Antropologicum* 24 (2000), 529–39.

Belcastro, Giovanna, Rastelli, Elisa, Mariotti, Valentina, Consiglio, Chiara, Facchini, Fiorenzo, Bonfiglioni, Benedetta, 'Continuity and Discontinuity of the Life-Style in Central Italy during the Roman Imperial Age–Early Middle Ages Transition: Diet, Health, and Behaviour', *American Journal of Physical Anthropology* 132 (2007), 381–94.

Betts, Eleanor, 'Towards a Multisensory Experience of Movement in the City of Rome', in R. Laurence and D. Newsome (eds), *Rome, Ostia and Pompeii: Movement and Space* (Oxford, 2011), 118–32.

Betts, Eleanor (ed.), *Senses of Empire: Multisensory Approaches to Roman Culture* (Abingdon, forthcoming).

Boivin, Nicole, 'Grasping the Elusive and Unknowable: Material Culture in Ritual Practice', *Material Religion* 5/3 (2009), 266–87.

Bruce, Patricia, 'Constructions of Disability (Ancient and Modern): The Impact of Religious Beliefs on the Experience of Disability', *Neotestamentica* 44/2 (2010), 253–81.

Catalano, Paola, Minozzi, Simona, and Pantano, Walter, 'Le necropoli romane di età imperiale: Un contributo all'interpretazione del popolamento e della qualità della vita nell'antica Roma', in L. Quilici and S. Quilici Gigli (eds), *Atlante tematico di topografia antica* 10 (2001), 127–37.

Catalano, P., Amicucci, G., Renassi, V., Caldarini, C., Caprara, M., Carboni, L., Colonnelli, G., De Angelis, F., Di Giannantonio, S., Minozzi, S., Pantano, W., and Porreca, F., 'Gli insiemi funerari d'epoca imperiale: l'indagine antropologica di campo', in M. A. Tomei (ed.), *Roma: Memorie dal sottosuolo. Ritrovamenti archeologici 1980/2006* (Rome, 2006), 560–6.

Chidester, David, 'The American Touch: Tactile Imagery in American Religion and Politics', in C. Classen (ed.), *The Book of Touch* (Oxford and New York, 2005), 49–65.

Ciaghi, Silvia, *Le terrecotte figurate da Cales del Museo nazionale di Napoli: Sacro, stile, committenza* (Rome, 1993).

Comella, Annamaria, 'Tipologia e diffusione dei complessi votivi in Italia in epoca medio – e tardo – repubblicana', *Mélanges de l'École française de Rome, Antiquité* 93 (1981), 717–803.

Comella, Annamaria, *Il deposito votivo presso l'Ara della Regina*. Materiali del Museo Archeologico Nazionale di Tarquinia 4 (Rome, 1982).

Cucina, A., Vargili, R., Mancinelli, D., Ricci, R., Santandrea, E., Catalano, P., and Coppa A., 'The Necropolis of Vallerano (Rome, 2nd–3rd Century AD): An Anthropological Perspective on the Ancient Romans in the *Suburbium*', *International Journal of Osteoarchaeology* 16 (2006), 104–17.

Deris, Sara, 'Examining the Hephaestus Myth through a Disability Studies Perspective', *Prandium: The Journal of Historical Studies* 2/1 (2013), 11–18.

Desmond, Jane, 'Embodying Difference: Issues in Dance and Cultural Studies', *Cultural Critique* (Winter 1994), 33–63.

Dillon, Matthew, 'The Didactic Nature of the Epidaurian *Iamata*', *Zeitschrift für Papyrologie und Epigraphik* 101 (1994), 239–60.

Draycott, Jane, and Graham, Emma-Jayne (eds), *Bodies of Evidence: Ancient Anatomical Votives Past, Present and Future* (Abingdon, forthcoming).

Dunbabin, Katherine, '*Ipsa deae vestigia* ... Footprints Divine and Human on Greco-Roman Monuments', *Journal of Roman Archaeology* 3 (1990), 85–109.

Edelstein, Emma J., and Edelstein, Ludwig, *Asclepius: Collection and Interpretation of the Testimonies*. 2 vols (Baltimore, MD, 1945).

Edensor, Tim, 'Walking in the British Countryside: Reflexivity, Embodied Practices and Ways to Escape', *Body and Society* 6/3–4 (2000), 81–106.

Edwards, Martha Lynn [= Rose, Martha Lynn], 'Constructions of Physical Disability in the Ancient Greek World: The Community Concept', in D. T. Mitchell and S. L. Snyder (eds), *The Body and Physical Difference: Discourses of Disability* (Ann Arbor, MI, 1997), 35–50.

Favro, Diane, 'The Street Triumphant: The Urban Impact of Roman Triumphal Parades', in Z. Çelik, D. Favro and R. Ingersoll (eds), *Streets: Critical Perspectives on Public Space* (Berkeley-Los Angeles, CA, London, 1994), 151–64.

Favro, Diane, and Johanson, Christopher, 'Death in Motion: Funeral Processions in the Roman Forum', *Journal of the Society of Architectural Historians* 69/1 (2010), 12–37.

Fenelli, Maria, 'Contributo per lo studio del votivo anatomico: i votivi anatomici di Lavinio', *Archeologia Classica* 27 (1975), 206–52.

Ferrea, Laura, and Pinna, Antonella, 'Il deposito votivo', in F. Coarelli (ed), *Fregellae 2: Il santuario di Esculapio* (Rome, 1986), 89–144.

Forsén, Björn, *Griechische Gliederweihungen: Eine Untersuchung zu ihrer Typologie und ihrer religions- und sozialgeschichtlichen Bedeutung* (Helsinki, 1996).

Garland, Robert, *The Eye of the Beholder: Deformity and Disability in the Graeco-Roman World* (London, 1995).

Garrison, Daniel (ed.), *A Cultural History of the Human Body in Antiquity* (New York, 2010).

Glinister, Fay, 'What is a Sanctuary?', *Cahiers du Centre Gustave Glotz* 8 (1997), 61–80.

Glinister, Fay, 'Reconsidering "Religious Romanization"', in C. E. Schultz and P. B. Harvey (eds), *Religion in Republican Italy* (Cambridge, 2006) 10–33.

Graham, Emma-Jayne, 'Disparate Lives or Disparate Deaths? Post-Mortem Treatment of the Body and the Articulation of Difference', in C. Laes, C. F. Goodey and M. L. Rose (eds), *Disabilities in Roman Antiquity. Disparate Bodies* A Capite ad Calcem (Leiden, 2013), 249–74.

Graham, Emma-Jayne, 'Holding the Baby? Sensory Dissonance and the Ambiguities of Votive Objects', in E. Betts (ed.), *Senses of the Empire: Multisensory Approaches to Roman Culture* (Abingdon, forthcoming).

Honkasalo, Marja-Liisa, 'Space and Embodied Experience: Rethinking the Body in Pain', *Body and Society* 4/2 (1998), 35–57.

Hopkins, Andrew, and Wyke, Maria (eds), *Roman Bodies: Antiquity to the Eighteenth Century* (London, 2005).

Howes, David, 'Sensation', *Material Religion* 7/1 (2011), 92–9.

Hughes, Jessica, 'Fragmentation as Metaphor in the Classical Healing Sanctuary', *Social History of Medicine* 21/2 (2008), 217–36.

Hughes, Jessica, 'Dissecting the Classical Hybrid', in K. Rebay-Salisbury, M. L. S. Sørenson and J. Hughes (eds), *Body Parts and Bodies Whole: Changing Perspectives and Meanings* (Oxford, 2010), 101–10.

Hughes, Jessica, *Votive Body Parts in Greek and Roman Religion* (Cambridge, forthcoming).

Ingold, Tim, 'Culture on the Ground: The World Perceived through the Feet', *Journal of Material Culture* 9/3 (2004), 315–40.

Jenkyns, Richard, *God, Space and the City in the Roman Imagination* (Oxford, 2013).

Kelley, Nicole, 'Deformity and Disability in Greece and Rome', in H. Avalos, S. J. Melcher and J. Schipper (eds), *This Abled Body: Rethinking Disabilities in Biblical Studies* (Atlanta, GA, 2007), 31–47.

Laurence, Ray, and Newsome, David (eds), *Rome, Ostia, Pompeii: Movement and Space* (Oxford, 2011).

Leary, Jim (ed.), *Past Mobilities: Archaeological Approaches to Movement and Mobility* (Farnham, 2014a).

Leary, Jim, 'Past Mobility: An Introduction', in J. Leary (ed.), *Archaeological Approaches to Movement and Mobility* (Farnham, 2014b), 1–19.

LiDonnici, Lynn R., 'Compositional Background of the Epidaurian *Iamata*', *American Journal of Philology* 113/1 (1992), 25–41.

Morgan, David, 'Preface', in D. Morgan (ed.), *Religion and Material Culture: The Matter of Belief* (London and New York, 2010), pp. xii–xiv.

Musco, Stefano, Catalano, Paola, Caspio, Angela, Pantano, Walter, and Killgrove, Kristina, 'Le complexe archéologique de Casal Bertone', in P. Catalano, J. Scheid and S. Verger (eds), *Rome et ses morts*. Les Dossiers d'archéologie 330 (Dijon, 2008), 32–9.

Oberhelman, Steven M., 'Anatomical Votive Reliefs as Evidence for Specialization at Healing Sanctuaries in the Ancient Mediterranean World', *Athens Journal of Health* 1 (2014), 47–62.

Osborne, Robin, *The History Written on the Classical Greek Body* (Cambridge, 2011).

O'Sullivan, Timothy, *Walking in Roman Culture* (Cambridge, 2011).

Paine, Robert R., Vargiu, Rita, Signoretti, Carla, and Coppa, Alfredo, 'A Health Assessment for Imperial Roman Burials Recovered from the Necropolis of San Donato and Bivio CH, Urbino, Italy', *Journal of Anthropological Sciences* 87 (2009), 193–210.

Pensabene, Patrizio, Rizzo, Maria Antonietta, Roghi, Maria, and Talamo, Emilia, *Terrecotte votive dal Tevere*. Studi Miscellanei 25 (Rome, 1980).

Pestilli, Livio, 'Disabled Bodies: The (Mis)representation of the Lame in Antiquity and their Reappearance in Early Christian and Medieval Art', in A. Hopkins and M. Wyke (eds), *Roman Bodies: Antiquity to the Eighteenth Century* (London, 2005), 85–97.

Petsalis-Diomidis, Alexia, 'The Body in Space: Visual Dynamics in Graeco-Roman Healing Pilgrimage', in J. Elsner and I. Rutherford (eds), *Pilgrimage in Graeco-Roman and Early Christian Antiquity: Seeing the Gods* (Oxford, 2005), 183–218.

Petsalis-Diomidis, Alexia, 'Amphiaraos Present: Images and Healing Pilgrimage in Classical Greece', in R. Maniura and R. Shepherd (eds), *Presence: The Inherence of the Prototype within Images and Other Objects* (Farnham, 2006), 205–29.

Petsalis-Diomidis, Alexia, *Truly Beyond Wonders: Aelius Aristides and the Cult of Asklepios* (Oxford, 2010).

Potter, Timothy W., *Una stipe votiva da Ponte di Nona* (Rome, 1989).

Potter, Timothy W., and Wells, Calvin, 'A Republican Healing-Sanctuary at Ponte di Nona near Rome and the Classical Tradition of Votive Medicine', *Journal of the British Archaeological Association* 138 (1985), 23–47.

Rebay-Salisbury, Katharina, Stig Sørenson, Marie Louise, and Hughes, Jessica, (eds), *Body Parts and Bodies Whole: Changing Relations and Meanings* (Oxford, 2010).

Recke, Matthias, 'Science as Art: Etruscan Anatomical Votives', in J. M. Turfa (ed.), *The Etruscan World* (London and New York, 2013), 1068–85.

Renberg, Gil H., 'Public and Private Places of Worship in the Cult of Asclepius at Rome', *Memoirs of the American Academy in Rome* 51–2 (2006–7), 87–172.

Riddle, Christopher A., 'The Ontology of Impairment: Rethinking How we Define Disability', in M. Wappett and K. Arndt (eds), *Emerging Perspectives on Disability Studies* (New York, 2013a), 23–39.

Riddle, Christopher A., 'Defining Disability: Metaphysical Not Political', *Medical Health Care and Philosophy* 16 (2013b), 377–84.

Robb, John, and Harris, Oliver, *The Body in History: Europe from the Palaeolithic to the Future* (Cambridge, 2013).

Rose, Martha Lynn, *The Staff of Oedipus: Transforming Disability in Ancient Greece* (Ann Arbor, MI, 2003).

Rouse, William, and Denham, Henry, *Greek Votive Offerings: An Essay in the History of Greek Religion* (Cambridge, 1902).

Rynearson, Nicholas, 'Constructing and Deconstructing the Body in the Cult of Asklepios', *Stanford Journal of Archaeology* 2 (2003) <http://www.stanford.edu/dept/archaeology/journal/newdraft/2003_Journal/rynearson/paper.pdf>.

Samama, Evelyne, 'A King Walking with Pain? On the Textual and Iconographical Images of Philip II and Other Wounded Kings', in C. Laes, C. F. Goodey and M. L. Rose (eds), *Disabilities in Roman Antiquity: Disparate Bodies A Capite ad Calcem* (Leiden, 2013), 231–48.

Sawchuck, Kim, 'Impaired', in P. Adey, D. Bissell, K. Hannam, P. Merriman and M. Sheller (eds), *The Routledge Handbook of Mobilities* (London and New York, 2013), 409–20.

Scheidel, Walter, 'Physical Wellbeing in the Roman World (version 2.0)', *Princeton/Stanford Working Papers in Classics* (2010) <http://www.princeton.edu/~pswpc/pdfs/scheidel/091001.pdf>.

Science Museum, 'Votive Left Foot, Roman, 200 BCE–200 CE' (n.d.). <http://www.sciencemuseum.org.uk/online_science/explore_our_collections/objects/index/smxg-84642>.

Shakespeare, Tom, *Disability Rights and Wrongs* (London and New York, 2006).

Southwell-Wright, William, 'Past Perspectives: What Can Archaeology Offer Disability Studies?', in M. Wappett and K. Arndt (eds), *Emerging Perspectives on Disability Studies* (New York, 2013), 67–95.

Southwell-Wright, William, 'Perceptions of Infant Disability in Roman Britain', in M. Carroll, and E.-J. Graham (eds), *Infant Health and Death in Roman Italy and Beyond* (Ann Arbor, MI, 2014), 111–30.

Trentin, Lisa, 'Deformity in the Roman Imperial Court', *Greece and Rome* 58 (2011), 195–208.

Turfa, Jean MacIntosh, 'Anatomical Votives and Italian Medical Traditions', in R. D. De Puma and J. P. Small (eds), *Murlo and the Etruscans: Art and Society in Ancient Etruria* (Madison, WI, 1994), 224–40.

Turfa, Jean MacIntosh, [Weihgeschenke: Altitalien und Imperium Romanum 1. Italien.] B. Anatomical Votives', in *Thesaurus Cultus et Rituum Antiquorum (ThesCRA)*, I (Los Angeles, CA, 2004), 359–68.

Turfa, Jean MacIntosh, 'Was There Room for Healing in the Healing Sanctuaries?', *Archiv für Religionsgeschichte* 8 (2006), 63–80.

van Straten, Folkert T., 'Gifts for the Gods', in H. S. Versnel (ed), *Faith, Hope and Worship: Aspects of Religious Mentality in the Ancient World* (Leiden, 1981), 65–151.

Vlahogiannis, Nicholas, 'Disabling Bodies', in D. Monserrat (ed.), *Changing Bodies, Changing Meanings: Studies on the Human Body in Antiquity* (London and New York, 1998), 13–36.

Vlahogiannis, Nicholas, 'Curing Disability', in H. King (ed.), *Health in Antiquity* (London and New York, 2005), 180–91.

Woolford, Kirk, and Dunn, Stuart, 'Micro Mobilities and Affordances of Past Places', in J. Leary (ed.), *Archaeological Approaches to Movement and Mobility* (Farnham, 2014), 113–28.

Yegül, Fikret K., 'The Street Experience of Ancient Ephesus', in Z. Çelik, D. Favro and R. Ingersoll (eds), *Streets: Critical Perspectives on Public Space* (Berkeley-Los Angeles, CA, and London, 1994), 95–110.

19

MENTAL DISABILITY?

Galen on mental health

Chiara Thumiger

Introduction

The move of applying a modern concept and social experience, that of disability, with its premise of cultural construction and historical specificity[1] to another culture, privileges by its investigatory nature the point of view of an anthropological observer, as opposed to an internal perspective that foregrounds the point of view of the subject, in our case the ancient men and women. The first posture necessarily pulls away from the reality of the observed individuals (in our case, ancient ideas and practices) to test its own parameters and meanings against them, and uncover new elements of relevance, including elements of contrast to its own world and intellectual system. It is in this spirit that a contemporary codified standpoint reflecting, at least in part, the assumptions of the modern observer can be a useful point of reference for historians. I propose to return to the definition of 'disability' offered by the World Health Organization, which was discussed in the Introduction to this volume, not as an anachronistic superimposition of our own cultural parameters as more evolved or truthful to the nature of human life than those of ancient parameters, but as a way to enrich our understanding of the differences that separate us from them, and possibly appreciate their lasting relevance to current debates.

The WHO definition emphasizes *impairments*, *activity limitations* and *participation restrictions* as part of the human experience of disability, focusing thus on the body, on society's reactions to certain conditions and on the need for interventions to remove respective barriers. As such, this definition covers mental impairments only in a derivative way. At the centre, in fact, are the physiology and structures of the human body and their variations, framed within the activities and interactions of life. Mental disability is only a particular case within this whole, and notably one which ancient medical literature barely considers in ways on which we could superimpose our own modern constructs, (e.g.) discussions of what used to be called 'retardation' in modern or contemporary medicine – 'mental disability'. In this sense we are setting ourselves out onto an anachronistic path as we inquire into mental disability in ancient sources.

Nonetheless, the WHO definition offers guidance to a search for elements of mental disability in an ancient thinker like Galen. All three expressions 'impairment', 'activity limitation' and 'restriction', first of all, indicate a permanent or long-lasting state of things that characterize an individual in his or her life and interactions with the world outside. This enduring quality of mental disability, by which mental health is deeply embedded into the nature of each individual

– physiological and psychological: the state of one's bodily functions, as well as character and personality – is one with which Galenic discussions of mental wellbeing and mental alteration are partly consonant. This is not a general datum when it comes to ancient medicine: Galen marks a clear departure from previous Greco-Roman medical literature, especially Hippocratic, in which mental alteration was fundamentally observed as an episodic and acute pathological event, devoid of personal and ethical colouring (Thumiger 2015, 2016).

Galen is thus highly innovative as a doctor and as a medical author in his attention to this level of experience qua medical matter, and a key figure in our inquiry. Even though a discussion of disability in our terms is, obviously, missing from his work, Galen shows a sophisticated awareness of issues that are very close to the debate in which scholars of disability studies engage today. Such points of debate include the idea of (dis)ability as a matter of degree rather than kind, and qualified by a multiplicity of natural factors; the cooperation, or simultaneous influence, of nature and nurture; specifically regarding mental health, the power of education and self-improvement strategies (as well as the limits of these powers) in the face of misfortune or against the constraints of one's biological innate (or acquired, but irreversible) perceived deficiencies.

In this chapter I shall survey Galen's views about flaws in the health of the mind as a lasting and ethical matter. As a contribution to the formation of a concept of (dis)ability, and mental (dis) ability in particular, I look at his ethical writings, but also at his more strictly medical discussions of the body and the mutual dependence between its physiology and the life of the mind.[2]

'Mental'

The topic of this chapter necessitates, first of all, a definition of 'mind' and mental health as they are understood by Galen in his work, as his understanding departs substantially from current medical and popular understandings. We cannot dwell here on the problems posed by the shifting mind–body distinction as historical phenomena in ancient philosophy and medicine (see Thumiger 2017 for a methodological survey). There are broadly two senses to mental life and health in Galen's writings: (1) A eudaimonistic concept sees mental health as the flourishing of individual spiritual, ethical and rational life. We may call this the 'software' of mental life. (2) A biological concept looks at mental life as dependent on certain physiologies of the body: the function and condition of key organs and systems (e.g. the brain and nerves) and the balance of elemental qualities and humours in the body as determinant of mental life and its health. We may call this the 'hardware' of mental life.

To each of these two correspond different etiologies as well as therapeutic and preventive strategies: within the first concept, philosophical training and education are fundamental and have much power to improve the life of the individual. Testimony to this is found especially in *The Diagnosis and Treatment of the Affections and Errors Peculiar to Each Person's Soul* (*Aff. pecc. dig.*) and *Avoiding Distress* (*Ind.*). On the other hand, within the second concept, it is the innate factors and the 'hardware' of bodily states that prevail. To an extent, these can be influenced by healing regimens and therapies, but there are limitations to what can be done to correct them, and individual willpower has little influence on it, if at all. Evidence to this second outlook is found in particular in *The Doctrines of Hippocrates and Plato* (*PHP*) and *The Capacities of the Soul Depend on the Mixtures of the Body* (*QAM*), as well as in *On Mixtures* (*Mixt.*) (which we shall not discuss here: on the topic see van der Eijk 2015).

The combination – often the juxtaposition – of these two narratives and philosophical frameworks is found explicitly in Galen for the first time in surviving Greek medical literature. It is true that from early on philosophers interrogated the physiological materiality of the body as a limit and measure to the powers of the soul. The discussion of *akrasia*, 'incontinence', offered by Aristotle in *EN* 7 (1148b15–1149a20) associated inclinations of the soul to bodily flaws: taste for immoderate pleasures, for instance, can intervene 'in some cases because of defects, in others because of character/habit, and in yet other cases because of a depravation of nature'; deviant behaviours may come about because of a disease, like *mania*; be 'morbid' (with an unclear distinction); or derive from habit; we further read that 'there are some insane people who are by nature entirely deprived of reason (...) some are so because of diseases, like the epileptic, or because of a morbid derangement' (on this passage see extensively van der Eijk 2013: 323–6; Sassi 2013: 423). In a comparable way, in *Phaedrus* 265a9–10 Plato had spoken of 'a madness that comes from human diseases' (μανία ὑπὸ νοσημάτων ἀνθρωπίνων) which is opposed to the four types of 'divine madness', and in *Timaeus* 86b1–7 the philosopher introduced a discussion of μανία and the diseases of the soul, using the label 'the diseases of the soul *that happen through the disposition of the body*'.[3]

These philosophical reflections established a tradition in which a combination of education and spiritual practices, alongside biological and innate factors, participate in the determination of mental health. When we turn to medicine, however, the whole tradition of 5th- and 4th-century BCE medical texts (Hippocratic mostly), roughly contemporary with these Platonic and Aristotelian observations, ignores the spiritual and ethical aspect completely. Integration of these two levels as part of the sphere of medicine is found for the first time in Galen.

A good illustration of the simultaneous presence of biological and spiritually or culturally constructed factors in Galen's discussion is offered by the reflections on human character in *PHP*, one of Galen's most important psychological works and the physician's most developed discussion of the bodily foundations of mental life, which he identified with the functioning of the brain and neural system. In *PHP* 3.3 (5.249 Kühn = De Lacy 185–90) Galen draws on many mythological and poetic examples of mental performance to corroborate his view of the soul as tripartite, and to anchor the fundamental agreement between the doctrines of Hippocrates and Plato that overarch his agenda in this work. While doing so he identifies factors that have an influence, for him, on the mental sphere: innate specifics such as ethnicity and gender, biological variations such as age, but also constructed aspects like culture and education: 'indeed among the Scythians and Gauls and many other barbaric peoples, anger is stronger than reason; and among us this is the case with the young and the uneducated'. Later in this book, he concentrates on one example in particular, the tragic heroine Medea as she is represented by Euripides. (On Galen's treatment of Medea's famous psychological portrayal against Crisippus, see Gill 1983, 2010: 211 and 287). Medea resolves to kill her own children after what is represented in the tragedy as an internal struggle between a line of action, a deliberate plan (βουλεύματα), various sets of considerations (pity, love, hope in a better future) and a devouring θυμός, a furious drive for revenge that keeps resurfacing and finally prevails (1079). Against Medea's surrender to rage, Galen juxtaposes the example of Odysseus and his mental debate as he faces the outrageous crimes of the suitors against his household. His lust for immediate revenge clashes against his awareness of better plans, and patience and reason finally prevail.

The assessments of these two characters, and especially Galen's interest in the manifestations of Medea's inner struggle, illustrate well the interplay, in the physician's view, between cognitive elements that we can take as culturally and personally constructed through education, exercise and will – strong emotions, rationality – and the hardware of individual biological features. Galen adds that

> one should mention here the case of Medea in Euripides and that of the Homeric Odysseus, in which the parts of the soul fight against one another showing clearly that

[the soul] is not one, and that the best part prevails in the wisest person, and the worst one prevails in the uneducated, barbarian one.

(Galen, PHP 3.3.7; 5.306 Kühn = De Lacy 188.17–190.4)

This struggle between θυμός and λογισμός in Medea is then explored in detail:

... being repeatedly driven up and down by the two of them [θυμός and λογισμός], when [Medea] has yielded to her θυμός, at that time Euripides has her say:

'I understand the evils I am going to do,
But anger prevails over my counsels'

Of course she knows the magnitude of the evils she is going to do, being instructed by reason; but she says that her anger overpowers her reason, and therefore she is forcibly led by anger to the deed, quite the opposite of Odysseus, who checked his anger with reason. Euripides has made Medea an example of barbarians and uneducated persons, in whom anger is stronger than reason; but among Greek and educated people, such as Odysseus, as the poet presents him, reason prevails over anger. In many instances reason is so much stronger than the spirited part of the soul that a conflict never arises between them; the one rules, the other is ruled. In many other instances anger is so much more powerful than reason that it rules and governs everywhere; this is seen in many barbarians, in children who are naturally inclined to anger, and in no few beasts and beastlike men.

(Galen, PHP 3.3.13–20; 5.306 Kühn = De Lacy 188.17–190.4)

The comparison between these two mental and ethical constitutions, however fictional, shows us a number of important features that return variously in Galen's reflections on the reality of human mental strength and weakness:

1 The identification of the health and power of the ψυχή in its core with its ability to keep strong drives under check and apply rational deliberation. This 'hegemonic', rational part of the soul,[4] in which these faculties reside, seems to represent in point of fact *the* soul *tout court* or at least its fundamental part (see the discussion in Singer 2013: 31).
2 The coexistence of factors of voluntary ethics *and* of biological determination ('this is seen in many barbarians, in children who are naturally inclined to anger, and in no few beasts and beastlike men').
3 The existence of a mixture of innate and acquired factors that are part of the person's character: birth[5] (Greek, barbarian, but also other innate qualities regardless of ethnicity) and education.
4 The role played by circumstances, highly exceptional in the case of both mythological examples (Odysseus' outrage at the suitors' pillaging of his household; Medea's extraordinary ordeal).

The use of Medea and Odysseus as examples of variations in mental fortitude, contextualized into a discussion of the brain and neural system, sets the terms of discussion along lines that are instructive for a history of the concept of mental disability. There are environmental elements, innate factors, and training and education variables, as well as extenuating conditions that combine to determine the outcome of an individual in terms of mental powers, here identified with sound decision-making and 'finding the good ways of living life'.

The 'software' of mental life: anger and its therapy

It is no coincidence that in Galen's discussion of the emotional part of the soul both Medea and Odysseus are battling against their θυμός, a term which encapsulates our 'fury' or 'anger', an intense and precipitous drive to action. Not only is θυμός a traditional concept in Greek culture for strong and destructive inner forces; anger is also the one emotion which Greek medicine considered as strongly linked to physiology and pathological in kind, and as such it had been discussed already by the Hippocratic authors. In Galen too, thus, anger is the natural candidate to identify a flaw in a person's soul as matter of medical concern, as well a strong cultural marker of mental weakness.[6]

Anger appears in several of Galen's psychological works, cast as an uncontrollable emotion which has a physiological component. Psychologically, it resides in the *thumoeides* part of the *psyche,* whereas the *hegemonikon*, the rational part of the soul strives to control it. Although other texts address the topic of anger and its management,[7] the treatise *Aff. pecc. dig.* is the one which offers the most focused discussion of this passion as capable of interfering with daily life and as a hindrance to one's performance and wellbeing. In the discussion offered by this treatise anger appears to belong to the constitution of the individual soul. Although it is curable, or at least improvable, it is also chronic and structural to the person. The rootedness of the disposition to anger is well illustrated by the second book of the treatise, devoted to the exploration of the difficulty of self-knowledge: it is impossible, states Galen, to have complete awareness of one's own typical errors and affections. For instance, one's tendency to act uncontrollably under the influence of anger, fear or distress, or to react beyond measure to the provocations of others are psycho-pathological traits, but are hardly perceived objectively by the person; this combination of unsound psychology and lack of awareness is a permanent state of affairs and lies far deeper than a bout of anger or a moment of weakness.

Improvement of these traits is possible, Galen insists. His suggestion involves the choice of a good 'supervisor' (*Aff. pecc. dig.* 3; 5.7–10 Kühn = de Boer 6.25–9.2) (see Harris 2001: 386–7; Gill forthcoming; Singer forthcoming; Devinant forthcoming), a close and trusted friend whose critical capacity and honesty, as well as his own moral qualities, are beyond doubt. The acquaintance that this supervisor must have with the person means he can advise and criticize his behaviour in a sincere and disinterested way; this coaching might be a long process, lasting for years or even the span of one's entire life. In the following chapter, Galen moves on to describe the manifestations of anger and the devastating effects it can have for the individual. Extreme examples of violent and self-debasing rage are cited: the angry man who, not managing to open the door in a hurry, began to bite the key, kick the door and curse the gods, foaming at the mouth (*Aff. pecc. dig.* 4; 5.16–20 Kühn = De Boer 12.11–14.24); the man who, through anger, struck his servant with a pen in his eye; and even the emperor Hadrian himself, who once caused his slave the loss of an eye in the same manner. Galen's therapy against these excesses is a form of self-scrutiny and ongoing effort, which can yield progress 'in the direction of dignity of life', but only 'in the third, in the fourth and fifth year'. This project of self-improvement is thus a very long and slow one; but it is a worthy investment of time (*Aff. pecc. dig.* 4; 5.21 Kühn = De Boer 15.13–15). Through good care, says Galen, we can ensure that our soul 'be not utterly disgusting, as was Thersites' body' (*Aff. pecc. dig.* 4; 5.15 Kühn = De Boer 11.24–5).

The comparison with the Homeric villain Thersites of *Iliad* 2.212–77 prominent for his crooked, ugly body and for his cowardly and corrupt nature, is significant. At stake here is more than an episodic behaviour to be corrected or avoided; rather, it is a rooted condition of the soul that impairs one's life, although one which can be challenged successfully 'even after the age of fifty' (*Aff. pecc. dig.* 4; 5.14 Kühn = De Boer 11.17). Thersites as paradigm of deep-seated baseness must have been commonplace in ancient culture; it interests us here because his is perhaps the first portrayal – and a very evident one – in ancient literature of bodily flaw that invites comparison with our concept of disability.[8] When a medical author or a philosopher uses Thersites as example of mental or spiritual damage, it is precisely because of the depth and rootedness of his blemishes that make him a paradigm of innate bodily defect accompanied by repulsive character. 'They are all Thersiteses of life', is Democritus' comment on the folly and hypocrisy of human beings in the fictional dialogue reported by the pseudo-Hippocratic *Epistula* 17:[9] the use of the expression in a popular text such as the Hippocratic pseudo-epigrapha testifies to this identification of the Homeric character with an impaired, ugly body and a lasting, rooted moral flaw.

The point made by Galen, that psychological flaws could be influenced even late in life is perhaps the most counterintuitive for us. Such optimism can be explained, at least in part, in the light of Galen's operating environment and audience, the world of the highly cultured and wealthy Roman elites, who had the potential leisure and intellectual instruments to embark on such projects and appreciate their value in the first place (about the social context of Galen's psychological works see Singer 2013: 4–9; more generally Mattern 2008: 14–20; Boudon-Millot 2012, esp. chs 6, 7; Mattern 2013: 99–138; on the wider social context, see Swain 2008; Van Hoof 2010 on the wider preoccupations of 'practical ethics' among the elites of the Roman Empire).

This faith in spiritual reformation reveals a first discrepancy between Galen's view and what our contemporary western audiences consider, or officially consider, a (mental) disability: a state of affairs in the abilities of an individual that is not to be unilaterally 'healed', but aided by a combination of exercises, personalized instruments (e.g. pharmacological, or prosthetic) and social policies.

Galen's optimistic faith in the possibility for the individual single-handedly to surpass or overcome a disability, however, is not as universal as his claims in *Aff. pecc. dig.* make it look. In this treatise, he is advertising his own self-improvement methodology as both necessary and effective. As we will see next, the recognition of hopelessness and incurability as far as certain mental flaws are concerned is also part of Galen's thought.

The 'hardware' of mental life: the body and its physiology

The WHO general definition of disability clearly foregrounds the question about the biologically determined basis of the dysfunction ('impairment is a problem in body function or structure'), or in other words of the failure in the body that is behind the perceived disability. When it comes to the sphere of mental health, the question cannot be separated from the debate about the relationship between mind and body and their mutual influence, by the time of Galen a long established medical and philosophical theme. The physician is especially interested in exploring the body and bodily malady as limit to mental powers. The relationship between these two spheres in Galenic thought is composite and adopts different angles in different works (on Galen's 'realism' in this respect see Gill, 2010: 160–7, 221–9).

In the ethical writings, not only as we have seen with *Aff. pecc. dig.*, but also in *On Avoiding Distress* (on which see Singer 2013; Vegetti 2013, Boudon-Millot and Jouanna 2002) Galen focuses mostly on the soul as the conscious seat of moral agency and source of rationality, whose training and nurture through philosophical practices safeguards the mental health of the individual. Thanks to these procedures a person can dominate anger and the extremes of its physiology, as we have seen, effectively proving that mental operations can have a direct influence on the state of the body. Other texts make an even stronger case for the influence of mental events on bodily health: Galen mentions cases in which λύπη, here a state of anxiety caused e.g. by social pressure or insecurity can very concretely cause bodily ailments;

elsewhere, he offers examples in which love sickness triggers a serious illness.[10] In *On Matters of Health* (*San. tu.*) 1.8.19–21 (6.41–2 Kühn = Koch 20.11–22) he makes an even more general claim: 'I have managed to restore not a few men who were ill because of the disposition of their soul (διὰ ὑπὸ τῆς ψυχῆς ἦθος) to health, by correcting the unbalance of their emotions', and goes as far as quoting Asclepius on this, citing the god's prescription of poetry and art as means to correct the temperature of the body:

> our ancestral god Asclepius ... prescribed for many patients [in emotional distress] to whom the motion of intense passions, having become more intense, had made the mixture of the body warmer than it should, to have odes written for them as well as to compose mimes and certain kinds of song ...

In *PHP* and most succinctly in *QAM* the traffic is inverted, and the bodily rooting and etiology of mental states and capacities come to the fore. In *PHP* Galen analyses the brain states and the neurological alterations that are behind mental pathologies, and in *QAM* he explores the statement that 'the capacities of the soul depend on the mixtures of the body', the clearest possible proclamation of a materialistic determinism in the sphere of psychology: the mental, i.e. the intellectual and ethical, qualities of an individual are dependent upon an underlying biology that effectively shapes it, or at least delimits the range of variations a soul can have.

Not only are physiological states that can come about through illness in point here; Galen also considers innateness a factor. In *Character Traits* he discusses human character and the non-rational elements that play a role as its spiritual as well as physiological determinants. At *Ch. Tr.* 1.28–30 (Kraus) we find a discussion of children that is exemplary for innateness of character difference: even at an early age children are said to differ from one another as far as disposition to anger, shame and other emotional reactions are concerned, as they 'all appear before they have been educated' (1.30 Kraus).[11] It follows that 'it is wrong [to say] that all affections come into being as a result of judgement and thought ... an affection ... is a bestial movement that comes about without the exercise of thought, consideration or firm judgement'. The innateness of such dispositions turns out to be another face of the same coin, the dependence of ethical traits upon the body; and while elsewhere Galen insists on the possibility that one can train one's anger, it is rather the non-cognitive, physiological disposition of it that he is accentuating here.

These clear statements appear indeed to pose open contradiction to the philosophical strategies proposed in the ethical writings, and even to the statements about the impact of the emotions on the states of the body. Galen is aware of this dissonance and the problems it poses. Towards the end of *QAM* he concludes his biological view of human mental life with the following reflection:

> This doctrine [that of the dependence of the capacities of the soul on the temperament of the body] therefore does not eliminate the good things that philosophy affords, but it is a good guide and illustration as far as these are concerned, even though it is to some extent ignored by some philosophers: for both those who think that all men are capable of virtue, and those who think that no one chooses justice per se, both have only grasped a half of human nature.
>
> *(Galen, QAM 11; 4.814 Kühn = Müller 73.6–10)*

Although there is room for philosophical improvement, Galen seems to suggest, the limit is set by the constraints of one's bodily characteristics. As a matter of fact, as we read on, it appears that the weight assigned to the body by Galen is more than 'a half', as the morality of each is said to be caused by 'temperaments of their bodies' *tout court*. What is sketched here, then, does not really appear to be a harmonization of a spiritualist view with a materialist datum, but the mutual extraneity of the two and the ultimate triumph of the second. So much so that at the very end Galen feels the need to take the natural objection – how could one possibly blame or hate a spiritually wicked person who is made so by his or her bodily characteristics? – and answer it bluntly (*QAM* 11; 4.814 Kühn = Müller 73.4):

> Not all men, in fact, are born enemies of justice, nor are all its friends, but either become so because of the temperaments of their bodies. In which way then, they say, can one justly approve, blame, hate, love a person who is good or bad not because of herself, but for the temperament, which clearly one derives from other causes? Because, we shall answer, it is in us all to desire the good, tend to it and cherish it and to hate the evil, shriek away from it and avoid it, before even pondering whether it is innate or not so. Surely, we do remove scorpions, tarantulas and vipers which are the way they are by nature and out of their own. Appropriately therefore we hate the wicked among men, without previously considering the reason that makes them so, and on the contrary we are attracted to the good ones and love them, regardless of whether they have become such by nature, because of the education they have received, or out of their own choice or customs. And we kill the *irremediably bad* for three good reasons: lest they do any harm, if they should live; so that they might instill fear in those similar to them, that they would be punished for the evil doings they will commit; and as a third reason, it is better for them to die, since they are so corrupt in their soul that they cannot be educated even by the Muses, nor can they receive any improvement from Socrates or Pythagoras.
>
> *(Galen QAM 11; 4.814 Kühn = Müller 73–4)*

There are evident problems in the notion of the 'irremediably bad' (τοὺς ἀνιάτους πονερούς) put forth here, although Galen does not seem to tackle this incongruity openly anywhere.[12] Severe defects in one's body are just accepted as a fact of existence that is beyond change: this is the first, important contradiction in Galen's philosophical programme of active care of the self.

Triggers: the role of environment and chance

Further restrictions to this programme result from the many triggers, the external circumstances that contribute to shaping an individual's soul beyond his or her control, corroborating its strengths or precipitating its weaknesses.

We have seen already how, in the opposition of Medea and Odysseus, Galen had observed the difference made by received education for the outcome of the two individuals under similar challenges. As one expects, this humanistic element of influence is given more space in the ethical works. Galen celebrates the importance of one's family as repository of models for the development of a good soul, and at *Ind.* (18.20–20.1 BJP) and *Aff. pecc. dig.* 8 (5.40–3 Kühn = De Boer 27.11–29.17) he returns to the example of his virtuous father and his morally flawed mother as contrasting influences on his own mental capacities as a child (on family, see Singer 2013: 272). Likewise, proper training and acquaintance with good friends can make an important difference, as we have seen in the example of the 'supervisor' in *Aff. pecc. dig.*

Parallel to these environmental and educational factors there are triggers in the hardest sense of the term: the impact of *tyche*, fortune and circumstances. Galen does not fully thematize this aspect, but does recognize its importance, effectively inserting a third player between the hard fact of bodily physiology and the more impalpable sphere of ethical agency:

the fortuitous coincidence of events that can undo a soul or promote its improvement. Against these, of course, men have but limited powers: in *On Avoiding Distress*, after having described the promises of philosophical self-training to improve the soul and strengthen it against life's adversities, he recognizes nonetheless the menace posed by existential obstacles:

> It amazes me, that Mousonios, like they report, often used to say 'oh Zeus, send me an adversity'. For all the time I pray for exactly the opposite, 'oh Zeus, please do not send me any adversity that might be capable of hurting me'. And so, also with regards to the health of the body, I always pray that it should remain healthy, as I have no interest in showing off spiritual strength with a broken head. Rather, even though I think it is right to exercise one's imagination envisaging all sorts of frightful events, so that we become able to bear such things with proportion, surely I would not wish to myself to bump into any that might be capable of hurting me.
>
> *(Galen, Ind. 73–6, BJP 22)*

We can perhaps look back and recognize the irrational element of *tyche* here: Zeus. This is fundamentally the same element Galen was preoccupied with in his rhetorical question at the end of *QAM*, in which he dismissed human questioning of nature's justice – how can one hate a physiologically wicked person? The figure of 'Zeus' as giver of good or bad life circumstances allows Galen to bypass the contradiction between the optimistic faith in philosophical reformation and the pessimistic implications of physiological determinism: both are appropriate, but under varying circumstances. No metaphysical query is admitted and the justice of such 'damnation' of the 'irreparably bad' is not posed as a problem. In the face of this position, Galen's admission that he himself might be too weak in the face of the most extreme adversities helps us requalify the statement – repugnant to modern humanism, whether Christian or secular – of the irreparability of extreme cases of wickedness, and read it in a more universal, existential light: there are conjunctures under which virtually all could be defeated in body or soul.

Gradualism, health and (dis)ability

Inserting environmental and familial circumstances and fortuitous triggers into the picture is one way to curtail the apparent contradiction between spiritualism and physiological determinism in Galen's writing. No human condition, no matter how optimal, can be considered a possession to be held forever but is in continuous need of tending and forever at risk;[13] this hard fact balances both physiological and spiritualist views about the mind.

A further element which offers mitigation to the gap between the two perspectives, and one that has underlain our discussions so far is gradualism, the recognition of the existence of degrees in an individual's virtues and mental flaws, and more generally in the definition of bodily health and lack thereof. Galen's gradualist view on 'health', ὑγιεία as a theoretical concept emerges clearly in the first book of his treatise *Matters of Health* (*De sanitate tuenda, San. tu.*, especially in 1.5). Here Galen proposes that the concept of health itself should be endowed with relativity as far as clinical practice is concerned,[14] a stance which in many respects can be placed in dialogue with current discussions of disability. In particular, gradualism in matters of health echoes the challenge to 'ableism' and 'disableism' moved by those critics who reject the binary view of humanity that posits a normative ideal of 'able body' as perfect standard, against which real individuals are measured.[15] Health as a whole is under scrutiny here, with no specific focus on the mental; the general, theoretical points apply however also to the issues posed by mental health and wellbeing.

Chiara Thumiger

Galen begins by rejecting the usefulness of a monolithic idea of health as an absolute state of perfection devoid of nuances. His preferred composite view of health is fundamental to his understanding of medicine as both discipline and practice: it effectively provides legitimization to the medical profession and gives sense to it as pragmatic activity, not a philosophical celebration of an abstract perfection. Likewise, lack of health, says Galen, can be defined in many different ways: 'what is imperfect and wanting (i.e. disorder, disease) has *latitude* (πλάτος)' (*San. tu.* 4; 6.11 Kühn = 8.2 Koch). Let us unpack what Galen is stating here. There are various ways in which health and disorder can be understood: health is a kind of symmetry, of good balance reflected in the various constitutions of the individual (in different seasons, at different ages, under different circumstances and so on), and in the various functions of his or her body (e.g., sight and hearing; the ability to run fast; etc.). What follows is Galen's view that there are disparate functions, constitutions, symmetries and ultimately 'healths' in each individual, depending on what aspects one considers (e.g. sight), and when, and under what circumstances. It is thus only possible to speak of the healthy working of a function at a given time, not of one all-comprising health: the same individual can be healthy in one respect and not in another, healthy at one time and not at another.

Many passages in these arguments are pertinent to a reflection on the notions of (dis)ability and the fallacy of (dis)ableism: if one fails to relativize health one falls into the paradox, Galen states clearly, of viewing the whole of humanity as sick, since most individuals fail to meet the perfect standard:

> for we are [all] afflicted no little by pain; but that condition in which we do not suffer pain, and are not impeded in the activities of life, we call health; and if anyone wishes to call it by any other name, he will accomplish nothing more than those who call life 'perpetual suffering' (…) when they declare that the constitutions of healthy bodies are the same as those of the sick, we no longer praise them nor do we accept their doctrine; for it were far better to allow sufficient latitude to health, than for us all to be beset with ceaseless maladies.
>
> *(Galen, San. tu. 5; 6.18 Kühn = Koch 10.15–20)*

One wonders who Galen's target is in this polemical invective against the absurdity of positing a humanity sick in its entirety, and in defence of a less ambitious definition of health as 'not suffering too much pain', and 'being able to carry out the activities of life'. The only possible referent for such a claim, and a notable one, is precisely relevant to the sphere of mental health: the Stoic idea of a 'madness of all mankind', an ethical-philosophical topos according to which most mankind is flawed, and as such is mad'.[16] Galen appears, then, determined to distance himself from grand claims about mankind's widespread ethical and mental deficiency, above which only a very few 'superhuman' sages could lift themselves, to propose a less ambitious programme: bodily as well as psychological and spiritual self-improvement is possible, day by day, for each according to his or her own needs and possibilities, and all degrees of functionality can be considered 'health' as long as life is reasonably free of pain and basic functions of survival are guaranteed to an acceptable level.

If we look back at the problematic clash, in Galen's doctrine, between nature and training, bodily constraint and voluntary spiritual flourishing, from this relativist and gradualist perspective, and we apply it in full to the sphere of mental life, we can begin, perhaps, to reconcile the two: the resignation of *QAM* (which is implicit also in *PHP* and other Galenic physiologies of mental life) and the activism supported by the ethical writings. (Mental) health turns out to be approached best aspect by aspect, person by person, circumstance by circumstance, life-stage by life-stage. In this sense, when in *Matters of Health* Galen says that Achilles and Thersites are both healthy – albeit in different ways and functions (*San. tu.* 1.5; 6.16 Kühn = Koch 9.32–4) – this feeds into our discussion on the topic of disability and health, and especially of moral baseness and health, as Thersites is conventionally a symbol for both. One can be 'disabled' and at the same time healthy *in some respect*; and its reverse is also true, that one can have exceptional capacities at a given time compared to the rest of humanity and still enjoy a lesser health *by one's own standards*. Galen spoke in *QAM* of the 'irremediably bad' (τοὺς ἀνιάτους πονεροὺς), a level of disability simply too severe to be overcome, saying that on the destinies of such people it is not worth spending too much thought or effort. We might however take this extreme category of 'absolutely bad' to be symmetrical to the 'perfect Stoic sage' or 'perfectly healthy individual', categories which exist almost exclusively in the abstract, about which theorizing or preoccupying oneself brings no reward, at least from a medical point of view.

Confirmation of the gradualist and relativist synthesis between Galen's two parallel lines of argument, the power of exercise and will on the one hand, and the constraints of the material world on the other (one's body and the overarching contingencies of luck) is finally found in the epistle *On Avoiding Distress*. This work is occasioned by a personal circumstance: the exceptional downturn suffered by Galen as he lost many of his most treasured possessions – books, rare pharmaceutical ingredients – in the 192 CE fire in Rome that destroyed the warehouse where they were kept. Here Galen targets precisely the balance between all these forces (*Ind.* 75–6, 22–3 BJP):

> I feel I have a precise and sharp sense of what are the capacities of my body and soul; so, I would not want any external affection to reach such a level as to destroy my health, or any misfortune to grow starker than the capacities of my soul. Still, I do not neglect to look after their [of body and soul, n.d.t.] good state, always striving, for what I can, to impress in them enough strength as to be able to contrast afflictions as they come. For I do not reckon my body to have the strength of Heracles, or my soul the fortitude that some say the wise possess, but I think it better not to neglect any exercise as long as it is in my power.
>
> *(Galen, Ind. 75–6, 22–3 BJP)*

Conclusion

We began by observing that both the term 'mental' and the concept of 'disability' need qualification and can be only be examined with reference to ancient medicine through an anachronistic lens. For Galen in particular, when it comes to the 'mental' sphere, impairment as lasting disability (as opposed to acute pathology such as e.g. the disease *phrenitis*) is generally framed as a moral-behavioural flaw: his discussions return time and again to the ethics of self-control and to voluntary self-improvement as antidotes to moral vileness and lack of rationality. When it comes to 'disability', Galen's discussions on the composite, relative and graded nature of human health seem to suggest a rejection of what we might call (dis)ableist paradigms in favour of a pluralist view in which different individuals enjoy different skills, strengths and weaknesses, and can improve on them in various ways and at different times.

The Galenic reflection is indeed very sophisticated, and has much to contribute to current debates in disability studies. On the other hand, before cheering too enthusiastically at the ancient physician's estrangement from ableist dogmas, we should remind ourselves, once again, of what his milieu and his audience were as he addresses his ethical ideal of mental soundness. His audience was not a socially varied landscape in terms of class, gender and age, but a rather definite target, composed of individuals very similar to himself – the rich members of the Roman leading classes, cultivated and wealthy, free and male (on the scope of such philosophical therapy see also Gill forthcoming, and cf. Gevaert in this volume on the impact of Stoicism). It is impossible for us to extract what Galen would have suggested for the improvement of the cognitive capacities of, say, an individual with Down's Syndrome, or for the soothing of the hallucinations and fears in a patient one would nowadays identify as schizophrenic, or afflicted by post-traumatic stress disorder. We cannot know, in other words, what he might have contributed to the health of disabled individuals or people with chronic mental illness as we define them. His interlocutor in this sphere remains the cognitively able individual in need of philosophical therapy, whose conscious mental life and ethical choices are engaged rationally and without mediation. Nonetheless, the exploration of intertwined aspects of character and education in relation to the health of the individual in Galen's work, his recognition of the power of luck in human affairs and his commitment to a view of human health as composite, comparative and to an important extent contingent can be placed into profitable dialogue with current debates on disability, especially as a warning against and antidote to normative and absolutist definitions of human perfection.

Acknowledgements

I would like to thank the Alexander von Humboldt Stiftung who financed my research and Philip van der Eijk for his continuous support. I benefited very much from the discussions with various colleagues in Berlin in the context of our Wednesday Galenic reading groups over the past years, and from the comments by Christian Laes to the first draft of this chapter.

Abbreviations

[Ps. Hippocrates]

Ep.	*Letters (Epistolae)*

Galen

Aff. pecc. dig.	*The Diagnosis and Treatment of the Affections and Errors Peculiar to Each Person's Soul* (*De propriorum animi cuiuslibet affectuum dignotione et curatione*)
BJP	*Oeuvres*, IV. *Ne pas se chagriner*, ed. V. Boudon-Millot and J. Jouanna, with A. Pietrobelli (Paris: Les Belles Lettres, 2002)
Ind.	*Avoiding Distress* (*De Indolentia*)
PHP	*The Doctrines of Hippocrates and Plato* (*De placitis Hippocratis et Platonis*)
QAM	*The Capacities of the Soul Depend on the Mixtures of the Body* (*Quod animi mores temperamenta corporis sequantur*)
San. tu.	*On Matters of Health* (*De sanitate tuenda*)
Mixt.	*On Mixtures* (*De temperamentis libri III*)

Notes

1 On disability in the ancient world, see Garland 1995, Rose 2003; for a methodological discussion, Laes et al. 2013b: 1–15; on mental disability and the problem it poses to the historian, Goodey and Rose 2013, Goodey 2011 on the concept of 'intelligence' as historical product, Laes 2014: 50–91; Laes in this volume p. 4–6 on (dis)ability vs. impairment *vis-à-vis* social construction.

2 On Galen and mental health in general see Heiberg 1927: 31–6, García Ballester 1988, Pigeaud 1988, Hankinson 1991, Stok 1996 on the wider Roman context, Godderis 2008, Gill 2010, Nutton 2013, Boudon-Millot 2013, Holmes 2013, Clark and Rose 2013; the general introduction in Singer 2013: 1–41; McDonald 2014 on *phrenitis*.

3 See Thumiger 2017 on these philosophical antecedents. For a discussion of the *Timaeus* passage and its influence on later philosophical tradition as well as Galenic ideas about mind and body see Gill 2000; Robinson 2000; Sassi 2013 for Plato on (medical) insanity; van der Eijk 2013: 316–21; Ahonen 2014: 43–51.

4 Galen adopts the Platonic representation of the soul as tripartite, as explained in *PHP*: the *logistikon*, the *thumoeides* (*PHP* 1–3) and the *epithumêtikon* (*PHP* 6) rule the rational, the emotional and the appetitive part respectively. See Tieleman 1996: pp. xxiv–xxix; Gill 2010: 103–24; Schiefsky 2012; Singer 2013: 21–2. Cf. also *Character Traits* 2–4, esp. 2.38.10–39.23 Kr.

5 Racial prejudice and ethnic stereotyping at the expenses of the non-European (the Eastern especially) is a well-known Greek cultural feature: see Hall 1991, Isaac 2004: 50, 86, 153. In Greek medicine the attitude is evident as early as the Hippocratic *Airs, Waters, Places* and its stigmatization of Eastern characters as cowardly and soft among the other things (*Aer.* 23. 3-4, 2, 84, 8 – 86, Littre = Jouanna 243.2–244.7).

6 See Harris 2001: 88–130 and 339–400 on philosophical approaches to restraining rage, as well as Galen on anger; von Staden 2011 on Galen and the previous medical tradition, Thumiger 2017 on the Hippocratic texts and classical medicine.

7 *PHP*, as we have seen, in a different frame; cf. also *Ch. Traits* I. 29-30 Kr. (Singer 142–3) on innate anger. On the therapy of the emotions in Galen see Gill 2010: 246–80; King 2013 on grief; Gill forthcoming.

8 On this figure, cf. Garland 1995: 81; Rose 2003: 12, 43; Laes *et al.* 2013b: 7; Goodey and Rose 2013: 18, 26; Laes 2014: 65–6, 179, 239, n. 673.

9 The broader context: 'in war they seem to approve courage, but they are bested daily by lust, by greed, by all the passions they are sick with. They are all Thersiteses of life' (καὶ δοκέουσι μὲν ἐν πολέμῳ ἀνδρείην ἐπαινεῖσθαι, νικῶνται δὲ καθ' ἡμέρην ὑπὸ τῆς ἀσελγείης, ὑπὸ τῆς φιλαργυρίης, ὑπὸ τῶν παθέων πάντων ἃ νοσέουσι. Θερσῖται δ' εἰσὶ τοῦ βίου πάντες, *Ep.* 17, Smith 82.20–2 = 9.364 Littré, tr. by Smith, with adjustments).

10 On these see Mattern 2015: 211 with n. 30 on erotic passion.

11 On anger in children in Galen's discussions on the topic see von Staden 2011: 66, n. 7. On innateness see also *QAM* 2 (4.768 Kühn = Müller 32–3).

12 On this see: Gill 2010: 140–67; Singer 2013: 23–30; Singer forthcoming; Devinant forthcoming.

13 Galen observes in *San. tu.* 5 (6.60 Kühn = Koch 14.25–8), that 'if ever the best constitution existed, it would not remain unchanged for an instant'; those who argue for it 'do not realize that they are arguing about something which either never exists in the animal body or, if ever it should exist, does not last any length of time'.

14 *San. tu.* 1.1 (6.1–79 Kühn = Koch 1–37); see Grimaudo 2008: 64–71. On Galen and gradualism in mental health see Lewis *et al.* 2016.

15 Campbell 2009: 3–76 for a survey of the theoretical discussion.

16 See Ahonen 2014: 107–12 for a survey of this idea. At *Aff. pecc. dig.* 3 (5.10–11 Kühn = De Boer 8.11–9.12) Galen discusses the idea that 'only the wise man is completely free of error' – the ethical equivalent to the idea of health as perfect ideal – to reject it decisively: appeal to such ideals of unattainable perfection easily become excuses to be indulgent towards friends who commit mistakes, and generally to give up on more realistic targets, such as the gradual self-improvement he is advocating for.

Texts and translations used

Hippocrates. *Pseudepigraphic Writings: Letters, Embassy, Speech from the Altar, Decree* (*Ep.*), ed. and tr. W. D. Smith, *Studies in Ancient Medicine*, 2 (Leiden: Brill, 1990).

Galen. *De sanitate tuenda*, ed. K. Koch. *CMG* V.4, 2 (Leipzig/Berlin: Akademie Verlag, 1932).

Galen. *Oeuvres*, IV. *Ne pas se chagriner,* ed. V. Boudon-Millot and J. Jouanna, with A. Pietrobelli (Paris: Les Belles Lettres, 2002).

Galen. *Scripta Minora*, ed. I. Marquardt, I. Müller and G. Helmreich (Leipzig: Teubner), 118–93 (repr. Amsterdam: Hakkert, 1967).

Galen. *Character Traits. De Moribus*, ed. P. Kraus, Kitāb al-aḫlāq li-Gālīnūs. *Bull. Fac. Arts Egypt Univ.* 5 (1937), 1–51.

Galen. *De Placitis Hippocratis et Platonis,* ed. and tr. P. De Lacy, 3 vols (Berlin: Akademie Verlag, 2005).

Galen. *Psychological Writings: Avoiding Distress, Character Traits, The Diagnosis and Treatment of the Affections and Errors Peculiar to Each Person's Soul, The Capacities of the Soul Depend on the Mixtures of the Body,* tr. V. Nutton, D. Davies and P. N. Singer, with the collaboration of P. Tassinari (Cambridge: Cambridge University Press, 2013).

Bibliography

Ahonen, Marke, *Mental Disorders in Ancient Philosophy* (Berlin and New York, 2014).

Boudon-Millot, Veronique, *Galien de Pergame: Un médecin grec à Rome* (Paris, 2012).

Boudon-Millot, Veronique, 'What is a Mental Illness, and How Can it be Treated? Galen's Reply as a Doctor and as a Philosopher', in W. V. Harris (ed.), *Mental Disorders in the Classical World* (Leiden, 2013), 129–45.

Campbell, Fiona Kumari, *Contours of Ableism: The Production of Disability and Abledness* (London, 2009).

Clark, Patricia Ann, and Rose, Martha Lynn, 'Psychiatric Disability in the Galenic Medical Matrix', in C. Laes *et al.* (eds), *Disabilities in Roman Antiquity* (Leiden, 2013), 45–72.

Devinant, Julien, 'Galen's Cases, Psychiatric Illness and Psychological Suffering', in C. Thumiger and P. N. Singer (eds) *Medical Conceptions of Mental Illness from Celsus to Caelius Aurelianus* (Leiden, forthcoming).

García-Ballester, Luis, 'Soul and Body, Disease of the Soul and Disease of the Body in Galen's Medical Thought', in P. Manuli and M. Vegetti (eds), *Le opere psicologiche di Galeno* (Naples, 1988), 117–52.

Garland, Robert, *The Eye of the Beholder: Deformity and Disability in the Graeco-Roman World* (Ithaca, NY, 1995).

Gill, Christopher, 'Did Chrisippus Understand Medea?', *Phronesis* 28/2 (1983), 136–49.

Gill, Christopher, 'Peace of Mind and Being Yourself: Panaetius to Plutarch', *Aufstieg und Niedergang der römischen Welt* 2/36/7 (Berlin, 1994), 4599–4640.

Gill, Christopher, 'The Body's Fault? Plato's *Timaeus* on Psychic Illness', in M. R. Wright (ed.), *Reason and Necessity* (London, 2000), 59–84.

Gill, Christopher, *The Structured Self in Hellenistic and Roman Thought* (Oxford, 2006).

Gill, Christopher, *Naturalistic Psychology in Galen and Stoicism* (Oxford, 2010).

Gill, Christopher, 'Philosophical Therapy as Preventive Psychological Medicine', in W. V. Harris (ed.), *Mental Disorders in the Classical World* (Leiden, 2013), 339–60.

Gill, Christopher, 'Philosophical Psychological Therapy: Did it Have Any Impact on Medical Practice?', in C. Thumiger and P. N. Singer (eds) *Medical Conceptions of Mental Illness from Celsus to Caelius Aurelianus* (Leiden, forthcoming)..

Godderis, Jan, *Galenos van Pergamon over de passies en de vergissingen van de ziel* (Leuven, 2008).

Goodey, Chris F., *A History of Intelligence and 'Intellectual Disability': The Shaping of Psychology in Early Modern Europe* (Farnham, 2011).

Goodey, Chris F., and Rose, Martha Lynn, 'Mental States, Bodily Dispositions and Table Manners: A Guide to Reading "Intellectual" Disability from Homer to Late Antiquity', in C. Laes *et al.* (eds), *Disabilities in Roman Antiquity* (Leiden, 2013), 17–44.

Grimaudo, Sabrina, *Difendere la salute: Igiene e disciplina del soggetto nel De Sanitate Tuenda di Galeno* (Naples, 2008).

Hall, Edith, *Inventing the Barbarian: Greek Self-Definition through Tragedy* (Oxford, 1991).

Hankinson, Jim, 'Galen's Anatomy of the Soul', *Phronesis* 36 (1991), 197–233.

Harris, William V., *Restraining Rage: The Ideology of Anger Control in Classical Antiquity* (Cambridge, MA, 2001).

Harris, William V. (ed.), *Mental Disorders in the Classical World* (Leiden, 2013).

Heiberg, Johan Ludvig, *Geisteskrankheiten im klassischen Altertum* (Berlin, 1927).

Holmes, Brooke, 'Disturbing Connections: Sympathetic Affections, Mental Disorder, and the Elusive Soul in Galen', in W. V. Harris (ed.), *Mental Disorders in the Classical World* (Leiden, 2013), 147–76.

Isaac, Benjamin Henri, *The Invention of Racism in Classical Antiquity* (Princeton, NJ, 2004).

King, Daniel, 'Galen and Grief: The Construction of Grief in Galen's Clinical Work', in A. Chaniotis and P. Ducrey (eds), *Unveiling Emotions*, II. *Emotions in Greece and Rome: Texts, Images, Material Culture* (Stuttgart, 2013), 251–72.

Laes, Christian, *Beperkt? Gehandicapten in het Romeinse Rijk* (Leuven, 2014).

Laes, Christian, Goodey, Chris F., and Rose, Martha Lynn (eds), *Disabilities in Roman Antiquity: Disparate Bodies A Capite ad Calcem* (Leiden, 2013a).

Laes, Christian, Goodey, Chris F., and Rose, Martha Lynn, 'Approaching Disabilities A Capite ad Calcem: Hidden Themes in Roman Antiquity', in C. Laes *et al.*, *Disabilities in Roman Antiquity* (Leiden, 2013b), 1–15.

Lewis, Orly, Thumiger, Chiara, and van der Eijk, Philip, 'Gradualism and Mental Health in Ancient Medicine', in G. Keil, L. Keuck and R. Hauswald (eds), *Gradualist Approaches to Mental Health and Disease* (Oxford, 2016).

McDonald, Glenda, 'Galen on Mental Illness: A Physiological Approach to *Phrenitis*', in P. Adamson, R. Hansberger and J. Wilberding (eds), *Philosophical Themes in Galen* (London, 2014), 135–52.

Manuli, Paola, and Vegetti, Mario (eds), *Le opere psicologiche di Galeno* (Naples, 1988).

Mattern, Susan P., *Galen and the Rhetoric of Healing* (Baltimore, MD, 2008).

Mattern, Susan P., *Prince of Medicine: Galen in the Roman Empire* (Oxford, 2013).

Mattern, Susan P., 'Galen's Anxious Patients: *Lypē* as Anxiety Disorder', in G. Petridou and C. Thumiger (eds), *Homo Patiens* (Leiden, 2015), 203–23.

Nutton, Vivian, *Ancient Medicine* (Oxford, 2004).

Nutton, Vivian, 'Galenic Madness', in W.V. Harris (ed.), *Mental Disorders in the Classical World* (Leiden, 2013), 119–27.

Petridou, Georgia, and Thumiger, Chiara (eds), *Homo Patiens: Approaches to the Patient in the Ancient World* (Leiden, 2015).

Pigeaud, Jackie, 'La psychopathologie de Galien', in P. Manuli and M. Vegetti (eds), *Le opere psicologiche di Galeno* (Naples, 1988),153–83.

Robinson, Thomas M., The Defining Features of Mind–Body Dualism in the Writings of Plato', in J. P. Wright and P. Potter (eds), *Psyche and Soma: Physicians and Metaphysicians on the Mind-Body Problem from Antiquity to Enlightenment* (Oxford, 2000), 37–55.

Rose, Martha Lynn, *The Staff of Oedipus: Transforming Disability in Ancient Greece* (Ann Arbor, MI, 2003).

Sassi, Maria Michela, 'Mental Illness, Moral Error, and Responsibility in Late Plato', in W. V. Harris (ed.), *Mental Disorders in the Classical World* (Leiden, 2013), 413–26.

Schiefsky, Mark J., 'Galen and the Tripartite Soul', in R. Barney, T. Brennan and C. Brittain (eds), *Plato and the Divided Self* (Cambridge, 2012), 331–49.

Singer, Peter N., *Galen: Psychological Writings. Avoiding Distress, Character Traits, The Diagnosis and Treatment of the Affections and Errors Peculiar to Each Person's Soul, The Capacities of the Soul Depend on the Mixtures of the Body*, tr. with introduction and notes by V. Nutton, D. Davies and P. N. Singer, with the collaboration of P. Tassinari (Cambridge, 2013).

Singer, Peter N., 'Galen's Approaches to Mental Disturbance', in Chiara Thumiger and Peter N. Singer *Medical Conceptions of Mental Illness from Celsus to Caelius Aurelianus* (Leiden, forthcoming).

Stok, Fabio, 'Follia e malattie mentali nella medicina dell'età romana', *Aufstieg und Niedergang der römischen Welt* 2/37/3 (1996), 2282–2410.

Swain, Simon, 'Social Stress and Political Pressure: On Melancholy in Context', in P. E. Pormann (ed.), *Rufus of Ephesus: On Melancholy* (Tübingen, 2008), 113–38.

Thumiger, Chiara, 'Happiness and Flourishing in Ancient Medicine', *Acta Classica* 6 (2015), 106–24.

Thumiger, Chiara, *The Life and Health of the Mind in Early Greek Medical Thought* (Cambridge, 2017).

Thumiger, Chiara, and Singer, Peter N. (eds), *Medical Conceptions of Mental Illness from Celsus to Caelius Aurelianus* (Leiden, forthcoming).

Tieleman, Teun, *Galen and Chrysippus on the Soul: Argument and Refutation in the De Placitis, Books II–III* (Leuven, 1996).

van der Eijk, Philip, 'Cure and (In)curability of Mental Disorders in Ancient Medical and Philosophical Thought', in W. V. Harris (ed.), *Mental Disorders in the Classical World* (Leiden, 2013), 307–38.

van der Eijk, Philip, 'Galen on the Assessment of Bodily Mixtures', in B. Holmes and K.-D. Fischer (eds), *The Frontiers of Ancient Science: Essays in Honor of Heinrich von Staden* (Berlin, 2015), 675–98.

Van Hoof, Lieve, *Plutarch's Practical Ethics* (Oxford, 2010).

Vegetti, Mario (ed.), *Galeno, Nuovi scritti autobiografici: Introduzione, traduzione e commento* (Roma, 2013).

von Staden, Heinrich, 'The Physiology and Therapy of Anger: Galen on Medicine, the Soul, and Nature', in F. Opwis and D. Reisman (eds), *Islamic Philosophy, Science, Culture, and Religion: Studies in Honor of Dimitri Gutas* (Leiden, 2011), 63–87.

20

MADNESS AND MAD PATIENTS ACCORDING TO CAELIUS AURELIANUS

Danielle Gourevitch

Introduction: the classification of mental diseases

Some time during the 5th–6th century CE, Caelius Aurelianus, an African of Sicca in Numidia who was a Roman physician and writer, set out to offer the public of his time both a translation from Greek to Latin and an adaptation of his famous predecessor's great treaty. In fact, Soranus of Ephesus (2nd century CE), who was not the father but certainly the master of the methodic school of medicine, wrote on gynaecological and paediatric medicine, and composed *Acute Diseases* (*Celeres* or *Acutae Passiones*) and *Chronic Diseases* (*Tardae* or *Chronicae Passiones*). The translation of Soranus' treatises is the more valuable for us since the original Greek version is lost.

In this chapter, I will first highlight some examples of madness in Caelius' work – referring to such categories as acute (*Ac.*) and chronic (*Chron.*) – so that the reader can understand the problematic issues and style of the author. The principle of his classification is that 'of all acute diseases some occur with fever and others without fever' (*Ac.* 1.3), while 'chronic diseases resemble acute only during the time of an attack' (*Chron.* 1.1). Of course, in acute diseases the situation is more striking and dramatic, and especially in cases of phrenitis. Or in Caelius' own words, among acute diseases with fever, 'phrenitis deserves most attention' (*phrenitis praeponenda*; *Ac.* 1.3), and so we shall take his advice.

Some acute madness

Phrenitis is defined several times in Caelius' work; two examples follow:

> We know definitely that phrenitis occurs with fever, not merely frequently but always, and that it never can occur without fever.
>
> *(Ac. 1.5)*

We say that phrenitis is an acute mental derangement accompanied by acute fever, a futile groping of the hands, seemingly in the effort to grasp something with the fingers (Greek *crocydismos* or *carphologia*) and a small, thick, pulse.

(Ac. 1.21)

Some distinguishing features within the cases are to be drawn, for example:

Similar and kindred to phrenitis in respect to loss of reason (*ex ipsa alienatione*), are mania (*furor*), commonly called *insania*, melancholy (*melancholia*), pleurisy (*pleuritis*) and pneumonia (*peripneumonia*). These diseases in periods of exacerbation very often produce mental aberration (*alienatio*). Also resembling phrenitis is the loss of reason due to the drinking of mandragora or henbane.

(Ac. 1.42)

All the diseases that cause loss of reason (*alienatio*) because of the pain (*ex dolore*) at the time of an attack may best be distinguished from phrenitis in the following way. When the pains in these diseases become intense, the mental derangements are aggravated and increased; but when the pains are mitigated, the derangement is lessened, for it is not serious and is easily cleared up. But the loss of reason in phrenitis, even if it does occur with concomitant pain, still if not always increase in attacks, decreased in remissions, but is found to be more abiding and persistent.

(Ac. 1.43)

There are two types of phrenitis:

one involving a state of stricture, the other a combination of stricture and looseness. For it is proper to make distinctions in such a way that different types of a disease are shown not by differences in symptoms but by a general and invariable indication.

(Ac. 1.52)

Phrenitis may well be the most important acute disease, but worse conditions exist. As for lethargy:

it receives its name from the loss of memory which the disease involves (…) And it is a more serious disease than phrenitis, just as is complete loss of vision compared with partial impairment.

(Ac. 2.1)

Some cases of chronic madness

In book 1, madness is considered in chapter 5, *de furore sive insania, quam Graeci manian vocant*:

Mania is an impairment of reason (*alienatio*); it is chronic and without fever and in these respects may be distinguished from phrenitis. For mania is not an acute disease nor is it observed to occur with fever; or, if fever is present in a case of mania, the case may be distinguished from phrenitis by consideration of time, for in mania the madness precedes any supervening fever and the patient does not have a small pulse (…) Mania occurs more frequently in young and middle-aged men, rarely in old men, and most infrequently in children and women. Sometimes it strikes suddenly, at other times it takes hold gradually. Sometimes it arises from hidden causes, at other times from observable causes, such as exposure to intense heat, the taking of severe cold, indigestion, frequent and uncontrolled drunkenness, continual sleeplessness, excesses of venery, anger, grief, anxiety or superstitious fear, a shock or blow, intense training of the senses and the mind in study, business or other ambitious pursuits, the drinking of drugs, especially those intended to excite love, the removal of long-standing haemorrhoids or varicose veins, and, finally, the suppression of the menses in women (*abstinentia solitae purgationis*).

(Chron. 1.146–7)

In other terms, chronic madness and acute madness can be terribly disabling; certain categories of people are more liable to suffer from it and some epidemiology could be determined.

Words and terminology

Now we turn our attention to the most important words to name or describe madness and its symptoms.[1] These will be dealt with in alphabetical order.[2]

As a general category, the patients are called *aegri* or *aegrotantes*. The diseases of course have more precise names, either Latin, Greek in the Latin alphabet, or a mixture of both languages according to various schemes; these terms in their turn give a derivate name to the patients' various diagnoses (*furor*, and *furiosus* or *furens*, for instance). But Caelius' nomenclature is not always clear or coherent.

Alienatio or **alienatio mentis** (stemming from the verb *alienare*, or the even stronger *abalienare*) seems to refer to several diseases, notably *phrenitis* (*Ac.* 1.21).[3] Etymologically the substantive is derived from *alienus*: patients become others, and are not themselves any more. The appearance of the patients is varied; sometimes they are as cheerful as happy children (*cum risu atque puerili saltatione*), sometimes they shout out their grief or are silent in their anxiety (*cum maerore atque exclamatione, vel silentio atque timore*; *Ac.* 1.52).

Catalepsis, a Greek word for *apprehensio vel oppressio*, could be replaced by *catocha/ catoche*, or *cataleptica passio*. Patients are called *catalyptici*. Catalepsy is a disease mostly of the senses, often to be understood as a sudden seizure (*Chron.* 1.3)

Deliratio, according to Caelius, is very similar to *alienatio*, yet the word itself is quite different, for the *delirans* patient does not follow a straight furrow (*lira*), while the *alienus* is no longer himself (*Ac.* 1.80).

Dementia refers to a partial loss of the capacity to think. The noun *amentia*, which etymologically refers to a total loss of intellectual capacity, occurs only once in Caelius (*Chron.* 1.49).

Furor refers to an acute and agitated madness without fever. But the use of this and similar words is not always coherent: *vulgo insania* (*Chron.* 1.15), *furor sine insania* or *mania* (*Chron.* 1.144), and so on.

Hydrophobia literally refers to fear of water. It owes its name to its main symptom, and Caelius deems it appropriate to explain this to Latin speakers: 'it refers to a strong fear of water, since the Greeks call fear "phobon" and water "hydor"' (*est enim vehemens timor aquae: nam Graeci timorem phobon vocant, aquam hydor appellant*; *Ac.* 3.98). But according to another definition, it also refers to heavy lust and at the same time fear of drinking (*Est agnitio hydrophobiae appetentia vehemens atque timor potus*; *Ac.* 3.101, see Gaide 1998). Caelius wonders whether it should be considered a disease of the soul or of the body (*utrum animae an corporis passio sit hydrophobia*; *Ac.* 3.109). In any case, he did not consider it a new disease (*non novam esse hydrophobicam* *passionem, Ac.* 3.125). The exact meaning of the word had always been somewhat ambiguous, hence the existence of synonyms. The meaning was not clear to the Romans because the word was originally Greek; Caelius, therefore, explained it: '*pheugydron,* for he who shies away from water' (*pheugydron siquidem aquam fugat*), '*cynolysson* for a disease which arises from the rabies by a dog bite' (*ex rabie canina morbum conceptum*; *Ac* 3.125).[4]

Insania, a word immediately clear to English-speaking people ('insane'), was commonly used to denote *furor* (cf. supra) but, contrary to what we might expect, the proper word used by doctors seems to have been *furor*.

Lethargia or *lethargus* was in general not differentiated from *catalepsis* (*Ac.* 2.10.57–8), or if it was, the differentiation was only in words not in facts. The followers of Asclepiades made this distinction, though they were not clear about the real difference between the two concepts: *(catalepsin) a lethargo discreverunt et nomine adjecto catalepsin vocaverunt et quidem nihil ei novitatis ascribentes.* That is to say, the name had changed, but it did not really refer to anything new.

Mania: nobody in Antiquity seems to have realized that the word might have something to do with the Greek μάντις, nor did Caelius (Casewitz 1991; Chandler 2009; Pigeaud 2010). In fact he tried in vain to discover the true etymology of the word: 'the Greeks have called it mania, and this name may refer to many different meanings' (*Graeci maniam (...) vocaverunt, ex quo nomine multae possunt significationes ostendi*; *Chron.* 1.144). Anyway it is a chronic impairment of reason without fever (*alienatio tardans sine febribus*) and *mania* is sometimes difficult to differentiate from *phrenitis* (*Chron.* 1.15) and is more frequent in men (*Chron.* 1.147).

Melancholia, a Greek loan-word, is also considered a chronic disease (*Chron.* 1.183; see Godderis 2000; Kazantzidis 2013). 'It derives its name from the fact that the patient often vomits black bile', not 'from the notion that black bile is (its) cause' (*Chron.* 1.181). The mental and psychological symptoms are serious, and again the disease is more frequent in men (*frequentat in masculis magis*; *Chron.* 1.181). As for melancholy:

> when it is actually present, symptoms are as follows: mental anguish and distress (*animi anxietas atque difficultas*), dejection, silence, animosity towards members of the household (*odio conviventium*), sometimes a desire to live and at other times a longing for death, suspicion on the part of the patient that a plot is being hatched against him (*suspicionibus velut insidiarum*), weeping without reason, meaningless muttering, and, again, occasional joviality.
>
> *(Chron. 1.181)*

Phrenitis, a Greek word built upon the name of the supposedly affected part (φρήν, φρενός), both the place where thought is produced, and thought itself (*nomen ... sumpsit a difficultate mentis; ... phrenas enim Graece mentes vocaverunt; quarum ... impedimentum phrenetica ingerit passio*; *Ac.* 1.4) (Centanni 1987; Gourevitch 1998). Already in the Hippocratic corpus, phrenitis referred to delirium with a high fever, then differentiated from μανία and μελαγχολία. In phrenitis, we see an interesting example of patients putting themselves and others in physical danger (*Ac.* 1.35). Some lines in Caelian seem very much to describe an actual patient, as for instance a person who is

> in such a state of anger that he jumps up in a rage and can scarcely be held back, is wrathful at everyone, shouts, beats himself or tears his own clothing and that of his neighbours, or seeks to hide in fear, or weeps, or fails to answer those who speak to him, while he speaks not only with those who are not present, but with the dead, ...

and asks for neither food nor drink, or when he does take food falls violently upon it and gulps it down unchewed, or else chews it but does not swallow it, keeping it in his mouth and after a while spitting it out.

(Ac. 1.35)

In such cases, we are strongly reminded of Galenic records, such as the case of the phrenetic who first threw out of the window some beautiful vases and then the servant who was in charge of him (Galen, *De locis affectis* 4.2 (8.225–6 Kühn); Gourevitch 1993 and Thumiger in this volume).

Tales of madness and mythological allusions

Indeed, Caelius Aurelianus also presents some case stories, but not many. Were these about 'real' patients whom Caelius met or treated? Or are these anecdotes mere tales of madness, stories taken over from predecessors in a game of learned allusions? Or are they a mixture of illness and culture? (See Mattern 2008 on the 'rhetoric of healing' with Galen.)

Lyssa or *rabies* with one of its main symptoms *hydrophobia* – generally but not necessarily due to the bite of a rabid dog – has a long story. Caelius (*Ac.* 3.121) alludes to Homer and offers a naturalistic interpretation of the myth of Tantalus, who had betrayed the gods and remained punished forever in Tartarus, where he could neither eat nor drink, the fruit and water disappearing whenever he reached for them. This is the mythological presentation: in reality, Caelius argues, Tantalus displayed the symptoms of a hydrophobic! And 'Homer himself recognized this disease, for he alludes to it figuratively (*per figuram*) when he speaks of (him)' (Caelius here refers to Homer, *Od.* 9.582). In the same chapter follows a similar explanation for Teucer 'who, after killing eight men, could not strike Hector' since, Caelius said, he could 'not kill this mad dog' (*hunc interficere non posse rabidum canem*) (here he refers to Homer, *Il.* 8.296). Teucer had been driven to this, stirred to mighty wrath (*iracundia moto*); burned or not with black bile, he certainly had many imitators. In *Ac.* 3.121 another literary allusion follows, that of the drunkard of Menander in an unidentified play: the playwright 'introduces an angry old man and draws a picture of *hydrophobia*, ascribing it to excessive drinking of wine and indicating that those who drink until they become ill are no longer able to drink' (Hilton 2009).

In a passage about the sickroom, Hercules and Orestes become the protagonists: 'Hercules, when he looked upon his sons and wife, saw the faces of his enemies and Orestes was terrified by the countenance of Electra, whom he mistook for a Fury' (*Ac.* 1.122). The words *vultus* and *visis/visibus* are interesting for the visual delusions based on the appearance of the human face. Seneca in his *Hercules Furens* considered the poor hero not guilty of crime, since he had been driven to kill his wife and children by error, as he was unable to recognize his family and friends (*Herc. Fur.* 1236), and Amphitryon, Hercules' supposed human father, insisted that this disaster did not imply any fault: *casus hic culpa caret* (*Herc. Fur.* 1201), a very beautiful formula still perceptible in the French sentence, though certainly less succinct: 'il n'y a ni crime ni délit, lorsque le prévenu était en état de démence au temps de l'action'.

It is a pity that Caelius has nothing to say about Ulysses' companions after Circe had poisoned them and turned them into pigs. But mythology is always close to his mind and to that of his audience. If love is a form of insanity according to some (*amorem generaliter furorem vocaverunt*), Medea is never very far away:

In the rich mythology of the Greeks there is story that a woman (*femina*, [her name is not mentioned here]) of divine descent, harried by human fates (*humanis fatis*) and beset by the grim pangs of vengeance, kills her offspring with her own hand.

(Chron. 1.177)

One may ask why Caelius refers to Greek mythology, and not to the Roman interpretation by Seneca in his famous tragedy, which was probably better known in that time (Pigeaud 1981b: 2). This is one of many textual instances that leads us to question the Romanization of Soranus by Caelius. Surely, he translated Soranus, but he also sometimes changes practical details, because he wants to make sure his readers will understand.

And if the text chosen by Drabkin is correct (he actually believes that the lover referred to is a man and not a god), the case story of a man in love with Proserpina, 'who sought to enter the lower world, thinking he could rightly take to wife a goddess wedded to another', becomes important medically. Another man longed for the nymph Amphitrite and 'threw himself in the sea' to meet her (*Chron.* 1.177). Caelius realized that the content of delirium is marked culturally and historically.

Social disability

Undoubtedly, Caelius Aurelianus considered such people as 'sick', as he did other persons for whom he did not need mythological allusions to describe their condition. He mentions several disturbed men, beginning with a *furens* who

> fancied himself a sparrow, another a cock, another an earthen vessel, another a brick, another a god, another an orator, another a tragic actor, another a comic actor, another a stalk of grain and asserted he was the centre of the universe, and another cried like a baby and begged to be carried in the arms (*alius se sustentandum manu poscebat, vagiens ut infans*).
>
> (*Chron. 1.152*)

In fact, these strange anecdotes very much reminiscent of similar cases reported by Galen (e.g. the patient who was afraid Atlas might drop the sky in Comm. 2 in *Hippocratis De humoribus* 30; 16.325 Kühn – see Laes 2014: 81 and Thumiger in this volume). All of these persons were certainly 'socially disabled', as their madness in all likelihood prevented them from performing 'normally' in everyday life, not that ancient doctors bothered about the topic of social inclusion or exclusion. Aretaeus of Cappadocia mentions the story of the artisan who dealt perfectly with customers and personnel, but who turned utterly mad, behaving strangely and full of anxiety whenever he went outside his workshop. Here, social historians would distinguish the man's ability to perfectly perform in professional matters and his obvious social disability. To Aretaeus, the case is just another telling anecdote about the chronic strange behaviour of a mad person (Aretaeus, *De causis et signis diuturnorum morborum* 1.6.6; Laes 2014: 187–8).

But Caelius also tells the sad story of a woman who became disabled from an occupational disease, namely rabies (Gourevitch 1999). In fact, she was a poor needlewoman, who had to repair even old and dirty garments:

> Once when a seamstress was preparing to repair, the cloak of a man (*chlamidem* [a surprising word in a Roman context, either in Italy or in Africa]) rent by the bites of a rabid animal, she adjusted the threads along the needle, using her tongue, and then as she sewed she licked the edges that were being joined, in order to make the passage of the needle easier. It is reported that two days later she was stricken by rabies.[5]
>
> (*Ac. 3.100*)

In such a disease the latency has no fixed pattern, but a lapse of two days seems short. Richer, idle women were no safer, as we see in the woman who 'became ill of hydrophobia when her face was slightly scratched by a small puppy' (*Ac.* 3.99). These two case stories are probably not genuinely Caelian, since they are introduced by the same verb *memoratur* as in Soranian anecdotes (Urso 2000b), or as parts of a common stock.

Caelius Aurelianus and 'everyday life'

We know little about Caelius' patients, his daily practice, whether or how his ideas had an impact in everyday reality, and how he himself was influenced by the world around him. However, such questions are worth asking, and some possibilities may be raised.

Caelius certainly must have been acquainted with juridic literature, where cases of persons irresponsible for their actions are mentioned, for instance the case of the young man, Aelius, who had murdered his mother, under the reign of Marcus Aurelius and Commodus. The judges wondered whether the possible culprit was pretending madness or not, in order to avoid punishment, and whether, if really insane, he suffered from continuous or episodic madness. An official rescript was considered necessary, and the rescript again was sent to Scapula Tertullus. It was eventually decided that by necessity it was better to keep him apart from human society by sending him out of town. If the patient had no place to go, then prison would suit the situation. Aelius' guardians pose another problem in this situation: Aelius was sick before the crime and already had guardians, who did not do their job even though they were responsible for him. If guilt is to be punished, it is not that of the ward, but that of his guardians (*Dig.* 1.18.4; cf. Toohey in this volume).

A terrible news story engendering the same social and legal problems had happened earlier, in the reign of emperor Tiberius (this was the source of inspiration for Néraudau 1991). According to Tacitus (*Ann.* 3.22) the praetor Plautus Silvanus had murdered his wife, for reasons we are not told. Love? Or that false love that jealousy is? Or any other reason? She was hurled down from their bedroom to the garden. First, Silvanus pretended he had been sleeping deeply all the time, and knew nothing. Yet the proof of a violent fight was discovered by the emperor himself when he visited the place. The grandmother of the guilty husband sent him a sword, hoping he would be courageous enough to commit suicide. He was not. He chose to have his veins cut by a third party, and died. But madness was to play its part in the story: poor Fabia Numantina, his first wife, in order to have Silvanus' *memoria* redeemed, was accused of having enchanted him with her spells and philters to take revenge on his unfaithfulness and desertion! The emperor was very glad that everything was settled before formal judgment.

A similar story might be attested on a codex in Berlin, from Hermopolis, dated 359 CE (*BGU* 4.1024 or *P. Aktenbuch*[6]), a frightening tale of phrenitis provides an interesting example of danger, love and death (Poethke *et al.* 2012). A man loved his girlfriend excessively and killed her (Πρός τινα φ[ιλοῦν]τα τὴν ἑαυ[το]ῦ φίλην σφοδρὰν ἔρωτα... Φό[νο]υ κατα[σ]ημαινομένου α[ἰτίαν] | τὴν ἐπικει[μ]ένην [σ]ου (read σοι) [μ]ανίαν [λέγεις] ἔρωτος). This was a case of real mania, and such a mental state was the cause of the deed (at least if αἰτία is correct)! Unfortunately, he had happened to see her in the company of another man; he could not resist his anger (μ[ὴ κατέχ]ων τὴ[ν ὀ]ργὴν), and drew some sort of a sword and killed her. He soon regretted it, that is, he feared for his own fate, not for hers, and he tried to be excused on the basis of madness, or on his silliness (ἀβελ[τε]ρείαν ὑποθήματος). And it worked, more or less: he was not sentenced to death but only sent to a mine (*damnatio in metallum*), for ἐν μετάλλῳ he would have plenty of time to realize that wrath is a bad counsellor! *Ira brevis furor est*, according to the poet Horace (*Epist.* 1.2.62). Both ancient philosophers and doctors have been concerned with the problem of anger (Van Hoof 2010) and so was Caelius.

Egypt is not so far from North Africa and Caelius may have heard of similar stories to the one that follows, but this took place some time after his death, and is recorded in a private letter of the 6th century, written and found in Oxyrhynchus (Maresch and Packman 1990). On the verso is the address and the usual salutations; the text is one of the rather rare instances of a love letter on papyrus. The text is lacunar, but it is possible to understand that the lover's mind became obsessed day and night by his sweetheart. Since the man sends his regards to the brother, mother (?), and 'everybody with you', I gather he is the husband. His heart is burnt by a love-fever: τὴν καρδίαν μου ὁ πυρε[τὸς τῆ]ς ἐρ[ωτικῆς] | [μανίας. Some of the writing on the papyrus is corrupt but Πυρετὸς is certain, and is the proper medical term for a pathological heat or fever. The man was always in search of her sweet face (ζητῶν τὸ γλυκύτατόν σου πρόσωπον) and right breast: the choice of the right breast (βυζεὶν = βυζ(ί)ον) seems to be commonplace, ever since archaic Greek times. In any case, the problem is erotic: this, too, is sure. However, the adjective ἐρ[ωτικῆς] might also be followed by the word λύπη ('pain') as is the case in Thucydides 6.59. Next, Aphrodite and her torches arrive, and probably Eros and his arrows, which makes the reader wonder about the fate of the poor man's heart: was it burnt (καίει or μαραίνει)? Did it melt (τήκει)? Was it destroyed (διαφθείρει)? Whatever happened, his case is special, for his bad state (ἥκισεν) is due to love (ἐ]κ τῆς σοῦ φιλί[ας); and not to another sort of incapacitation (οὐχὶ δὲ ἐκ τῆς ἀδυνα[μίας μου).[7]

This leaves us with the intriguing question of whether or not ancient doctors considered love sickness a curable (mental) disease. Galen believed it was (*De praenotione ad Posthumum* 6 (14.631–3 Kühn)) and Caelius mentions the phenomenon too (*Chron* 1.177, cf. supra). All this sounds quite modern: the DSM V lists symptoms associated with love sickness as a mental disease (Laes 2014: 87–8; cf. Pigeaud 1981b).

Social therapies: places and methods

This is not the place to scrutinize medical therapies, drugs and foods as causes or cures of madness, for they depend on the same methods and principles as in any other disease according to the methodic doctrine (Gourevitch 1991a). But, still in accordance with the same scientific philosophy, there are some specificities in the treatment of mental patients, which are mainly based on social contexts: the place, organization and decoration of the sick room (*locus aptandus est, Chron.* 1.58), the choice of the visitors and of the themes of conversation, and music therapy.

The place of the sick room in the house is especially important when the patient is nervous and agitated, as for instance in case of phrenitis (*Chron.* 1.9 passim); it should be out of the way (*in loco omni ex parte devio, Chron.* 1.58), that is to say away from any human voice (*ne aliqua transeuntium voce pulsentur, Chron.* 1.58) or any passage or entrance (*hominum ingressu, Chron.* 1.60).

Windows, light and darkness are a matter of serious thought, for light has a relaxing property, and darkness an astringent property. In the first place, windows should be high (fenestris altioribus) to prevent patients from jumping out if unguarded (*Chron.* 1.58), and larger or smaller according to the specific case. Some light is needed, but not too much, according to each patient's needs. In some extreme cases, we see instructions to 'cover the patient's eyes', or 'admit a small amount of soft light' (*Chron.* 1.61), whether daylight (*aetheriae*) or lamplight (*lucernae*), skilfully arranged towards the patient's face. The same skill of arrangement is needed if shade or darkness is necessary (*Chron.* 1.62). In all cases, the good doctor will never excite his patients, and may even yield to their desires for a certain time 'for the sake of soothing their madness' (*Chron.* 1.63, *aliquando mitigandi furoris causa aegrorum voluntati serviendum*).

Temperature and air: the room should be neither too hot, nor too cold, according to the type of the disease and to common sense: cold constricts, heat inflames, and a small room with a low ceiling might be suffocating (*suffocabilis, Chron.* 1.58).

Decoration is to be carefully thought out, for paintings might cause some sorts of apparitions, or phantasmata, which might excite the patients (*Chron.* 1.59); patients might not be able to differentiate the paintings from real things. There should be no bright colours, either, for 'colours will jump out … and strike the vision' (*percutient visum*). This is a very interesting theory on the mechanics of vision between the object to the eye, which can be seen also in Soranus' instructions on choosing how to have a beautiful baby (Gourevitch 1987 and 2004).

Furniture: Spreads and covers that are too colourful should be avoided, for the same reasons (*Chron.* 1.59) and the bed should be 'firmly fixed in place on all sides' (*firme locatus*) which 'will remain stationary (*immobilis*) when the patient tosses about restlessly or of necessity has to be confined by bonds (*necessitate cogente devincti*)' (*Chron.* 1.60 – note the Latin verb *devincire* which is more brutal, or more realistic, than simple *vincire* which is more frequent, its usage already established by the time of Celsus). Also, soft beddings and covers are needed (*stramenta mollia atque operimenta*), in order not to aggravate the patient's condition (*asper, asperare*).

The doctor and the medical team (*servientes,* or *ministri*): Also in the chapter about phrenitis, the duties and capacities of the medical attendants are nicely described (*Ac.* 1.64). We never hear of female *ancillae* in the process, but this absence is certainly not enough to formulate a theory of gendered medicine. We have been told already that the attendants had to be morally and physically strong enough to bind the patients, to guard them and to watch over them to prevent them from harming themselves or others: for instance, they might jump out of the window the very minute they are left alone without attendants (*latuerunt, Chron.* 1.58). We now admire their patience, their sympathy and their skill:

> The attendants will have to endure the crazy whims of the patient and deal skilfully and ingeniously with them, agreeing to some and rejecting others, sympathetically, however, to avoid exciting him by frequent opposition.
>
> *(Ac. 1.64)*

The most terrible part of the task of the attendants (*Chron.* 1.65) is binding the patient, in the absence of almost any efficient medicine: an excessive *furor* can make the patient 'jump off the bed'. In this case, a larger team is needed (*plurimis ministris*) to stop him, but always acting with great self-control, and remaining gentle (*lenitate*). Such a restraint may be for a long time, and therefore it will be necessary to add bindings or, better, to replace bindings with servants, especially if the patients hates the sight of the restraints: *ligationibus utimur*, one must always try to avoid hurting the patient, and to prevent a swelling, by using wool (*lana*) or clothing (*veste*) between the ropes (*vinculis*) and the body.

Another difficulty for these men is alleviating the dryness of the patient's tongue (*Chron.* 1.66): a soft sponge first dipped in warm water will be squeezed, with caution (*non sine cautione*), 'for patients, under the compulsion of mental derangement (*alienatione coacti aegri*) have often bitten the fingers holding the sponge'. Soothing the thirst and moistening the skin and head is part of the normal methodic practice, as we know, but for mental patients, the substances mixed in the water must be absolutely without odour, lest it might 'aggravate the mental derangement (*alienatio*)'.

Visitors as medicines: Passers-by, servants and members of the family may be a nuisance, and we already know that the doctor should be on the lookout for them, because he should be very cautious about visitors. Although some are welcome, others may be deeply unwelcome, and in such a case the team should not 'permit people who were disliked by the patient before he became ill to enter the sickroom'. But some visitors may be considered medicinal and it is again the responsibility of the team (verbs in the first person of the plural *prohibemus, permittimus*) to allow those 'who are regarded by the patient with awe and veneration to enter', but not too often (*per intervalla*), for familiarity and repetition might spoil the psychological effect (*Chron.* 1.65).

Music is sometimes recommended for *mania* (*de furore sive insania quam Graeci manian vocant, Chron.* 1.175–6), with a very sophisticated distinction: melodies on pipes (*decantionibus tibiarum*) should be in the pleasant Phrygian mode (*modulatio*) for depressed patients (*qui ex maestitudine in furore noscuntur*), and in the grave Dorian mode when the mind is impaired by laughter and childish hilarity (*cachinnus*, from Gr. καχάζειν, a pleasant expressive verb, with its imitative reduplication of the first syllable). Such musical nuances are just ridiculous, according to Caelius, as some other stupid procedures (*experimentis inanibus Chron.* 1.178), such as induced love or venesection or hunger or flogging, and so on.

Hope for rehabilitation

Whatever the malady, there is hope for rehabilitation, owing to correct medicines and social interventions, both in acute and in chronic diseases. First, in the case of phrenitis, according to the methodic system, care should take place at the right time. The doctor will take

> measures that the patient may be restored from a condition of mental derangement (*ab alienatione mentis*) to a state of complete sanity. For in most cases patients remain in a state of sadness, anger, or aberration right up to the return of physical health. It is necessary therefore to use grave and serious language to those whose state has been of hilarity (...) But those who are in a state of sadness or anger must be soothed with gentle encouragement and pleasant and cheerful language (…) It is not surprising that those who are not yet cured of a disease should suffer a relapse when their mental state has, so to speak, dealt a wound to their sickbed (*cum animae qualitas sua ... cubilia quadam vulneratione afficerit*).
>
> *(Ac. 1.98–9)*

Anyway the doctor is also to be careful to take into consideration the idiosyncrasies of any of his patients, as far as the light in the room is concerned, for instance: 'since some patients avoid and dislike light, and others darkness, we should have to put the former in a dark place and the latter in a bright place' (*Ac* 1.121).

Hydrophobia can be a very interesting case of 'traitement moral de la folie', as the French psychiatrist François Leuret (1797–1851) put it. Caelius knew that

> those who are greedy for the purple (*purpuram cupientes*) or for statues, military glory, royal power, or wealth are said to be affected not by a disease of the veins, sinews or arteries, but by a disease of the soul (*animae passione*).
>
> *(Ac. 3.109)*

In the same way, in hydrophobia it was not so important to compel the patient to drink, but to make him long to drink. Specifically, the cure for hydrophobia 'consists not in getting the patient to drink, but in getting him to drink voluntarily (*ut bibere velint*)' (*Ac.* 3.133).[8]

In chronic diseases as well it is important to be humble enough to deal kindly with the wishes of the patient, for instance in mania 'patients often are found to dislike darkness'. In such a case the doctor or the assistant should not insist on keeping him in a dark room (*Chron.* 1.171).

In some rare but fascinating instances, Caelius informs us about the social status of his patients, who invariably seem to have belonged to the literate and cultivated upper class.

Indeed, regarding the encouragement of patients towards rehabilitation, there is a strong social prejudice *de facto*, or at least a distortion, against the poor, who have no literate conversation skills and can rarely, if ever, participate in refined exchanges. In a therapy based on dialogue, what can be done in the case of a patient who *litteras nescit* (that is, unacquainted with literature, or even illiterate?). The doctor has a solution, though it may seem impractical to us:

> Give him problems appropriate with his particular craft (*ejus artis*), e.g. agricultural problems if he is a farmer [*rusticus,* writes Caelius – which might simply indicate a man of the country, without any special gift or skill], problems in navigation if he is a pilot (*gubernator*).
>
> *(Chron. 1.165)*

And even if the patient suffering from mania is without any skill at all, causing his rehabilitation to be both more difficult and less desirable socially, the doctor should not give up, but

> ask him questions on commonplace matters, or let him play checkers (*calculorum ludus,* probably any game on a check board). Such a game can exercise his mind, particularly if he plays with a more experienced (*peritior*) opponent
>
> *(Chron. 1.165)*

During the same period of rehabilitation, just before the former patient might cope again with reality and duty, a trainer might be useful (*alipta*), and a bit of travel, for the sake of a treatment of everyday life, thanks to 'natural water (*naturalibus aquis*), (…) particularly those free from any pungent odour', or for mere pleasure: 'a trip abroad by land or sea and various mental diversions (*animi avocamentis*) are helpful in affording relaxation of the mind (*mentis laxatio*)' (*Chron.* 1.170).

Conclusion

At times, readers of Caelius Aurelianus are surprised by what is not treated. Thus, the modern audience might be surprised not to find anything similar to Emperor Claudius' situation, i.e. general deficiencies, coupled with ugliness, probably related to obstetrical problems. In the famous case of the emperor, Claudius was considered, in his childhood, to be a shame for his family (Gourevitch 2006). Nor do we see instances in Caelius' works of an incapacitating lack of judgement. We do not see mental problems in old age, such as the loss of memory. Absent are mentally deficient children or adult patients, or people with other partial deficiencies such as a mute boy who was dear to his grandmother all the same (Gourevitch 1991c). Or pretending and faking illness which may become a social plague, in civic life as well as in ordinary daily life (Gourevitch 1975, 2009) – later on, the monastic rules mention the same problem (cf. Kuuliala in this volume). Or Down's Syndrome. We know all these conditions were present, and that the ancients were aware of them, when we read other medical texts, or by looking at certain works of art (Grmek and Gourevitch 1998).

On the other hand, the emphasis on humane care and empathy for the mad patient is very touching all through Caelius' book. Incantations and amulets have nothing to do with real cures (*incantationibus, ligamentis*), and benevolence is always necessary, especially to cope with agitated patients. The doctor tries not to hurt, refuses to flog (*flagellare, Chron.* 1.175 and 178), for it is nonsense to whip reason into someone (*ut quasi iudicio mentis pulso resipiant, Chron.* 1.175). In the 1st century CE, Celsus thought differently about this matter (Celsus, *De med.* 3.18.21–2) and the history of psychiatry up to the 20th century reveals many examples of similar drastic treatment such as shock therapy. Of course the probability of rehabilitation is minor if the disease is chronic, but to Caelius the real doctor has to try, using medication, sequestration as a necessity and not as a punishment, and almost any kind of human communication.

Medication being inefficient for the most part, one doctor is not enough; on the contrary, a whole team is required, which makes the treatment of people of less affluence very problematic. One can only speculate about the problem of a poor insane murderer, having no place to go except prison, since there were no hospitals. Judges and lawyers, being interested mostly in patrimony, business matters and (political) responsibility, did not usually ask for medical advice, instead making up their minds themselves (Israelowich 2014 and see Toohey in this volume).

Surely, animalization and dehumanization of the mad patient were methods Caelius utterly disapproved of. Thus he protests that it is not the task of the doctor 'to calm his mad patients by continual fasting' (*furentes jugi abstinentia mitigari, Chron.* 1.171–2). He admonishes his reader not to do as these bad physicians who 'prescribe a starvation diet (*immodicam abstinentiam* = from food), *quam Graeci limanchiam vocant*, not realizing that excessive abstention from food impairs the bodily power'. Such writers and doctors

> seem to be madmen themselves, rather than the physicians of madmen (*insanire potius quam curare*). Thus they say that we must consider as analogous the case of wild beasts (*ferarum similitudinem*), who when food is denied are supposed to lose their ferocity and grow tame (*mansuescunt*).
>
> *(Chron. 1.171–2)*

Has this particular focus on a humane approach towards suffering patients something to do with Christianity? Or is it a Caelian touch on an approach which was already codified in the original Greek version by Soranus (Mazzini 1999a, b)? Hard to tell, but certainly true doctors, according to St Augustine (354–430),[9] far from behaving like *phrenetici*, refrain from getting angry with their dangerous patients even if the latter try to hurt them. They practise medicine at their own risk, ready to die as Christ did on the holy cross. Caelius indeed may have read some pages by Augustine. Nevertheless, this constant effort may be just the consequence of sharing the 'milk of human kindness', in a world where *medicus* had long before become *medicus amicus* (Mudry 2006) – a view which was already largely sustained by Celsus in the 1st century CE.

Notes

1 Excluding 'special pathologies' such as epilepsy, sexual diseases and hysterical suffocation (Gourevitch 1996, 1998), passive homosexuality in men and in women (*Chron.* 4.9: *de mollibus sive subactis*, who suffer from a *mentis passio*, as well as the women called *tribades*, Schrijvers 1985; Gourevitch 1995; Boehringer 2007), erotic dreams (*somnus venereus* or *oneirogmos, Chron.* 5.80) and perversions (Gourevitch 1982, 1983; Pigeaud 1981a), other bad dreams (*incubo, -onis Chron.* 1.54) and excessive drinking, especially of wine: *cum saepe ex vinolentia furor atque insania generentur* (*Chron.* 1.175, on which see Gourevitch 2013b).
2 Useful accounts are Pélicier 1989; Rénier 1950; Gourevitch 1991b; Stok 1995, 1999; Urso 1999; Laes 2014: 78–83. For more details concerning the differences between *vitium* and *morbus*, see Gourevitch 2013a.
3 Also *furor* or *insania, melancholia, pleuritis, peripneumonia*, and in cases of poisoning with *mandragora* and *altercum* or henbane (possibly a plant which causes one to be 'another person', or which incites chronic quarrelling (*altercari*).
4 For the discussions about the duration of the incubation, see Galen, *Comm. 3 in Hippocratis Praed. Lib* 1.50 (16.621 Kühn).
5 Cf. supra footnote 4 for the duration of the incubation.

6 It is a *codex miscellaneus*, i.e. containing texts of various types, among which seven judicial reports, of a high literary level; ours is the fourth. It belonged to a certain Aurelius Philammon, otherwise unknown.

7 It is my pleasurre to thank our young colleague from Liege, Antonio Ricciardetto, for his great knowledge and kind help. For papyri from Egypt, see also Rosalie David in this volume.

8 This raises the question whether Caelius considered hydrophobia a 'moral disease', a 'disease of the soul'. In *Ac.* 1.109–11, which is titled 'Utrumne animae an corporis passio sit hydrophobia', he concludes that 'hydrophobia derives from a bodily force and is therefore a bodily disease (*corporis passio*) though it also attacks the psychic nature (*animae qualitatem*), as do mania and melancholia'.

9 'Sermons de Mayence 61', *Revue des études augustiniennes* 37 (1991), 70, par. 18. See Gourevitch 1997, 1998; and Claes and Dupont in this volume.

Editions and translations

Caelius Aurelianus, *On Acute Diseases and on Chronic Diseases*, ed. and tr. Israel E. Drabkin (Chicago, IL, 1950).

Caelius Aurelianus, *Celerum Passionum libri III, Tardarum Passionum libri V*, ed. G. Bendz, tr. into German by I. Pappe, CML 6/1 (Berolini, 1990).

Throughout this chapter, I have used Drabkin's translation, though I have sometimes slightly modified it.

Bibliography

Boehringer, Sandra, *L'homosexualité féminine dans l'Antiquité grecque et romaine* (Paris, 2007).

Bosman, Philip (ed.), *Mania in the Greco-Roman World* (Pretoria, 2009)

Casewitz, Michel, '*Mantis*: Le vrai sens', *Revue des Études Grecques* 105 (1991), 1–18.

Centanni, Monica, 'Nomi del male: Phrenitis e epilepsia nel corpus Galenicum', *Museum Patavinum* 5 (1987), 47–79.

Chandler, Cleve E., 'Madness in Homer and the Verb μαίνομαι', in P. Bosman (ed.), *Mania in the Greco-Roman World* (Pretoria, 2009), 8–18.

Cilliers, Louise, and Retief, François P., 'Mental Illness in the Greco-Roman Era', in P. Bosman (ed.), *Mania in the Greco-Roman World* (Pretoria, 2009), 130–40.

Gaide, Françoise, 'La rage dans les textes médicaux latins antiques: noms, description, étiologie, traitements', in C. Deroux (ed.), *Maladie et maladies dans les textes latins antiques et médiévaux* (Brussels, 1998), 29–41.

Godderis, Jan, *Kan men een hemel klaren, even zwart als drek? Historische, psychiatrische en fenomenologisch-antropologische beschouwingen over depressie en melancholie* (Leuven, 2000).

Gourevitch, Danielle, 'À propos de la simulation dans l'Antiquité: Galien et sa monographie princeps, *Quomodo morbum simulantes sint deprehendendi libellus*', *Médecine légale et expertise médicale* 1 (1975), 13–18.

Gourevitch, Danielle, 'Quelques fantasmes érotiques et perversions d'objets dans la littérature gréco-romaine', *Mélanges École Française de Rome. Antiquité* 94/2 (1982), 823–42.

Gourevitch, Danielle, 'À propos d'une image de bestialité', *Littérature, médecine, société* 5 (1983), 115–29.

Gourevitch, Danielle, 'La psychiatrie de l'Antiquité gréco-romaine', in J. Postel and C. Quetel (eds), *Nouvelle histoire de la psychiatrie* (Toulouse, 1983), 13–30.

Gourevitch, Danielle, 'Se mettre à trois pour faire un bel enfant, ou l'imprégnation par le regard', *L'Evolution psychiatrique* 3 (1987), 559–63.

Gourevitch, Danielle, 'La pratique méthodique: Définition de la maladie, indication et traitement', in P. Mudry and J. Pigeaud (eds), *Les écoles médicales à Rome* (Geneva, 1991a), 51–81.

Gourevitch, Danielle, 'Les mots pour dire la folie en Latin: À propos de passages de Celse et de Célius Aurélien', *L'Évolution psychiatrique* 56 (1991b), 561–8.

Gourevitch, Danielle, 'Un enfant muet de naissance s'exprime par le dessin : À propos d'un cas rapporté par Pline l'Ancien', *L'Évolution psychiatrique* 56 (1991c), 889–93.

Gourevitch, Danielle, 'Affectif et cognitif: Étude de quelques cas galéniques', in H. Grivois (ed), *Affectif et cognitif dans la psychose* (Paris, 1993), 27–37.

Gourevitch, Danielle, 'Women Who Suffer from a Man's Disease: The Example of Satyriasis and the Debate on Affections Specific to the Sexes', in R. Hawley and B. Levick (eds), *Women in Antiquity: New Assessments* (London and New York, 1995), 149–65.

Gourevitch, Danielle, 'La lune et les règles des femmes', in B. Backhouche, A. Moreau and J.-C. Turpin (eds), *Les astres: Actes du colloque international de Montpellier* (Montpellier, 1996), II. 85–99.

Gourevitch, Danielle, 'Le malade dangereux à Rome', in T. Albernhe (ed.), *Criminologie et psychiatrie* (Paris, 1997), 478–83.

Gourevitch, Danielle, 'La première mort de l'hystérie', in C. Deroux (ed.), *Maladie et maladies dans les textes latins antiques et médiévaux* (Brussels, 1998), 62–9.

Gourevitch, Danielle, 'Cherchez la femme', in P. Mudry (ed.), *Le traité des Maladies aiguës et des maladies chroniques de Caelius Aurelianus: Nouvelles approches* (Nantes, 1999), 177–206.

Gourevitch, Danielle, 'Soranos, adieu Soranos', *Cahiers de la villa Kérylos* 15 (2004), 135–61.

Gourevitch, Danielle, 'Sommes-nous tous des ânes, ou la pathographie est-elle une discipline ridicule? Quelques exemples en histoire ancienne', in P. Charlier (ed.), *Actes du Ier colloque International de Pathographie* (Paris, 2006), 285–99.

Gourevitch, Danielle, 'Il simulatore vorrebbe ingannare il medico, secondo Galeno e altre fonti', *I Quaderni del Ramo d'Oro on-line* 2 (2009), 92–100.

Gourevitch, Danielle, 'La stérilité féminine dans le monde romain: vitium ou morbus, état ou maladie?', *Histoire des Sciences Médicales* 47, 2 (2013a), 219–31.

Gourevitch, Danielle, 'Two Historical Cases of Acute Alcoholism in the Roman Empire', in C. Laes, C. F. Goodey and M. L. Rose (eds), *Disparate Bodies in Roman Antiquity* A Capite ad Calcem (Leiden, 2013b), 73–87.

Gourevitch, Danielle, and Gourevitch, Michel, 'Chronique anachronique, III. Simulation', *L'Évolution psychiatrique* 46 (1981), 203–9.

Gourevitch, Danielle, and Gourevitch, Michel, 'Le phrénétique chez Augustin', in G. Madec (ed.), *Augustin prédicateur (395–411)* (Paris, 1998), 505–17.

Grmek, Mirko, and Gourevitch, Danielle, *Les maladies dans l'art antique* (Paris, 1998).

Harris, William V., *Restraining Rage: The Ideology of Anger Control in Classical Antiquity* (Cambridge, MA, 2001).

Hilton, John L., '*Furor, dementia, rabie:* Social Displacement, Madness and Religion in the *Metamophoses* of Apuleius', in P. Bosman (ed.), *Mania in the Greco-Roman World* (Pretoria, 2009), 84–105.

Horstmanshoff, Manfred, 'Les émotions chez Caelius Aurelianus', in P. Mudry (ed.), *Le traité des maladies aiguës et des maladies chroniques: Nouvelles approches* (Nantes, 1999), 259–90.

Israelowich, Ido, 'Physicians as Figures of Authority in the Roman Courts and the Attitude towards Mental Diseases in the Roman Courts during the High Empire', *Historia* 63/4 (2014), 445–62.

Kazantzidis, George, '"Quem nos furorem, μελαγχολίαν illi vocant": Cicero on Melancholy', in W. V. Harris (ed.), *Mental Disorders in the Classical World* (Leiden and Boston, MA, 2013), 245–64.

Laes, Christian, *Beperkt? Gehandicapten in het Romeinse Rijk* (Leuven, 2014).

Maresch, Klaus, and Packman, Zola M., *Papyri from the Washington University Collection, St. Louis, Missouri*, Part II (Opladen, 1990) (= Pap. Colon. XVIII = *P.Wash.Univ.* II 108).

Mattern, Susan P., *Galen and the Rhetoric of Healing* (Baltimore, MD, 2008).

Mazzini, Innocenzo, 'Elementi Celiani in Celio Aureliano', in P. Mudry (ed.), *Le Traité des maladies aiguës et des maladies chroniques de Caelius Aurelianus: Nouvelles approches* (Nantes, 1999a), 27–46.

Mazzini, Innocenzo, 'Sorano e Celio Aureliano di fronte alla terapia ippocratica', in I. Garofalo, A. Lami, D. Manetti and A. Roselli (eds), *Aspetti della terapia nel Corpus Hippocraticum* (Florence, 1999b), 419–30.

Mudry, Philippe, '*Medicus amicus*, un trait romain dans la médecine antique', in B. Maire (ed.), *Medicina, soror philosophiae* (Lausanne, 2006), 479–82.

Nardi, Enzo, 'Furor et insania', *Studi Romani* 13 (1990), 237–43.

Néraudau, Jean-Pierre, *Le mystère du jardin romain* (Paris, 1991).

Pélicier, Yves, 'Les sources classiques du vocabulaire de la folie', in *Du banal au merveilleux: Mélanges offerts à Lucien Jerphagnon* (Fontenay, 1989), 253–73.

Pigeaud, Jackie, 'Le rêve érotique dans l'Antiquité gréco-romaine: L'oneirogmos', *Littérature, Médecine, Société*, 3 (1981a), 10–23.

Pigeaud, Jackie, *La Maladie de l'âme: Étude sur la relation de l'âme et du corps dans la tradition médico-philosophique antique* (Paris, 1981b).

Pigeaud, Jackie, *Folie et cures de la folie chez les médecins de l'Antiquité gréco-romaine: La manie* (Paris, 2010²).

Poethke, Gunther, Prignitz, Sebastian, and Vaelske, Veit, *Das Aktenbuch des Aurelios Philammon: Prozessberichte, Annona militaris und Magie in BGU IV 1024–1027* (Berlin and Boston, MA, 2012).

Rénier, Eric, 'Observation sur la terminologie de l'aliénation mentale', *Revue internationale des droits de l'Antiquité* 5 (1950), 429–55.

Schrijvers, Piet H., *Eine medizinische Erklärung der männlichen Homosexualität aus der Antike* (Amsterdam, 1985).

Stok, Fabio, 'Il lessico della follia tra lingua tecnica e metafora', in P. Colice Radici (ed.), *Atti del II seminario di studi sui lessici tecnici greci e latini* (Messina, 1995), 499–508.

Stok, Fabio, 'Follia e malattie mentali nella medicina dell'età romana', in *ANRW* II/37/2 (Berlin, 1996), 2282–2409.

Stok, Fabio, 'Struttura e modelli dei trattati de Celio Aureliano', in P. Mudry (ed.), *Le traité des maladies aiguës et des maladies chroniques: Nouvelles approches* (Nantes, 1999), 1–26.

Stok, Fabio, 'Note sul lessico della patologia in Celio Aureliano', in S. Sconocchia and L. Toneatto (eds), *Lingue tecniche del greco e del latino*, III (Bologna, 2000), 147–67.

Van Hoof, Lieve, *Plutarch's Practical Ethics: The Social Dynamics of Philosophy* (Oxford, 2010).

Urso, Anna-Maria, 'La formalizazzione di un vocabolario nosologico latino nelle *Passiones celeres* e *tardae* di Celio Aureliano', in P. Radici Colace (ed.) *Atti del secondo seminario internazionale sui lessici tecnici Greci e Latini* (Naples, 1995), 449–508.

Urso, Anna-Maria, 'Il vocabolario nosologico di Celio Celio Aureliano fra tradizione e innovazione', in P. Mudry (ed.), *Le traité des maladies aiguës et des maladies chroniques: Nouvelles approches* (Nantes, 1999), 213–58.

Urso, Anna-Maria, 'Definizioni diagnostiche e prescrizioni terapeutiche nella trattatistica medica latina: Celio Aureliano e il problema della *perspicuitas*', in S. Sconocchia and L. Toneatto (eds), *Lingue tecniche del greco e del latino*, III (Bologna, 2000a), 179–91.

Urso, Anna-Maria, 'Autorità e autonomia nelle *Passiones celeres et tardae* di Celio Aureliano', in P. Radici Colace and A. Zumbo (eds), *Atti del seminario internazionale di studi e letteratura scientifica Greca e Latina* (Messina, 2000b), 397–421.

Urso, Anna-Maria, 'La letteratura medica latina dell'Africa tardoantica: Consuntivo degli studi', *Lettre d'informations: Médecine antique et médiévale* NS 4 (2005), 1–40.

21

DISABILITY IN THE ROMAN *DIGEST*

Peter Toohey

Not a great deal has been published concerning physical or mental disability in the Roman *Digest*. What has been tends to focus on mental disability. It is possible that the *Digest* contains more on the subject of disability, in the broadest of senses, than most ancient works, even the literary and the medical. I have, therefore, attempted to provide a sampling of some of what seem to me to be the more intriguing passages within the *Digest* on this subject. What emerges is a vivid picture of how the Roman legal system may have understood and adjudicated some of the societal problems relating to disability.

The term 'disability' needs to be used with circumspection. Its use might imply that the *Digest*, or the Romans themselves, had a unitary vision of disability. They did not, although their understanding of some of the elements of what today would be considered as 'disability' is strikingly consistent. Whence does this consistency emerge? Despite the fact that the *Digest* offers a compilation of the work of many jurists and a compilation that was drawn from a broad chronological base, it is consistent enough in its treatment, for example, of madness or of being deaf or dumb. I presume that this consistency results because, when the *Digest* contemplates and meditates upon the various conditions relating to disability, it is reflecting on real-life situations that are of a common and limited type and that persist through time. These were conditions, furthermore, with which the jurists and the readers of the *Digest* would have been familiar from their daily lives.

While the *Digest* does display elements of what might be termed a unitary understanding of disability, it achieves this by producing what might be judged to be an *instrumental* definition of disability. Disability, that is to say, is a visible or clearly perceptible physical or mental condition that renders a person at a disadvantage or problematical before the law.[1] In our society we favour what might be termed, for want of a better designation, an *existential* understanding of disability. It is a physical or a mental condition that renders societal inclusion and function difficult for an individual to sustain. One of the great problems for the existential understanding of disability is this: when does a disability constitute for an individual a minority status? When does a disability render a person at a disadvantage and when does a disability render a person simply different? Is blindness, for example, a disability or does it rather confer minority status on a blind person? There is no such a problem for the jurists of the *Digest*. The question with which they are concerned seems only to be this: does a visible or clearly perceptible disability place a person at disadvantage or render them problematical before the law?

Some terms and descriptions in the *Digest* referring to disability

How do you say 'disability' in the Latin of the *Digest*? There are many terms associated with its physical or mental manifestations that are to be found in the legal text, but there is no single word that would match our term. To illustrate I will accumulate here the most prominent terms and descriptions for disability and disabilities – those at least with which I am familiar. These words are used in discussions within the *Digest* of individuals whose legal status is, at times, sufficiently uncertain as to require judicial attention. The *Digest* is a practical document and for this reason there are very few passages that could be said to express emotional reactions to the situation in which these individuals find themselves. I will follow this precedent and in this chapter I will simply attempt to report the manner by which physical or mental disability appears to be discussed by the jurists within the *Digest*.

The term *debilis* (or verbal forms such as *debilitatus*, or nominal forms such as *debilitas*) is used periodically. It is close in meaning to 'disabled' but can in addition mean 'incapacitated', something which can be temporary or permanent. In one passage the term *debilis* means almost what a modern speaker of English might hope of it. *Digest* 1.16.9.5 notes that the proconsul (here the officiating magistrate) will allow use of counsel by 'women, *pupilli* [minors under the care of a guardian], those under a disability [*alias debilibus*], or those who are out of their mind [*qui suae mentis non sunt*]'. The *Digest* means here that these individuals may let someone else to speak for them. From the manner in which the *debiles* are distinguished from women, wards and the mad and from the fact that speech seems to be at issue with this group, it looks very much like *debilis* refers just to the deaf and the dumb. The descriptive noun *casus* (misfortune – the misfortune that renders a person deaf or blind, for example) can be used in a similar manner. One passage concerns those who may make application to a magistrate on matters of law (the deaf are disallowed from such applications) notes:

> On grounds of disability (*propter casus*), [Nerva the Younger] forbids a deaf person (*surdus*) without any hearing at all to make application before him. For no one was allowed to make application who was unable to hear the praetor's decree. This would have been dangerous even for the applicant himself; for if he had not heard the praetor's decree, he would have been punished as contumacious for not obeying it ...
>
> *(Digest 3.1.1.3)*

In *Digest* 3.1.1.5 *casus* stands in for blindness (*casum: dum caecum utrisque luminibus orbatum praetor repellit*).

The less specific terms *infirmitas* (weakness or disability), *infirmus* (invalid) or *valetudinarius* (invalid) are also to be found, as is the descriptor *morbus perpetuus* (unending illness). There are more specific designations. The two terms *surdus* (deaf), and *mutus* (mute or dumb) appear frequently in the *Digest* and often in tandem.[2] *Caecus* (blind) and, less commonly, *eluscatus* (blinded – or in one of its other verbal forms) are also to be found. I believe that *furor* (it literally means 'madness') is the condition or disability to receive the most attention in the *Digest*. A person subject to *furor* may be designated by a very wide variety of terms. The mad individual is most commonly termed *furiosus* (mad/insane), a victim of *furor*. There are many other near synonyms, nouns or adjectives, such as *aegritudo, amentia, demens, dementia, fanaticus, fatuus, furens, furiosus, furor, furere, furoris infortunium, gaudens simplicitate, imbecillus, insanus, languor animi, vitium animi, lunaticus, melancholicus, morio, non compos mentis, non suae mentis, captus mente, valetudo mentis, integritas mentis, resipiscens, sanitas, vecors,* and *vesanus* (cf. Gourevitch in this volume for Latin medical vocabulary).[3] Except in the most obvious of senses (*fatuus, morio,* or *gaudens simplicitate,* for example, which seem to have the meaning of 'simple minded'), these terms for madness appear to be used more or less interchangeably. Whether the hermaphrodite (*hermaphroditus*) or the eunuch (*eunuchus*) were to be thought of in the same ambit as of the physically disabled, such as the deaf, the mute, the blind or the mentally disabled, I cannot say, for references to them are uncommon. There are other more precise descriptions of disabled individuals to be found such as the humpbacked (*gibberosus*), the hunchbacked (*curvus*), those affected with itching (*pruriginosus*) or those afflicted with scabies (*scabiosus*). There are some other puzzling terms that are found to be associated with discussions of the legal standing of the disabled. Such are, for example, *protervus* (reckless, but with hints of mental unbalance) and *prodigus* (wasteful in the financial sense, again with hints of mental unbalance – a spendthrift). The *protervus* or the *prodigus* individual is often discussed in the same passages as are the physically or mentally disabled.

A variety of disabilities, described if not necessarily named, occur that are discussed in *Digest* 21.1.9–16. The passage lists and discusses, in addition to being mute, disabilities such as having lacerations of the limb, being short or dim sighted, being blighted with 'warts or polypuses in the nose', or with 'imbalance, or the fact that one leg is shorter than the other', with limps, being a habitual bed-wetter (this is not the result of drink or laziness), being a man born 'with fingers joined together', or being born with congenitally swollen tonsils. A female slave 'who regularly produces stillborn issue' is diseased, 'just as is a woman who is so tight that she cannot fulfil the function of a woman', or one 'one who menstruates twice within a month … [or one who] never menstruates, unless this latter be by reason of her age'. I will return to some of these conditions in my brief discussion of slavery.

The *Digest,* you might conclude from the foregoing, is very good at the specifics, the visibilities of disability and how disability may represent a financial burden, but it does not bother very much with any overarching notion of disability or with its psychological implications. That is the case and it is perhaps to be expected from such a practical and precise document. There are, however, a few passages that give some sort of an idea of what the jurists of the *Digest* might have said, had they been asked what constitutes disability.

Is there a concept of disability in the *Digest*?

An indication of the way the Roman law code may have thought of those suffering a permanent or serious physical or mental incapacity is provided in a very interesting passage. Here, in a discussion of who could and who could not be appointed a judge (*iudex*), the *Digest* explains:

> not everybody may be appointed a judge by those with the right to appoint judges. For some are prevented by statute (*lex*) from becoming judges, some by nature (*natura*), and some by custom (*mores*). For example, the deaf and the dumb *(surdus mutus)*,[4] the permanently insane (*perpetuus furiosus*), and the *impubes* [a person under the age of puberty, 14 for a boy] through lack of *iudicium* (judgement?) are prevented by nature (*natura*). A person expelled from the senate is prevented by statute (*lex*). Women and slaves are prevented by custom (*mores*), not because they lack *iudicium* but because it is accepted that they do not perform civic duties.
>
> *(Digest 5.1.12.2)*[5]

The deaf, the dumb, the permanently insane, the prepubescent, those who have been expelled from the senate for malefaction, and women and slaves are treated alike as far as the law is concerned (although *Digest* 5.1.6 specifies 'a blind man can act as a judge'). But Paulinus, the jurist being reported in the passage, can make clear distinctions. Women, for example, may suffer some of the legal disadvantages of the disabled, but they should not be confused with them, for their exclusion is the result of custom (*mores*). Nor should those who have fallen foul of the law. Their exclusion, based on malefaction, is the result of a statute (*lex*). What is perplexing, however, is the lumping together of the deaf, dumb, the *impubes*, and the *perpetuus furiosus*. Paulinus suggests that the deaf and the dumb lack *iudicium*, whatever that word means, just as do the insane and the young. It is easy enough to understand why Paulinus considered that the insane and the *impubes* lacked reliable *iudicium* (mental perturbation on the one hand and youth and inexperience on the other). But why did he think of the dumb and the deaf as somehow lacking in *iudicium*?

The following passage, which cites the jurist Ulpian, may make Paulinus' logic more clear. This passage concerns verbal contracts or stipulations (*stipulationes*), which were a very important part of Roman law. The *Digest* devotes the whole of its book 45 to these. This is what Ulpian tells us:

> A stipulation can only be effected when both parties can speak, and therefore neither a mute (*mutus*) nor a deaf person (*surdus*) nor an *infans* [a child under 7, deemed incapable of rational speech] can contract a stipulation; nor, indeed, can someone who is not present (*nec absens quidem*), since they both should be able to hear. If, therefore, such a person wishes to make a stipulation, he does so through a slave who is present and acquires an action on a stipulation.
>
> *(Digest 45.1.1pr)*

This passage may make it more comprehensible why, in the first of our two passages, the deaf and the mute are likened to the *furiosus* and to the *impubes*. Perhaps, when he says that the four all lack *iudicium*, what Paulinus means has not so much to do with mental capacity or judgement, as it does with an inability to make intentions clear through speech. It appears that the sense in which Ulpian and the *Digest* more generally, or at least sometimes, understand *iudicium* may closely linked to the capacity for speech, or even the capacity to render judgement in speech. Thus the deaf, the mute, the *infans*, the *impubes* and the madman can be understood to be deficient in *iudicium*, the capacity to express judgement in speech. This may enable a tentative definition for what the *Digest* might have thought of as 'disability'. It relates not so much to the actual nature of disability as to the inability, by nature (*natura*), of being able to communicate *iudicium*, or judgement, through articulated speech. This tentative definition addresses the concern of the *Digest* that was noted at the beginning of this chapter. The concern of the jurists seems to have been this: does a visible disability or clearly perceptible disability place a person at disadvantage before the law? It does indeed, or even worse, as is suggested by Laes 2011. This is because the judgements of the *Digest* were formulated by a 'small minority of the urban well-to-do in a literary culture, in which speech, language, and reason were closely intertwined'. Being unable to speak may have even 'implied being deprived of reason [so *iudicium* in this context]'. The lack of *iudicium*, the inability, that is, to communicate judgement through speech, is a clearly perceptible disability, whether the person was or was not deprived of reason (*si quod agatur intellegant* – Digest 37.3.2). A person labouring under such a disadvantage requires special assistance when coming before the law. It is worth noting as well that this also partially answers the query that I raised concerning the disability status of hermaphrodites and eunuchs. Provided they were not slaves, their ability to use speech and to communicate is in no way impeded by their status. As far as the *Digest* is concerned they are people before the law like any other – see *Digest* 1.5.10 (hermaphrodites) and 1.7.40 (eunuchs).

It would be misleading, however, to press this definition too far. The unexpected notion of being absent or away is a surprisingly important one and may also contribute to the way that the *Digest* understood what we term disability. In a discussion of how complicit in a master's murder a slave is by inactivity, Ulpian notes a deaf slave is also to be countered among the [mentally defective] (*inter imbecillos*) or among those who are not under the same roof, because, as those who hear nothing because of distance (*spatium*), he hears nothing because of a deficiency (*per morbum*).

(Digest 29.5.3.8)

The blind, incidentally, are let off as well, as are the dumb, because they cannot rouse the alarm by shouting, and also the 'lunatics' (*furiosi*). Elsewhere the *Digest* likens the situation in which the deaf, the dumb, the *furiosus* and the *impubes* find themselves to that of someone who is absent (*absens*) and therefore cannot speak for themselves. The disability of the *absentes*, as we would understand it, can only be a metaphorical one, for they are not lacking in *iudicium* by nature (*natura*) but by constraint or distance (*spatio*). But it is worth stressing that the linking of disability with being absent is a powerful one in the *Digest*. It occurs on a number of occasions. Julian likens a madman to someone who is absent (*absens*) – or even asleep (*quiescens*):

A lunatic (*furiosus*) is not understood to make a codicil, because he is not understood to perform any other legal act, as in all circumstances and in every respect he is treated like someone absent or asleep. (*Furiosus non intellegitur codicillos facere, quia nec aliud quicquam agere intellegitur, cum per omnia et in omnibus absentis vel quiescentis loco habetur.*)

(Digest 29.7.2.3)

The *absentia* of the *furiosus* is to be comprehended as being like that of, for example, a soldier on duty overseas and whose affairs need to be managed by another person. Paulus provides what may be the most straightforward statement on this use of *absens* (*Digest* 50.17.124): 'Someone who is mad (*furiosus*) is in the same position as someone who is absent, as Pomponius writes in the first book of his *Letters.*' There are as well a certain number of other passages which pair the madman, in a legal setting, with an individual who is *absens* because he has been taken captive by the enemy (*Digest* 23.4.8 and compare *Digest* 41.2.1.3): 'when a son marries where his father is insane (*furens*) or has been captured by the enemy (*ab hostibus capto*) or where a daughter does so, there is no alternative to entering into a pact on the dowry with these people themselves'.

The inability of the disabled to represent themselves through speech and their being 'absent' are, as you might suspect, far from being the whole story. All disabilities were not equal and all disabilities do not seem to have been equal before the law. It would be confusing, therefore, to press these two helpful definitions too far. We learn elsewhere in the *Digest* that, on the matter of offering freedom to slaves, the deaf and the dumb had different rights to the insane – or at least their relatives did. At *Digest* 40.2.10 and 40.9.1 we hear that 'the son of a deaf or dumb father can manumit by his command, but the son of a lunatic cannot manumit'. The reason for this adjudication is, presumably, because the insane have lost the capacity for reason (*consilium*). This is made clear at *Digest* 48.8.12 (compare 6.1.60) where it is explained that 'an infant (*infans*) or a madman (*furiosus*) who kills a man is not liable under the *Lex Cornelia*, the one being protected by innocence of intent (*innocentia consilii*), the other excused by the misfortune of his condition (*fati infelicitas*)'. The madman is let off the hook in this case because he has no sense (no capacity for *consilium*) of what he is doing.

This sliding scale of responsibility, as it is attributed to those with disabilities, can also be seen in the case of the blind (*caeci*). They certainly do have the power of speech. But they are both present and 'absent'. An understanding of disability that focuses primarily on speech is not necessarily applicable to the blind for, if they have their wits (*si quod agatur intellegant* – *Digest* 37.3.2), then they can speak for themselves. The jurists take this into account, but significant gestures in legal communication can be lost on the blind, as the following long but very helpful passage makes clear:

> Next comes an edict against those who are not to make application [to the magistrate] on behalf of others. In this edict the praetor debarred on grounds of sex and disability (*casus*). He also blacklisted exceptionally disreputable persons (...). On ground of disability (*casus*), the praetor rejects the man blind in both eyes, obviously because he cannot see and respect the magistrate's *insignia*. Labeo also has the story of Publilius, the blind father of Nonius Asprenas, when he wished to make application, being left in the lurch by Brutus turning away his chair. But although a blind man cannot make application on behalf of someone else, yet he keeps his senatorial rank and can also act as a judge. Could he then hold magistracies? This needs discussion. There is certainly an example of a man who did so. Appius Claudius, though blind, took part in councils of state, and in the senate expressed a very stern view of Pyrrhus's prisoners of war. But it is better to say that the blind man can retain a magistracy already entered upon but is absolutely forbidden to seek another one. There are many examples in support of this opinion.
>
> *(Digest 3.1.1.5)*

As you can see from this passage, the problems faced by the blind are practical and related to miscommunication. They are not comparable to those faced by the deaf and the dumb or the insane – or the *absentes*. The blind might not recognize a magistrate's insignia, or more importantly, like Publilius, they may misconstrue the judicial circumstances in which they find themselves.

A cluster of people cannot easily represent themselves before the law – women, children, the *debiles* (perhaps the deaf and the mute), sometimes the blind, the extravagant (*prodigi* and the *protervi*), the simple minded, and even those who are unborn or are overseas on military service or are captives of the enemy. All of these display an inability in communicating (and receiving) judgement through speech or gesture. Some of the members of this group are to all intents and purposes 'absent'. The legal treatment accorded to these individuals places them in a position that might match what we would understand as being due to the disabled. According to the *Digest* these people suffer a clearly perceptible disability. These individuals require special protection or special treatment in legal circumstances because they cannot properly protect themselves. But the Romans, as we see them in the *Digest,* were very practical and unsentimental people. They are not interested in overarching notions of disability, in the way that modern legislators may be, but rather they are interested in specific impediments that an individual may suffer that would render their appearance in a court difficult to adjudicate fairly. The Romans of the *Digest* seem to have an unarticulated but real enough concept of disability. It is one that may relate to the inability of individuals to communicate properly and to be present.

The legal standing of people with 'disabilities'

To follow are just a few of the areas to which special attention is paid in the *Digest* to those whom we would say are suffering from a disability. Here I am not using the term disability in the strict sense described above. Here I am concerned more broadly with all of the categories mentioned. My list is certainly not intended to be comprehensive.

Guardians and tutors for the free who are disabled

Those who were deemed incapable of managing their own affairs had a *curator*, a legal guardian, appointed to look after their wellbeing and their finances. (If it was an *impubes* who needed this assistance the manager was called a *tutor*.) The curator offered the *iudicium*, the reasoned communication that these individuals were unable to offer often because of their 'absence'. The curator became the voice of those whom we readily recognize as suffering disability (the insane, the blind, the deaf and the dumb) as well as those whom we do not so readily recognize as suffering from disability (women, children, the unborn, people who are away or are prisoners of war).

A curator was appointed 'by a parent or by the decision of the majority of their tutors or by a person having jurisdiction over such matters [a praetor]' (*Digest* 3.1.3 and 3.1.4). They could be appointed to someone who was underage (an *adulescens*; *Digest* 3.1.3.3) or someone who is 'unable to look after their own affairs because of chronic illness' (*infirmitas*), such as the dumb (*mutus*), the deaf (*surdus*), the spendthrift (*Digest* 3.1.3.3–4) or the insane. The use of the curator is one of the most practical modes by which those suffering disabilities in Rome were cared for. Comparable procedures existed in ancient Greece (such was the purport of the *dikè paranoias*, see Clark 1993: 156–74; Vaughan 1919: 59–72; and Rose and Dillon in this volume) and in classical Arabic law, according to Michael Dols in his great book (Dols 1992: 428–30 also discusses Roman law; on the links between curatorships and madness there is also assistance to be derived from Tristán 2000 and Pulitano 2002; Trenchard-Smith 2010 cites Sesto 1956; see also Gourevitch in this volume). The distinction between Greece and Rome seems to have resided in the fact that for the Roman the appointment of a curator was a legal right.

The details of the responsibilities of the curator are discussed periodically in the *Digest* concerning the *furiosus* (but less so concerning other disabilities). The *Digest* explains of curatorship (linking it with the comparable tutelage) the following:

> Equally, tutelage is a personal *munus* [public service], the care of a grown-up or of a madman (*furiosi*), likewise of a spendthrift (*prodigi*), a dumb person or of an unborn child, even to the extent of providing food, drink, shelter, and so on. But in addition, there is a curator provided for the good of someone who is away (*absens*), by whose activity usucapion is prevented and who sees that debtors are not released.
>
> *(Digest 50.4.1.4)*

The curator was appointed by a legal magistrate, a praetor – it was a duty that could not be shirked and it could be expensive:

> Moreover, those who are already administering three tutelages or three curatorships or three tutorships and curatorships all told, which are still in existence, that is, where the *pupilli* are not yet of age, are exempt from a fourth tutelage or curatorship. Indeed, a curator of a lunatic (*furiosi*) rather than of a minor can count this last among the number of curatorships (...)
>
> *(Digest 27.1.2.9)*

And it was a duty that could have serious legal ramifications:

> After the death of a lunatic (*furiosus*), an action on a judgment will not be granted against the curator who managed his affairs, any more than it will be granted against

tutors, as long as it is certain that no renewal of debts was made with his consent after he had resigned his office, and that no obligation was transferred to the curator or tutor.

(Digest 26.9.5)

A curator could be a member of the family, a son, for example, but it was usually not. Dols (1992: 428) maintains that a husband, for example, could not act for his mentally impaired wife. If an individual was under the age of 25 and did not have a parent, then the praetor could appoint a tutor whose responsibilities match that of a curator. A tutor, if the circumstances required it, could be appointed for an unborn child.

A madman required the use of a curator in the furthering of all legal transactions and contracts. But this is not always the case for the deaf and dumb. We have noted earlier (*Digest* 40.2.10, 40.9.1) that 'the son of a deaf or dumb father can manumit by his command, but the son of a lunatic cannot manumit'. *Digest* 44.7.48 indicates that 'in any transactions in which speech is not required but consent is sufficient, such as hire, sale, and other like contracts, a deaf person (*surdus*) can also take part seeing that he is able to take part and consent.'

Disabled individuals who did require the use of a curator or tutor when completing contracts or transactions were provided with some legal protection. In *Digest* 42.5.16–22. there is a discussion of who gains first access to the funds of a debtor when his assets have been sold off – what and who constitutes a preferred or privileged creditor amongst those who have a just claim against the debtor. The first example concerns the dowry of an affianced woman, when her marriage is called off. Her dowry occupies this position of being a privileged debt ('for it is a matter of public concern that, when she [the woman] reaches an adult age, she may properly enter into a marriage'). And so it is for those who are acting as financial managers for those who, because of age or *disability*, are attempting to recoup a debt for their client. Debts for these individuals are preferred, that is to say they move to the front of the queue when claims are being made against the debtor's estate:

> If a person who is not a tutor in fact conducts affairs as though he were a tutor, the privilege [of moving to the front of the debt queue] operates; and it is of no consequence whether he personally be the debtor or the heir or other successor of the debtor. The *pupillus* himself also has the preferred position but not his heirs. It is also highly appropriate that others for whom curators are appointed on the ground that they are *debilis* or spendthrifts (*prodigi*), 20 (…) or deaf mutes (*surdo muto*), 21 (…) or weak minded (*fatuo*), 22 (…) should have the same position of preference.
>
> *(Digest 42.5.19.1)*

Paradoxically the disabled could themselves be required to act as curators or tutors.

> bodily infirmity (*corporis debilitas*) provides an excuse from those *munera* (public services) that are discharged merely by bodily activity. But those which can be carried out by the mental application of a sensible man (*consilio prudentis viri*) or with the patrimony of a man who is sufficiently well endowed for this purpose are not remitted except for clear and agreed demonstrable reasons.
>
> *(Digest 50.5.2.7a)*

I presume that the reference to patrimony means that, for example, a deaf or a dumb individual could pay to have someone carry out the *munera* for them. *Digest* 50.5.2.7a could not apply to madmen, however, because they lacked *consilium*. If their condition were intermittent however they could presumably undertake such *munera* in their periods of sanity.

The law is here very strange to our ears for the deaf and the dumb, despite their being potentially liable to curatorships and tutorships, were not allowed to make wills (see Küster 1991; Laes 2014; Buckland 2007: 288):

> A person in parental power has not the right to make a will, and this is so much the case that even if his father gives him permission, he still cannot thereby lawfully make a will. 1. Deaf or dumb persons cannot make a will; but if someone has become dumb or deaf after making a will, because of illness or some other accident, the will nevertheless remains valid.
>
> *(Digest 28.1.6)*

The main exception to this rule (*Digest* 29.1.4 'It is settled that by military law a deaf and a dumb person can make a will if he is still with the colors before dismissal as unfit for service') seems only to strengthen the force of the exclusion. The deaf and dumb were, however, entitled to own property (*Digest* 37.3.2): dumb, deaf or blind persons can receive *bonorum possessio* (a legal variant of ownership) if they can understand the transaction.

Slavery and disability

But not all groups in Rome were afforded the protection of a 'legal voice', of a curator in other words. These are the voiceless, the slaves of Rome. The un-free were just as liable to suffer from some or another *perpetuus morbus* as were the free. Does the *Digest* have anything to tell us about this unfortunate group? The *Digest* does indeed, but its focus is on work and 'workability' as it relates to the disabled slave. The discussion concerns those conditions 'whereby the usability of a slave is reduced' (*ex quo quis minus aptus usui sit*, 21.1.5). These are the instances of disability that render a person problematical, rather than at a disadvantage before the law (the advantages and disadvantages relating to the individual slave are not considered).

What happens if you should buy a slave who is, unknown to you, subject to a disability that may interfere with their work or their usefulness to your enterprise? What happens if a recently purchased slave is, unbeknownst to you, suffering a condition 'whereby [their] (…) usability (…) is reduced'? You would know if they were blind, deaf or dumb, but you might not know if they were subject to *furor*. If a slave with one or another disability ('diseases', *morbi*, or 'defects', *vitia*) is purchased and the disability is not made apparent by the vendor, then the purchaser may be entitled to rescission, or their money back. In such cases what is at issue before the law is not the rights and needs of the disabled slave, but the rights and needs of their purchaser. Under what conditions may the purchaser get his money back if he has bought a slave who is suffering from one or another of the disabilities mentioned earlier in my chapter (humpbacked, hunchbacked and so on)?

There are a number of conditions that limit what constitutes a refundable disability. The following long passage makes clear some of the niceties of the sometimes imponderable logic of the *Digest* on the matter of mental defects in a purchased slave:

> So if there be any defect (*vitium*) or disease (*morbus*) which impairs the usefulness and serviceability of the slave, that is ground for rescission (…) 9. The question is raised in Vivian whether a slave who, from time to time, associates with religious fanatics (*fanaticos*) and joins in their utterances is, nonetheless, to be regarded as healthy (*sanus*). Vivian says that he is; for he says that we should still regard as sane those with minor mental defects (*animi vitia*) (…) 10. Vivian says further that although, at some

time in the past, a slave indulged in Bacchanalian revels around the shrines and uttered responses in consonance therewith, it is still the case that if he does it no longer, there is no defect in him and there will be no more liability in respect of him than if he once had a fever; but if he persists still in that bad habit, cavorting around the shrines and uttering virtually demented ravings (*ut circa fana bacchari soleret et quasi demens responsa daret*), even though this be the consequence of excess and thus a defect, it is a still a mental, not a physical, defect, and so constitutes no ground for a rescission (…) 11. Vivian says the same in respect of slaves who are excessively timorous, greedy or avaricious, quick tempered. 21.1.2 (…) [or] prone to fits of depression. 21.1.4pr. (…) For all these defects, for which he says that rescission is not applicable, Vivian would give the action on purchase.1. But if a physical affliction should have mental consequences, say that the slave raves in consequence of his fever or wanders through the city quarters, talking nonsense in the manner of the insane, there is, in such cases, a mental defect flowing from a physical one, and consequently, rescission will be possible.

(*Digest 21.1.1.8–21.1.4.1*)[6]

Pomponius speaks of runaway or wandering slaves, whom he thought could be also mad. In a longish discussion of the grounds according to which the sale of a slave could be judged as invalid he notes:

Generally, the rule which we appear to observe is that the expression 'defect and disease' (*vitii morbique*) applies only in respect of physical defects; a vendor is liable in respect of a defect of the mind (*animi vitium*), only if he undertakes liability for it, otherwise not. Hence, the express reservation of the wandering or runaway slave; for their defects are of the mind, not of physical (*hoc enim animi vitium est, non corporis*).

(*Digest 21.1.4.3*)

The mental defects of slaves can extend beyond such actions as wandering or running away. Venuleius at *Digest* 21.1.65pr highlights as *vitia mentis* such unexpected activities as being 'addicted to watching the games or studying works of art or lying' (*si ludos adsidue velit spectare aut tabulas pictas studiose intueatur, sive etiam mendax ... teneatur*).

Much of this discussion in the *Digest* hinges on the distinction between a *morbus* (a disease) and a *vitium* (a defect). It leads to an interesting distinction between the natures of disability. Gourevitch 2013 and Lanza 2004 maintain that a disability that does not interfere with the purpose for which a slave has been purchased is a *vitium* or defect, while one that does interfere is to be thought of as a *morbus*. The presence of the latter in a new slave may have entitled you to a refund from the purchaser.

Marriage

The attitude of the *Digest* to disability is by and large matter of fact. But there is often considerable sympathy displayed towards the mentally disabled. I have attempted to demonstrate this in 'Madness in the *Digest*' (2013). Here I would like to offer just one instance of this benign attitude. The *Digest* provides a very vivid and, for once, an emotional portrait of marriage as it might be experienced by the disabled, in this case by the insane. In this instance the portrait is of a *furor* that develops after a marriage has been contracted (Evans Grubbs 2002: 190). The madness can only countenanced if it occurs within a marriage, for diagnosable madness prevented a marriage from taking place in the first place. This is made clear at *Digest* 23.1.8:

'It must be obvious that insanity *(furor)* is an impediment to betrothal, but if it arises afterward, it will not invalidate it.' The passage from which I will now quote offers advice and rulings on the rights within marriage of a wife or a husband who has succumbed to insanity:

> Let us see what is to be done if a husband or a wife becomes insane *(furere)* within a marriage. There can be no doubt that the person in the grip of insanity *(furore detenta est)* cannot repudiate the marriage, because that person is not in their senses. What if a woman is repudiated in these circumstances? If there were lucid intervals during the madness *(intervallum furor habeat)* or the disease is permanent but bearable for those connected with her, then the marriage ought not to be dissolved at all. Where a person who is aware of the situation and is of sound mind repudiates the other person who is insane *(furenti)* in the way we described above, that person will be to blame for the dissolution of the marriage. For what could be more generous than a husband and wife sharing in each other's misfortunes *(quid enim tam humanum est, quam ut fortuitis casibus mulieris maritum vel uxorem viri participem esse)*?
>
> *(Digest 24.3.22.7)*

There are, however, grounds for a husband's seeking a divorce. These are directly related to the level of violence to which the madwoman is prone. So we hear:

> But if the insane person is so violent, savage and dangerous *(propter saevitiam furoris)* that there is no hope of recovery and it is terrible for her attendants and if the other party fears for his safety and is tempted by the desire to have children because he has none, this person will be allowed, if of sane mind, to repudiate the other party who is insane *(furenti)*, so that the marriage will be ended without blame attaching to anyone and neither of them will suffer damage.
>
> *(Digest 24.3.22.7)*

In some instances, however, the husband may be unwilling to seek a divorce even in an intolerable situation. This may be because he has designs on the misuse of her dowry. In a case such as this recourse should be had to the curator or to other family members, such as the woman's father who can attempt to recover the dowry either for himself or for the daughter:

> But suppose the woman has the most savage form of insanity *(in saevissimo furore muliere constituta)* and the husband does not want to end the marriage because he is too cunning for this, but treats his wife's misfortune with scorn and shows her no sympathy but clearly does not give her proper care, but misuses her dowry. Here the insane woman's curator or her relatives can go to court, to force the husband to give all this sort of support to the woman, to provide for her, to give her medicines, and to omit nothing a husband should do for his wife as far as the amount of the dowry allows. But if it is clear that he is about to squander the dowry and not enjoy it as a man should, the dowry should be sequestered, and the wife should have enough for the maintaining of herself and her household. All dotal pacts which the parties entered into at the time of marriage action must continue in their former condition and are dependent on the recovery of the health of the wife. Again, the father of the insane woman *(furiosae)* can legally bring an action to recover the dowry himself or for his daughter. For although the insane woman cannot repudiate, her father can certainly do so.
>
> *(Digest 24.3.22.8–9)*

The passage finishes with a bizarre twist. What if the daughter's father himself goes mad after a divorce has taken place? I am not sure whether the advice here is an example of wilful speculation, or whether it offers some sort of evidence that madness ran in some Roman families. At any rate, here is the jurists' advice:

> If after the marriage has been dissolved the father becomes insane (*furiosus*), his curator can bring an action to recover the dowry with his daughter's consent, or where there is no curator the daughter can bring it, but she must give security that her act will be ratified. It has also been decided where a father is captured by the enemy (*ab hostibus captus sit*), an action to recover the dowry should be granted to the daughter.
>
> *(Digest 24.3.22.10–11)*

Conclusion

For the Romans of the centuries that are dealt with by the *Digest* disabilities of the various types surveyed here seem to have been primarily a legal problem. A contrast could be made to the 19th, 20th and 21st centuries where disability is, I think it is fair to say, primarily seen as a medical problem – while perhaps for the 17th and 18th centuries it was viewed a social problem. Most recently the societal approaches to disability seem designed, in post-Enlightenment fashion, with an eye to provide for an individual's entitlement to personal fulfilment regardless of their status. Perhaps disability is moving into new conceptual territory.

The Roman *Digest* was concerned with little more than what seemed fair and practical from a legal point of view. I suspect that this was the prevailing attitude at Rome. Perhaps this was because medicine mattered less as a solution in Antiquity. As we can see from Galen or Aretaeus or Caelius Aurelianus, there was very little that could be done by physicians to cure or even to mitigate mental disorder or disabilities such as being deaf or dumb (see Gourevitch in this volume). And very little could be done from a social point of view either when such disabilities (I am thinking of madness here) lead to violent behaviour. There were no hospitals, no prisons to speak of, and, effectively, no police force. But there was a highly articulated legal code whose role was the resolution, not the control, of difficult social issues. There was, as we have seen, a code that could deal with such problems as might arise from disability: those relating to marriage, inheritance, slave ownership, property and personal damages, and so forth.

The *Digest* seems to display what I have termed as an *instrumental* understanding of disability. Disability is a visible or clearly perceptible physical or mental condition that renders a person at a disadvantage or problematical before the law. Roman law shows little interest in the totalizing notions of our society and its concern with an *existential* understanding of disability. The Roman *Digest* pays no attention to the capacity of disability to render societal inclusion and societal function difficult for an individual to sustain. Nor does it exhibit any interest in what we would term minority status. Whether blindness, for example, is a disability or evidence of minority status was not a problem for the jurists of the *Digest*. The Romans, as we see them in the *Digest,* were very practical and unsentimental people. They are not interested in overarching notions of disability, in the way that modern legislators may be, but rather they are interested in specific impediments in the face of the law. If the disability applied to a slave, then they were interested in the ways his or her disability could be accounted for in court. They seem to have had, despite this, a nascent sense of a concept of disability. It was something that in some instances we readily recognize as disability (insanity, blindness, being deaf and dumb), but in others not (women, children, the unborn, people who are away or prisoners of war). Their world was, as Laes 2011 emphasizes, an oral one. It is fitting that their concept is one that may relate to the inability of individuals to communicate properly and this related to a sense of their being in some manner 'absent'.

Notes

1 Mental illness e.g. was a visible condition in almost all of the ancient contexts that I have encountered. Certainly this is the case for the *Digest*. The jurists and the magistrates were in no doubt of a person's mental disability because that person showed it. They could only be fooled when a person feigned madness.

2 See also n. 4 for the apparent combination, *surdus mutus*, 'deaf mute'. For a very useful discussion on this topic see Laes 2011.

3 Nardi 1983: 18–45 has an extensive discussion of this topic. Stok 1996: 2296–2303 is also of considerable assistance.

4 Or does the passage refer to a deaf-mute? The *surdus mutus* combination occurs approximately five times in the *Digest*. The combination *surdus et mutus* is more common, where it seems to mean 'the deaf and the dumb'. *Surdus* and *mutus* are linked periodically without a connector to terms such as *caecus* (*mutus surdus caecus* at *Digest* 23.3.73pr. e.g. where it means, presumably, 'the mute, the deaf, and the blind').

5 *Non autem omnes iudices dari possunt ab his qui iudicis dandi ius habent: quidam enim lege impediuntur ne iudices sint, quidam natura, quidam moribus. natura, ut surdus mutus: et perpetuo furiosus et impubes, quia iudicio carent. lege impeditur, qui senatu motus est. moribus feminae et servi, non quia non habent iudicium, sed quia receptum est, ut civilibus officiis non fungantur.*

6 Parlamento 2001 expands on the notion of *vitium animi* and aims to show that the puzzling figure of the 'melancholic slave' in the lines to follow this passage should be understood in terms of Hippocratic (and Galenic) medicine and Cicero's *Tusculans* 3.5.11 as the victim of a *vitium animi* rather than a *vitium corporis*.

Bibliography

There is on the topic of mental disability Margaret Trenchard-Smith's 2010 excellent and very thorough chapter, and my own on madness in the *Digest* (Toohey 2013). Trenchard-Smith's essay looks forward to comparisons with Byzantine law. Mine looks backwards, hoping to use the *Digest* to elucidate 'classical' Roman attitudes towards madness, especially those to be seen in medicine. Trenchard-Smith, given her 'medieval' remit and Byzantine interests, is also and understandably less concerned to emphasize the importance of law for 'an understanding of Roman social history' – hence we stress different implications of the juridical evidence. Stok 1996 provides a useful synoptic reading of madness in Roman Antiquity. Scull 2015 is now on every list. Notable also are Nardi 1983, DiLiberto 1984 and King 2000. There is a long examination of the madman in Roman law in Semelaigne 1869: 215–28 (also covered is 'Hippocratic medicine', Erasistratus, Asclepiades, Celsus, Aretaeus, Caelius Aurelianus and Galen). There are also the standard handbooks such as those of Buckland 2007 or Kaser 1989. Laes 2014 has many useful remarks on the law and disabilities relating to disabled new-borns, mental disabilities, the blind, the deaf and deaf-mutes, the speech impaired and the mobility impaired (see also Laes 2011). Küster 1991 should also be consulted.

Buckland, William W., *A Text-Book of Roman Law from Augustus to Justinian*, 3rd edn rev. by Peter Stein, repr. (Cambridge, 2007³).

Clark, Patricia Ann, 'The Balance of the Mind: The Experience and Perception of Mental Illness in Antiquity' (unpublished PhD, University of Washington, 1993).

DiLiberto, Oliviero, *Studi sulle origini della 'cura furiosi'* (Naples, 1984).

Dols, Michael, *Majnun: The Madman in the Medieval Islamic World* (Oxford, 1992).

Evans Grubbs, Judith, *Women and the Law in the Roman Empire: A Sourcebook on Marriage, Divorce, and Widowhood* (London and New York, 2002).

Gourevitch, Danielle, 'La stérilité féminine dans le monde romain: *Vitium* ou *morbus*, état ou maladie?', *Histoire des Sciences Médicales* 47/2 (2013), 219–31.

Harris, William V. (ed.), *Mental Disorders in the Classical World* (Leiden, 2013).

Johnston, David, *Roman Law in Context* (Cambridge, 1999).

Kaser, Max, *Römisches Privatrecht: Ein Studienbuch*, 15th edn (Munich, 1989).

King, Peter, 'The "Cognitio" into Insanity' (unpublished PhD, University of North Carolina, Chapel Hill, 2000).

Krause, Jens-Uwe, *Gefängnisse im Römische Reich* (Stuttgart, 1996).

Küster, Axel, *Blinde und Taubstumme im römischen Recht* (Cologne, 1991).

Laes, Christian, 'Silent Witnesses: Deaf-Mutes in Graeco-Roman Antiquity', *Classical World* 104/4 (2011), 451–73.

Laes, Christian, *Beperkt? Gehandicapten in het Romeinse rijk* (Leuven, 2014).

Lanza, Carlo, '*Res se moventes* e *morbus vitiumve*', *Studia et Documenta Historiae et Iuris* 70 (2004), 54–162.

Leibrand, Werner, and Wettley, Annemarie, *Der Wahnsinn: Geschichte der abendländischen Psychopathologie* (Freiburg and Munich, 1961).

Nardi, Enzo, *Squilibrio deficienza mentale in dritto romano* (Milan, 1983).

O'Brien-Moore, Ainsworth, *Madness in Ancient Literature* (Weimar, 1924).

Parlamento, Enrica, '*Servus melancholicus*: I *vitia animi* nella giurisprudenza classica', *Rivista di Diritto Romano* 1 (2001), 1–20.

Pulitano, Francesca, *Studi sulla prodigalità nel diritto romano* (Milan, 2002).

Scull, Andrew, *Madness in Civilization: A Cultural History of Insanity* (Princeton, NJ, 2015).

Semelaigne, Armand, *Études historiques sur l'aliénation mentale dans l'antiquité* (Paris, 1869).

Sesto, Genaro J., *Guardianship of the Mentally Ill in Ecclesiatical Trials: A Canonical Commentary with Historical Notes* (Washington, DC, 1956).

Stok, Fabio, 'Follia e malattie mentali nella medicina dell' età romana', *ANRW* II/37/3, (Berlin and New York, 1996), 2282–2409.

Toohey, Peter, 'Madness in the *Digest*', in W. V. Harris (ed.), *Mental Disorders in the Classical World* (Leiden, 2013), 441–60

Trenchard-Smith, Margaret, 'Insanity, Exculpation and Disempowerment in Byzantine Law', in W. J. Turner (ed.), *Madness in Medieval Law and Custom* (Leiden and Boston, MA, 2010), 39–56.

Tristán, Paula Domínguez, *El 'prodigus' y su condición jurídica en derecho romano clásico* (Barcelona, 2000).

Vaughan, Agnes Carr, *Madness in Greek Thought and Custom* (Baltimore, MD, 1919).

Watson, Alan, *The 'Digest' of Justinian*, 4 vols (Philadelphia, 1998).

IV

The late ancient world

22

HYSTERICAL WOMEN?

Gender and disability in early Christian narrative

Anna Rebecca Solevåg

... for she said, 'If I but touch his clothes, I will be made well [σωθήσομαι]'.

(Mark 5: 28)

... as well as some women who had been cured of evil spirits (πνευμάτων πονηρῶν) and infirmities (ἀσθενειῶν): Mary, called Magdalene, from whom seven demons (δαιμόνια) had gone out, and Joanna, the wife of Herod's steward Chuza, and Susanna, and many others, who provided (διηκόνουν) for them out of their resources.

(Luke 8: 2–3)

Introduction

The two quotations that introduce this chapter are taken from stories about women with impairments and their encounters with Jesus. The first story, which is told in similar versions in the Gospels of Matthew, Mark and Luke, is about a woman who had a gynaecological condition resulting in continual bleeding for twelve years. The other is about Mary Magdalene, Jesus' close associate and helper, who apparently had seven demons and was healed by Jesus. Christianity has often been called a religion of healing, and in early Christian narratives, we meet disabled and sick characters mostly in stories about the healing miracles by Jesus and the apostles. This article will look at such early Christian narratives from the perspective of gender.

One principal objective is to survey what disabilities or ailments women have in early Christian narratives. How are their illnesses and impairments described? Are they similar to men's? If not, in what way do they differ? I will argue that women's disabilities in early Christian narratives are gendered in the following way: while male characters with disabilities often belong to the typical categories of 'blind, deaf and lame', female characters have disabilities that were conceived of as typically 'womanly', or in other ways tied to gender and/or sexuality. In other words, there is a certain 'hysterical' i.e. 'womblike' quality to female disabled characters.

A second aim is to probe deeper and ask, what difference does gender make? Drawing on ancient ideas about gender, I show how notions about gender coloured ideas about disability and ability, illness and health. I also look at the gendered roles of patient and healer in search of traces of women as agents of healing in early Christian narratives. Finally, I ask about the particular Christian meanings given to disability, illness and suffering. Here I briefly discuss the doctrine of the resurrection of the body and how it relates to ideas about disability and gender.

In an oral culture like the ancient Mediterranean, storytelling was a part of everyday life. Disability scholars David Mitchell and Sharon Snyder have pointed out that disability often functions as 'narrative prosthesis' in literature. Disability engenders narrative because difference requires an explanation: 'the very need for a story is called into being when something has gone amiss with the known world – the tale seeks to comprehend that which has stepped out of line' (Mitchell and Snyder 2001: 53). I have chosen to focus on three clusters of narratives that early Christian writers produced the New Testament Gospels and Acts, the Apocryphal Acts of the Apostles and the Martyr Acts. In these tales we meet embodied female characters and sense the efforts at making meaning of disability, illness and bodily suffering.

Suzanne Dixon has shown that women were portrayed differently in different genres in Antiquity (Dixon 2001). While inscriptions highly praised women as wives and mothers, the satirical works of Sallust and Juvenal scorned women for their promiscuity and moral decay (Dixon 2001: 17–18). To our knowledge, virtually all literary sources preserved from Antiquity are male-authored. For Dixon, this calls for caution, as references to women 'amount to male-centered fantasies and moral statements of what women should or should not be' (2001: 16). Following Dixon, I do not think that the selected sources depict women particularly truthfully. Each of these narrative genres has a particular style and a particular purpose. What I am interested in is documenting the representations of women and their disabilities occurring in these texts and discussing possible reasons for these particular representations.

Disability studies scholars often define disability as 'loss or limitation of opportunities to take part in the normal life of the community on an equal level with others due to physical and social barriers' (Goodley 2011: 8). As the Introduction to this volume makes clear, disability is a concept that has been constructed differently in different time periods and cultures. The ancients had no term that is equivalent to our 'disability', but there were, of course, categories of impairment and illness. Research on disability in Antiquity is such a new topic that there does not yet exist a definition of what disability was in that cultural context (Laes *et al.* 2013a: 5–6). The sources we have preserved from Antiquity may not be adequate to distinguish medical impairment from social discrimination, but close readings of textual representations of disability provide a good starting point (Moss and Schipper 2011: 6).

Women with disabilities in early Christian narrative

Women in the New Testament healing stories

In the Gospels (Matthew, Mark, Luke and John) and in the Acts of the Apostles, there are altogether about fifty healing stories. Sixteen of these concern women. Some of these are parallel stories, so there are only nine unique narratives. The following list notes the literary character, her illness/disability and citation:

1 Peter's mother-in-law, healed from a fever (Matt. 8: 14–15//Mark 1: 29–31//Luke 4: 38–9)
2 Jairus' daughter, illness/death (Matt. 9: 18–26//Mark 5: 21–43//Luke 8: 40–56)
3 Woman, flow of blood (Matt. 9: 18–26//Mark 5: 21–43//Luke 8: 40–56)
4 Syrophoenician/Canaanite girl, demon-possessed (Matt. 15: 21–18//Mark 7: 24–30)
5 Elisabeth, mother of John the Baptist, barrenness (Luke 1: 5–25)
6 Mary Magdalene and Jesus' female disciples, demon possession and illnesses (Luke 8: 2–3)
7 Woman, crippling demon (Luke 13: 10–17)

8   Tabitha, illness/death (Acts 9: 32–41)
9   Slave woman, spirit of divination (Acts 16: 16–18)

From this list we can see that Matthew and Mark told the exact same stories about women healed by Jesus. Luke skips the story about the Syrophoenician/Canaanite woman, but adds one of his own, a story about a woman bent over from a crippling demon. He also tells two stories about women miraculously healed that are not typical healing stories. These are the brief mention of the healing of Mary Magdalene and the women who followed Jesus, and an elaborate story, as part of his birth narrative, about how Elisabeth, the mother of John the Baptist, became pregnant by divine intervention after suffering from barrenness all her life.

It should be noted that the Gospel of John is conspicuously absent from this list. John has fewer healing stories than the Synoptic writers (i.e. Matthew, Mark and Luke). He only recounts three healing stories in his Gospel (not counting the resurrection of Lazarus), all of which are longer, more elaborate and with clear symbolic overtones (the royal official's son, 4: 46–54; the ill man at Betzatha, 5: 1–9; the man born blind, 9: 1–7). John's Gospel is much more symbolic than the Synoptics, and these healing stories are probably thought to be more representative of Jesus' ministry and 'signs' than the Synoptic narratives (Culpepper 1987: 72–3; Pilch 2000: 124).

Comparing the list above to healing stories involving male characters, several observations can be made. First, the list of ailments is quite different. Three recurring categories when Jesus heals men are the categories of blind, deaf and lame. Rebecca Raphael has even named these three disabilities 'the biblical trilogy of disability' (Raphael 2009: 13). Interestingly, none of these categories come to the fore in the healings of women. Leprosy and demon possession are also frequent and particularly significant illnesses in the healing stories of the New Testament (for leprosy, see e.g. Matt. 8: 2; Mark 14: 3; Luke 17: 12). Of these five illness categories, only demon possession can be found on our list. The other recurring illness is, I will argue, gynaecological problems.

At least four of our stories are concerned with demon possession, possibly five. Luke's account of the healing of Peter's mother-in-law has affinities with the stories about demon possession. Jesus rebukes (ἐπετίμησεν, 4:35) the fever, using terminology connected with exorcism (see e.g. Mark 9: 25; Luke 9: 42), rather than with healing of other ailments (such as θεραπεύω, σώζω and ἰάομαι). Most people in the ancient world believed that the gods could cause illness, either directly through divine intervention or by the more specialized means of possession (Avalos 1999: 62–3). Δαιμόνιον is the Greek term for an inferior divine being (Liddell and Scott 1940 s.v.), and the polytheistic religions of the era all accommodated the idea that gods, lesser gods and spirits could possess a person for good or for bad (Martin 1995: 155). Among the pagan writers that mention demon possession are Lucian and Plutarch (Lucian, *Philops.* 8–16; Plutarch, *De superstitione* 7, 168c). Demon possession occurs frequently in Jewish and early Christian sources, as these religious traditions, having a more dualistic worldview, connected demon possession more closely with Satan and evil forces (see e.g. Mark 3: 22–7). The medical writers of Antiquity, however, viewed illness as a problem of imbalance rather than invasion by demons or other foreign bodies (Hipp., *De morbo sacro*; Martin 1995: 146–53; Moss 2010: 512–14; cf. Kellenberger in this volume)

Several of the stories seem to be concerned with fertility and barrenness. Many commentators have observed that the intertwined stories about Jairus' daughter and the woman with the flow of blood are both ultimately concerned with the two women's capacity to reproduce (Wainwright 2006: 114–15; Collins 2007: 280–4). Elisabeth's miraculous pregnancy is another example. From this story we also learn that a certain amount of shame was connected with barrenness. 'This is what the Lord has done for me when he looked favourably on me and took away the disgrace I have endured among my people' (Luke 1: 25) is Elisabeth's surprised but happy exclamation upon discovering that she is pregnant.

A second observation is that many of the healed women are named, known or part of the group around Jesus or the community of Christ-believers. Examples include Mary Magdalene, Elisabeth, Tabitha and Peter's mother-in-law. Some who are not named are still placed in a family relationship as daughters (the Syropheonician and Jairus' daughter). In contrast, the male characters who are healed are usually nameless strangers with no significant family relations and no prior or subsequent ties to the Jesus movement. The only exception is the blind man Barthimeus, who is named in Mark (10: 46–52) and becomes a follower of Jesus in all the Synoptics (Matt. 20: 29–34; Luke 18: 35–43).

Thirdly, there is a focus on service (διακονία): Peter's mother-in-law serves Jesus and the disciples as soon as she has been healed; the women healed from demon possession, Mary Magdalene among them, all serve Jesus and the disciples through their own means; Tabitha is known for her service to the church, sewing garments and housing widows.

Finally, the space of these healings is interesting to consider. Several of the healing stories concerning women seem to take place in domestic space, like the healing of Peter's mother-in-law, Jairus' daughter and Tabitha. The house was women's space, the place for women's household chores (exemplified by Peter's mother-in-law and Tabitha) and for marriage and childbearing (Elisabeth and Jairus' daughter). Yet Jesus is also sought out by women in public (male) space. Both the woman with the flow of blood and the Syrophoenician mother with the possessed daughter, as well as Luke's bent woman approach Jesus in search of healing. By stealth, the woman with the flow of blood approaches Jesus from behind, intending to touch the hem of his garment without Jesus' knowledge, (Mark 5: 27); others approach with the proper amount of respect and submission, by falling to their knees and addressing Jesus as κύριε, master or lord. Interestingly, it is the unnamed women without a connection to the Jesus group who approach Jesus in public. Below I will discuss these observations in light of ancient Mediterranean views on gender and disability, but first I turn to the Apocryphal Acts' and the Martyr Acts' representations of women with disabilities.

Women healed and converted in the Apocryphal Acts

Women play an important role in the narratives of the Apocryphal Acts of the 2nd century. There are five Apocryphal Acts that date back to the 2nd and 3rd centuries, the Acts of John, the Acts of Andrew, the Acts of Paul (and Thecla), the Acts of Peter and the Acts of Thomas. With the exception of Acts of Thomas, only fragments of these works survive (Klauck 2008: 2–3). These texts revolve around the missionary journeys of one particular apostle, culminating in his martyrdom (or natural death in the case of John, see Acts John 20). Many of the same literary topoi and theological themes recur in these narratives, the importance of female sexual renunciation being one of them. Healing as well as preaching is part of each apostle's *modus operandi* in these texts, in which we come across several healings of women.

In the Acts of John, the healing stories are closely related to conversion. There is an almost automatic effect: healing miracles engender conversion (see e.g. Act John 22, 30, 33). Women are among John's patrons and converts. The first miracle John performs is the healing of a woman, Cleopatra, who is paralysed, or perhaps suffering from a mental illness (παραπλήγου, 19). The terms παραπλήξ and παραπλήσσω can connote paralysis as well as madness or derangement (Liddelland Scott 1940 *s.v.*). John also heals a stadium full of old women, some of whom are paralysed (παραλυτικὰς, 30), others sick with other ailments (ἄλλας νοσούσας, 30). The women have been gathered in the theatre for this purpose, and the healing becomes a spectacle for the people of the city, in order that they may convert and believe in Christ (30–6).

In the Acts of Peter, women who encounter the apostles (both Paul and Peter feature in the narrative) are exposed to unhealing as well as healing. In a fragment only preserved in Coptic (Cod. Berol. 8502.4, henceforth BG 4), Peter heals and then 'unheals' his daughter, who is paralysed. The reason he gives is that the daughter would 'harm many souls, if her body remains healthy' (BG 4.131.3–4. English translation from Parrott 1979). The girl became paralysed at age 10, when she was abducted by a man who wanted to take her in marriage and God miraculously preserved the girl 'from defilement and pollution' through paralysis (BG 4.135.12–13). Peter's daughter, who is lying in a corner, is referred to as paralysed (*sēq*) and crippled (*essosht*) (BG 4.129.4–5). Later in the story we learn that her paralysis has affected one whole side of her body and that she is 'dried up' (*shooue*, BG 4.135.7–9). The Acts of Peter also contain another story about divinely sanctioned infliction of paralysis. The apostle Paul curses a congregant, Rufina, who attends the eucharist but is an adulterer. The woman not only becomes paralysed (*contorminata cecidit,* Acts Pet 2), 'on the left side from head to foot' (English translation from Elliott 1993), similar to Peter's daughter. Rufina is also rendered mute (Acts Pet 2).

Similarly to the Acts of John, there is also a mass healing of older women in the Acts of Peter. A group of believing widows, who are blind, approach Peter at a worship gathering demanding to be healed, because the apostle has already healed one woman in their group. As Peter prays for them, the women all have visions of Jesus, seeing him in different forms. Peter uses the incident to preach on different ways of seeing (Acts Pet 21). The most important is to see with one's mind and not with one's eyes: to see Jesus Christ. In any case, it seems that the widows are healed.

In the Acts of Thomas, there are two elaborate stories about demon-possessed women who are healed by the apostle. Both incidents are clearly related to sexuality and to the theme of sexual renunciation that permeates the narrative. During his missionary journey in India, Thomas is approached by a beautiful woman asking for healing. She is tormented by a demon who comes to her every night and has intercourse with her (Acts Thom 43). Thomas expels the demon, but it turns up later in the story, this time with a son, possessing another woman and her grown daughter (Acts Thom 62–71). The demons incessantly throw the women to the ground and strip them naked, thus they need to be kept locked up at home.

The Acts of Andrew and the Acts of Paul and Thecla contain fewer healing stories altogether, and none concerning women. Let me still briefly mention the Acts of Paul and Thecla, as this apocryphal acts has been an important text in the research history on gender and women's place in early Christianity (see e.g. Burrus 1987; Cooper 1996; Levine and Robbins 2006). Thecla, Paul's convert, fights successfully in the arena twice. On the second occasion, she is helped by the women spectators at the games, who shout and throw aromatic herbs into the arena so that the animals are hypnotized (Acts Paul 35).

Compared to the New Testament, women's impairments in the Apocryphal Acts come closer to the 'biblical trilogy' of blind, deaf and lame. We have blind widows, and several instances of paralysis (Rufina, Peter's daughter and possibly Cleopatra). Similar to the Gospels, demon possession also turns up in the Apocryphal Acts as an illness that befalls women. Another pattern observed in the New Testament narratives, that women were named and in family relationships, continues in the Apocryphal Acts. With the exception of the mass healings of old women in the Acts of Peter and the Acts of John, the women encountered are presented as wives or daughters and often named.

Gender and suffering in the Martyr Acts

The broken rather than the healed body is in focus in the martyrdom accounts. Since this is unusual for early Christian texts, these narratives may give us a somewhat different perspective on the configuration of gender and disability in early Christianity. Women appear in many of the early Christian martyrdoms. Where women are given narrative space, we find some recurring themes. Women martyrs, in contrast to men, are often charged with madness and superstition in their hearings. In the *Martyrdom of Saints Agapê, Irenê, and Chinê at Saloniki*, the magistrate calls the Christian women's refusal to eat sacrificial food 'insanity' (μανία, 3.2). This 'diagnosis' is repeated, as the women resist encouragements to sacrifice to the Roman gods (μανία, 3.7; 5.1 ἀπόνοια, 6.2). Crispina, likewise, is charged with folly and superstition (*vanitas … animi, superstitione, Martyrdom of Saint Crispina* 1.6) and asked to desist from her foolish frame of mind (*sensu tuo stulto*).

Moreover, categories of femininity and infirmity overlap in these narratives. Blandina is called weak (ἀσθενής, Letter of the Churches of Lyons and Vienne 18), and later in the narrative 'tiny, weak and insignificant' (μικρὰ καὶ ἀσθενὴς καὶ εὐκαταφρόνετος, 42) (English translation from Musurillo 1972). Yet, she is masculinized through her imitation of Christ and called a 'mighty and invincible athlete' (μέγαν καὶ ἀκαταγώνιστον ἀθλητὴν, 42). Crispina is threatened with disfigurement (*deformatio, Martyrdom of Saint Crispina* 3.1), which turns out to be a threat not of torture or broken bones, but of having her hair cut and head shaved. In the *Martyrdom of Perpetua and Felicitas*, Perpetua has visions of becoming an athletic male (10.1–15), but as the two women fight in the arena it is their femininity that is highlighted. Perpetua is called a delicate young girl (*puellam delicatam*, 20.2) and Felicitas is described as 'a woman fresh from childbirth with the milk still dripping from her breasts' (20.2).

There is a titillating focus on the scantily clad or completely naked bodies of the women. Agathonicê is undressed and the spectators marvel at her beauty (*Acts of Carpus, Papylus and Agathonicê*, Latin rec. 6.4), and Perpetua tries to cover her thighs with the short tunic she is given (*Martyrdom of Perpetua and Felicitas* 20.4). Irenê is taken to a brothel, naked, as punishment for keeping Christian writings, but her virginity is miraculously preserved (*Martyrdom of Saints Agapê, Irenê, and Chinê at Saloniki* 5.8–6.2). Sabina, likewise is threatened with being put in a brothel (*Martyrdom of Pionius* 7.6). In the *Martyrdom of Potomiaena and Basilides*, Potomiaena is handed over to be sexually violated by gladiators, but a soldier prevents it. The martyr is killed 'by boiling pitch … slowly poured over different parts of her body, from her toes to the top of her head' (4).

Finally, there is a component of motherhood in many of these martyrdom narratives. Most of the female martyrs are explicitly mothers who chose martyrdom despite admonitions to pity their children (e.g. *Martyrdom of Perpetua and Felicitas*, 5.3, *Acts of Carpus, Papylus and Agathonicê*, Latin rec. 6.2, Greek rec. 43). Blandina, although not explicitly a mother, is described as 'a noble mother encouraging her children' due to her mothering role towards the other martyrs (*Letter of the Churches of Lyons and Vienne* 55). The motherhood theme is particularly elaborated in the *Martyrdom of Perpetua and Felicitas*, which even includes a childbearing scene. Felicitas, a female slave among the confessors, gives birth in prison, seemingly without any help, as the guards reproach her for her foolishness. Her suffering is particularly harsh, according to the narrator 'because of the natural difficulty of an eight months' delivery' (15.5).

What difference does gender make?

The convergence of gender and disability in Antiquity

In Antiquity, women were subordinate to men in all areas of society. Religious myth, tradition, philosophy, law and medicine undergirded ideas about women's inferiority in physique, mental capacity, moral ability and civic accomplishment. A woman was, according to Aristotle by default disabled (cf. Beal in this volume for a similar thought in the Hittite records). In *On the Generation of Animals* he states that women are characterized by inability (ἀδυναμία) as men are characterized by ability (*Gen. An.* 766a, see also *Gen. An.* 728a). Galen, too, states that women are a less developed, somewhat truncated version of humankind when he claims that women are imperfect (ἀτελές) and mutilated (ἀνάπηρον, *De usu part.*, 14.2; 4.143–4 Kühn). Greek medical thought for the most part constructed the female body as weaker, colder and more porous than the male (Dean-Jones 1994: 115, 118–19). Women were both anatomically inferior and pathologically dependent on the male body (Garland 1995: 170–2).

Thomas Laqueur has argued that gender difference was, in Antiquity, perceived as a 'sliding scale' of one all-encompassing sex, rather than of male and female as stark opposites. Laqueur states that 'men and women were arrayed according to their degree of metaphysical perfection, their vital heat, along an axis whose telos was male' (Laqueur 1992: 5–6). Woman was an inferior version of man, not quite fully formed, lacking in perfection. The quotations from Galen and Aristotle illustrate that their main idea about the female is not grounded in difference, but in lack or deficiency. Laqueur's 'one-sex model' of gender difference in Antiquity has been very influential but is also contested (King 2013; Solevåg 2013: 70–2). Although this model may not have been the only existing gender model in Antiquity, its notion of the female as inherently weak and deficient is interesting when it comes to the intersection of gender and disability. To be weak (ἀσθενής) was a label commonly used for sick, chronically ill and disabled people (Rose 2003: 13). This construction of disability as weakness and lack thus overlaps with the construction of women as men's weaker, less able counterparts. In Candida Moss's words, while the healthy body was seen as 'impermeable, dry, hot, hard, regulated and masculine', the sickly body was 'drippy, leaky, moist, uncontrolled, feminine, soft and porous' (Moss 2010: 514).

With these gender ideas in mind, the ancient world has often been called patriarchal. A more nuanced way of understanding the hierarchical structure of ancient Mediterranean society is through the term *kyriarchal*. This neologism, coined by New Testament scholar Elisabeth Schüssler Fiorenza, underscores the importance of the male head of the household, the *kyrios* or *paterfamilias* and stresses that domination was not only gender-based, but more intersectional, including slaves, children and other subordinates (Schüssler Fiorenza 1999: 9). From a perspective of disability, the kyriarchal model is helpful in order to understand what constituted disability in the ancient world. Depending on a person's location in society, a certain impairment could be more or less disabling. For a free man of the ruling class, it was of utmost importance to be able to hear and speak. In the oral culture of the Roman Empire, male citizens were expected to declare publicly their name and properties for the census and to utter oaths. Hence, deaf and deaf-mute people were generally excluded from office-holding (Laes 2013: 153). Carts, litters and donkeys were used to transport the sick, the injured and people permanently unable to walk (Rose 2003: 24–5). Hence a motor impairment would be less disabling if a person could afford to hold slaves to transport him or her, more so if transport was less accessible yet necessary in order to earn a living.

Free women's role was first and foremost to bear legitimate children. Hence, it has been argued that barrenness was the most disabling impairment for a married woman (Edwards 1996: 91). The focus on fertility as the most important aspect of women's health is clear in the medical literature. When women are considered in the medical texts, it is first and foremost their reproductive capacity that is scrutinized. In Ann Ellis Hanson's words, the gynaecologies of Antiquity are 'pronatalistic', that is, their intent is to protect women's fertility and to aid the bearing of a more perfect child (Hanson 1990: 316). According to the Hippocratic writers, women's health was best when they had intercourse on a regular basis and bore children (Hanson 1990: 319). Intercourse would 'irrigate' the womb with sperm, so that it would not become desiccated and migrate in search of moisture. Pregnancy similarly anchored the womb and secured the menstrual blood to be put to use as nourishment for the fetus (Dean-Jones 1994: 121). Lack of these conditions could result in a 'wandering womb'. One of the symptoms the wandering womb could cause was a suffocating feeling, ὑστερικός πνίξ, which was accompanied by madness (Soranus, *Gyn.* 2.26, Galenus, *De methodo medendi* 1.15; 11.47 Kühn). The medical literature thus constructs women as closer to the irrational than men (Dean-Jones 1994: 115), and it was their particular sexual organs and womb (and also breasts) that rendered them vulnerable to madness; it was, literally, in their nature to be hysterical.

Slave women could be used for reproductive labour, as childbearers, wet-nurses or midwives, but could also be used for other forms of work, such as hard labour, household chores and as maids. In the medical literature this is reflected in the fact that when slave women are mentioned, the issue is less often reproductive than when free women are discussed (Demand 1998: 83).

Gender, illness and suffering in early Christian narrative

With these gender constructs and power relations in mind, how can we understand the representation of sick, disabled and suffering women in the narratives presented above? Why are there no blind, deaf or lame women in the New Testament narratives? I argue that this is because men, in the kyriarchal gender paradigm, are thought of as more representative of humanity than women. The healing of a blind man represents the healing of any blind person, whereas the healing of a woman does not have the same implication. This can explain why the Gospel of John, which only narrates three healing stories, devotes all three healings to the healing of men. The fact that the male healing stories more often concern nameless strangers enhances this generic quality about male healings. The disabled characters 'become' their disability when they are called 'the blind man', ὁ τυφλός (e.g. John 9: 17), 'the lame man' ὁ παραλυτικός (e.g. Mark 2: 3), etc.

While the healing stories concerning male characters say something about the cultural assumptions about disability, the healings of women reveal more about gender. Rebecca Raphael has shown that barrenness is the most common disability for women in Genesis (Raphael 2009: 54). This pattern of gendered disability is continued in the New Testament. The stories about Elisabeth, Jairus' daughter and the woman with the flow of blood all show the childbearing drive of Greco-Roman society in general and the medical writers in particular. In the Markan version, the woman with the flow of blood has explicitly sought doctors in search of healing for her medical problem (Mark 5: 26). Moss argues that Mark's description follows the ancient medical model of the porous and leaky body (Moss 2010: 514).

Although both women and men are healed or exorcised from demon possession in the New Testament, one may wonder if women, according to these narratives, are more susceptible. This is particularly apparent in Luke, where several women are connected to demon possession, including Peter's mother-in-law, the women from Galilee who follow Jesus and the woman who is bent by a 'crippling demon'. Elaine Wainwright suggests that this labelling of women may be an attempt to domesticate and colonize the service of women in the Christ-believing communities (Wainwright 2006: 106).

In the Apocryphal Acts, the healing stories concerning women are gendered in somewhat different configurations. These narratives are focused on sexual renunciation, hence in conflict with the Greco-Roman drive towards reproduction. The Greco-Roman view, indeed, is turned on its head. Barrenness is not among the disabilities healed, but many of the healings are closely connected with the theme of sexual renunciation and thus focus on the 'problem' of the female body. The demons in the Acts of Andrew are sexually aggressive, forcing the women who are possessed away from the ascetic lifestyle they have chosen. Moreover, the illness of Cleopatra, if interpreted as madness, may also be linked to gynaecological theories that connected women to the irrational. If, on the other hand, this is a motor impairment, it is similar to Rufina's ailment as well as that of Peter's daughter. Even a mobility impairment could be read as a gynaecological problem. Meghan Henning has shown that paralysis, in the medical literature, could be seen as 'a visible symptom of a set of internal problems with the female reproductive system' (Henning 2015: 317). She argues that Peter's daughter's paralysis would imply to the ancient reader that she was infertile and therefore prospective suitors would be deterred (Henning 2015: 318–19). These two women are unhealed, rather than healed. Although Rufina's unhealing is a punishment, Peter's daughter is unhealed as a protection against sexual violence or even, as Henning argues, marriage.

In both the Acts of Peter and the Acts of Thomas, the impairments that befall these women happen when they are outside the home. The women who become possessed in the Acts of Thomas have been to the baths and are walking along the aqueducts. Peter's daughter was first seen by Ptolemy, her suitor and abductor, when she was at the baths. Such stories underscore not only how sexually vulnerable women were outside the protective unit of the household, but also how sexual violence and disability overlap in these stories – the one causes the other.

In addition to these upper-class female characters, who are named, and who are important in the story due to their sexual renunciation and patronage, we also meet, twice, a group of unnamed older women who receive healing. In the Apocryphal Acts, old women and widows are consistently constructed as sick, disabled and in need of care, similar to Tabitha and the widows she cared for (Acts 9: 39). It was, of course, a fact of life that old people were ill, but early Christian texts construct a gender difference. Old women are presented as particularly infirm and needy, while old men, the presbyters, are presented as leaders of the church (see e.g. 1 Tim. 5: 1–15). The ailments of their bodies very seldom come to the fore, to the contrary they are described as strong and healthy despite old age (*Martyrdom of Polycarp* 7.8, 8.3, 9.1).

When it comes to our final group of texts, the Martyr Acts, I want to comment on two of the observations made earlier: motherhood and madness. The focus on motherhood in the Martyr Acts, again shows how important childbearing was considered to be in the Roman Empire. That the women martyrs were mothers made their sacrifice even more difficult and admirable in the eyes of the ancient Christian reader. In the *Martydom of Perpetua and Felicitas*, the physical toll of childbearing is likened to the suffering of martyrdom (15.6). But martyrdom superseded childbearing as the ultimate suffering for a Christian woman (Tert., *Fug.* 9). The women are depicted as Christ-like in their suffering, but not all in the same way. In these texts the difference between slave and free becomes significant. Perpetua, the free woman, is presented as masculine in the arena, and even has a vision of having a male body, whereas the slave women's female bodies (Blandina and Felicitas) are drawn in a different way, their suffering is compared to childbirth, and they do not 'become male' (Solevåg 2013: 230–5).

That women martyrs were accused of being mad is an example of how women were constructed as closer to the irrational than men. Their deviant religion and denouncement of civic piety – considered aberrant behaviour – is attributed to a deranged mind. Although demon possession is not the same as madness, they seem both to be similarly constructed as women's ailments in these texts. As noted, madness in women was given a gynaecological explanation by the medical writers. Similarly, the understanding of women's sexual organs as independently wandering – an 'animal within' – overlaps with the idea of demon possession as an external force entering and taking over the body. Deviant or erratic behaviour that in the invasion paradigm was attributed to demon possession could be explained by madness, among followers of the balance paradigm.

In all of the three text groups, then, we find a recurrence of what could be called a 'female dyad of disability': gynaecological/reproductive issues and demon possession/madness.

The male healer and the female patient

Early Christian narratives constructed Jesus and the apostles as healers (see e.g. Matt. 9: 35; Mark 2: 17; Acts 3: 6–8; Acts Andr 2; Acts Pet 29). Elaine Wainwright has brought attention to the fact that in the New Testament no women are healers, only healed (Wainwright 2006: 1–2). What do we find if we extend this research question to the texts in our survey? Are women represented as healers in any of these texts?

Moss has argued that within the Gospels we can find a story of a woman who acts as a healer. The woman with the flow of blood is in the Markan version presented as initiating her own healing by pulling power from Jesus, and thus reversing the power dynamics between patient and healer (Moss 2010: 515–16). The women in the Apocryphal Acts and Martyr Acts are, like women in the New Testament, never called doctor (f. ἰατρίνη) or even midwife (μαῖα), although we know that women served in these functions during the time period (Wainwright 2006: 50–62). Like the woman with the flow of blood, there are some hints also in the Apocryphal Acts and Martyr Acts about women performing a healing role. In the Acts of John, some women are given power to raise dead in Jesus' name (Act John 24, 83). This narrative 'democratizes' healing and miracle work, extending it beyond the circle of apostles. Women do become, then, vehicles for the restoration of bodies in this text.

As noted, the women spectators in the Acts of Paul and Thecla use aromatic herbs to anaesthetize wild animals. This is a subtle reminder that women were in possession of herbs and other *pharmaka* that were used for healing purposes (cf. the Gospel stories of the woman who anointed Jesus and the women at the tomb, also in possession of aromatic herbs, Mark 14: 3, 16: 1). Although Thecla's ministry in the Acts of Paul and Thecla is clearly focused on preaching the word of God, the cult around St Thecla soon became a popular healing cult, with a much visited pilgrimage site (4th–6th century) in Seleucia in Asia Minor (Davis 2001: 36). A longer version of the Acts' ending, dating to from the 4th century, describes how all the sick of Seleucia are brought to the mountain where Thecla resided. Thecla's prowess in healing drives the physicians in the region out of business, and assuming that she acquires her healing powers through the virgin goddess Artemis, the physicians try to rape her. Miraculously, Thecla escapes into the rock and is taken directly into heaven (Elliott 1993: 372–4). A later work, the *Life and Miracles of St Thecla* (c.444/8) gives an account of the healings and other miracles Thecla performed (Davis 2001: 41).

Perpetua, in the *Martyrdom of Perpetua and Felicitas*, prays for her brother while she is in prison. The brother had died from cancer of the face as a child, and Perpetua has two visions of him. First, she sees him suffering and unable to drink from a fountain which is too tall for him, and with the wound he had when he died still on his face (*Martyrdom of Perpetua and Felicitas* 7.4). Confident that she is privileged as a confessor, she prays for him for a number of days (7.9). In a second vision she sees him again, clean, refreshed and a scar where the wound had been (8.1). Perpetua has posthumously 'healed' her brother and transferred him from a place of suffering to a place of bliss (8.4).

Female healing is, then, a rare phenomenon in the Apocryphal and Martyr Acts, as well as in the New Testament. But the anecdotal evidence we have from these early Christian texts tell us that women were in possession of *pharmaka*, were considered efficient petitioners and intermediaries in prayers for healing, and that female saints established the locus of healing shrines.

In the New Testament we saw a focus on service by women, διακονία, in connection with the healing narratives. The construction of women as recipients rather than ministers of healing correlates with the increasing domestication of women that we see in early Christian texts. In order to counteract public opinion criticizing the 'hysterical' women who belonged to this new and strange sect (see Orig. *C. Cels.* 2.60; 3.55; *Martyrdom of Saints Agapê, Irenê and*

Chinê at Saloniki 3.2) early Christian writers represented Christian women as in compliance with the Greco-Roman ideals of public and private, honour and shame (MacDonald 1996: 252–5). The texts may therefore downplay the healing functions that women possibly had within the communities of belief as an extension of their diaconal role, for example through caring for the sick, disabled and elderly, and assisting at births (Osiek and MacDonald 2006: 66–7).

Conclusion: gender, disability and early Christian meaning making

In this survey I have looked at some early Christian representations of disability, illness and suffering in light of ancient Mediterranean gender constructions. In addition to such a contextualization one might also ask what kinds of specifically *Christian* meanings were given to disability, suffering and healing? How was disability *theologized* in early Christian narrative? As noted, healing stories as well as martyrdoms take on a certain flavour when women are in focus. But there are some general trends that can also be seen through the texts surveyed here. Healings are often seen as a sign of what is to come, that is, the resurrection of the body for all believers (Ireneus, *Adversus Haeresus* 5.13.1). The healings of women in the New Testament are, similar to male healings, signs of the impending arrival of the kingdom of God. As the first epigraph of this chapter shows, healing overlaps with salvation, a term used for both in the Gospels is σώζω. In the Apocryphal Acts, healing accompanies conversion, the first step towards resurrection. Healing miracles and resurrection miracles also overlap in these narratives (Acts John 19–23; Acts Pet 27). The apocryphal attention to the virgin body and the preservation of it functions as an analogy to the perfect female body in heaven – with virginity preserved for the heavenly groom, Christ (Clark 2008). Finally, in the Martyr Acts, the resurrection of the body becomes the vindication of the martyrs' gruesome death and bodily destruction. These texts often invoke the reward of the martyrs, eternal life and present images of the body in the resurrection, for example in Perpetua's visions.

Most church fathers taught that all believers would be resurrected with perfect bodies, without any disabilities or blemishes (see e.g. Theophilus, *Letter to Autolycus* 2.26; Pseudo-Justine, *On the Resurrection* 4; Augustine, *City of God* 22.21). As Moss notes, 'the eradication of deformity (...) is a notable feature of the emerging doctrine on the resurrection' (Moss 2011: 1011). Augustine, however, retains a place for the scars of martyrs' in the resurrection (*City of God* 22.19.1149), as discussed by Kristi Upson-Saia and Moss (Upson-Saia 2011; Moss 2011: 1010–11).

Interestingly, our texts also show some differing voices that are not in unison with the choir of praise for the perfected risen body. The Acts of Peter preserves a place for the unhealed in the Christian community, and even a particular gift of 'seeing' for the blind widows. To be able-bodied is not necessarily better in the salvation economy of this text. Likewise, in Perpetua's vision of her brother, the boy still has a scar after he is healed and transferred to heaven. He has not risen with a perfect body, but still retains a sign of his suffering, similar to Augustine's allowance for martyrs.

With such a variety of textual sources surveyed, one can only make broad strokes in a conclusion. More research is needed in order to understand the representations and theological uses of disability in each of these early Christian narratives. Such research is useful, not only because it will expand our knowledge of the history of disability (Kudlick 2003), but also because it expands our insight into texts that have been foundational in the development of Christian doctrine on illness and disability and still are influential in many Christian communities (Betcher 2007: vii–viii; 2013).

Bibliography

Avalos, Hector, *Health Care and the Rise of Christianity* (Peabody, MA, 1999).
Betcher, Sharon V., *Spirit and the Politics of Disablement* (Minneapolis, MN, 2007).
Betcher, Sharon V., 'Disability and the Terror of the Miracle Tradition', in S. Alkier and A. Weissenrieder (eds), *Miracles Revisited: New Testament Miracle Stories and their Concepts of Reality* (Berlin, 2013), 161–82.
Burrus, Virginia, *Chastity as Autonomy: Women in the Stories of Apocryphal Acts* (Lewiston, 1987).
Clark, Elizabeth A., 'The Celibate Bridegroom and His Virginal Brides: Metaphor and the Marriage of Jesus in Early Christian Ascetic Exegesis', *Church History* 77/1 (2008), 1–25.
Collins, Adela Yarbro, *Mark: A Commentary* (Minneapolis, MN, 2007).
Cooper, Kate, *The Virgin and the Bride: Idealized Womanhood in Late Antiquity* (Cambridge, MA, 1996).
Culpepper, R. Alan, *Anatomy of the Fourth Gospel: A Study in Literary Design* (Philadelphia, PA, 1987).
Davis, Stephen J., *The Cult of Saint Thecla: A Tradition of Women's Piety in Late Antiquity* (Oxford, 2001).
Dean-Jones, Lesley, *Women's Bodies in Classical Greek Science* (Oxford, 1994).
Demand, Nancy, 'Women and Slaves as Hippocratic Patients', in S. R. Joshel and S. Murnaghan (eds), *Women and Slaves in Greco-Roman Culture: Differential Equations* (London, 1998), 69–84.
Dixon, Suzanne, *Reading Roman Women: Sources, Genres and Real Life* (London, 2001).
Edwards, Martha Lynn [= Rose, Martha Lynn], 'The Cultural Context of Deformity in the Greek World: Let there be a Law that No Deformed Child shall be Reared', *Ancient History Bulletin* 10 (1996), 79–92.
Elliott, John K., *The Apocryphal New Testament: A Collection of Apocryphal Christian Literature in an English Translation* (Oxford, 1993).
Garland, Robert, *The Eye of the Beholder: Deformity and Disability in the Graeco-Roman World* (Ithaca, NY, 1995).
Goodley, Dan, *Disability Studies: An Interdisciplinary Introduction* (Los Angeles, CA, 2011).
Hanson, Ann Ellis, 'The Medical Writers' Woman', in D. M. Halperin, J. J. Winkler and F. I. Zeitlin (eds), *Before Sexuality: The Construction of Erotic Experience in the Ancient Greek World* (Princeton, 1990), 309–37.
Henning, Meghan, 'Paralysis and Sexuality in Medical Literature and the Acts of Peter', *Journal of Late Antiquity* 8 (2015), 306–21.
King, Helen, *The One-Sex Body on Trial: The Classical and Early Modern Evidence* (Farnham, 2013).
Klauck, Hans-Josef, *The Apocryphal Acts of the Apostles: An Introduction* (Waco, TX, 2008).
Kudlick, Catherine J., 'Disability History: Why we Need Another "Other"', *American Historical Review* 108 (2003), 763–93.
Laes, Christian, 'Silent History? Speech Impairment in Roman Antiquity', in C. Laes *et al.* (eds), *Disabilities in Roman Antiquity* (Leiden, 2013a), 145–80.
Laes, Christian, Goodey, Chris F., and Rose, Martha Lynn, 'Approaching Disabilities *A Capite ad Calcem*: Hidden Themes in Roman Antiquity', in C. Laes *et al.*, *Disabilities in Roman Antiquity* (Leiden, 2013b), 1–15.
Laes, Christian, Goodey, Chris F., and Rose, Martha Lynn (eds), *Disabilities in Roman Antiquity: Disparate Bodies A Capite ad Calcem* (Leiden, 2013).
Laqueur, Thomas, *Making Sex: Body and Gender from the Greeks to Freud* (Cambridge, MA, 1992).
Levine, Amy-Jill, with Maria Mayo Robbins, *A Feminist Companion to the New Testament Apocrypha* (London, 2006).
Liddell, Henry George, and Scott, Robert, *A Greek-English Lexicon*, rev. Henry Stuart Jones and Roderick McKenzie (Oxford, 1940).
MacDonald, Margaret Y., *Early Christian Women and Pagan Opinion: The Power of the Hysterical Woman* (Cambridge, 1996).
Martin, Dale B., *The Corinthian Body* (New Haven, 1995).
Mitchell, David T., and Snyder Sharon L., *Narrative Prosthesis: Disability and the Dependencies of Discourse* (Ann Arbor, MI, 2001).
Moss, Candida R., 'The Man with the Flow of Power: Porous Bodies in Mark 5:25–34', *Journal of Biblical Literature* 129 (2010), 507–19.
Moss, Candida R. 'Heavenly Healing: Eschatological Cleansing and the Resurrection of the Dead in the Early Church', *Journal of the American Academy of Religion* 79 (2011), 991–1017.
Moss, Candida R., and Schipper, Jeremy, *Disability Studies and Biblical Literature* (Basingstoke, 2011).
Musurillo, Herbert, *The Acts of the Christian Martyrs* (Oxford, 1972).

Osiek, Carolyn, and MacDonald, Margaret Y., *A Woman's Place: House Churches in Earliest Christianity* (Minneapolis, MN, 2006).

Parrott, Douglas M., *Nag Hammadi Codices V, 2–5 and VI: with Papyrus Berolinensis 8502* (Leiden, 1979).

Pilch, John J., *Healing in the New Testament: Insights from Medical and Mediterranean Anthropology* (Minneapolis, MN, 2000).

Raphael, Rebecca, *Biblical Corpora: Representations of Disability in Hebrew Biblical Literature* (London, 2009).

Rose, Martha Lynn, *The Staff of Oedipus: Transforming Disability in Ancient Greece* (Ann Arbor, MI, 2003).

Schüssler, Fiorenza, Elisabeth, *Rhetoric and Ethic: The Politics of Biblical Studies* (Minneapolis, MN, 1999).

Solevåg, Anna Rebecca, *Birthing Salvation: Gender and Class in Early Christian Childbearing Discourse* (Leiden, 2013).

Upson-Saia, Kristi, 'Resurrecting Deformity: Augustine on Wounded and Scarred Bodies in the Heavenly Realm', in D. Schumm and M. Stoltzfus (eds), *Disability in Judaism, Christianity and Islam* (New York, 2011), 93–122.

Wainwright, Elaine M., *Women Healing/Healing Women: The Genderization of Healing in Early Christianity* (London, 2006).

23

AUGUSTINE'S SERMONS AND DISABILITY

Martin Claes and Anthony Dupont

Introduction

The responsibility accompanying the social position that Augustine bore as a man of letters, pedagogue and bishop resounds in his words as preacher, words through which he allowed a variety of intellectual and spiritual sources to speak to the contemporary life of late classical North Africa (for a general introduction in Augustine's life and thinking, see Lancel 1999; Brown 2000; van der Meer 1961). By virtue of these tasks and responsibilities, both corporeal and spiritual disability were regularly the subject of his thinking and speaking (Brown 1988; Rassinier 1991). Although Augustine's speaking on this subject is inextricably bound up with his longing for spiritual fulfilment through philosophy and religion, it is striking that, in spite of the high degree of abstraction of his subjects, the comforting and encouraging words of a close friend, mother and shepherd continually resonate through his preaching. He preaches for example on the incarnation using the following imagery:

> So what did our mother Wisdom do? She became weak in the flesh, in order to gather chicks together, in order to lay eggs and hatch them. But *the weakness of God is stronger than men* (1 Cor. 1: 25).
>
> *(Sermo 305A.6, tr. E. Hill 1997: 328)*

As a man of letters, he addressed a group of scholarly men who bore responsibility for others through their position in society. As a teacher of rhetoric, he had a specific interest in the way in which (young) people can grow in wisdom through knowledge and insight. This made it possible for them, as jurist or politician, to analyse and articulate their own or others' social problems. As shepherd of the church, he had an immediate and specific responsibility for the care of the sick and the poor in the community to which he was appointed.

Although it is difficult to grasp the intensity and variety of the effect of Augustine's theological writings, his sermons belong to the genre that has perhaps touched the greatest number of people, most certainly among his contemporaries.

> From his writing assuredly it is manifest that this priest, beloved and acceptable to God, lived uprightly and soberly in the faith, hope and love of the Catholic Church

in so far as he was permitted to see it by the light of truth, and those who read his works on divine subjects profit thereby. But I believe that they were able to derive greater good from him who heard and saw him as he spoke in person in the church, and especially those who knew well his manner of life among men.

(Possidius, Vita Augustini 31, tr. H. T. Weiskotten)

His hearers were in the first place the faithful of the cathedral city of Hippo, but were not limited to the Christian circle of listeners. His multifarious audience in the port town Carthage and his former occupation as professor in rhetoric testify to this. In addition to his direct contact with his audience as pulpit orator, there was also the written influence: his sermons began to have a life of their own in the church. Some of Augustine's sermons were written down by stenographers (*notarii*) who were present during the liturgical celebrations. In the form of collections of sermons, these served in their turn as models for preaching elsewhere in North Africa and Rome (see various contributions in Pollmann and Otten 2013).

Augustine knew the importance of the care for the sick from his own experience. He frequently mentioned his own struggles with illness or disease. He made reference in his early works for example to lung problems (*Contr. ac.* 3.7.15; *De ord.* 1.2.5: 'pectoris doloris'), and as a child he had suffered from a life-threatening illness (*Conf.* 1.1.17). Neither was he, in the death of his son Adeodatus and his mother Monica, spared from losing friends and family members (*Conf.* 9.6.14; 9.11.27). In *sermo* 20B (published only in 1994), Augustine mentions that he has only just recovered from illness and has to keep the sermon short because of his lesions.

I know your eagerness, brothers and sisters, but it is also necessary for you to spare my fragile state of health. No, I don't want to refuse your holinesses the ministry of my preaching, whatever it may be like, so that I may serve the Lord, who has restored me to health. However, we still have to deal gently with the more recent scar, which is not yet, perhaps, completely healed.

(Sermo 20B.11, tr. E. Hill 1997: 34)

In one of his latest writings, directed against one of his fiercest opponents, the 'Pelagian' Julian of Aeclanum, Augustine gives an overview of both physical and mental disabilities:

For it is necessary that you feel sorrow when you do not find any answer and you do not want to change your view which is so bad. For it forces you by an unavoidable necessity to locate in a place of such great happiness and beauty the blind, the one-eyed, those with inflamed eyes, the deaf, the mute, the lame, the deformed, the crippled, the worm-infested, the lepers, the paralytics, the epileptics, and those suffering from all kinds of other defects, and at times monstrous because of a terribly ugliness and horrible strangeness in their members never seen before. What shall I say of the defects of minds because of which certain people are by nature lustful, others prone to anger, others timid, and still others forgetful, some insensitive, stupid, and so feebleminded that a person would prefer to live with some animals than with such human beings? Add the groans of mothers in childbirth, the wailing of the newborn, the pains of the suffering, the struggles of the ill, the many torments of the dying, and the many more dangers of the living.

(Contra Iulianum opus imperfectum 6.16 (8), tr. Teske 1999: 641–2, CSEL 85.2.345, see also Laes et al. 2013: 1)[1]

Augustine situates this catalogue of human suffering within his doctrine of original sin. All these disabilities are a direct consequence of Adam's fall in paradise, and the participation of all of mankind in the sin and guilt of the first man. Consequently, Augustine is not blind to the reality of human disability, but at the same time, on a figurative or spiritual level, it always refers to a 'deeper' reality, the 'root' of all disabilities, namely (original) sin. The latter will become a refrain in our study of the presence of the issue of disabilities in Augustine's preaching.

In the context of his preaching, Augustine used the words: *aeger* (sick), *infirmitas* (infirmity), *morbus* (disease), *medicus* (doctor), *medicina* (medicine), *medicamentum* (medicine), *sanare* (to heal), *sanus* (healthy), *salus* (health). We will concisely present this medicinal vocabulary next. In light of the strong intertwining of Augustine's speaking of these terms and his use of imagery to indicate a spiritual condition or process, attention will be given in the following section to three metaphors that Augustine used in his preaching. After that we will consider how Augustine perceives his own sermons as having healing powers.

Augustine's medicinal terminology

Sickness and illness: aeger (aegrotus), infirmus (infirmitas) and morbus

When Augustine speaks of specific care for souls in a pastoral context, he often chooses the words *aeger* (*aegrotus*) and *infirmus* to indicate the sick in every sort of situation (Eijkenboom 1960: 126–30, 152–6; cf. also Kuuliala *et al.* 2015: 5–7 on defining *infirmitas* and the impossibility of discerning it from temporary illness). Augustine shows for example understanding and empathy in his sermons when he explains that, for a person who is ill, a short time can seem very long:

> It is your illness that makes the time seem to pass slowly, when in reality it is swift. Think what the demands of the sick are like. They think nothing so long-drawn-out as the mixing of a drink for them when they are thirsty. The attendants are working fast to minimize the distress of the sick person, yet he or she is demanding, 'When is it coming? Isn't it cooked yet? When will they give it to me?' You are just the same: the people serving you are hurrying as much as they can, but your illness makes you think their rapid work slow.
>
> *(Enn. in Ps. 36, Sermo 1.10.2, tr. Boulding 2000: 98–9; PL 36.361)*[2]

Sometimes, in Augustine's perspective, the illness is a form of martyrdom, especially in the struggle to resist the false hope that comes from medical charlatanism (*Sermo* 286.7; PL 38. 1300).[3] Augustine often links his reflections on *aeger* and *infirmus* with humankind's spiritual condition. He considered this as being weak and as 'an illness requiring healing' (*Sermo* 9.9; PL 36.600: *Nam quid es, homo, nisi aeger sanandus?*). Augustine remarks in *Sermo* 9 that the illness hates itself, in its condition of illness, just as the sinner does. The same applies to the doctor, who hates the patient's fever, but not the patient. The sick person needs in turn to trust and to agree with the doctor and to value his instruction increasingly as the healing progresses.[4] In addition to the words *infirmus* and *aegritudo*, Augustine sometimes uses *morbus* to indicate a specific ailment. These words do not only have a negative connotation for him. They have the beneficial purpose of bringing the sick (sinner) back onto the right path: Where do the indispositions come from? Where do the contagious illnesses and diseases come from? All of them are obviously corrections from the hand of God, according to the *Doctor gratiae*.[5] Of course, this brings in the well-known problem of the theodicy and the responsibility of God who is essentially good (Belser Watts and Lehmhaus p. 441–2 in this volume on Jewish thought; Kellenberger p. 53 and 58 for the matter of theodicy in the Old Testament tradition).

The practice of medicine, physician and medicine: medicina, medicus, medicamentum

Where the word *medicina* is used by Augustine to indicate the discipline of medicine in particular, with the word *medicus* he refers especially to the doctor as practician of the medical art (Eijkenboom 1960: 70–125; Bochet 2010). The fact that Augustine compares Christ to a doctor and to medicine (*medicamentum*) indicates that Augustine followed the example of a large group of church fathers who had a predominantly positive opinion of doctors, medical science and the medicine of which they made use (Dörnemann 2003: 288–98). In this way he concurred with the numerous places in the Bible where both Yahweh and Christ are called doctor and healer (Exod. 15: 26; Gen. 50: 2; Jes. Sir. 38: 1–15; Matt. 9: 12–13; Mark. 7: 33; Mark 1: 29–31; Gal. 4: 12–14; 2 Cor. 12: 9–10). Augustine must have had a reasonably broad knowledge of the medical science of his time. This was primarily at the service of his spiritual exposition of the developments and the condition of the human soul, but his familiarity with the dynamic in relation to the illnesses, symptoms, diagnosis and recovery is indicative of more than a superficial interest in this field of study.

In Augustine's time, the image of medical science was to a great extent determined by the writings of Galen (Nutton 2012). In addition, Augustine praises the ancient Greek physician Soranus as the inventor of the medical practice (*Contra Iul.* 51). Their theoretical background was to a great extent determi-ned by the physiologist Hippocrates and combined elements, mixtures and humours (Nutton 2012). Furthermore, North Africa had a lively cult of the god Asclepius. This cult lived on in the Asclepion of Pergamon, a school and sacred place with an altar dedicated to Zeus. Knowledge of herbal therapies, mud baths, fasting and therapies based on dreams was accumulated here and passed on.

Although these medical practices interwoven with pagan religions were the source of much debate between Christians and non-Christian contemporaries in Augustine's time, medical practice had gained a fairly good reputation (Origen, *Contra Celsum* 3.24 and 7.6 for pagan views; Arbesmann 1954; Honecker 1985; Doucet 1989 for a Christian reaction). They were united in the care of the sick and the needy (Dörnemann 2003: 288–98). There is nothing to indicate that Augustine distanced himself from contemporary medical practices and ideas. Methods that in his perspective were related to magic or the worship of heathen gods were the exception to this. In Augustine's opinion they gave false hope and were misleading. This indicates that patients in their daily life probably regularly resorted to magical and astrological remedies and that practice at times knew no clear boundaries between 'real medical science' or 'superstition' (cf. Amundsen and Ferngren 1986: 55).

In this context, we need to mention Augustine's 'late' acceptance of miraculous healings, healings at the intercession of the very popular martyr saints in North Africa. Augustine was originally convinced that no miracles took place after the era of the New Testament. He changes that opinion after 415, when the relics of the proto-martyr Stephen were discovered. After that discovery, Augustine accepted that also in his time miracles happened at the intercession of saints (Lancel 1999: 648–58). Augustine, despite this change in attitude, never changed his role as a critical theologian into a mere acceptance of the habits of the masses. The discovery of the Stephen relics did not imply a substantial change in Augustine's theology of martyrdom. The concern to aim the attention of the faithful to God and Christ remains the same: not the martyrs themselves but Christ through them performs the healing miracle. *Sermones ad populum* 320–3 testify to the fact that a certain Paul and Palladia were miraculously healed in the chapel dedicated to Stephen in Hippo, in the presence of Augustine. They suffered from trembling limbs. In this collection of sermons Augustine also gives account of similar miraculous healings taking place at the Stephen shrines in the Italian Ancona and the African Uzalis (cf. Dupont 2006). A more extended description of healings centred around Stephen relics can be found in Augustine's work *De civitate Dei*, composed between 413 and 427. From the twenty-four stories about the healing from mostly physical diseases, there is only one which explicitly warns against the failure of a superstitious *remedium.* It is the story of Petronia who wore a ring on her body which contained a kidney stone from an ox as a therapy for a severe disease. Its medical malfunctioning was demonstrated in a miraculous way on her journey towards the Stephen shrine in Uzalis. The sick woman Petronia interprets the miracle as a sign of her future healing by intercession of St Stephen (*De civitate Dei* 22.8). The majority of these stories focus on testimonials to the healing power of Christ, who works in and through the saints and martyrs. It is the aim of Augustine in these healing narratives to make clear to his audience that these contemporary miracles confirm and explain the main topics of the revealed faith, such as salvation and the future eschatological resurrection of all people (see also the anthology in Brock 2012).

Health: sanare, sanus, salus

When Augustine gives a description of the work of a doctor, he often uses the word *sanare* in the technical and profane meaning of healing. The frequently occurring Gospel stories of healing offer Augustine the occasion, in imitation of the Latin men of letters such as Cicero, Seneca and Livy, to describe the technical process of healing using this word. Its meaning is closely connected to that of the words *sanus* and *sanitas.* Augustine indicates in this way the condition of health. Just as Augustine indicates the healing process in the language of the day with the word *sanare*, he uses *sanus* for the condition of health as it was understood in daily usage. He points out that we are usually not aware of this condition, rather of its opposite.

> Our guts, our innards, which are called intestines, how do we know about them? And then, precisely, it's good, when we don't feel them. When we don't feel them, after all, when we are unaware of them, is when we are healthy.
>
> *(Sermo 277.8; PL 38.1262; tr. Hill 1997: 38)*

Augustine links health to the virtue of moderation. Moreover, Augustine regularly urges his audience to be patient and forbearing during their healing process:

> A surgeon unsheathes the knife to operate on the wound, and says to the sick person, 'Be patient now, bear up, you must endure this'. He requires patience under the pain, but promises health when the painful time is past.
>
> *(Enn. in Ps. 91.1.21; PL 37.1171; tr. Boulding 2002: 345)*[6]

Furthermore, with the word *salus*, Augustine also indicates the health that humankind and animals have in common and more specifically also the health for which people long when they ask for Christ's intervention (Eijkenboom 1960: 5–7). Augustine had himself been ill. Perhaps he was greeted with a hearty applause or other approving looks when he started to preach *sermo* 20B:

> I cannot thank the Lord God enough, nor your graces in his presence, for these joyful congratulations, which pour out, I can see very well, from the fountain of your love for me.
>
> *(Sermo 20B.1; tr. Hill 1997: 29)*

Being ill at that time was also evidently a social occurrence in which isolation and reintegration played a role. It reflects the warm relationship between Augustine and his community. A few sentences further in *sermon* 20B, Augustine broadens the anxious experience of his own physical limitations by pointing out, through a discourse on the spiritual dimension, the close relationship between physical suffering and the spiritual growth process, the guidance of which he considers to be his responsibility as shepherd.

> Nor should you be surprised that we suffer such things in this body. It is fitting, after all, that we should suffer; nor can what the Lord wills ever in any instance be unjust.
>
> *(Sermo 20B.1; tr. Hill 1997: 29)*

What follows demonstrates that Augustine possessed a detailed knowledge of the dynamics of the therapeutic process that took place between the physician and the patient.

> Note the prudent sick man, who values good health and looks forward to its restoration, prefers to ask the doctor for what he fancies at this moment, so that if the doctor refuses, he will forgo what would give him pleasure, but trust the doctor to give him back his health.
>
> *(Sermo 20B.4; tr. E. Hill 1997: 31)*

The medical knowledge serves the rhetorical goal of the analogy: the explanation of the relationship between illness and spiritual growth. Through references to for example martyrdom, Augustine puts the pure physical deliverance hoped for by many into the broader context of eschatological salvation. He used the latter as an example to indicate that eternal salvation and redemption have a higher priority than physical, temporal health. The martyrs testified formerly in an exemplary way through such a radical choice.[7]

Although the vocabulary pertaining to health has in the first instance a profane meaning, Augustine uses it regularly in comparative and figurative language to indicate the condition of the human spirit or of humankind in general. He regularly seeks in this way to explain Jesus' spiritual influence on people by means of images taken from medical practice. One example of this is his explanation of Jesus' healing of the man born blind, which for Augustine relates to the healing and restoring of the inner sight.

> The Physician who heals our interior eyes, enabling them to see that eternal light which is himself.
>
> *(Enn. in Ps. 36, Sermo 2.8.19; PL 36.368; tr. Boulding 2000: 109)*

> The doctor concentrates on curing the patient's old fever ... it was only by being taught humility [by the fact that the physician visits the sick patient, symbolizing God becoming human in Christ] that the patients would be healed of their pride.
>
> *(Enn. in Ps. 35.17.21; PL 36.353; tr. Boulding 2000: 87)*

Characteristic of Augustine's view of physical suffering is the explanation he offers in his sermons on the Gospel of John, for example in *Tractatus in Johannis evangelium* 3.14. In this sermon, Augustine urges his listeners to bear and endure illness and adversity as a forbearing patient. Those who are ill are encouraged to undergo whatever has happened to them as a therapy of the divine physician, where the patient Christ is an example for the sick.

> This grace was not in the Old Testament (...) but it prepared the way for that Physician who was to come with grace and truth; as a physician who, about to come to anyone to

cure him, might first send his servant that he might find the sick man bound. (...) The Lord comes, cures with somewhat bitter and sharp medicines: for He says to the sick, Bear; He says, Endure; He says, Love not the world, have patience, let the fire of continence cure you, let your wounds endure the sword of persecutions. Were you greatly terrified although bound? He, free and unbound, drank what He gave to you; He first suffered that He might console you, saying, as it were, that which you fear to suffer for yourself, I first suffer for you. This is grace, and great grace. Who can praise it in a worthy manner?

(Tract. in Ioh. ev. 3.14; tr. Schaff 1888/1991: 23)

The reading and exploration of the preceding texts show to a great extent that physical suffering is in particular used as a metaphor in Augustine's preaching for the weakness and incapacity of the whole of humankind. In his preaching, Augustine focused especially on making his listeners aware of this, to subsequently point them to Christ as physician. Through using this imagery, Augustine succeeds in making the dimension of spiritual healing and growth accessible to his listeners in language they can understand. Augustine does not ignore physical disability in this context, but integrates it into an encompassing plan of salvation. The latter tendency is clearly illustrated by Augustine's metaphorical use of medical imagery in his preaching, which will be the subject of closer reflection in the following section.

Three medical metaphors

Augustine took the Bible as the departure point of his preaching, and he frequently quotes at length from the Bible (Bright 1999). Not infrequently, Augustine's sentences are a concatenation of quotations and his own text. The Bible is a rich source of images and metaphors for the preacher of Hippo, who as a rhetor appreciated their didactic value. Augustine had recourse to three medical metaphors: Christ as physician, broken humanity, the Christian community as Body of Christ.

Christus medicus: about a physician who is also the medicine

The *Christus-medicus* imagery is frequently found in Augustine's sermons (Eijkenboom 1960; Bochet 2005; Kolbet 2010). Augustine, in his use of the *Christus-medicus* metaphor, represents a long tradition that has its foundations in the many stories of healing in the Gospels. In early Christian literature, Christ is often identified as *soter* and *iatros*: saviour and physician. Although the image usually refers to Christ, Augustine often makes a comparison in his sermons between the activities of God as Father and that of a physician. This form of comparison is found in particular in his theological writings (Dörnemann 2003: 311; Honecker 1985: 315).

Even more frequently, Augustine applies the term *medicus* to Christ as humble physician. The healing process is here an attractive image for the divine incarnation. God becoming man in Christ as a sign of humility, indicating that this humility is the most powerful medicine. Augustine encourages his flock in this way. He warns them that pride is the primary cause of spiritual suffering and incapacity. Original sin, brought about through pride, is the form of incapacity that is inherent to human existence since the fall. Augustine compares this original sin to the condition of a high fever where foolish humankind turns in raving madness against the advice of the Physician.

For a Physician was He, and to cure the madman had He come. As a Physician cares not what he may hear from the madman; but how the madman may recover and become sane; nor even if he receive a blow from the madman, cares he; but while he to him gives new wounds, he cures his old fever: so also the Lord came to the sick man, to the madman came He, that whatever He might hear, whatever He might suffer, He should despise; by this very thing teaching us humility, that being taught by humility, we might be healed from pride.

(Enn. in Ps. 35.17; tr. Boulding 2000: 87, PL 36.353)[8]

The mad mentioned above refer, according to Augustine, to the Jews who did not recognize Christ as their saviour. Not only the Jews, however, need a physician. Christ figures in his sermons also as an eye doctor who heals humankind from an eye disease (the inability to see the law; *Tract. in Ioh.* 44.17.4) and frees him from the swelling of pride (*Enn. in Ps.* 18, *Enn.* 2.15.26; PL 36.163).

At times Augustine links the imagery of *Christus medicus* with the term *salvator*, saviour. In this context, Christ is both physician and medicine. Among those things identified as medicine by Augustine, are the eucharist (*Tract. in Joh.* 6.15.8; PL 35.1432) and baptism (*Sermo* 30.5; PL 38.190). In the numerous variations of this imagery in his preaching, Augustine seems to relate the metaphor of *medicamentum* particularly to Christ himself: the humility of his incarnation reveals humility as the best antidote against pride, the source of all illness/sin. Augustine is in this way able, for his community, to call to mind the theological subject matter of the process of incarnation and salvation in clear and recognizable images and personal experiences. The medical terminology is in this context always used to serve the theological reading and explanation.

Brokenness: Augustine's anthropology of disability

Augustine indicates in his preaching that he is aware of the powerlessness and brokenness of humankind. To clarify the consequences of this in the pastoral setting in which he worked, he makes use of the medical metaphor of the *morbus mortalitatis*: the illness of mortality or *infirmitas humana*, the human weakness. In Augustine's view, in its unsaved condition, humankind is disabled and wanting.

[This condition] is a kind of natural illness, because the pain imposed as a punishment has become an aspect of nature to us. What was a penalty to our first parents is for us a natural condition.

(Enn in Ps. 37.5; tr. Boulding 2000: 109)[9]

In general, he considers physical and mental suffering, disability and mortality as not natural, as not intended in God's original plan. They are the penal consequences of Adam's original sin. They have become, in the same way as hunger and thirst, an inseparable part of our daily existence, as they weakened our human nature. The expression *infirmitas humana* was often used by Augustine in his polemic with the Pelagians on will and grace to clarify the workings and consequences of original sin (*Sermo* 374.16; Bartelink 1991). The brokenness affects all of humankind and is presented by Augustine as a patient stretched out over the whole world. Augustine points his congregation to a solution for this broken condition through comparing incarnation and salvation to the working of a physician.

The human race is sick, not with a physical disease, but with sins. It's laid low over the whole wide world, from the east to the furthest west, one gigantic invalid. To heal this gigantic invalid there came down the all-powerful doctor. He humbled himself to the level of mortal flesh, as though to the level of the sick person's bed.

(Sermo 87.13; tr. Hill 1991: 315)

In his anthropology, Augustine takes his point of departure partially from Neoplatonism (the immaterial and immortal soul) and Stoic philosophy (virtue ethics), but as time goes on he develops his own personal Christian synthesis. In this view, after the fall – Adam and Eve having been the first to sin – human beings are characterized by a *defectus* or defect. Only Christ can save humankind from this metaphysical infirmity (Dupont 2012) – for which Augustine freely uses the aforementioned vocabulary of being sick, of infirmity and disability. He focused in this context not only on an individual's physical or mental disability. As mentioned, this disability involves the totality of humankind. Augustine believed in the necessity of a universal liberation from original sin through Christ the physician. Brokenness and disability were in this way raised by Augustine above the purely individual perspective and broadened into a theological interpretation of salvation and liberation. He is able to proclaim this anthropological view in a way understandable to his audience through applying the imagery of disability to the whole of humankind. Augustine was deeply convinced that God created mankind well, and that man's original good nature was not destroyed by original sin, however it is tainted by it (*natura uitiata*). Hence Augustine sees the complete restoration of the human condition, expressed in the transformation to a perfect body, not taking place during the earthly existence. This bodily perfection is an eschatological reality, reserved for the afterlife. Augustine explains this process of transformation in more detail in his *De civitate Dei* when he examines biblical passages such as Luke 21: 18 (Not a hair of your head shall perish) in the context of the eschatological rising of deceased infants in a perfect and mature body.

> What, therefore, are we to say of infants, if not that they will not rise in that tiny body in which they died, but will receive, by the wondrous and most rapid operation of God, that body which they would have received in any case by the slower passage of time?
> *(De civitate Dei 22.14, tr. Dyson 1998: 1142)*

Characteristic for Augustine is the Christological focus of his view on this process of transformation. It is the wholeness of the eschatological Christ which functions for Augustine as a model for the eschatological restoration of each (imperfect or even disabled) human person (*De civitate Dei* 22.15). That this idea was essential for Augustine is demonstrated when he stretches this view on the eschatological restoration into details in his exploration on the physical consequences of this theory in *De civitate Dei* 22.16–17.[10] The Pauline promise that humans are destined to be conformed to the image of the son of God (Rom. 8: 29) provides Augustine with scriptural arguments for his reflections on age and gender of the eschatological human body. Certainly, this view has its consequences for Augustine's ideas on disability during earthly lifetime, as it situates the universal human condition of brokenness within a universal perspective of salvation and eternity. Christ, as a healer and an exemplary human person, becomes normative for all human suffering and disability (cf. Brock 2012).

That Augustine liked to make use of medical terminology when discussing this mental-spiritual disability becomes apparent in his frequent use of the word *dolor* (pain) to indicate the universal incapacity. This came about through the action of one individual, Adam, and became a universal and inseparable part of human existence (*Sermo* 57.11, *Sermo* 88.7, *Enn. in Ps.* 57.20). Although Augustine generally considers the pain and discomfort of this earthly life as a negative phenomenon, he regularly emphasizes that suffering and discomfort are also a sign of becoming liberated from them. After this life, men and women can experience liberation through the intervention of Christ the Physician. Pain is the indication that a bitter medicine or a painful therapy, such as amputation, is working well, and that the healing process has begun. Again, this raises the question whether this form of theodicy could still be relevant today.

Community: the church as body

Influenced by Paul's thought, Augustine was very familiar with the use of the classic image of the human body to reflect on the dynamics and relationship of the church and the world as an organic whole. The way Augustine deals with 1 Cor. 12: 12–25 is characterized by a strong emphasis on the unity of the church and society with the argument that 'we were baptized into one body in a single Spirit, Jews as well as Greeks, slaves as well as free men, and we were all given the same Spirit to drink'. Suffering and disability are reason for extra care and attention because 'when one member suffers, all members share in that suffering; if one member is honoured, all other members share in that joy'. The latter Pauline claim, implies a direct relation between the ecclesial community, as body, and Christ himself. He is the head of the body, and is mentioned in *De civitate Dei* 22.156 as the norm for the resurrected body of all human persons (Brock 2012). He is both intercessor before God the Father and Physician for the earthly sick in need. The relationship in the community is both spiritual (praying to God/Christ for healing) and material in the reciprocal care for each other.

> Paul the apostle, who knew that he belonged with all the other members to the body of the priest, does commend himself to the prayers of the Church, because *the members care for each other; and if one member is glorified, all the members rejoice with it, and if one member suffers, all the members suffer with it* (1 Cor. 12: 25–6). The head intercedes for all the members, the members should intercede for each other under the head.
>
> *(Sermo 198.57; tr. Hill. 1997: 224)*

Care and compassion for the sick acquires in this way a transcendental dimension that makes God's salvific action present in the community. It is simultaneously a source of spiritual power and tangible care for the neighbour. The practice of neighbourly love is in Augustine's sermons often an image of the individual spiritual process of growth, but also of the community as an organic whole. Hence, neighbourly love and care for the sick and the poor were closely linked to prayer and fasting (*sermones* 206–8), an integral part of mankind's (individual and collective) growth. Although Augustine's sermons show him to be an enthusiastic caretaker of souls and expositor of the Bible, the same sermons also speak of an involved leader who is never solely concerned with spiritual welfare. He regularly urges his listeners to care for the poor and the sick in the community (*sermo* 302–3). This daily lived practice of neighbourly love, *caritas*, is the sole touchstone for him of the spiritual exegesis of the Bible (*De doc. chr.* 1.27.58; 3.15.54).

Characteristic of Augustine's view of community is the almost literal interpretation of the Pauline metaphor of the spiritual body in the abovementioned letter to the Corinthians (van Bavel 1957). Community growth leads in Augustine's opinion to a growth process of increasing uniformity with the body of Christ. God's Word in the Bible and the tangible signs of the sacraments of baptism and the eucharist make these spiritual realities visual and substantial. Augustine defines that Christ includes both Christ as the *caput* and the whole *corpus*, the church, all its members. Only by incorporating all believers – the members of his body – can Christ be considered as whole, as being the *totus Christus*. The specificity of Augustine's *totus Christus* intuition is that he sees Christ identifying himself with his followers, also in their mortal and even sinful condition. *Enarratio* 142.3 states: 'Christ therefore suffers in my flesh, as it still struggles on earth'.

Augustine's use of medical terms as psychagogy

Augustine's sermons are very rhetorical. They are intended not only to please (*delectare*) and convince (*docere*) his hearers, but above all to move them (*movere*) and to bring about change in their lives (*conversio*; see Cicero, *De oratore* 27.115 for similar thought on the function of oratory). As spiritual leader, Augustine wanted to contribute through his preaching to an improvement of the quality of (Christian) life in his community. Augustine himself describes his ideal and practice of the Christian rhetor in *De doctrina Christiana* 4.

Through using medical images in a rhetorical way, Augustine chose to link up with a widespread philosophical tradition with old roots. The process of acquiring knowledge and insight was clarified in this tradition through comparing the relationship between the philosopher and the student to that of a physician and his patient. Discussions and debates in such a context have the aim of liberating the hearer from misunderstandings, incorrect insights and vices. These are considered as illnesses of the spirit that keep the listener from a virtuous attitude to life and happiness. This tradition of self-therapy through conversation with a physician goes back to ancient philosophical practices (see Hadot 1987; Nussbaum 1994; Rabbow 1954; Kolbet 2010. See also the contributions by Gevaert on the Stoa, and by Thumiger and Gourevitch on ancient medical practice in this volume).

As pulpit orator, Augustine developed within this tradition his own protreptic rhetorical style. He not only passes on knowledge and insight through his sermons, but is intent on bringing about a change in the life and thinking of his hearers. The medical terminology is helpful to activate and guide the psychological process of change, just as a doctor activates and guides the process of healing with a patient. Sermons, in his view, have a psychagogical function. Augustine considers his own sermons as a primary therapy for the healing of the soul. Not only tangible signs (sacraments), but also words and arguments have here a therapeutic function, intended to bring the listener to a change in outlook and lifestyle. Physical and mental disability are in this perspective applied to a person and community's way of life. They are the image for the actual (deficient) condition of the human person, but also refer to a perspective of hope and expectation as path and goal that can offer people encouragement.

Conclusion

In conclusion, we return to the question of the way in which Augustine's view of disability can contribute to an understanding of the social culture in patristic North Africa. What is in the first place striking in this context is that Augustine holds up the practice of the care of the sick and the poor as a touchstone for the interpretation of biblical and theological concepts such as salvation, sin and incarnation. The practice of care for one's neighbour coincides in his opinion with the process of spiritual growth that he has in mind for his community. The community is related in an organic way to the spiritual body of Christ and through its spiritual growth is becoming more and more identical with the eschatological reality of Christ. This had also its consequences for Augustine's view on human suffering as explained more elaborately in his reflections on the wounds of the martyrs and perfected resurrected human body after the model of the risen Christ in *De civitate Dei* 22. Care for one's neighbour and for the sick was therefore no ancillary activity, but was a central task of the community. Second, we have noted that the medical terminology had an important rhetorical function in Augustine's preaching. It almost always refers however to the dynamics of the spiritual process of individual and communal healing for which Augustine considers himself responsible. His preaching is rhetorically forceful and has a psychagogical character. Finally, it is evident that the organic mutual commitment was central to Augustine's view of community. From his actions and speaking as bishop, it regularly comes to the fore that he nonetheless felt himself, in his community and as person, to be strongly connected with the surrounding social and intellectual culture.

Physical and spiritual disability in Augustine's preaching are inseparably linked to human existence. Disability is in his view undesired, but inescapable for every person. Augustine preached regularly on physical and spiritual disability and he turns his reflections on these matters into an exhortation to care for one another in the daily life of the community. In his sermons the metaphorical function of physical and spiritual disability dominates. A person is for Augustine more than his physical stature but is also an intellectual and spiritual being who can be healed and can grow in wisdom and insight. He considered the latter as his most important vocation as shepherd and bishop. It will come therefore as no surprise that he devoted the greatest portion of his consideration of disability to the clarification of the human healing process as being of a spiritual nature.

Notes

1 Contra Iulianum opus imperfectum 6.16: *Necesse est enim ut doleatis, quando quid respondeatis non inuenitis et tam prauam sententiam mutare non uultis, quae uos ineuitabili necessitate compellit in loco tantae beatitudinis et pulchritudinis constituere caecos luscos lippos surdos mutos claudos deformes distortos, tineosos leprosos paralyticos epilepticos et aliis diuersis generibus uitiosos atque aliquando etiam nimia foeditate et membrorum horribili nouitate monstrosos. Quid dicam de uitiis animorum, quibus sunt quidam natura libidinosi, quidam iracundi, quidam meticulosi, quidam obliuiosi, quidam tardicordes, quidam excordes atque ita fatui ut malit homo cum quibusdam pecoribus quam cum talibus hominibus uiuere? Adde gemitus parientium fletusque nascentium, cruciatus dolentium, labores languentium, tormenta multa morientium et pericula multo plura uiuentium.* On a related note, for Augustine's thinking on deafness and muteness (e.g. in *De magistro* 3.5 and *De quantitate animae* 18.31), see King 1996 and Laes 2011; and concerning mental disabilities (esp. in his polemics with Julian of Aeclanum), see Kellenberger 2011.

2 *Infirmitas facit diu videri quod cito est. Quodomo inveniuntus desideria aegrotorum? Nihil tamdiu, quam ut calyx sitienti temperetur. Utique festinatur a suis, ne forte offendatur informus. Quando fiet? Quando coquetur? Quando dabitur? Celeritas est in illis qui tibi seruiunt, sed infirmitas tua diuturnum putat quod cito agitur.*

3 *Ante dies lectus est quidam libellus, ubi cuidam aegrotae quae doloribus acerrimis torquebatur, cum dixisset, ferre non possum; [...] Fit martyr in lecto, coronante illo qui pro illo pependit in ligno.*

4 *Sermo* 9.9 (PL 36.600): *Aegrum attendite. Aeger aegrotatem se odit qualis est: inde incipit concordare cum medico. Quia et medicus odit quam qualis est: nam ideo vult sanum esse, quia odit eum febrientem: est et medicus febris persecutor, ut sit hominis liberator.*

5 *Sermo* 5.2 (PL 38.54): *Ecce quomodo Deus diligit homines. Attendamus fratres; numquid non illos flagellat? Numquid non illos corripit? Si non illos corripit, unde fames? Unde aegritudines? Unde pestilentiae et morbi? Omnes enim istae correptiones Dei sunt.*

6 *Medicus exserit ferrum ad secandum vulnera, et dicit ei quem secturus est: Patiens esto, sustine, tolera; in doloribus exigit patientiam, sed post dolores promittit salutem.*

7 In *De civitate Dei* 22.19 Augustine illustrates his admiration for the martyrs and their testimony of faith, when he states that 'the love we bear for the blessed martyrs makes us desire to see in the kingdom of heaven the marks of the wounds which they received for Christ's name; and it may be that we shall indeed see them. For this will not be a deformity, but a badge of honor, and the beauty of their virtue – a beauty which is in the body, but not of the body – will shine forth in it ... ' For Augustine's claim that the wounds of the martyrs are healed by God in the afterlife, but remain as enduring scars to underline the identity of the martyrs, see Belser Watts 2015; Upson-Saia 2011.

8 *Medicus enim erat. et phreneticum curare venerat. Quomodo medicus non curat quidquid audiat a phrenetico, sed quomodo convalescat et fiat sanus phreneticus, nec si et pugnum ab illo accipiat curat; ille illi facit nova vulnera, ille veterem febrem sanat; sic et Dominus ad aegrotum venit, ad phreneticum venit, ut quidquid audiret, quidquid passus esset contemneret hoc ipso eos docens humilitatem, ut humilitate docti sanerentur a superbia.*

9 *Iste naturalis quidam morbus est, quia natura nobis facta est poena et vindicta, primo homini quod erat poena natura nobis est.*

10 *De civitate Dei* 22.16: *Resurgent itaque omnes tam magni corpore, quam uel erant uel futuri erant aetate iuuenali; quamuis nihil oberit, etiamsi erit infantilis uel senilis corporis forma, ubi*

nec mentis nec ipsius corporis ulla remanebit infirmitas. See also *De civitate Dei* 22.17: *Sed mihi melius sapere uidentur, qui utrumque sexum resurrecturum esse non dubitant. Non enim libido ibi erit, quae confusionis est causa. Nam priusquam peccassent, nudi erant, et non confundebantur uir et femina. Corporibus ergo illis uitia detrahentur, natura seruabitur.*

Bibliography

Translations

Augustine, *Expositions on the Psalms 33–50*, tr. Maria Boulding (New York, 2000).

Augustine, *Expositions on the Psalms 73–98*, tr. Maria Boulding (New York, 2002).

Augustine, *Homilies on the Gospel of John; Homilies on the First Epistle of John; Soliloquies.* Nicene and Post-Nicene Fathers, First Series, Vol. 7, ed. and tr. by Philip Schaff (Buffalo, NY, 1888/1991)

Augustine, *The City of God Against the Pagans*, ed. and tr. Robert W. Dyson (Cambridge, 1998).

Augustine, *Sermons (51–94) on the New Testament*, tr. Edmund Hill (New York, 1991).

Augustine, *Newly Discovered Sermons*, tr. Edmund Hill (New York, 1997).

Augustine, *Sermons (273–305A) on the Saints*, tr. Edmund Hill (New York, 1997).

Augustine, *Answer to the Pelagians*, III. *Unfinished Work in Answer to Julian*, tr. Roland J. Teske (Hyde Park, NY, 1999).

Weiskotten, Herbert Theberath, *The Life of Saint Augustine: A Translation of the Sancti Augustini Vita by Possidius Bishop of Calama* (New York, 2008).

Secondary sources

Amundsen, Darrel W., and Ferngren, Gary B., 'The Early Christian Tradition', in R. L. Numbers and D. W. Amundsen (eds), *Caring and Curing: Health and Medicine in the Western Religious Traditions* (Baltimore, MD, and London, 1986), 40–64.

André, Jean-Marie, 'Saint Augustin et la culture médicale gréco-romaine', in *La cultura scientific-naturalistica nei Padri della chiesa (I–V sec.)* (Rome, 2007), 597–604.

Arbesmann, Rudolph, 'The Concept of "Christus Medicus" in St. Augustine', *Traditio* 10 (1954), 1–28.

Bartelink, Gerard, 'Fragilitas (infirmitas) humana chez Augustin', *Augustiniana* 41 (1991), 815–28.

Belser Watts, Julia, 'Disability, Animality, and Enslavement in Rabbinic Narratives of Bodily Restoration and Resurrection', *Journal of Late Antiquity* 8/2 (2015), 288–305.

Bochet, Isabelle, 'Maladie de l'âme et thérapeutique scripturaire selon Saint Augustin', in V. Boudon-Millot and B. Pouderon (eds), *Les Pères de l'Eglise face à la science médicale de leur temps* (Paris, 2005), 379–400.

Bochet, Isabelle, 'Medicina, medicus', *Augustinus-Lexikon* 3 (2010), c. 1230–4.

Bright, Pamela (ed. and tr.), *Augustine and the Bible* (Notre Dame, IN, 1999).

Brock, Brian, 'Augustine's Hierarchies of Human Wholeness and their Healing', in B. Brock and J. Swinton (eds), *Disability in the Christian Tradition: A Reader* (Grand Rapids, MI, and Cambridge, 2012), 65–100.

Brown, Peter, *The Body and Society: Men, Woman and Sexual Renunciation in Early Christianity* (New York, 1988).

Brown, Peter, *Augustine of Hippo: A Biography* (Berkeley, CA, 1967); 2nd edn: new edn with an epilogue (London, 2000²).

Dolbeau, Francois, 'Un sermon inédit de Saint Augustin sur la santé corporelle partiellement cite chez Barthélemy d'Urbino', *Revue des Etudes Augustinienne* 40 (1994), 279–303.

Dörnemann, Michael, *Krankheit und Heilung in der Theologie der frühen Kirchenväter* (Tübingen, 2003).

Doucet, Dominique, 'Le thème du médicin dans les premiers dialogues philosophiques de Saint Augustin', *Augustiniana* 39 (1989), 447–64.

Dupont, Anthony, '*Imitatio Christi, Imitatio Stephani.* Augustine's Thinking on Martyrdom Based on his Sermons on the Protomartyr Stephen', *Augustiniana* 56/1–2 (2006), 29–61.

Dupont, Anthony, *Gratia in Augustine's Sermones ad Populum during the Pelagian Controversy* (Leiden, 2012).

Eijkenboom, Petrus Cornelis Josephus, *Het Christus-Medicusmotief in de preken van Sint Augustinus* (Assen, 1960).

Ferngren, Gary B., and Amundsen, Darrel W., 'Medicine and Christianity in the Roman Empire: Compatibilities and Tension', *ANRW* II/37/3 (1996), 2957–80.

Griffith, Susan, 'Medical Imagery in the New Sermons of Augustine', *Studia Patristica* 43 (2006), 107–12.

Hadot, Pierre, *Exercises spirituels et philosophie antique* (Paris, 1987).

Honecker, Martin, 'Christus medicus', *Kerygma und Dogma* 31 (1985), 307–23.

Kellenberger, Edgar, 'Augustin und die Menschen mit einer geistigen Behinderung: Der Theologe als Beobachter und Herausgeforderter', *Theologische Zeitschrift* 67 (2011), 25–36.

King, Lesley A., '*Surditas*: The Understandings of the Deaf and Deafness in the Writing of Augustine, Jerome and Bede' (unpublished PhD, Boston University, 1996).

Kolbet, Paul, *Augustine and the Cure of the Souls: Revising a Classical Ideal* (Notre Dame, IN, 2010).

Kuuliala, Jenni, Krötzl, Christian, and Mustakallio, Katariina, 'Introduction: *Infirmitas* in Antiquity and the Middle Ages', in C. Krötzl, K. Mustakallio and J. Kuuliala (eds), *Infirmity in Antiquity and the Middle Ages: Social and Cultural Approaches to Health, Weakness and Care* (Farnham, 2015), 1–15.

Laes, Christian, 'Silent Witnesses: Deaf-Mutes in Graeco-Roman Antiquity', *Classical World* 104/4 (2011), 451–73.

Laes, Christian, Goodey, Chris F., and Rose, Martha Lynn, 'Approaching Disabilities *a capite ad calcem*: Hidden Themes in Roman Antiquity', in C. Laes, C. F. Goodey and M. L. Rose (eds), *Disabilities in Roman Antiquity: Disparate Bodies A Capite ad Calcem* (Leiden, 2013), 1–16.

Lancel, Serge, *Saint Augustin* (Paris, 1999).

Nussbaum, Martha C., *The Therapy of Desire: Theory and Practice in Hellenistic Ethics* (Princeton, NJ, 1994).

Nutton, Vivian, 'Physiologia from Galen to Jacob Bording', in M. Horstmanshoff, H. King and C. Zittel (eds), *Blood, Sweat and Tears: The Changing Concepts of Physiology from Antiquity into Early Modern Europe* (Leiden and Boston, MA, 2012), 27–40.

Pollmann, Karla, and Otten, Willemien (eds), *The Oxford Guide to the Historical Reception of Augustine*, 3 vols (Oxford, 2013).

Rabbow, Paul, *Seelenführung. Methodik der Exerzitien in der Antike* (Munich, 1954).

Rassinier, Jean-Paul, 'Le vocabulaire médical de Saint Augustin: Approche quantitative et qualitative', in G. Sabbah (ed.), *Le latin médical : La constitution d'un language scientifique* (Saint-Etienne, 1991), 380–2.

Rist, John, *Augustine: Ancient Thought Baptized* (Cambridge, 1994).

Upson-Saia, Kristi, 'Resurrecting Deformity: Augustine on Wounded and Scarred Bodies in the Heavenly Realm', in D. Schumm and M. Stoltzfus (eds), *Disability in Judaism, Christianity, and Islam: Sacred Texts, Historical Traditions, and Social Analysis* (New York, 2011), 93–122.

van Bavel, Tars, 'L'humanité du Christ comme "lac parvulorum" et comme "via" dans la spiritualité du Saint Augustin', *Augustiniana* 7 (1957), 245–81.

van der Meer, Frits, *Augustine the Bishop: The Life and Work of a Father of the Church* (London, 1961).

24

INFIRMITAS IN MONASTIC RULES

Jenni Kuuliala

Introduction

During late Antiquity, with the rise of Christianity, asceticism started to gain increasing popularity as an alternative lifestyle, vocation, and family strategy. From the 3rd century CE, monasticism had a great influence on the shaping of the new religious and intellectual culture of Europe. The early monasteries, first in Egypt and later elsewhere, became centres for healing, and they had important roles in the economy of their areas (see e.g. Crislip 2005: esp. 1-38; Dunn 2003; Harmless 2004; Kardong 2010; Layton, 2014; Leyerle and Young 2013; de Vogüé 1991-2008; Vuolanto 2015).

The most defining factor of the monastic lifestyle was the dedication of one's time and thoughts to following God, and the growing popularity of monasticism provided an alternative lifestyle in a very tangible way. Before Christianity, the idea of deliberately or decisively staying unmarried was not a valid life-choice, but once the ascetic lifestyle started to gain ground in the contemporary culture, it spread quickly and became institutionalized in the monastic regulations of the late ancient and early medieval orders. The rules moderated the extremes of ascetic lifestyle, stressing work, prayer and order (see e.g. Elm 1994: 2–3; Risse 1999: 91–2). Choosing life in a monastic order – or making an oblation of a child to one – can also be seen as a family decision, tradition or even survival strategy, securing memory, God's grace or spiritual and bodily protection (see Vuolanto 2005: 120–2, 2015; Jong 1996).

It is impossible to know how often people chose monastic lifestyle or became oblates because of – at least in part – health problems, or as a result of difficulties in secular life, whether in work or in marriage prospects, as hinted at by Jerome, who complained about parents dedicating their 'deformed and crippled daughters' (*deformes et aliquo membro debiles filias*) to virginity (Hieron, *Ep.* 130.6; see also Laes 2013). Presumably, however, the monastery was also considered a shelter during periods of infirmity caused by old age, illness or impairments. Moreover, those already living in monastic communities would likely acquire impairments or suffer illnesses at some time in their life.

As the early monastic communities were searching for their path and grew in popularity they needed to find ways to regulate their communal lifestyle. In this the care of the *infirmi* was of crucial importance, regardless of whether those affected by illness or impairments had acquired their health issues before or after taking their vows.

This chapter focuses on monastic rules from the late 4th to the early 7th centuries. These texts have received substantial academic interest for several decades, and their origins, influence and transmission have been analysed by several scholars. It is not my intention to join in that discussion, which has been undertaken by those better qualified, but to focus on one particular set of aspects of the early monastic rules: their ideas, views and advice offered about the *infirmi*. Infirmity here treated excludes self-afflicted ailments; austerity, fasting and abstinence are discussed only when relevant to the caretaking of the infirm. The main emphasis is on the most widespread rules with the greatest impact on western monasticism, but other early rules will be referred to when appropriate.[1] First we will discuss how the status, care and concessions of the *infirmi* were arranged and regulated, and secondly analyse how these rules relate to the discussion of bodily impairments in late Antiquity.

Caring for the infirm

The ancient and early medieval monastic rules focus on the harmony of communal lifestyle. One of the most influential, and one of the 'original' rules, known as the *Asketikon*, was written by St Basil the Great or Basil of Caesarea (330–79) in the 370s. The rule differs stylistically from the others, for instead of being a rulebook, it consists of a list of questions and answers, distributed into long responses (hereafter LR) and short responses (hereafter SR), many of which concern the scriptures (Kardong 2010: pp. xi, xiii, 1–14; Clarke 1913). Although Basil is a more influential figure in the eastern church, his rule was important in the development of western monasticism. St Benedict of Nursia (c.480–547), whose rule became the most definitive from the Carolingian period until the early twelfth century and beyond, is therefore also the best-studied figure (see esp. Elm 1994: 8–10; Moyse 1982; de Vogüé 1971, 1977, 1985, 1991). St Benedict recommends Basil's *Asketikon* to be read for topics over which his authority does not extend (*Regula Benedicti* 73.5). Basil stresses the importance of living together with other brothers to facilitate everyday physical necessities but also because the Gospels state that we should care for other people. Following the right path was also easier as a community (Kardong 2010: 38; *Asketikon* LR 3.59–67, 7.1–37). St Augustine of Hippo, who in c.395 wrote another set of rules greatly shaping western monasticism,[2] specifies that the purpose of those coming to live together is to live harmoniously, intent upon God, and with one heart and one soul. The common good takes over the individual good, and the individual good profits the common good (*Praeceptum* 1.2–3, 5.2). This is in accordance with his other opinions concerning the communal nature of Christianity, and the other rules present similar ideas (Kardong 2010: 176–7; Puzicha 1990: 31). Those choosing the monastic lifestyle were supposed to give away everything they owned and fully yield to the community and the authority of the abbot or abbess. This did not, however, mean that the individual would be forgotten. St Benedict stresses the importance of obedience and communality, attempting to eliminate the excessive individualism of earlier asceticism. At the same time, the rule is thoroughly considerate towards the needs of an individual monk, which benefited the common good (see e.g. de Dreuille 2000: 120–130).

The idea of working for the common good and for Christ himself is distinctively present in the rules concerning the treatment of the *infirmi*. St Basil mostly concentrates on how those presiding should take care so that the infirm do not view their situation as an excuse for enslaving themselves to pleasures, but instead to use their circumstances to grow as lovers of God and Christ, and their love perfected through patience (*Asketikon* SR 160). In the later rules, the focus changes (de Vogüé 1971: 1087). The anonymous early 5th-century author of the Rule of the Master states that the brothers who want to show that they are charitable should console and serve the infirm, showing them brotherly love.[3] The passage refers to the famous paragraph of the acts of mercy in Matthew

25: 36, *infirmus fui et visitatis me*, and appears in an almost identical form in *Regula Benedicti* and in works that cite it, which additionally refer to Matthew 25: 40: *Quod fecistis uni de his minimis mihi fecistis.*[4] The Master addresses the chapter to healthy individuals, all of whom should visit the ill as an act of mercy. For Benedict, however, the citation from Matthew is a 'scriptural evidence of two axioms' – the care of the sick must come first, and they must be served like Christ (de Vogüé 1971, 1976: 1080–1). Equally, the 7th-century *Regula Cuiusdam ad Virgines* (PL 88.1065) expresses compassion for the infirm by stating that they must lack nothing, as they are already carrying the *poena* in their infirm flesh (on the rule, see Diem 2011).

Charity towards the sick was an important religio-cultural idea that had started to gain more ground with the rise of Christianity, into which monastics most likely were socialized before entering a monastery. The concept became more regulated especially under the Benedictine rule (Crislip 2005: 69–70). Some, though not all later rules, repeat Benedict's statement verbatim, and the view is reflected clearly in the ways they address the caretaking of *infirmi*. As an example, St Donatus of Besançon's (d. 660) 7th-century rule, which is largely based on Benedict and has been called the 'oldest witness to the text' (Diem 2012: 4–5), takes this aspect directly from him (Donatus of Besançon, *Regula ad Virgines* PL 87.276 and 279). After all, by 600, Pope Gregory I was promoting Benedict's rule as the basis for all monastic communities, and the rules written during that time include many of its key elements, combining them with passages and ideas from other rules (McNamara *et al.* 1996: 9–10).

When addressing the treatment of those in ill-health, the rules usually refer to *infirmi* or *egrotantes*, only occasionally giving further instructions regarding different types of conditions or defining someone as *infirmus*. In the Pachomian system and in Shenoute's 5th-century White Monastery, the elders and the overseers were responsible for the initial diagnosis, which included distinguishing between a real and a feigned illness (*Pachomia Latina*, ch. 40),[5] and similar practices likely existed in other monastic communities (cf. Gourevitch in this volume). In the *Rule of the Four Fathers* (11.15–18), written by the founders of the Lérins monastery in c.410, for example, it is specified that those presiding are to make the decisions about the caretaking of the infirm. St Augustine advises that one should take complaints about bodily pain seriously (*Praeceptum* 5.6), which presumably results from failures in providing for those who complained because of suspicions of malingering (Crislip 2005: 88–9). *Regula Magistri* takes an entirely different approach: the chapter on brothers who are ill is mostly concerned about spotting the ones who are feigning their maladies (de Vogüé 1971: 1076). Those feigning illness were to be put on a strict diet that was hard to swallow, so that hunger would make them give up their pretence (*Regula Magistri* 69.1–4). For the Master, fever seems to be an indicator of the severity of a condition, and in this way, his opinion differs from that of Augustine, who writes that the care of the sick and the convalescing shall be assigned to someone who can personally obtain from the storeroom what they need 'even though they are not running a fever' (*Praeceptum* 5.8).

The harsh tone of the Master's text (see e.g. Kardong 1996: 306) is justified, according to Adalbert de Vogüé (1971: 1076–7), by its views concerning obligatory work and prayer, also echoing primitive Christian ideas concerning hospitals and their guests. In any case, the 'illness' these brothers had was of a spiritual nature (Yearl 2007: 182). Nothing in the corresponding part of Benedict's rule refers to the Master's concern with feigning illnesses (*Regula Benedicti* 52–3). Concerning the authority of Benedict's rule, his view most likely was more important for the everyday experience of the *infirmi*. There is, however, later evidence of how the problem of feigning an illness was handled in a monastic setting, so the topic continued to be of some importance. It was ordered in the monastery of Cluny, founded in 910, that if someone in the infirmary got caught in 'idle talk' and thus likely did not feel ill, he would face corporal punishment (Yearl 2007: 189).

Perhaps the greatest invention of early monasticism concerning the *infirmi* was the infirmaries.[6] The earliest known reference to a monastic infirmary comes from the Greek *Life of Pachomius* from c.324. Apparently, in those times the infirmaries were spatially removed from the rest of the community, in order to keep what was happening in them out of the sight of healthy monastics (Crislip 2005: 11–12; *Pachomia Latina*, ch. 5). St Basil's rule also discusses the hospice and whether or not people with bodily infirmities should be transferred there (*Asketikon* SR 286, 430, SR 155). These hospices could be maintained by the community itself, and therefore the question could refer to transferring a chronically ill brother or sister from 'inside' the community to a church-sponsored hospice 'outside' (*Asketikon* 430, n. 759). Augustine does not offer much guidance on the physical surroundings of the infirm. St Caesarius of Arles, however, who wrote the first rule specifically addressed to female monastics in 512, was largely influenced by Augustine, and another, more impersonal rule for monks (Clark 1983: 141; de Vogüé and Correau 1988: esp. 43–5, 47–8, 68–70), instructs that the needs of those who 'are truly old and infirm' (*vero senes sunt et infirmae*) should be provided for in one room instead of giving them private, partitioned rooms. He allowed them, however, to have a separate pantry and kitchen, if the abbess judged it necessary (Caesarius of Arles, *Statuta Sanctarum Virginum* 9.1–3, 32.1–4). There is the possibility that Caesarius' writings echo the idea that one's infirmity had to be 'real' before receiving special treatment. Caesarius borrows from the Pachomian rule, promoting the idea that nobody was allowed to choose his room, just as nobody was allowed to choose his work. The views also reflect the rule's general tendency to emphasize female monastic enclosure (Caesarius of Arles, *Statuta Sanctarum Virginum* 187, n. 9; Diem 2102: 30–1; Diem 2014: 197, 199–200; Foot 2000; Schulenburg 1984).

Benedict also instructs that a specific *cella* must be reserved for the *infirmi* (*Regula Benedicti* 36.7), which Adalbert de Vogüé (1971: 1090) reads to imply that the Benedictine infirmaries were more sophisticated than those of Augustine. After the monastic writings of the 4th-century Egyptian coenobitic communities, the Benedictine rule is indeed the most detailed one concerning the care of the sick and the fraternal relations among those taking care of them. This has been seen as an inspiration that transformed Benedictine monasteries 'into some of the most important centres driving progress in medical science' (d'Aronco 2007: 235), and influenced the organization of the infirmaries in other monastic communities, which borrowed from his rule. As an example of this, St Donatus and the writer of *Regula Cuiusdam ad Virgines* also mandate that the *infirmi* must each be given a *cella* of his own (Donatus of Besançon, *Regula ad Virgines* PL 87.279; *Regula Cuiusdam ad Virgines* PL 88.1065).

Another practical aspect of caretaking was the regulations concerning those nursing the infirm, often the cellarers (Crislip 2005: 17). The western rules give them, relatively, a lot of attention, focusing on some of their tasks and the required characteristics. For Augustine, their most important task was to obtain from the pantry what is necessary, and he further states that the ones in charge of the pantry should serve the others with no grumbling (*Praeceptum* 5.8–9). Similarly, one of the Lerinian works, *Regula Orientalis* (25.8–9), from the late 400s, emphasizes that the cellarer must provide the infirm everything they need. Instead of concentrating on attitudes towards ill-health, as in St Basil's *Asketikon*, Benedict focuses on the relations between the patients and those nursing them (de Vogüé 1971: 1084–5). Because taking care of the *infirmi* is to be done in a manner honouring God, the abbot must take care that they lack nothing, and they must be placed in the care of a God-fearing and attentive brother. The infirm themselves are in turn not supposed to strain those taking care of them with vain demands (*Regula Benedicti* 36.7). These views are repeated in other rules. Quoting Augustine, Caesarius of Arles writes that the sick and the feeble should be placed in the care of a devoted and remorseful sister who is able to serve the ill with kindness (Caesarius of Arles,

Statuta Sanctarum Virginum 32.1–2; see also Donatus of Besançon, *Regula ad Virgines* PL 87.279; *Regula Cuiusdam ad Virgines* PL 88.1057).

Medicine and treatment

There is evidence of controversies regarding 'secular' medical care in the 4th-century Egyptian and Cappadocian monasteries, where some monastics and ascetics refused to practise such treatment, and criticized it. This prompted St Basil to write the longest chapter of his rule about medical care (see Crislip 2005: 26–8; Yearl 2007: 181–2). Basil wrote in favour of Hippocratic/ Galenic medicine: because our bodies are prone to suffering, medical art is permitted by God. He also combined the discussion about the primary reasons for bodily afflictions with the justification for medicine. The fall resulted in bodily pain, but humankind was also provided help, in some measures at least, as he adds, by the art of medicine. (*Asketikon* LR 55.1). This is an important viewpoint concerning the question of infirmity in monasteries and in the late antique world at large. The issue is addressed further elsewhere (cf. Efthymiadis in this volume). Here it is sufficient to say that although many late antique writers were of the opinion that sin was the cause of bodily suffering, and used this concept in their *exempla* and other texts (Laes 2011a: 44–6), this did not result in general ill-treatment of the infirm. Bodily conditions were a burden of the *whole* mankind, a part of our shared defectiveness. The infirm were not held responsible for their bodily conditions, nor were they responsible for their recovery. Those matters belonged to the whole community (see also Crislip 2005: 75).

In his more practical advice on medical care, Basil makes some distinction between acute and chronic conditions, which is exceptional in the rules. He states that, especially in the case of chronic conditions, when varying and painful treatments are being sought, one should 'amend the sins of the soul' by prayers and repentance. Moreover, he warns against trusting in doctors too much, and gives advice on infirmities caused by various factors. Medicine may be useful for conditions caused by faulty lifestyle or with other bodily origins, but not for the ones that are due to sin. Here Basil refers to the statement in Proverbs 3.12 that God chastises those he loves, and to 1 Corinthians 11: 30–2, according to which we are chastened by the Lord so that we may not be condemned along with the world (*Asketikon* LR 55.3–5).

Basil's opinions on medicine are exceptionally detailed in comparison to the rules written after his time, which mainly address the question of bathing. Augustine's rule is relatively liberal in this respect, stressing the importance of good monastic hygiene and health, even allowing the monks to go to public baths, albeit in groups. He continues by warning that if a person with bodily pain desires treatment, a physician should be consulted if there is any doubt about the treatment's benefits. Even if the sick person did not want to bathe, the physician's advice must be followed (*Praeceptum* 5.5–7). Although the two recensions of Augustine's rule (those addressed to monks and nuns) do not differ significantly from each other concerning nursing the infirm, the passage on bathing in *Regula Benedicti* (36.8) appears to be inspired precisely by the female version of Augustine's rule, stating that a bath is to be prepared daily for the infirm and more rarely for the young and the healthy (de Vogüé 1971: 1089–90). Caesarius of Arles (*Statuta Sanctarum Virginum* 31.1–3) specifies that one must bathe when the physician so orders, even if the patient herself is against the idea. If the infirmity does not require bathing, then it is not permitted. Donatus of Besançon's *Regula ad Virgines* (PL 87.279–80), which combined the Benedictine rule and that of Caesarius with Columbanian ideals (Diem 2012: 10–13), repeats these principles.

The attention paid to bathing in the monastic rules is a well-known consequence of the earlier bathing culture and the suspicions the early Christian writers had towards it. Bathing, an essential element of Greco-Roman medicine and lifestyle, came to indicate *luxuria*, evidencing carnal love and softness, which, interestingly, did not prevent the early bishops from building private baths (Rapp 2005: 210 – on bathing, see e.g. Fagan 2002; Yegül 2009; Zytka 2013). The ascetics could even strive to avoid washing themselves altogether, and illness could be used as an ascetic practice in which one refused treatment (Coon 2011: 121; Crislip 2005: 92–9, 2013: 62–3). In terms of the views on bathing, all of the rules were unanimous in that the sick and infirm were allowed and even required to bathe if the physician so advised. This is one of the instances where the rules clearly state the responsibilities of the *infirmi*. Alongside the idea that they must not burden their caregivers, succumbing to treatment only reluctantly was no better, as it weakened the communal spirit. Gaining health benefited both the individual and the community.

Diet and concessions

In addition to obedience and communality, the monastic rules overall emphasize poverty, which was one of the keystones of monasticism, having its basis in the Bible and in the apocryphal *Acts of Thomas*, first adopted by the early ascetics (Allen *et al.* 2009; Brown 2002: esp. 36–42; Carner 2002: 57–81, 120–53; Maxwell 2006: 69–74, 127–8, 132–3). In their discussions of poverty, the rules stress the idea that everyone should get provisions based on their individual needs, albeit always supervised by the abbot or abbess (*Praeceptum* 1.5; *Regula Benedicti* 34.1; *Regula Orientalis* 39.2; Caesarius of Arles, *Statuta Sanctarum Virginum* 28.1–4). Therefore, the special needs of the infirm – usually including also children and those affected by old age – were recognized. This also pertains to the monastic diet and meat consumption, one of the most regulated aspects of the monastic lifestyle, and the one in which the *infirmi* were most frequently given concessions, although the rules do not specify how diets for specific infirmities and illnesses were determined (Bazell 1999: 186–9; Crislip 2005: 30, 74–5; Schulenburg 1998: 374–89; Harlow and Smith 2001; Zimmermann 1973). This is specified, for example, in *Regula Cuiusdam ad Virgines* (PL 88.1062), which states that everyone should be given an equal amount of food, except those weakened by age or by bodily illness, and those new to monastic life.

The ideological background for the importance of diet lies in the ideas about discipline of the human body, which had been expressed already by the early ascetics. The body had to be humbled by praying, vigils, fasting and physical labour, because it was involved in the soul's transformation (Risse 1999: 75). As mentioned above, however, the monastic rules, although sharing the same background, aimed at regulating these practices. The possibility of bodily infirmity played an important role here as a basis for some of the regulations. Fasting was important, but only to the point one's health permitted. Augustine specified that the sick (*aegroti*) were allowed to take food in between meals. Understanding everyone's needs was important within the community: if one is treated differently because of health affected by a former lifestyle, others should not be annoyed by the discrepancy. Those who can get along with less should feel grateful (*Praeceptum* 3.1, 3).

Both the Master (*Regula Magistri* 28.13–26) and Benedict (*Regula Benedicti* 37.1–3) also regulate dietary allowances. The Master allows the *infirmi* to break the fast because their bodily weakness (*fragilitatem corporis*) prevents them from doing what they want, for 'the spirit is willing, but the flesh is weak' (Matt. 26: 41). Thus, the *infirmi* were not to be blamed for their specific needs, but the Master also warns against feigning infirmity out of the desire for a meal. The Master and Benedict give similar allowances for children and those weakened by old age (Clark 2011: 118–19), whereas Donatus of Besançon, who had a somewhat more flexible attitude towards fasting, did not (Diem 2012: 17). Commonly the rules forbidding meat consumption allowed it for the infirm in order to improve their state, which further underlines the practical take on the religious aspects of health (e.g. Aurelian of Arles, *Regula ad Monachos*

PL 68.393–4, Aurelian of Arles, *Regula Virgines* PL 68.403–4). *Regula Benedicti* (36.9, 39.11) specifies that this exception pertains only to the very weak (*infirmis omnino debilibus, omnino debiles aegrotos*), making a rare categorization of different levels of infirmity and their special treatment. The writer's background might influence these usually unanimous views: *Regula Coenobialis* (PL 80.210–211) of St Columbanus (d. 615), influenced by the ascetic spirituality of early Irish Christianity (Clark 2011: 19), forbade meat to anybody, because giving up the abstinence would only lead to vice, whereas his contemporary Donatus let the abbess decide (Donatus of Besançon, *Regula ad Virgines* PL 87.280). Even Columbanus's *Regula Coenobialis* (PL 80.222), however, made allowances for the *infirmi* concerning abstinence.

Similarly, the needs the infirm had for wine were taken into account. The daily portion in Benedict's rule (*Regula Benedicti* 40.3) was such that it would be sufficient for them, and Caesarius of Arles (*Statuta Sanctarum Virginum* 30.7) specifies that it is the abbess's duty to distribute the rarely available good wine to the infirm and to those with more refined educations. Augustine, whose views Caesarius follows, parallels the infirm equally with those weakened by the comforts of their earlier life (*Praeceptum* 5.4–5). Those unable to tolerate the prescribed abstinence were to be treated with understanding, but the goal was a situation in which such allowances were unnecessary. Although the infirm monks and nuns were not considered to be responsible for their condition, on the ideological level, bodily weakness could secure a more comfortable lifestyle, but it prevented one from fully pursuing the monastic ideals.

Labour

When the monastic system developed, work and worship became the most institutionalized characteristics of the new lifestyle. Manual labour was vital for providing for the monastery, albeit less so in the case of the Merovingian female communities possibly sustained by outsiders (Diem 2012: 12–13). It also served an important spiritual purpose (Crislip 2005: 71–2), preventing idleness, which, as formulated by Benedict, is the enemy of the soul (*Regula Benedicti* 48.1; *Asketikon* SR 69; Clark 2011: 105). Manual work and worship overlap in the rules, especially concerning the treatment of the *infirmi*. Already by the time of the early Egyptian communities, allowances were being made for the infirm regarding attending the oratories and performing manual labour. The sick were not stigmatized for their inabilities, nor pushed to meet the obligations of monastic worship (Crislip 2005: 71–4). Of the later rules, the Master's daily programme is subordinated to the spiritual life. At the same time, in Benedict's rule the work of the infirm is discussed in the chapter about manual labour and *lectio divina*, omitting the hours of the office (de Vogüé 1971: 590–604; Murphy 2013). The question of the work of the *infirmi* intermingles with their attending the *lectio divina* and, though not explicitly remarked, presumably also with the liturgy of the hours.

The topic of *infirmitas* and religious service is briefly addressed in the Master's advice on detecting the fraudulent monastics. If a brother complaining about pain without fever wanted to avoid excommunication, he had to attend the oratories regularly, although allowed to do so on a mattress. If he did not go to work but attended the orations, he would escape excommunication, though he would get a smaller daily ration than those working (*Regula Magistri* 69.9–11). As for manual labour, the Master further states that the 'delicate fathers and the infirm' (*fratribus delicatis et infirmis*) must be given work that helps them to serve God and does not kill (*non occidantur*) them (*Regula Magistri* 50.75). The Benedictine rule also specifies that the infirm or delicate brothers must be given such occupation that they are not overwhelmed or tempted to leave because of it (*ut nec otiose sint nec uiolentia laboris opprimantur aut effugentur*) (*Regula Benedicti* 48.24), being also concerned with the morale of the infirm and the possible effects of working too hard (de Vogüé 1971: 1122–3). Both writers are in accordance about the work of the *infirmi*, concluding the respective chapters with a pronouncement similar to that concerning the fasting of the young: the abbot must take their weakness into account (*Regula Magistri* 28.26, 50.78; *Regula Benedicti* 37.2, 48.25). As pointed out by de Vogüé (1971: 1117–19), here again both writers associate weakness with children, the old and the infirm. Concerning the early Egyptian regulations, Andrew Crislip (2005: 71–2) writes that the exceptions concerning manual labour and 'God's work' did not only pertain to the acutely ill, but also to those with chronic conditions. The same can be said about the rules of the Master and Benedict, who also take the 'delicate' brothers into account.

An interesting set of rules by the Master and Benedict concerns the work of those whose intellectual capacities were not up to the requirements of reading. The former (*Regula Magistri* 50.75–6) writes that brothers who are 'hard-headed' and simple (*duricordes vero et simplices*) and therefore cannot or do not want to learn their letters, should be given large tasks, albeit with moderation. Interestingly, Benedict states that if someone is so indifferent and idle that he does not want to or cannot meditate or read (*ita neglegens et desidiosus fuerit ut non vellit aut non possit meditare aut legere*), he must be given other work (*Regula Benedicti* 48.23). While the Master therefore considers the illiteracy of such monks more a weakness than a flaw, Benedict views their illiteracy in harsher tones, being mainly concerned over the dangers of idleness (de Vogüé 1971: 1120–3). *Lectio divina* was a vital religious practice and keystone of monastic life, underlined in *Regula Benedicti*, which perhaps explains the tone of the rule. This aspect of work tailored to inabilities may have been gender-specific as well as prone to change over time. As discussed by Albrecht Diem (2012: 19–20), in Donatus of Besançon's rule literacy already had a different role. It does not mean that nuns' reading skills would have disappeared (see e.g. McKitterick 1994), but rather that learning and literacy were privileges or even duties of the elite, presumably concerning mostly those entering the monastery early enough to be suitably educated. Therefore, it is possible that in their context illiteracy was not viewed as problematic in the same way Benedict perceived it to be. In the Master's and Benedict's rules, the word *infirmi* is not used for the illiterate, but from the monastic/religious point of view, the physically weak were more 'able' than the illiterate – perhaps even less 'disabled'. This concept will be discussed in the remaining pages of this chapter.

Monastic infirmity and disability

Thus far I have consciously avoided using the word 'disability'. The term, and its modern sociological and political connotations also promoted by the World Health Organization, would have been completely alien to the writers of the early monastic rules. The same obviously pertains to all pre-modern eras and writers, as recently discussed by several scholars (see e.g. Kuuliala *et al.* 2015; Laes *et al.*, 2013a; Metzler 2006: 2–3; Rose 2003: 1–3). The most accepted and employed theory of 'disability', the social model, rests on the idea that bodily or mental impairment (another modern, highly ambivalent term) leads to the disablement of the individual within any given society and its discriminating attitudes and preferences (Linton 1998; on criticism e.g. Shakespeare 2006). As in other ancient and medieval texts, so the monastic rules usually use the word *infirmus* when discussing situations we might label as disability, but the term could refer to conditions of illnesses of various aetiologies. There was variation in the terminology, though: *infirmus* could be replaced with *aegroti*, 'sick', and sometimes the writers talk about 'bodily fragility' (*fragilitatem corporis*) or *imbecillitate*. Often these terms were used synonymously. Can we, then, read a discourse on 'disability' in these texts?

In his innovative analysis on the 'sick role' in early Egyptian coenobitic monasticism, Andrew Crislip concludes that the sick monastics were not held responsible for their conditions, and they were not expected to recover on their own except in the case of illnesses of demonic origin. The Egyptian writers even outspokenly condemned those scorning the sick, which presumably also included chronic or permanent infirmities. However, the need of help to convalesce justified the access to benefits and behavioural exemptions (Crislip 2005: 76–8, 89–90, 179, n. 55). Although such statements do not appear verbatim in the other rules under scrutiny here, the importance of high-quality treatment of the *infirmi* is emphasized by the demand for diligent caretaking in the name of God and Christ. The rules portray infirmity as a matter-of-fact state of human existence that had to be handled in a manner that would honour God and benefit the whole community. In this light, one can hardly read the infirm as systematically 'disabled' by their communities. After all, physical pain was not something that a human could avoid (see Cohen 2010: 228), hence neither were the functional limitations it could bring about.

The rules do stress the importance of convalescence, however, and allowances were often made with this goal in mind. As stated by Augustine, the *infirmi* should return to their 'happier ways' *(feliciorem consuetudinem)* after fully recovering. He is referring to the general monastic lifestyle but also explains how these ways are better for God's servants as it means that they need less *(Praeceptum* 3.5, 3.18). The idea was repeated by Caesarius of Arles in *Statuta Sanctarum Virginum* (22.3–4), and in his much briefer *Regula Monachorum* (17.1) Caesarius, as well as his contemporary Aurelian of Arles's *Regula ad Virgines* (PL 68.403), instructed that the *infirmi* must be treated in a way that will facilitate their rapid convalescence. Benedict shared Augustine's view in his discussion of the dietary allowances *(Regula Benedicti* 36.9). These statements present the authors' concern that bodily infirmity could prevent the monastics from fulfilling their social and religious roles, both by being a physical obstacle and by tempting the monk or nun to succumb to a worldly and comfortable lifestyle – this perhaps being the most serious impediment physical infirmity could produce. As discussed by Riccardo Cristiani (2003: 20–9), when regulating the treatment of the monastics who violated the rule, the writers frequently use vocabulary related to infirmity. The wrongdoer was often 'infirm' or 'sick', and the abbot or abbess was a physician, whose task was to provide *medicamina*. Although the infirm were not blamed for their conditions, the connection of bodily suffering and sin remained prevalent, even if in the background.[7]

The fulfilment of social expectations in one's social sphere has been seen as one of the aspects defining 'disability' in pre-modern societies. This was, however, highly dependent on social status and also gender, although the latter may have had less significance in the monastic setting, where procreation and supporting a family were not issues. What was a disability for one person was not for another, and people from different social groups required different skills and abilities (see e.g. Laes 2011b; Trentin 2013). What is equally essential when discussing the 'disability' of bodily infirmity in early monastic rules is the wide spectrum of bodily conditions to which the rules most likely referred. They caused different symptoms; some were temporal; some were chronic; some were fatal; others resulted in relapse or in remission: each brought a unique challenge to the infirm monastic's life.

The allowances provided for the *infirmi* may have led to the need for distinction among infirmities, as presented by the Master, but few of the rules make any categorizations by the duration of an infirmity. Andrew Crislip writes that the 'temporary nature of the sick role is implicit' in the sources. Yet the length of time needed to convalesce was not mentioned, and according to Crislip, the convalescence of those with chronic conditions was regulated differently than those with passing illnesses. Those with chronic conditions, however, received care, and their stigmatization was condemned (Crislip 2005: 81–4, 182 n. 82). Crislip is referring here mostly to the Pachomian dietary regulations to support his argument, as well as to the writings concerning scorn mentioned above. The difficulty with this kind of an approach, however, especially concerning the relatively short rules under scrutiny here, is the lack of exact medical vocabulary. At the same time, many milder chronic conditions, such as indistinct mobility impairments, would hardly show in the monastic regulations in any case. What counted as (temporary) sickness and what a chronic condition in late Antiquity does not conform to our often wavering modern diagnostic techniques, where many conditions are labelled as both disabilities and illnesses. It is thus reasonable to expect that the chronic nature of infirmity was fluid and negotiable, although ultimately defined by the abbot or abbess. After all, cure was equally a communal matter (Horn 2013). Occasionally the rules do, however, specify that the regulations concern *both* (temporarily) sick people and otherwise weak people. Augustine's categorization, where he addresses the chapter on the care of the infirm to concern those who are 'sick, whether recovering from illness, or having any feebleness, also without fever' (*aegrotantium cura, sive post aegritudinem reficiendorum, sive aliqua imbecillitate, etiam sine febribus laborantium*) (*Praeceptum* 5.8–9, repeated in Caesarius of Arles, *Statuta Sanctarum Virginum* 32.1) is illuminating from this point of view, for the word *imbecillitate* can be interpreted to concern all kinds of debilitating bodily conditions. Similarly, St Basil's discussion on the human body's vulnerability to suffering is revealing. He set the example for the later (Benedictine) communities by stating the idea that bearing chronic conditions could serve as an example for those who do not endure any adversity, and in the case of saints, the purpose of illness was to demonstrate their human nature (*Asketikon* LR 55.3–5).

When it comes to everyday practices and views, monastic rules – like normative sources in general – are tricky. In addition to our ignorance concerning the usage of the less-known ones, the texts do not reveal the actual reasons behind many of the guidelines. For example, was the caretaking of the *infirmi* and their special allowances delineated because the communities were unwilling to endure this task, or did the infirm themselves continue refusing treatment? Why do the rules only handle quite a small portion of the different aspects of the allowances and caretaking, and why do some of them omit the topic altogether? Albrecht Diem has pointed out that monastic rules must be read against each other instead of by a synthetic approach, as the latter does not do justice to the source evidence or the dynamics of early medieval monasticism. Furthermore, although the Benedictine rule became the definitive one, in the course of the 6th and 7th centuries there was, especially in the Columbian communities, discussion over whether or not it should even become a part of their programme (Diem 2012: 10, 36–8). There are indeed many aspects of monastic lifestyle in which the rules do differ from each other, often in the sense that the Columbian ones promote stricter asceticism and discipline, which evidently led to the preference of the more moderate *Regula Benedicti* (Diem 2012: 36).

On the whole, the rules are relatively unanimous in the big picture about regulating the care of the *infirmi*. It appears that these rules did not play a major role in the varying constructions of monastic ideals and therefore could have unanimous principles (on the discourses in Merovingian Gaul, see Diem 2014). The biggest difference among the rules is whether or not the topic ended up being regulated at all – and if so, which aspects. For example, the lack of rules concerning female monastics' physical labour and infirmity by Donatus of Besançon can be seen to derive from the ways in which those monasteries' subsistence was organized. Otherwise gender does not seem to have played a major role in the regulations about the infirm, partly because during the period under discussion here, male and female monastic ideals were mostly compatible (Diem 2014: 193). On the other hand, that for example Columbanus's *Regula Monachorum* and *Regula Coenobialis* do not address the caretaking does not mean that he would have left the *infirmi* without support, but is just one manifestation of his focus on the monks' inner life and penitence (see Meens 2014: 53–7). Concerning everyday life in the monastic communities, the Master's interest in spotting frauds is a striking difference, but as it did not find its way into the other rules, its influence appears to have been of only moderate importance. Somewhat surprisingly, perhaps the most distinct and 'disabling' regulation is to be found in Benedict's discussion of the illiterate, whom he does not even define as *infirmi*. Whether or not his statement actually refers to what we would label as 'intellectual disability' is impossible to deduce (cf. Kellenberger in this volume). It is nevertheless a fine example of the importance of the demands of a monastic social role. In other cases, (physical) infirmity, when not leading to wilful idleness, was not a threat to the monastic lifestyle, but rather enabled the community to serve Christ.

Conclusion

As a whole, the early monastic rules regulate the position and caretaking of the *infirmi* by following the biblical Acts of Mercy, therefore the weak were supposed to be taken care of as if Christ himself was being served. The abbot or abbess was the one in charge, to make sure that they lacked nothing. Additionally, the infirm were granted allowances, especially concerning monastic diet and labour, and their caretaking was to be such that convalescence was achieved. However, there were no diagnostic means – and, presumably, not even the need – to make clear distinctions between illness and impairment in the modern sense, and the rules' emphasis on fairness and reason, as well as the idea that all people should be provided what they need, implicitly also include prolonged conditions. The fluctuating vocabulary concerning infirmity is indeed revealing: it appears that besides the occasional emphases that certain allowances were only addressed to the 'very weak', strict categorizations were not needed, but the importance of individual needs stressed in all the rules comprised the guiding principle.

Although the monastic rules are normative sources written to regulate life within a given community, their theological background and aim must not be overlooked. The grounds for the guidelines are always to be found in the theological thinking of the writers. Caretaking of the *infirmi* was an aspect of monastic lifestyle, which all the communities had to handle one way or another, but it too had a firm basis in the Bible, and the sick and the weak can be seen as instruments by whom their communities could demonstrate their charity. Nevertheless, caring for the *infirmi* was an essential aspect of Christian monasticism at large, but the details of it were not of crucial importance in shaping and developing monasticism as were regulating enclosure, vigils or chastity. Therefore, the rules remained relatively compatible in their regulations. The grounds set in the early rules, the Benedictine one especially, were the basis on which the later monastic communities built. These rules had fundamental significance in shaping medieval health-care and treatment of the infirm, regardless of the type of their physical condition.

Acknowledgements

This chapter has been written with the support of the University of Bremen and the European Union FP7 COFUND under grant agreement n° 600411. I wish to thank Jan Ulrich Büttner for his help with the paper, as well as Albrecht Diem for sending me some research articles of his.

Notes

1 The earliest rule having strong influence on western monasticism was that of St Pachomius from c.320, translated into Latin by St Jerome and apparently known by the later writers. On Pachomius's life, see e.g. Rousseau 1985; Harmless 2004: ch. 5. The treatment of the infirm in the Pachomian (and Shenoutan) rules has been extensively analysed in Crislip 2005. Therefore, it will

be relatively briefly addressed here. It is worth pointing out that we know of the less prominent rules mostly through Benedict of Aniane's (d. 821) preservation work. (For a survey, see de Vogüé 1985.) Therefore, aside from the rules whose setting and background are best documented, often we do not know if they were actually in use and, if so, how widely. See e.g. Diem 2012: 1–3.

2 The first title specifying Augustine as the writer of the rule, commonly known as *Praeceptum*, appears in 430. Textual criticism and comparisons, however, provide strong evidence for his authorship. See Lawless 1987: 123–35; Verheijen 1967. There exist versions of the *Rule* addressed to both nuns and monks, which has led to some discussion concerning the original audience of the text. According to George Lawless, the different families of the text indicate that the *Rule* and the *Rule for Nuns* 'clearly developed along independent lines'. The *Rule for Nuns* therefore appears to be an adaptation of the one written for monks. See Lawless 1987: 137–9.

3 *Regula Magistri* 70.1–3: 'Fratres, qui se voluerint ostendere, quod pleni sint caritate, ad certamen aegrotos fratres uisitent, consolentur et serviant, ut caritas fraternalis in necessitate probetur et dominicam vocem factis adimpleant dicentis: *Infirmus fui et visitastis me*.' The similarities and differences between the rules of the Master and Benedict are extensively analysed in de Vogüé 1971. De Vogüé's theory of the chronology was challenged in Dunn 1990, which led to further discussion on the topic. See Dyer 2000; Clark 2011: 15–16. It is not known if the rule as it stands was ever used in a monastery.

4 *Regula Benedicti* 36.1–4: 'Infirmorum cura ante omnia et super omnia adhibenda est, ut sicut revera Christo ita eis serviatur, quia ipse dixit: *Infirmus fui et uisitastis me*, et: *Quod fecistis uni de his minimis mihi fecistis*. Sed et ipsi infirmi considerent in honorem Dei sibi servire, et non superfluitate sua contristent fratres suos servientes sibi'. Earlier in the rule Benedict lists all the acts of mercy, of which visiting the *infirmi* is one. Ibid. 3.1–31. See also Donatus of Besançon, *Regula ad virgines*, PL 87.279; *Regula cuiusdam ad Virgines*, PL 88.1065.

5 There are other types of early monastic writings referring to the methods of discerning e.g. possession from other types of afflictions. The biographers of Pachomius portray him as interested in the nature of various sicknesses, which enabled the correct treatment for everyone (Crislip 2005: 19–21). On Shenoute and White Monastery, see also e.g. Layton 2014; Schroeder 2013.

6 Interestingly, the Lerinian *Third Rule of the Fathers* (12.1–3) even specifies that the infirm are *not* allowed to leave the monastery, but must be treated there.

7 The authors had, however, somewhat different opinions on the matter. In Donatus of Besançon's rule, the nuns, as opposed to Benedict's monks, are actually able to cure themselves (Diem 2012: 33–5).

Bibliography

Primary sources

The Asketikon of St Basil the Great, ed. and tr. Anna M. Silvas (Oxford, 2005).

Augustine of Hippo and his Monastic Rule, ed. George Lawless (Oxford, 1987).

Aurelian of Arles, *Regula ad Monachos*, in *Patrologiae Cursus Completus*, ed. J. P. Migne, Series Latina, 68 (Paris, 1841–64), cols 387–96.

Aurelian of Arles, *Regula ad Virgines*, *Patrologiae Cursus Completus*, ed. J. P. Migne, Series Latina, 68 (Paris, 1841–64), cols 399-406.

Augustine's Rule: A Commentary by Adolar Zumkeller, O.S.A., tr. Matthew J. O'Connell, ed. John E. Rotelle (Villanova, PA, 1987).

Césaire d'Arles, *Œuvres monastiques*, I. *Œuvres pour les moniales*, ed. Adalbert de Vogüé and Joël Correau, Sources Chrétiennes 345 (Paris, 1988).

Césaire d'Arles, *Œuvres monastiques*, II. *Œuvres pour les monials*, ed. Joël Correau and Adalbert de Vogüé, Sources Chrétiennes 398 (Paris, 1994).

Columbanus, *Regula Coenobialis*, in *Patrologiae Cursus Completus*, ed. J. P. Migne, Series Latina, 80 (Paris, 1841–64), cols 210-224.

Donatus of Besançon, *Regula ad Virgines*, in *Patrologiae Cursus Completus*, ed. J. P. Migne, Series Latina, 87 (Paris, 1841–64), cols 273–93.

Kardong, Terrence (ed. and tr.), *Benedict's Rule: A Translation and Commentary* (Collegeville, MN, 1996).

'Pachomia Latina. Règle et épitres de S. Pachome, épitre de S. Théodore et "Liber" de S. Orsiesius: Texte Latin de S. Jérôme', ed. Amand Boon, *Bibliothèque de la Revue d'Histoire Ecclésiastique*, VII (Louvain, 1932).

Puzicha, Michaela (ed. and tr.), *Die Regeln der Väter* (Münsterschwarzach, 1990).
La Règle du Maître, I–II, ed. Adalbert de Vogüé, Sources Chrétiennes 105 (Paris, 1964).
La Règle de Saint Augustin, ed. Luc Verheijen (Paris, 1967).
La Règle de S. Benoît, I–VI, ed. Adalbert de Vogüe, Sources Chretiennes,181–5 (Paris, 1971–2).
Regula cuiusdam ad virgines, Patrologiae Cursus Completus, ed. J. P. Migne, Series Latina, 97 (Paris, 1841–64), cols 1953–70.
Regula Tarnatensis, ed. F. Villegas, 'La "Regula Monasterii Tarnatensis": Texte, sources et datation', in *Revue Bénédictine*, 84 (1974), 7–65.

Secondary sources

Allen, Pauline, Neil, Bronwen, and Mayer, Wendy, *Preaching Poverty in Late Antiquity: Perceptions and Realities* (Leipzig, 2009).
Aronco, Maria A. d', 'The Benedictine Rule and the Care of the Sick: The Plan of St Gall and Anglo-Saxon England', in B. S. Bowers (ed.), *The Medieval Hospital and Medical Practice* (Aldershot, 2007), 235–52.
Bazell, Dianne M., *Arnaldi de Villanova: Opera Medica Omnia – de Esu Carnium*, XI (Barcelona, 1999).
Brown, Peter, *Poverty and Leadership in the Later Roman Empire* (Hanover, 2002).
Carner, Daniel, *Wandering, Begging Monks: Spiritual Authority and the Promotion of Monasticism in Late Antiquity* (Los Angeles, CA, 2002).
Clark, Elizabeth A., *Women in the Early Church* (Collegeville, MN, 1983).
Clark, James, *The Benedictines in the Middle Ages* (Woodbridge, 2011).
Clarke, Lowther William Kemp, *St Basil the Great: A Study in Monasticism* (Cambridge, 2003 [1913]).
Cohen, Esther, *The Modulated Scream: Pain in Late Medieval Culture* (Chicago, IL, and London, 2010).
Coon, Lynda L., *Dark Age Bodies. Gender and Monastic Practice in the Early Medieval West* (Philadelphia, PA, 2011).
Crislip, Andrew T., *From Monastery to Hospital: Christian Monasticism and the Transformation of Health Care in Late Antiquity* (Ann Arbor, MI, 2005).
Crislip, Andrew T., *Thorns in the Flesh: Illness and Sanctity in Late Ancient Christianity* (Philadelphia, PA, 2013).
Cristiani, Riccardo, 'The Semantic Range of Medical Language in the Rule of Benedict', *American Benedictine Review* 54 (2003), 20–9.
Diem, Albrecht, 'Das Ende des monastischen Experiments: Liebe, Beichte und Schweigen in der Regula cuiusdam ad virgines (mit einer Übersetzung im Anhang)', in G. Melville and A. Müller (eds), *Female vita religiosa between Late Antiquity and the High Middle Ages: Structures, Developments and Spatial Contexts* (Münster and Berlin, 2011), 81–136.
Diem, Albrecht, 'New Ideas Expressed on Old Words: The *Regula Donati* on Female Monastic Life and Monastic Spirituality', *Viator* 43 (2012), 1–38.
Diem, Albrecht, '... *ut si professus fuerit se omnia impleturum, tunc excipiatur.* Observations on the Rules for Monks and Nuns of Caesarius and Aurelianus of Arles', in V. Zimmerl-Panagl, L. J. Dorfbauer and C. Weidmann (eds), *Edition und Erforschung lateinischer patristischer Texte . 150 Jahre CSEL. Festschrift für Kurt Smolak zum 70. Geburtstag* (Berlin, 2014), 191–224..
de Dreuille, Mayeul, *Seeking the Absolute Love: The Founders of Christian Monasticism* (New York, 1999).
de Dreuille, Mayeul, *The Rule of Saint Benedict and the Ascetic Traditions from Asia to the West* (Leominster, 2000).
Dunn, Marilyn, 'Mastering Benedict: Monastic Rules and their Authors in the Early Medieval West', *English Historical Review* 105 (1990), 567–94.
Dunn, Marilyn, *Emergence of Monasticism: From the Desert Fathers to the Early Middle Ages* (Oxford and Malden, MA, 2003).
Dyer, Joseph, 'Observations on the Divine Office in the Rule of the Master', in Margot E. Fassler and Rebecca A. Baltzer (eds), *The Divine Office in the Latin Middle Ages: Methodology and Source Studies* (Oxford, 2000), 74–98.
Elm, Susanna, *'Virgins of God': The Making of Asceticism in Late Antiquity* (Oxford, 1994).
Ferngren, Gary B., *Medicine and Health Care in Early Christianity* (Baltimore, MD, 2009).
Fagan, Garret, *Bathing in Public in the Roman World* (Ann Arbor, MI, 2002).
Foot, Sarah, *Veiled Women*, I–II. Studies in Early Medieval England (Aldershot, 2000).

Harlow, Mary, and Smith Wendy, 'Between Fasting and Feasting: The Literary and Archaebiological Evidence for Monastic Diet in Late Antique Egypt', *Antiquity* 75 (2001), 758–68.

Harmless, William, *Desert Christians: An Introduction to the Literature of Early Monasticism* (Oxford, 2004).

Horn, Cornelia B., 'A Nexus of Disability in Ancient Greet Miracle Stories: A Comparison of Accounts of Blindness from the Asklepieion in Epidauros and the Shrine of Thecla in Seleucia', in C. Laes *et al.* (eds), *Disabilities in Roman Antiquity* (Leiden, 2013), 115–43.

Jong, Mayke de, *In Samuel's Image: Child Oblation in the Early Medieval West* (Leiden, 1996).

Kardong, Terrence, *Pillars of Community: Four Rules of Pre-Benedictine Monastic Life* (Collegeville, MN, 2010).

Kuuliala, Jenni, Krötzl, Christian, and Mustakallio, Katariina, 'Introduction: Infirmitas in Antiquity and the Middle Ages', in C. Krötzl, K. Mustakallio and J. Kuuliala (eds), *Infirmity in Antiquity and the Middle Ages: Social and Cultural Approaches to Health, Weakness and Care* (Aldershot, 2015), 1–11.

Laes, Christian, 'Disabled Children in Gregory of Tours', in K. Mustakallio and C. Laes (eds), *The Dark Side of Childhood in Late Antiquity and the Middle Ages* (Oxford, 2011a), 39–62.

Laes, Christian, 'Silent Witnesses: Deaf-Mutes in Graeco-Roman Antiquity', *Classical World* 104 (2011b), 451–73.

Laes, Christian, 'Raising a Disabled Child: A Life Course Approach', in J. Evans-Grubbs and T. Parkin (eds), *Oxford Handbook of Childhood and Education in the Roman World* (Oxford, 2013), 125–46.

Laes, Christian, Goodey, Chris F., and Rose, Martha Lynn (eds), *Disabilities in Roman Antiquity: Disparate Bodies* A Capite ad Calcem (Leiden, 2013a).

Laes, Christian, Goodey, Chris F., and Rose, Martha Lynn, 'Approaching Disabilities *a capite ad calcem*: Hidden Themes in Roman Antiquity', in C. Laes *et al.* (ed.), *Disabilities in Roman Antiquity* (Leiden, 2013b), 1–15.

Layton, Bentley, *The Canons of our Fathers: Monastic Rules of Shenoute* (Oxford, 2014).

Leyerle, Blake, and Young, Robert Darling (eds), *Ascetic Culture: Essays in Honor of Philip Rousseau* (Notre Dame, IN, 2013).

Linton, Simi, *Claiming Disability: Knowledge and Identity* (New York, 1998).

McKitterick, Rosamond: *Books, Scribes and Learning in the Frankish Kingdoms, 6th–9th Centuries* (Aldershot, 1994).

McNamara, JoAnn, Halborg, John E., and Whatley, E. Gordon, 'Introduction', in J. McNamara, J. E. Halborg and E. G. Whatley (eds), *Sainted Women of the Dark Ages* (Durham, 1996).

Maxwell, Jaclyn L., *Christianization and Communication in Late Antiquity: John Chrysostom and his Congregation in Antioch* (Cambridge, 2006).

Meens, Rob, *Penance in Medieval Europe, 600–1200* (Cambridge, 2014).

Metzler, Irina, *Disability in Medieval Europe: Thinking about Physical Impairment during the High Middle Ages, c.1100–1400* (London and New York, 2006).

Moyse, G., 'Monachisme et réglementation monastique en Gaule avant Benoît d'Aniane', in *Sous la Règle de Saint Benoît: Structures monastiques et sociétés en France du Moyen Âge et à l'époque moderne* (Geneva, 1982), 3–19.

Murphy, James B., 'Opus Dei: Prayer of Labor? The Spirituality of Work in Saints Benedict and Escrivá', in L. Bruni and B. Sena (eds), *The Charismatic Principle in Social Life* (London, New York, 2013), 94–111.

Rapp, Claudia, *Holy Bishops in Late Antiquity: The Nature of Christian Leadership in an Age of Transition* (Berkeley-Los Angeles, CA, 2005).

Risse, Guenter B., *Mending Bodies, Saving Souls: A History of Hospitals* (Oxford, 1999).

Rose, Martha Lynn, *The Staff of Oedipus: Transforming Disability in Ancient Greece* (Ann Arbor, MI, 2003).

Rousseau, Philip, *Pachomius: The Making of a Community in Fourth-Century Egypt* (Berkeley-Los Angeles, CA, 1985 [1999]).

Schroeder, Caroline T., *Monastic Bodies: Discipline and Salvation in Shenoute of Atripe* (Philadelphia, PA, 2013).

Schulenburg, Jane Tibbetts, 'Strict Active Enclosure and its Effects on the Female Monastic Experience (ca. 500–1100)', in J. A. Nicholas and L. Thomas Shank (eds), *Distant Echoes, Medieval Monastic Women* (Kalamazoo, MI, 1984), 51–86.

Schulenburg, Jane Tibbetts, *Forgetful of their Sex: Female Sanctity and Society, ca. 500–1100* (Chicago, IL, and London, 1998).

Shakespeare, Tom, *Disability Rights and Wrongs* (London and New York, 2006).

Squatritti, Paolo, *Water and Society in Early Medieval Italy, AD 400–1000* (Cambridge, 1998).

Trentin, Lisa, 'Exploring Visual Impairment in Ancient Rome', in C. Laes *et al.* (eds), *Disabilities in Roman Antiquity* (Leiden, 2013), 89–114.

Verheijen, Luc, *La Règle de saint Augustin*, I. *Tradition manuscrite;* II. *Recherches historiques* (Paris, 1967).

de Vogüé, Adalbert, *La règle de Saint Benoît VI: Commentaire historique et critique.* Sources Chrétiennes 1986 (Paris, 1971).

de Vogüé, Adalbert, *La règle de Saint Benoît VII: Commentaire doctrinal et spiritual.* Sources Chrétiennes 1986 (Paris, 1977).

de Vogüé, Adalbert, *Les règles monastiques anciennes (400–700).* Typologie des sources 46 (Turnhout 1985).

de Vogüé, Adalbert, *Histoire littéraire du mouvement monastique dans l'antiquité*, 12 vols (Paris, 1991–2008).

Vuolanto, Ville, 'Children and Asceticism: Strategies of Continuity in the Late Fourth and Early Fifth Centuries', in K. Mustakallio , J. Hanska, H.-L. Sainio and V. Vuolanto (eds), *Hoping for Continuity: Childhood, Education and Death in Antiquity and the Middle Ages* (Rome, 2005), 119–32.

Vuolanto, Ville, *Children and Asceticism in Late Antiquity: Continuity, Family Dynamics and the Rise of Christianity* (Aldershot, 2015).

Yearl, M. K. K., 'Medieval Monastic Customaries on *Minuti* and *Infirmi*', in Barbara S. Bowers (ed.), *The Medieval Hospital and Medical Practice* (Aldershot, 2007), 175–94.

Yegül, Figret, *Bathing in the Roman World* (Cambridge, 2009).

Zimmermann, Gerd, *Ordensleben und Lebensstandard: Die Cura corporis in den Ordensvorschriften des abendländischen Hochmittelalter* (Münster, 1973).

Zytka, Michal Jacub, *Baths and Bathing in Late Antiquity* (Cardiff, 2013).

25

THE COPTIC AND ETHIOPIC TRADITIONS

Carol Downer

In the early Christian world, attitudes to disability were inevitably informed by biblical and especially New Testament teaching. Therefore, although we can still see at play Old Testament ideas in which the responsibility for sickness or incapacity lies with the sin of the person concerned or with that of his forebears, this attitude is overlaid or revolutionized by the teaching of Christ as represented in the New Testament. However, because this teaching related to individuals or individual situations where his discernment and purpose was obviously paramount in each case, his later followers could not have an absolute ruling and themselves would have to apply discernment in each situation. This is the picture that emerges from our chief sources for the Coptic and Ethiopic worlds. Much material will inevitably be drawn from instances of healing where an individual's previous illness or disability is made visible through the sources (Holman 2009: 153–70; Horn 2009: 171–97; Horn and Phenix 2009 passim).

First we have to indicate the time-frame we are dealing with when looking at the Coptic and Ethiopic tradition in Antiquity. We are on safer ground with the Coptic because much of the literature relevant to us, although collected orally at first, was originally composed in the 1st millennium CE or copied in monastic *scriptoria* from earlier manuscripts, giving us some idea of the chain of transmission. We have more difficulties with the Ethiopic because, though there doubtless existed a growing oral tradition after the relatively early foundation of Christianity in the 4th century in Ethiopia, much of the Miracle literature that provides our source material survives in Ge'ez from about a millennium later, as will be seen below.

Evidence from Ethiopia

Sir Wallis Budge in his introduction to *One Hundred and Ten Miracles of Our Lady Mary* (1933) states that the oldest Ethiopic manuscript in the British Museum collection of Miracles of the Virgin Mary, on which he is chiefly drawing, and probably the oldest extant in the National Libraries of Europe, Oriental 652, is no older than the 15th century. Budge had in 1900 already published a weighty volume of Lady Meux's manuscripts with forty of these miracles and 111 facsimiles of original coloured illustrations (in a limited edition of 300 copies, but now available to all in the Online Collection of St John's University and the College of St Benedict), *The Miracles of the Blessed Virgin Mary and her Mother Hanna and the Magical Prayers of Aheta Mîkâêl,* and followed this in 1922 with *Legends of Our Lady Mary the Perpetual Virgin and Her Mother Hanna,* which presented the translation of most of the preceding work in more manageable form with black and white photos of illustrations from the original manuscripts. As there is considerable overlap between these works, I shall mainly quote from *One Hundred and Ten Miracles*, which, with a description of the manuscripts, contains an introduction to the collections. In my text, the Arabic numerals are page references, and not sections of the Miracle.

Michael Knibb in the first of his 1995 Schweich lectures on the Ethiopic version of the Old Testament also discusses some of these difficulties. It is possible that the earliest translation of the Bible may have begun after the adoption of Christianity by Ezana in the mid-4th century, but most scholars now attribute it to the arrival of two distinct groups of monks from the eastern Empire in the latter part of the 5th and early 6th centuries. It seems that the translation of the scriptures into Ge'ez was completed by at latest mid-7th century, but almost all the manuscripts of the Old Testament in Ge'ez we possess are 15th century, with very few belonging to the 14th and none to the 13th. Christianity flourished in Ethiopia until 925 under twenty-two 'Solomonic' kings, resisting the incursions of Islam, but then a woman of Lasta, Judith 'the fire', maybe pagan or Jewish, overthrew the reigning king and established a rule which persisted till the late 13th century. Christianity now languished with little literature produced. Budge (1933: p. xxii) nevertheless believed that after the Bible was translated in the early period many miracle stories relating to the Virgin Mary and the saints would have been received, with oral transmission continuing even under persecution. None of the translations of these nor of ancient homilies on Mary, however, survived, so that we find our earliest extant collections in Ethiopia were made in the 14th or 15th centuries, when, after the restoration of the 'Solomonic' line through the efforts of St Takla Haymânôt (according to tradition, he converted the last of the Lasta kings to Christianity in 1270) literary activity again began to flourish, and many early Christian works were translated.

The *Life and Miracles of Takla Haymânôt* (Budge 1906) reveal many miracle stories similar to those we think existed before the literary silence which fell during the intervening regime, but these (and their illustrations) are more valuable for comparative purposes, since they must originate in the 13th century or later. Moreover, when we examine some of the legends of Mary closely, they appear to come from Europe or elsewhere and to have been imported into Ethiopia, probably in the 13th century. A little later there was also European influence on the iconography of the illuminations of these manuscripts, although they acquired a distinctive Ethiopic flavour. Budge comments that these still provide our only testimony to the daily life of the people among whom the artist lived, probably in the late 15th or early 16th century (Budge 1933: p. xxxviii). Although many Ethiopian miracle stories came also from Egypt, these have to be separated from accretions from Palestine, Europe or elsewhere, a gigantean task;[1] Budge has appended to the stories alternative versions he found in Latin or French, a useful tool. Stories believed to originate in Europe conversely sometimes prove to be of Egyptian origin, so we must trust that all these reveal a situation compatible with earlier conditions in Ethiopia, if they are to be considered as evidence.

Budge remarks (1933: 9) that we see Mary in many miracles healing physical injury, leprosy, erysipelas, diseases of the mouth, deafness, blindness, madness, etc, for Jews as well as Gentiles. Yet there is no healing of deafness cited amongst the 110 examples chosen, and in the one obvious example of 'diseases of the mouth', this occurred when the Virgin had actually caused the breaking of teeth and ensuing complications herself – she turned the loaves which certain thieves had stolen to stone, and then healed the damage done to their mouths, thus bringing the men to repentance (Miracle XI). Besides this, there are two examples of leprosy,[2] two of healing of blindness, two of the restoration of hands (V and Vᵃ), and one of the healing of a man who had been epileptic for fifty-six years, LXXII, this last when the Virgin was only 12 years old. Budge, who had perused many such miracle collections, perhaps had other stories in mind, though, tellingly, even in this collection, in LXX, we hear of a secret sapphire portrait being made of the Virgin, efficacious for wounds, lameness, blindness and leprosy, but with no specific mention of deafness.

Miracles concerning priests

In some stories such as that of the Virgin Mary and the Jew of Akhmim (Miracle III.8–9), almost certainly of Coptic origin, we see the Virgin Mary healing a fatal injury to the man's backbone, which would undoubtedly have paralysed him. As he was a Christian priest his continuing ministry depended on good health (he was 100 years old at the time), so she gave him renewed youth and 130 years more of life, obviously a happy outcome.

Another Egyptian priest aged 100, John Bakansî, from the church of Abu As-Sêfên (St Mercurius) in Cairo, was going blind. After a year of losing the sight in both eyes, he determined to carry out an oath. He would approach the icon of the Virgin when the other monks had retired after the midnight office and prostrate himself before it 300 times. After another year, the Virgin appeared to him out of the icon, took her breasts from inside her dress, and squeezed her breast-milk into his eyes, made the sign of the cross over him and returned into the icon. When he opened his eyes, he saw the icon burning with fire, and found fragrant milk in his eyes (interesting as a mother's milk is reputedly found medically helpful in healing infants' eye ailments).[3] The priest in this story (IV.47) was healed of his blindness, continuing to function until he was 120. Longevity seems expected in these Ethiopian tales although these priests are Egyptian, and perhaps there was a reminiscence of the extreme old age recorded of some Egyptian saints; Shenoute was said to have died at 118.

In XX.63–4, we hear the extraordinary tale of the Virgin and the old priest Katîr, who had ministered in his church in Elksûs for forty years, and had become infirm. The verger wished him gone, and was very angry, but the priest begged for a few days' grace until some monks arrived who might take him away, then, weeping, fell asleep. Meanwhile the verger had a vision of the Virgin accompanied by two shining beings that were commanded to beat his feet. She told him that henceforth he would be paralysed and the priest healed. So the priest continued to minister and the verger remained paralysed until he died. He seemed to have accepted this somewhat brutal punishment as he himself told the story of the apparition.

In the healing of Bishop Mercurius (XXIII.71) whose whole body was so covered with leprosy that his archbishop told him gently it was no longer seemly to minister as a priest while the disease was upon him, incubation before the Virgin Mary was again involved. I have not given much space to leprosy elsewhere, but the crippling effects of this disease in ancient society cannot be ignored. This case is noteworthy, however, in that the bishop had continued to function and did not seem physically disabled after leprosy struck, and in that the archbishop dared to touch him. One might imagine that there would be a question of Mercurius here falling short of the ritual purity normally required of a priest, particularly in the confessedly Judaeo-Christian Ethiopian Orthodox church; what does seem clear from these four stories about clerics is that the body of a priest had to be 'perfect' for him to minister at the altar. I am told that it still holds true today that disabled men may not become priests as they cannot represent Christ's 'perfect man' at the altar. Disabled and blind people may and do become religious, though doubtless there are practical considerations as they will need their brothers' or sisters' help in moving around monastic complexes.[4] Priests who have later become disabled may continue to function in a limited way according to their ability (cf. Metzler in this volume).

Other miracles

Another healing from Upper Egypt (XVI.53) was of a rich girl who had lost her sight as a result of smallpox and was taken by her parents to a great festival of the Virgin in a church in the country called Dalgâ.[5] Here again the girl was healed when the Virgin stepped out of her icon to breathe on her and sprinkle her with drops of milk from her breast. The girl and her mother had been asleep but the Virgin woke the girl to perform this miracle (Figure 25.1).

These stories are reminiscent of the incubation which often took place in martyrs' shrines in Egypt, just as in ancient times it had taken place in temples of the gods (Idris Bell 1953: 68–9). There is homely detail in the amazement of the overseer at the healing when he came in with the *prosphora* for the eucharist in the early morning, and in the praises of the people when they came later into the church. We find a similar scenario in XXIV.73 when the Virgin heals a poor woman with a broken foot.

The story of a Frankish man born with a lame foot (XXII.68–70) includes an unusual ingredient, important for the sense of guilt felt by the afflicted. This man would cover his leg with a cloth to avoid discovery, but one day the archbishop, perhaps discerning some spiritual

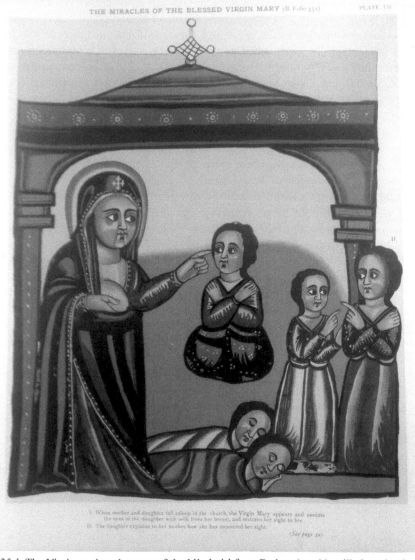

Figure 25.1 The Virgin anoints the eyes of the blind girl from Badramân with milk from her breast and restores her sight. From Ms. B (Budge 1900), eighteenth century. Cf. Budge 1933: pl. XXVIII, probably fifteenth century

disturbance, angrily recalled the congregation after its first dismissal from church, and then let them go again one by one until only the cripple was left. In tears the man prostrated himself before the icon of the Virgin, whereupon his foot was immediately loosened. The archbishop, amazed, beckoned to him and asked how long he had been in that state. The cripple told his life-story, adding 'When I came into the church this day, thou wast angry with all [the people] because of my sin'. He explained to the archbishop that when he dismissed the congregation one by one 'the lot went forth for me, and I alone was left'. The reasons for the archbishop's anger and subsequent amazement are left unclear. It may seem strange that cripples should either feel unworthy to enter a church or be excluded by the authorities on account of their incapacity. Two other European tales mentioned by Budge (1913: 68–9) may shed light on this: one records a man suffering from 'mal des ardents' – a cancerous disease of terrible virulence which struck northern Europe in 1128–9 and is often described by contemporary writers – who had his foot amputated in despair of a cure, but after praying in the cathedral fell asleep and found his whole foot restored by the Virgin, so that he walked away 'on his two feet'. (This suggests incidentally that others took the disabled man into church, or the amputee would have had to drag himself). Another mentions the Virgin curing a man turned out of Soissons Cathedral because of the smell of his putrefying foot. In the Ethiopian version neither infectious disease nor putrefaction are implied, so we must assume a perception of sin on the lame man's part.

Visual representation

In these Ethiopian tales the illustrations are numerous and graphic. We witness the breast-milk being squirted into the eyes of the blind and the stages of healing of the man with broken back portrayed in almost comic-strip fashion. In Coptic Egypt, healing is not so often found in wall paintings, perhaps because of a desire to avoid scenes of suffering, violence or cruelty even where the situation demands.

> We thus find lions drawn as if stripped of their savage character; the icons of martyrs do not express the pain and suffering they have endured. The elders of the deserts, despite (...) the severity of the struggle (...) reflect mirth and happiness [Figure 25.2]. Icons are distinguished by their simplicity (...) expressing internal quietude and calm or innocence.
>
> *(Coptic Icons 1998: I. 6)*

In the plastic arts, however, biblical healings are occasionally depicted. A 6th- or 7th-century comb from Deir Abū-Hinnis in Egypt, probably for liturgical use, depicts on one side the raising of Lazarus and the healing of a blind man who is carrying a stick bound with a ribbon or carved diagonally, which might be indicative of his disability (Gabra and Krauss 2007: 152, pl. 95; Youssef 2014). What is *not* usually visible is the portrayal of disabled people in the way that we find lame officials or dwarfs in funerary contexts in pharaonic Egypt (cf. David in this volume), where their representation in traditional poses indicates their being to some measure incorporated without prejudice into the fabric of (noble) society. An exception might be the portrayal of St John Kolobos at St Antony's Monastery (Figure 25.3, cf. Bolman 2002: 52, 82) where the base line against which the surrounding saints are set *rises* to accommodate his shorter stature. However, he was probably not actually a dwarf, or, if he was, was made priest which indicates his acceptability. Perhaps the norm in Christian Egypt is 'non-visibility' as disabled bodies seem unable to reflect the health and wholeness of God's perfect creation, although portrayal of blindness, e.g. by showing the eyes closed, may be acceptable as it was in later representations and in manuscripts (*Illustrations from Coptic Manuscripts* 2000: 122–3).

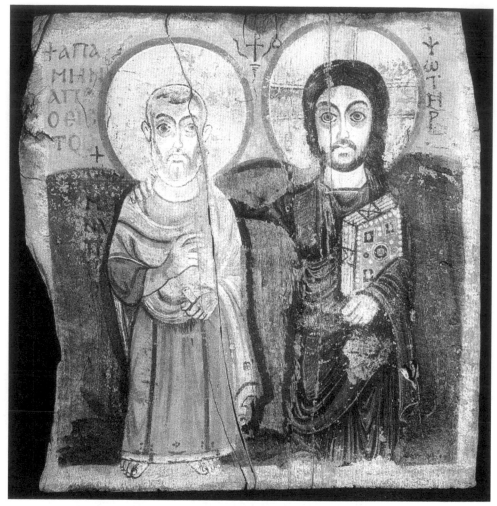

Figure 25.2 The ascetic Apa Mena is shown standing in perfect joy and serenity with Christ the Saviour. Panel from the monastery of Bawit, now in the Louvre, variously dated from 6th to 8th century. Encaustic and distemper on fig-wood.

Evidence from Coptic Egypt

Apophthegmata Patrum, Historia Monachorum in Aegypto, Palladius, John Cassian

Of necessity I shall draw primarily on literary sources for the 4th to 6th centuries CE which reflect the growth of monasticism, always a key focus for care of the sick and disabled. Increasing numbers of visitors were coming then to the Egyptian desert, attracted by accounts of the lives of the desert fathers and their sayings, known as the *Apophthegmata Patrum* (*AP*), which were doubtless heard in oral form before being early committed to writing, and reflect the heart of their teaching (Gould 1993: 5–9). The *Historia Monachorum in Aegypto* (*HMA*) is the fruit of one visit in 394/5, and Palladius' *Historia Lausiaca* (*HL*) of a longer stay between c.390 and 400, although Palladius wrote his account later, in about 420. John Cassian, in Egypt for the last decade of the 4th century, wrote two treatises witnessing to his experiences which much influenced the West. In *Conferences* 15, on *Divine Gifts*, he gives three examples of

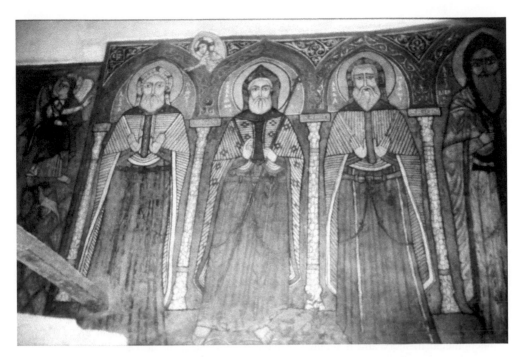

Figure 25.3 St John Kolobos (the Little) stands on a wavy line which represents a hill to make him level with his taller companions on either side, his friend Pishoi the Great on the left, and Sisoes on the right. From a programme of paintings in the Church of St Antony at the Red Sea, created in 1232/3 by a team of Coptic artists under a master named Theodore (Bolman 2002: 37). Photograph by Downer 1999.

charisms exercised by Abba Abraham the Simple, including raising a mummy from the dead, but ends by summing up succinctly the spirit of the desert on the issue of healing:

> We see therefore that the working of signs was never made much of by our fathers. On the contrary, although they possessed this by the grace of the Holy Spirit, they never wanted to exercise it unless perchance an extreme and unavoidable necessity forced them.
>
> *(Cassian, Conf. 2.3)*

The observations of these outsiders are extremely important as being more objective for evidence than those in the following hagiographical accounts, although there is much detail about daily life and disability in *all* our sources (Laes 2010).

St Antony

Not long after St Antony's death in 356, St Athanasius seems to have responded to requests for more information about his life, and wrote the narrative which had so much influence not only in the East, but in northern Europe, and was instrumental in St Augustine's own conversion from Manichaeism in 386. (Although the authorship of the *VA* has long been a matter of debate, it is generally now acknowledged as Athanasius' work.) One of Antony's great charisms was his gift of healing, so we must consider him a primary source for our topic. However, not even Antony's 'non-medical healing' was always successful (Crislip 2005: 25–6).

Pachomius, Theodore and Shenoute

St Antony may have been known as the Father of Monasticism, but even he saw that Pachomius had a genius for organization which he himself lacked: today Pachomius is recognized as the true founder of coenobitic monasticism in Egypt. Pachomius died ten years before Antony despite their great difference in age, and, to Antony's regret, they never actually met (G^1 or *First Greek Life of Pachomius*, 120). Here I use Veilleux's translations from the *Pachomian Koinonia* (3 vols, 1980–2) for healings by Pachomius and Theodore. The *Life* of Shenoute, later head of the White Monastery, was written by his successor, Besa.

Didymus and blindness

In *HL* 4, we hear of Didymus the Blind, whom Palladius met four times in all. This scholar had been blind since the age of 4, and by his own account had never learned to read or gone to school, yet rose to the heights of perfection. 'He was adorned with such a gift of knowledge, that it was said the passage of Scripture was fulfilled in him, "The Lord maketh the blind wise"' (LXX, Ps. 146: 8). His friend St Antony visited him three times in Alexandria. He was renowned for his scriptural exegesis of the Old and New Testaments, and is mentioned by the ecclesiastical historians Socrates, Sozomen and Theodoret; Sozomen 3.15 recounts that he taught himself to read with his fingers by tablets with letters engraved in them. He had a phenomenal memory and is reputed to have become head of the Catechetical School in Alexandria where his invention of a tactile reading system may have helped other blind people, although we hear little of such developments: one problem could have been lack of literacy amongst carers for the blind in antiquity. Didymus' overcoming of an incapacity generally thought to be one of the worst to befall humankind seems in this instance to be regarded as a gift of God in itself, and no one asked the question: 'Who sinned, this man or his parents?' as they did of the man born blind in John 9: 1.

In the *AP* (*Systematic Sayings*, Guy 7.60), a tale of blindness incurred through accident seems to reflect the judgement of God on the victim's recalcitrance but also God's purpose in preparing him ultimately to head the community. A father in a *coenobium* had an assistant who 'became negligent' and left the monastery. For three years the old man prayed for him to return and finally persuaded him. However, one day the assistant, sent to gather straw, became blinded in one eye. When finally his pain diminished, the old man sent him, still blind, to gather palms, but through the action of Satan, he was blinded in the other eye, and had to remain quiet in the monastery thereafter. The old man was much distressed by this but as time passed and his death approached he called the brethren to him and finally the blind man came to him distraught, asking to whose care he would entrust him. He was told by the elder to pray that he, the old man, might have power of persuasion before God for he hoped that on the Lord's Day the other would be able to convene the *synaxis*. The old man died and a few days later his assistant's sight was restored, and he became father of the monastery.

Deafness

This is one of the problems of this study, due to its very invisibility and infrequent mention, as previously seen in the case of the Ethiopian Miracles. Christian Laes in his careful study of deaf-mutes in Greco-Roman Antiquity, while recording known instances of deafness and muteness over an extended period, has also remarked on the problems of definition and identification, adding relevant legal and medical references (Laes 2011). Doubtless in late Antiquity deaf people suffered the sort of abuse they must always have done, being shouted at, rudely spoken to and treated as imbecilic because of their lack of understanding, though there is no obvious record of this. Those who lost their hearing imperceptibly as they grew older may have been better tolerated, but there seems little evidence of this either. Those born deaf would often have been mute as well, and there are occasional healings of such people. More frequent is the mention of healing of those who have become deaf and dumb through trauma of some kind. However, Guy 18.49 has an example of a young virgin struck dumb before an extended vision which was really 'an apocalypse'. She presumably regained her speech to tell the tale, so we must also consider the idea of dumbness as a figure of speech. There is a tale of a disciple (Guy 14.32) who had been told to be silent for five years by his spiritual father. The father sent him elsewhere at the end of this time, apparently without remembering to lift the ban on speaking, with the result that his penitent never spoke again in his life, and was thought to be dumb. Such imposed disability is not unusual amongst the desert fathers; although not a genuine physical impediment it is deserving of comment.

Others kept silent through saintliness, illness or depression. Chaîne 210 (= Guy 18.45.12) recounts the tale of an aged virgin who tells her life-story and way of asceticism to one of the monks. As a small child she had a saintly father who was nearly always ill and kept to his bed, but even when working was so silent that those who did not know him thought him dumb. In contrast her mother was flighty, wicked and devoted to pleasure. When the virgin, now on the brink of womanhood, lost her mother (the father having died previously) she had a dream presenting the 'two ways' to her, and after seeing her mother in hell-fire and father in heaven, naturally chose to follow the father's way. This story might strike one as illustrating one of the hidden 'disabilities': although much is made of the father's undoubted virtue, it is possible he also suffered from long-term depression or a disease such as multiple sclerosis.

Healing of other disabilities

Holy men, doctors and miracles

Numerous healings also are recorded in the *HMA*. John of Lycopolis told the brothers that an ascetic was good if he practised hospitality, gave alms and cared for the sick, implying a more immediate contact (*HMA* 1.62). Nevertheless, he did not usually perform cures publicly himself. In *HMA* 1.12 the wife of a senator who had lost her sight through cataracts asked her husband to take her to the saint. When told he never spoke to a woman, she begged only that he be informed of her plight and pray for her. He sent her some oil with which she bathed her eyes three times, and on the third day she regained her sight. Another woman, the wife of a tribune, according to a story we know from Rufinus' version of the *HMA* (*Lives* 143), begged to come to him but was permitted only to see him in a dream, and so received healing. Rufinus also mentions John's gift of lifting oppression (*Lives* 155).

In *HMA* 13.9, the visitors are told of another ascetic called John who always moved from place to place and lived only on holy communion which he received on Sundays. He would beg palm branches from the priest and weave harnesses for the beasts of burden. A cripple wanted to visit him for healing but as soon as he mounted the ass and his feet touched the harness made by John he was cured. We are told John sent other gifts to the sick and they were healed immediately. We note again the same reluctance to have direct contact or prayer with the sick that St John Cassian recorded.

In the case of Copres (*HMA* 10), many cures were worked before their eyes, though these are unspecified. However, Copres himself, when telling of the great wonders worked by Patermuthius, one of their fathers, adds (*HMA* 10.24), 'What wonder if we lesser men perform the little things that we do, healing the lame and the blind, which physicians also accomplish by their skills?' (Amundsen and Ferngren 1996). It is refreshing here to find mention of ordinary doctors, but there are hagiographic accounts also of doctors such as St Coluthus and Sts John and Cyrus the Unmercenaries, who gave their medical services for nothing. Coluthus, after offering a blind beggar his shirt, effected the man's cure from blindness (*Encomium* 49-52); soon he became assistant to the new bishop's son who was a deacon and taught him the practice of medicine (*Encomium* 54). Blows and inflammation of the eyes are mentioned as conditions which Coluthus healed in life, but he was martyred shortly afterwards and then his medical career took wing with the healing of another cripple and various instances of injustice. Sophronius, the monk and companion of John Moschus, was healed of an eye condition at the sanctuary of Cyrus and John just south of Alexandria, and wrote the account of all he had witnessed there. Although oils and other media are mentioned even in miraculous healings, it is rare to learn of the actual ingredients applied (PG 87.3: 3423–3675). In Chaîne (1960: no. 255), we hear of the use of burnt saffron as a possible cure for the gangrenous feet of Abba Dioscorus, and occasionally in other texts of treatment with *cassia*. Crislip (2005: 92–4) mentions how Amma Syncletica in the 4th century embraced illness as a positive ascetic practice although her body was eaten up with corruption: 'the heaviest stench governed her whole body so that the ones who served her suffered more than she did' (*V. Syncleticae* 111, tr. Castelli). She finally allowed the doctor to apply aloe, myrrh and myrtle wet with wine, 'feeling mercy for those who were with her', having previously refused all medical treatment. From this, we hear, the excessive stench was destroyed.

Theon in *HMA* 6.1, who had practised silence for thirty years, put his hand through his cell window and cured many sick people, some doubtless disabled, whilst Elias in *HMA* 7 worked many miracles every day amongst the sick who visited him. *HMA* 26 tells of John 'the father of hermitages' who performed many miracles 'and was especially successful at healing people with paralysis and gout', interesting specializations. At Nitria there lived Benjamin, an 80-year-old ascetic who had reached the heights of perfection and had an amazing gift of healing himself, but became so incredibly swollen with dropsy in his last days that the door had to be taken down to move his body when he died. Palladius (*HL* 12) tells the story 'that we might not be too surprised when some accident befalls just men', adding that Bishop Dioscorus, then priest of Mount Nitria, himself took the blessed Evagrius and the narrator of the story to Benjamin.

One poignant but curious tale in the *Sayings*, Poemen 7, tells of a child whose face, through the power of the devil, was turned backwards. The father, a relative of Abba Poemen, came to him, but when he saw all the old men gathered there he sat outside the monastery, weeping. One of the old men came out and asked him why he wept. The story emerged that Abba Poemen always turned him away for some reason: through fear of a charge of nepotism or through discernment perhaps. The old man wisely took the child to all the others in turn, asking them to make the sign of the cross over him, and lastly to Poemen, who at this stage could not refuse, and so the child was healed.

In the *AP* (*Sayings*, p. 110: Macarius 15), Abba Macarius finds a small paralytic child dumped by his father at the door of his cell. The father had retreated to a safe distance to see what would happen, but unsurprisingly the child, not knowing, cried his eyes out. The saint looked out to see what the disturbance was, asked the child what had happened and who had left him, and then told him to get up and run after his father. The child, who seemingly had never walked before, did as he was told and thus the miracle took place, and father and son walked home. For Macarius the power of God was never in question, but the actual healing must be low-key and incidental, never seeking to draw attention to anyone but God, as Cassian had noted.

More on women and girls

According to Rufinus, in another story told of the usually kindly Macarius, a small girl was brought to him with a body so diseased that her 'flesh was eaten away' with 'an innumerable host of worms', and the stench so bad no one could approach. He arranged for prayers to be said for seven days continuously, and then anointed her limbs with oil and restored her health, but in such a way that no femininity thereafter showed through and she would thus be freed for life from being able to beguile men with womanly deceits. At least she lived!

In SBo 41 (Veilleux 1980–2: I. 64–5) the wife of a councillor of Nitentori (Denderah) who like the woman in Matthew 9: 18–22 had been suffering from a flow of blood for a very long time, sought out Pachomius. The social implications were far-reaching, as in the Jewish and Christian worlds the menstruating woman was unclean, socially isolated and thus effectively disabled. Pachomius is persuaded by his friend Apa Dionysius to go outside the gatehouse with him 'on an important matter' and the woman, touching his habit from behind, is at once healed, as was the woman in Matthew 9. Because of his desire always to flee human glory, Pachomius becomes 'sad to death' at this. A similar story is told of Pisentius, Bishop of Coptos and also spiritual adviser at Jeme in the early 7th century, where a woman with uncontrollable menstrual flow touches the hem of his garment and is healed (Wilfong 2002: 37; Budge 1913: 32a–b for text and translation).

Animals

The delightful story of Macarius, the disciple of Antony, in *HMA* 21.15, shows how the fathers cured even the disabilities of animals. One day a mother hyena which occupied the cave next to his came and licked his feet while he was at prayer, and gently drew him by the hem of his tunic to her own cave where she showed him her cubs who had been born blind. He prayed over them and returned them to her with their sight restored. In gratitude she gave him a ram-skin, which he spread under him; this was the one that Palladius (*HL* 18) tells us was given to Melania after his death, though here in *HMA* one of the brothers still had it. Shenoute, too, showed his gentler side when, according to Besa's *Life* 161, he healed a camel which had just given birth of her unwillingness to feed her new-born. The foal was thus exceedingly weak, but the mother returned to her duties after being given a lecture by Shenoute and a bowl of water from the church basin. The saint here shows his concern for the livelihood of the villagers which must have depended greatly on the wellbeing of their animals. Many Egyptian saints display a great rapport for animals, but this cannot be said to be exclusively Egyptian (Bell 1992). The Ethiopian *Miracles of Takla Haymânôt* show a similar concern for livestock, with emphasis on birds and beasts with good breeding potential (cf. Budge 1906: Miracle XX: the resurrection of the widow of Angôt's *hen* from the soldier-thieves' pot!).

Hospitals

The New Testament is naturally a major source not only for the plight of the disabled or disturbed within the early Christian era, but also for attitudes to those with disability of any kind. Thus we see Christ healing the paralytic at the building by the Sheep Pool in Jerusalem called Bethzatha in the fifth chapter of the Gospel of St John. The variant of this name, Bethesda, 'House of Mercy', perhaps indicates this was a kind of hospital. Here lay a multitude of invalids, blind, lame and paralysed, waiting for the angel to ruffle the waters. Jesus asks this man who has been there for thirty-eight years whether he wants to be healed. 'Sir, I have no one to put me into the pool when the water is troubled, and while I am waiting another steps down before me,' he replies. 'Rise, take up your pallet, and walk', Jesus tells him. From this we learn something of the social conditions of the long-term disabled. If a paralysed man had no one to look after him, he normally stood no chance of healing, even in cases like this where a miraculous element was involved. However, there were five porticos here where such people seemingly could find shelter, along with others also hoping for help and healing.

In the *Historia Lausiaca* 6, 'On the Rich Virgin', we have evidence for a similar institution in late 4th-century Alexandria. The superintendent of this hospital for cripples knew a certain virgin who had not been weaned off worldly things and, under the pretext of family affection for her niece, to whom she had promised her money, was affected by pangs of avarice. This man, called Macarius, had previously been a stone-worker, and so approached the woman telling her of some brilliant jewels he had access to. She gave him £500 to choose her the best of these, not even asking to view them, though given the option. His 'jewels', it transpired, were the patients in the hospital for which he was responsible; so that when in due course the stones failed to materialize, she made inquiries, and was taken to see the living stones on which she had deposited her wealth. It is immediately apparent how similar this is to Act 2 in the *Acts of Thomas* (James 1975: 371) where Thomas promises to build the Indian king a fantastic palace (by which he means a heavenly dwelling-place) and uses the money laid down to buy food for the poor and destitute. Knowledge of this story may have inspired Macarius' action in the first place, as Clarke notes in his 1918 translation of *HL* 56–7. Here men and women were succoured on different floors, and may have been quite numerous.[6]

Another virgin mentioned in *HL* 67, Magna, was renowned for providing for hospitals, but in Galatia. There was doubtless similar provision in Egypt outside Alexandria, and we hear of care and healing of the sick at several points in the *HMA* where establishing of hospitals might be expected. In Oxyrhynchus, *HMA* 5, the magistrates of this profoundly Christian city had watchmen posted at the gates so that if needy strangers appeared, they might ensure their care, these probably including blind and disabled as well as the poor. Ordinary citizens competed to offer their homes to strangers. *HMA* 5.5 tells us 'each of us had our cloaks rent apart by people pulling us to make us go and stay with them'.

In *Sayings* (Ward 1975: 80, John the Dwarf 40), a young girl, Paësia, is left an orphan and decides to make her house into a hospice for the use of the fathers of Scetis, where for a while she serves them with her resources. Although she later falls away and is finally brought to repentance, the story gives an insight into the way such a household worked, with a door-keeper and her children also living there, the old woman presumably as house-keeper. Family members and friends would certainly look after their own disabled, and in *HL* 21 we even see Eulogius, a solitary and cripple himself, 'adopting' from the marketplace one more disabled than himself, with no feet or hands, and taking him home on a mule. He looked after him for the remaining fifteen years of their lives as he had vowed, not without considerable emotional difficulty: it seems the other cripple began to suffer from dementia, judging from his reported abusiveness. The nearby ascetics suggested Eulogius seek help from St. Antony. Both he and his protégé were reprimanded for nearly giving up on the other and were told that, as death was approaching each, they should return home and fulfil their promises to support each other to the end.

Demon possession

We hear in *VA* 48 of an importunate military officer, appropriately called Martianus, whose daughter is troubled by a demon, and who keeps calling on St. Antony for healing at a time when he wants to withdraw from everyone. He tells this man to go away and to call on Christ for himself: if he believes, the child will be healed (with possible allusion to the centurion's servant in Luke 7: 2 and Jairus' daughter in Luke 8: 41). The man eventually gets the message and calls out for help with the result that the child is healed at once. Similarly in *VA* 71 a mother brings a demoniac daughter to him in the street and this time Antony heals the child directly. Such scenes must have been familiar in a world without controlling drugs, but persist into our lifetimes. Forty years ago in Alexandria when walking in the streets with a Coptic priest, I witnessed a Muslim group bringing a disturbed man to the Christian, with much ringing of bells; the moment the priest prayed the man became quiet and the family took him away. This sort of occurrence is still apparently common today.

In one case of demon possession, a sick boy (perhaps suffering from anorexia) is tricked into taking bread that has been made by the brothers until the demon finally releases its hold, and the father is able to anoint him with blessed oil sent by Pachomius, to ensure a complete healing (SBo 44, Veilleux 1980–2: I. 68). When another person troubled by a demon (SBo 110, Veilleux 1980–2: I. 162–3) is successfully healed, the mention of his violent jerking might at first suggest a form of epilepsy, although Pachomius' prior examination of the body of this man to find the demon's point of entry and discovery of its place of subsequent residence in his neck tell us otherwise (see Knapton 2016). However, Pachomius frequently does actually treat the demon-possessed as sick, which is significant and perhaps indicative of some understanding of mental illness also.

In SBo 111 (Veilleux 1980–1982: I. 163–4) where Pachomius discerns the demon in a very humble man, he is given a word by an angel of the Lord to indicate that the sickness is the Lord's will for the patient and that he should not ask to be relieved of it since it is for his soul's salvation. Here it is unclear whether the demon is afflicting the sick person with mental or physical illness as the man seems to show no obvious signs of possession although Pachomius clearly recognizes the demon for what it is. Many such cases even if not physical were obviously debilitating and crippling and should certainly be classified as disability. Not all were seen as demon possession, however: there must have been many ordinary, everyday sicknesses and afflictions recognized in the Nile Valley. Pachomius and about 130 of his contemporaries died in 346 from a plague that was evidently accepted as a terrible illness with fearsome symptoms and high fever (SBo 130, Veilleux 1980–2: I. 175), but not demonic.[7]

Many sick and possessed persons were also brought to Theodore, Pachomius' eventual successor, that he might heal them through his gift of the grace of the Lord, we are told in SBo 151-152 (Veilleux 1980–2: I. 214). Here unfortunately two pages of the manuscript are missing so we have lost important detail about the nature of at least one cure. In G¹, 133, however, we are told again about Theodore:

> Whenever seculars came to him, either on the road or in the monastery, about someone possessed by the devil or otherwise suffering, he would tell them, 'Do not think that we can intercede with God on their behalf when we are sinners. If God in his mercy for his own creature wants to spare it, he has the power to do so, as he always shows his goodness to all'. And when they insisted very hard, asking him to pray, he would ask that the will of God and that which was expedient be done. And so the Lord would heal them.

We can assume from so general a statement that amongst the sick and possessed there would be physically disabled as well as those paralysed by mental illness and depression; this is not always explicit because of the attitude taken towards healing in the Pachomian communities. In Pachomius's own teaching, he is very clear that, for him, what is important is a right relationship with the Lord (SBo 45–6, Veilleux 1980–2: I. 68–9): he compares the healing of the spiritually blind, dumb or maimed to that of the physically impeded, and concludes that the former is far more important. However, we are told in S² Fragment 5.8 (Veilleux 1980–2:

I. 447–9) that when Theodore and two brothers were leaving the monastery on one occasion, Pachomius told them to expect miracles, quoting to them Luke 5: 17: 'And the power of the Lord made him heal'. In the same fragment, 9–11, we are told of Pachomius healing two men suffering from dropsy, and a man suffering paralysis after a snake bite: the latter's friends, after bringing their patient by wagon, desired Pachomius to rub him with oil. The man at once jumped up as Pachomius approached telling him not to trouble himself as he had been healed the moment he came towards him. Here we gain insight into the ways in which people became afflicted, and the kinds of transport available when they had to travel for help.

Martyrdoms

Although the way healings took place often revealed the self-effacing attitude of the fathers, this was not the case if pagan gods were to be defeated or shown up for what they were. Christ says in John 14: 12: 'All these things and greater you will do because I go to my Father'. Many Coptic martyrdoms therefore make great display about healing. One reason was often the growth of a special commemoration of a particular saint at their shrine. The recitation of a panegyric or account of a passion was 'a recognized moment in a ritual of power' (cf. Sabine G. MacCormack n. 73 in Brown 1981: 82). Brown, in discussing the lack of a passion for St Patroclus of Troyes, quotes Gregory of Tours, *GM* 63.81 who says that little reverence had been paid to this martyr because the story of his sufferings was not available. Brown observes that, without a *passio,* the *praesentia* of the saint lacked weight, and concludes by saying: 'Thus, of the Coptic passions of the martyrs, those that recount in the most grisly detail the break-up and miraculous reintegration of the martyr's body are precisely those associated with well-known healing shrines' (Brown 1981: 82).

The passion of St George, that most beloved of eastern saints (Budge 1888), illustrates the last point well, as does that of St Pteleme, the son of the decurion of Denderah, another military saint, who may be a prototype of St George, and had many miracles associated with his later cult (Downer 2004). As with St George his body was cut in two and the parts thrown out for the wild animals to devour, and like St George Pteleme was restored to life so that he might face down his persecutor, in this case the notorious Arianos, historical governor of the Thebaid, around whom also a hagiographic cycle later grew. Such destruction of the body at first might seem reminiscent of the dismemberment of Osiris in pharaonic legend, but among the Middle and Upper Egyptian millennialists of the 3rd and 4th centuries CE there seem also to have existed expectations of Old Testament heroes like Elijah and Enoch being similarly tortured and killed, only to be resurrected to defeat the 'Lawless One', as may be gleaned in the Coptic *Apocalypse of Elijah* 15 (Frankfurter 1992). This expectation of and teaching about martyrdom may well have arisen in the aftermath of the Decian Persecution.

Within the account of St Pteleme's passion, another healing took place, that of one of his torturers, who in the process of discovering whether Pteleme was still alive after his earlier sufferings had accidentally set fire to the saint's hair with the torch he was holding to his face. When Pteleme shook his head to put the fire out, the flame caught the torturer's eye and put it out. Later, when St Pteleme had been miraculously restored to life only to be thrust into a boiling cauldron for a further ordeal, he sat there scooping the water over himself, now apparently cool like that of a mountain stream, and thanking Arianos for allowing him a bath after so long a time. Dionysios, his former torturer, is standing by while this is going on and Pteleme says to him, 'Come, bathe your eye in the cauldron, so that you may receive your sight'. Dionysios, naturally reluctant, tells Pteleme that one eye will suffice: he would rather not risk the other! He is finally won over, jumps into the cauldron, and is immediately healed, but is taken out to be buried alive even before Pteleme's final demise. Interestingly, Dionysios cries to God that, although willing to die for the sake of His name, he wishes he had first received baptism. A heavenly voice reassures him he has already received baptism in the cauldron, and he dies happy. This whole incident provides an appealing humour in a narrative otherwise full of grim detail. The saints, as in the case of St George and St Pteleme, were often restored temporarily to full bodily strength following the complete destruction of their bodies from terrible and unbelievable tortures. Yet historical accuracy is not what these accounts are about: the form the narrative takes is the hagiographer's way of conveying a spiritual truth which is at the same time appealing to its audience. A good story is an excellent way of illustrating an argument.

Conclusions

The focus in this book is on disability, although our knowledge is generally informed by the accounts of miraculous healings in the lives of people suffering from short- or long-term conditions. We must remember, however, that, following biblical ideas, sickness was still generally thought to represent a spiritual disorder and thus healing brought about by a holy man represents, in this Christian era, a sign of the 're-creation of humanity through Christ' (Ferguson 1997: 512). We recall also the proviso mentioned earlier, that in each case discernment might be applied. Frequently the healings, inevitably indications of previous incapacity, take place without comment on the sinful state of the person healed. It is generally those who want to be healed that are the recipients of divine grace, but we should bear in mind the fact that many non-religious in late Antiquity may have made their living from begging as a result of their disability. Christ when healing a blind man asked him what he would like him to do for him. 'Lord, that I may see', was his response. This would seem the obvious answer until one considers the fearful question that might be engendered by the need to make a completely new start. Would one succeed in life as a 'whole' person? This issue was amusingly parodied in the film *Life of Brian* (1979) where the lepers prefer to stay lepers because of their lucrative 'charitable' racket. Even if highly capable despite one's disability, like Didymus, how easy would the change be should the disability suddenly be removed? A friend who has been profoundly deaf all her life, yet highly successful in her career in the world, recently had a 'miraculous' cochlear implant and, like others interviewed in recent programmes on this subject, said she found that hearing for the first time necessitated considerable adjustment on her part. Those in the Egyptian desert or in Ethiopia who experienced healing of disability of whatever duration were also empowered to change their lives, sometimes as a condition of their healing, or else were forced to continue in discomfort and misery. There were doubtless many such cases, but these are not what the literary accounts record.

Notes

1   Cf. Shoemaker 2002: 275–6 and references in nn.197–201 for the aid brought by Mary to many worldwide who sought her assistance when all the while she was 'preparing for her death in Bethlehem and Jerusalem'.
2   Apart from Bishop Mercurius (cf. XXIII, cited here p. 357), we hear of the Virgin healing another leper in LXXXIII.
3   In the West the 'milk of the Virgin's intercession' is sometimes referred to, while Bernard of Claivaux claimed healing as a child from three drops of milk from the Virgin's breast. The earliest known but disputed representation of the *Virgo Lactans* is apparently from a catacomb in Rome, but in Egypt it became a popular scene in monks' cells and churches. This subject has been extensively studied by Elizabeth S. Bolman in several articles, while in the book she edited on St Antony's Red Sea Monastery, 2002: 55–7, she suggests that our Ethiopian story may be relevant

to the portrayal of the Virgin and Child in the apse at St Antony's where the painting itself was perhaps used for protection and healing. Cf. Gabra and Krauss 2007: 41–2 and 64, on images of the *Virgo Lactans* at the ruined monasteries of St Jeremiah at Saqqara and St Apollo at Bawit .

4   I am grateful to Archdeacon TesfaMichael for his comments on ritual purity, to Fr Maximous el-Antony for this information about disability and priesthood, and to Michael Jones of ARCE for his observation about logistical difficulties for the disabled in monasteries.

5   A Dalga in Upper Egypt was recently in the news because of the kidnapping of a Christian girl there in 2015.

6   The orphanage in Prousa, Bithynia, mentioned by Theodore the Studite in Letter 211, gives an indication of possible numbers in such an institution, divided between 40 boys and 40 girls, for which inheritances and dowries were provided. See Miller 2003: 133. Whereas very small numbers had once been envisaged in such institutions, this of necessity changes our view and perhaps gives an indication of the possible size of provincial hospitals also. St Coluthus bought an *ergasterion* in Antinoe in which to care for needy strangers, which could indicate large numbers.

7   See also Crislip 2005: 22–5, on demonic and non-demonic illness, and Crislip 2005: 26–38, on religious and medical healing. We also find cited there fragments of a Coptic medical handbook with its herbal treatments from the Monastery of Apa Jeremias at Saqqara, and from Apa Thomas near Assiut fragments on a plastered wall that reveal similar herbal treatments and a papyrus showing that invocations in pharaonic style were still employed in healing alongside 'medical' ingredients. Surgery was also employed as in the case of Apa Stephen's cancer (*HL* 24).

Bibliography

List of abbreviations and editions

Finding passages of late ancient Greek, Coptic or Ethiopic texts can be quite a challenge, even to experienced classicists or ancient historians. However, other than for many Arabic texts (cf. Gaumer and Benkheira in this volume), there has been a tradition of one century of careful text editing, translating and commenting. In order to facilitate consultation for the readers of this volume, there is a list here of editions and translations under the abbreviations which I use in this chapter. The purpose of this list is purely practical: to enable readers not familiar with this research tradition to look up the primary sources. It is not intended to be exhaustive. Also, some books appear twice, as different abbreviations are of necessity used throughout the chapter. My thanks are due to Christian Laes for reordering the abbreviation and editions list and adding this note.

Acts of Thomas

James, Montague Rhodes, The Apocryphal New Testament (Oxford, 1924, corrected 1953. Reprinted 1975).

Apocalypse of Elijah

Coptic Text ed. and tr. Albert Pietersma, Susan Turner Cromstock and Harold W. Attridge (Chico, CA, 1981).

AP = Apophthegmata Patrum

Les Apophtegmes des Pères: Collection Systématique, 3 vols. Sources Chrétiennes 387, 474, 498. Introduction, critical edn, tr. and notes by Jean-Claude Guy (Paris, 1993, 2003, 2005).
Ward, Benedicta, *Sayings of the Desert Fathers: The Alphabetical Collection* (Fairacres, Oxford, 1975).
The Wisdom of the Desert Fathers. Systematic Sayings from the Anonymous Series of the Apophthegmata Patrum, tr. with an introduction by Benedicta Ward (Oxford, 1991).
Les Sentences des Pères du désert. Série des anonymes. 5 vols. French tr. Louis Regnault (Solesmes, 1985).

Besa

Besa, the Life of Shenoute. Introduction, translation and notes by David N. Bell (Kalamazoo, MI, 1983). Text of the Vita in *Sinuthii Archimandritae Vita et Opera Omnia I: Corpus Scriptorum Christianorum Orientalium 4* (Copt. a). Edd. J. Leipoldt and W. E. Crum (Paris, 1906).

Budge

Budge, E. A. Wallis (ed.), *The Martyrdom and Miracles of St George of Cappadocia* (London, 1888).

Budge, E. A. Wallis (ed.), *The Miracles of the Blessed Virgin Mary and her Mother Hanna and the Magical Prayers of Aheta Mîkâêl* (London, 1900).

Budge, E. A. Wallis (ed.), *The Life of Takla Haymânôt and the Miracles of Takla Haymânôt in the Version of Dabra Libanos* (London, 1906).

Budge, E. A. Wallis (ed.), *The Paradise of the Holy Fathers.* Vol. I containing the *Life of St Anthony* by Athanasius, Archbishop of Alexandria, *Histories of the Fathers* by Palladius, Bishop of Helenopolis, *The Rule of Pachomius,* and St Jerome's *History of the Fathers.* Vol. II containing The Counsels of the Holy Men and the Questions and Answers of the Ascetic Brethren, generally known as *The Sayings of the Fathers of Egypt* Translated out of the Syriac with Notes and Introduction by E. A. Wallis Budge (London, 1907).

Budge, E. A. Wallis (ed.), *Coptic Apocrypha in the Dialect of Upper Egypt* (London, 1913).

Budge, E. A. Wallis (ed.), *Legends of Our Lady Mary, the Perpetual Virgin, and Her Mother Hanna,* tr. from the Ethiopic Manuscripts collected by King Theodore at Makdala and now in the British Museum (London, 1922).

Budge, E. A. Wallis (ed.), *One Hundred and Ten Miracles of Our Lady Mary,* tr. from Ethiopic Manuscripts for the most part in the British Museum with extracts from some ancient European versions, and illustrations from paintings in manuscripts by Ethiopian artists (London, 1933).

Chaîne

Chaîne, Marius (ed.), *Le Manuscript de la Version Copte en Dialect Sahidique des 'Apophthegmata Patrum'* (Caïro, 1960).

Encomium = Encomium S. Coluthi

Encomium on St. Coluthus, attributed to Isaac of Antinoe. Ed. Stephen E. Thompson in *Encomiastica from the Pierpont Morgan Library.* CSCO 544 (Scriptores Coptici, Tomus 47), 46–83 (text); CSCO 545 (Scriptores Coptici, Tomus 48), 37–64 (translation).

Four Martyrdoms from the Pierpont Morgan Coptic Codices. Edd. E. A. E. Reymond and John W. B. Barns (Oxford, 1973). [The text and translation of the Martyrdom of St. Coluthus may be found on pp. 23–9, 139–43, 144–50, with Index, 229, Introduction, 9–19].

G¹ etc. = 1st and 2nd Greek Life of Pachomius

Pachomian Koinonia, 3 vols by Armand Veilleux (Kalamazoo, MI, 1980–2).

Guy

Les Apophtegmes des Pères, Collection Systématique, 3 vols. Sources Chrétiennes 387, 474, 498. Introduction, critical edn, tr. and notes by Jean-Claude Guy (Paris, 1993, 2003, 2005).

HL = Historia Lausiaca of Palladius

The Lausiac History of Palladius. Vol. I. A Critical Discussion together with notes on Early Egyptian Monachism. Vol. II. The Greek text edited with introduction and notes (Cambridge, 1898 and 1904).

HMA = *Historia Monachorum in Aegypto*

Historia Monachorum in Aegypto. Greek text ed. André-Jean Festugière (Brussels, 1961).
Ward, Benedicta, *The Lives of the Desert Fathers*, tr. Norman Russell with introduction by Benedicta
Ward (London and Oxford, 1981).

S¹, S² etc. = *the First and Second Sahidic Life of Pachomius*

Pachomian Koinonia, 3 vols by Armand Veilleux (Kalamazoo, 1980–2).

Sbo = *Bohairic Life of Pachomius*

Pachomian Koinonia, 3 vols by Armand Veilleux (Kalamazoo, MI, 1980–2).

VA = *Vita S. Antonii of Athanasius (PG 26.835–976)*

Life of St Antony. English tr. by Robert T. Meyer (London, 1950).
Life of Antony and Letter to Marcellinus. English tr. by Robert C. Gregg (New York, 1980).

V. Syncleticae = *Vita Syncleticae*

Vita Sanctae Syncleticae: 'The Life and Activity of the Blessed Teacher Syncletica'. English tr. by E. A.
Castelli, in V. L. Wimbush, *Ascetic Behavior in Graeco-Roman Antiquity. A Sourcebook* (Minneapolis,
1990) 265-311.

Secondary sources

Amundsen, Darrel W.,and Ferngren, Gary B., 'Disease and Disease Causality in the New Testament',
ANRW II/37/3 (1996), 2934–56.
Bell, David, *Holy Animals: A Book of Beastly Tales* (Kalamazoo, MI, 1992).
Bolman, Elizabeth S., *Monastic Visions: Wall Paintings in the Monastery of St. Antony at the Red Sea*
(New Haven, CT, and London, 2002).
Brown, Peter, *The Cult of the Saints* (Chicago, IL, and London, 1981).
Chitty, Derwas J., *The Desert a City* (New York, 1966).
Coptic Icons. 2 vols (Cairo, 1998) [no authors listed].
Crislip, Andrew T., *From Monastery to Hospital* (Ann Arbor, MI, 2005).
Downer, Carol, 'The Martyrdom of St Pteleme (Pierpont Morgan Coptic Manuscript M581): Edition,
Translation, and Commentary' (unpublished PhD, London, 2004).
Ferguson, Everett (ed.), *Encyclopedia of Early Christianity* (New York and London, 1997²).
Ferngren, Gary B., and Amundsen, Darrel W., 'Medicine and Christianity in the Roman Empire:
Compatibilities and Tension', *ANRW* II/37/3 (1996), 2957–80.
Frankfurter, David, *Elijah in Upper Egypt: The Apocalypse of Elijah and Early Egyptian Christianity*
(London, 1992).
Gabra, Gawdat, and Krauss, Marianne-Eaton, *Treasures of Coptic Art* (Cairo and New York, 2007).
Goehring, James E., and Timbie, Janet A. (eds), *The World of Early Egyptian Christianity: Language,
Literature and Social Context* (Washington, DC, 2007).
Gould, Graham, *The Desert Fathers on Monastic Community* (Oxford, 1993).
Holman, Susan R., 'Sick Children and Healing Saints: Medical Treatment of the Child', in C. B. Horn and
R. R. Phenix (eds), *Children in Late Ancient Christianity* (Tübingen, 2009), 143–70.
Horn, Cornelia B., and Phenix, Robert R. (eds), *Children in Late Ancient Christianity* (Tübingen, 2009).
Horn, Cornelia B., 'Approaches to the Study of Sick Children and their Healing: Christian Apocryphal
Acts, Gospels, and Cognate Literatures, in C. B. Horn and R. R. Phenix (eds), *Children in Late Ancient
Christianity* (Tübingen, 2009), 171–98.
Idris Bell, Harold, *Cults and Creeds in Graeco-Roman Egypt* (Liverpool, 1953).

Illustrations from Coptic Manuscripts (Cairo, 2000) [no authors listed].

James, Montague Rhodes, The Apocryphal New Testament (Oxford 1975; corrected reprint, first edition 1924).

Knapton, Sarah, 'Stimulating the 'Spock' Nerve in the Neck Can Halt Arthritis', in Daily Telegraph, 7 July (2016).

Knibb, Michael A., *Translating the Bible: The Ethiopic Version of the Old Testament* (Oxford, 1999).

Laes, Christian, 'Young and Old, Parents and Children: Social Relations in the Apophthegmata Patrum', in C. Krötzl and K. Mustakallio (eds), *De Amicitia: Social Networks and Relationships in Antiquity and the Middle Ages* (Rome, 2010), 115–34.

Laes, Christian, 'Silent Witnesses: Deaf-Mutes in Graeco-Roman Antiquity', *Classical World* 104/4 (2011), 451–473.

Miller, Timothy S., *The Orphans of Byzantium: Child Welfare in the Christian Empire* (Washington, DC, 2003).

Neil, Brownen, 'The Miracles of SS. Cyrus and John: The Greek Text and its Transmission', *Journal of the Australian Early Mediaeval Association* 2 (2006), 183–93.

Sellew, Philip, 'Thomas Christianity: Scholars in Quest of a Community', in J. N. Bremmer (ed.) *The Apocryphal Acts of Thomas* (Leuven, 2001), 11–35.

Shoemaker, Stephen J., *Ancient Traditions of the Virgin Mary's Dormition and Assumption* (Oxford, 2002).

Stathakopoulos, Dionysios (ed.), *The Kindness of Strangers: Charity in the Pre-Modern Mediterranean* (London, 2007).

Wilfong, Terry G, *Women of Jeme: Lives in a Coptic Town in Late Antique Egypt* (Ann Arbor, MI, 2002).

Youssef, Youhanna Nessim, 'The Liturgical Comb from Dayr Abū-Hinnis', in *Coptica 13* (2014), 41–9.

26

THE DISABILITY WITHIN

Sexual desire as disability in Syriac Christianity

John W. Martens

At various points in the biblical tradition, both in the Hebrew Bible (HB) and in the New Testament (NT), female barrenness is seen as a disability which impacts individuals and the broader community. After all, the first blessing in the HB is Genesis 1: 28, in which 'God blessed them, and God said to them, "Be fruitful and multiply, and fill the earth and subdue it"'. Examples of barrenness in the HB, which run counter to God's blessing, include Sarah, Rebekah, Hannah and Samson's mother; in the NT, the most significant example is Elizabeth, the mother of John the Baptist. Their disability is healed when God gives them all the blessing of a child.

And yet, by the time we come to the texts of the late antique Syriac Christian tradition, *Gospel of Thomas* (*GTh*), the *Acts of Judah Thomas* (*AJTh*), the *Liber Graduum* and Aphrahat's *Demonstrations*, it is fecundity and sexuality that are seen as disabilities, something which is an obstacle to salvation and which must be healed. In the earliest Syriac Christianity it was necessary to be celibate to receive baptism (Brock 1973: 7; Harvey 1990: 4–8; Murray 2004: 15, 1975: 58–79; Vööbus 1951: 9–58).

While this would change by the 4th century, the view of sexuality was not much altered for the religious elite. As described in the *Liber Graduum* and Aphrahat's *Demonstrations*, a place was made for married Christians, who were a majority, but it was the celibate who had conquered their sexual disability and by virtue of this already shared life with the angels in heaven. It is true that the modern, scholarly language of disability was not on the minds of Syriac Christians (cf. Solevåg in this volume) but the theological constructions of sexual desire had broad social repercussions in Syriac Christianity both for those for whom sexuality became a major disability for living the Christian life and for married Christians.

Notions of disability

Before examining the Syriac texts, it will be necessary to discuss how I understand disability and how it might apply to the Syriac Christian texts. Candida Moss and Jeremy Schipper write that 'when we discuss disability, we often discuss more than an exclusively medical or biological condition. We do not understand disability in medical terms alone' (Moss and

Schipper 2011: 2). Their point is that notions of disability depend upon social context and experience, including religious belief. In the context of ancient Judaism, infertility

> embodies perfectly the modern definition of a disability. One of the fundamental premises of critical disability theory is that what qualifies as a disability depends on the cultural ideas that we use to narrate and interpret physical, cognitive, and emotional differences. When we identify some of these differences as 'disabilities,' we are usually describing more than just a medical diagnosis. We are also accounting for political, religious, sexual, and legal factors, among others, related to the social and environment context in which these differences present themselves (…) Discussions of disability can help us to express a variety of cultural ideas, including ideas about gender, divine activity, marriage, family, and the eschaton.
>
> *(Baden and Moss 2015: 4–5)*

The religious factor named here is significant, since often stigmas 'based on various physical deformities, those associated with perceived blemishes of character, and those described as "tribal stigmas" (race, religion, nationhood) are broken down in religious contexts' (Baden and Moss 2015: 5). They might be 'broken down' in two ways, with some differences no longer being seen as disabilities, such as race or nationhood, while others, previously not seen as disability, such as sexuality, now understood as disabling.

Christianity began to challenge the assumption that barrenness was a disability and switched the code (Baden and Moss 2015: 6). Beginning with the teachings of Jesus and continuing with those of the Apostle Paul, early Christianity began to think of abstention from marriage and celibacy, in preparation for the eschaton, as the preferred path. While marriages were chosen by most people, an important point to which we will return, they were considered secondary in religious worthwhileness by the religious elite. It is not strange that some branches of Christianity would validate celibacy above all, to the extent that sexuality itself was seen as a burden, or obstacle in the way of salvation.

Amos Yong, for instance, has argued that the Ethiopian eunuch is disabled, since he is unable to procreate. Yong says that in the Ethiopian eunuch's conversion and baptism 'the redemption of disability doesn't necessarily consist in the healing of disabilities but involves the removal of those barriers – social, structural, economic, political, and religious/theological' which exclude those with disabilities (Yong 2011: 69). But we can take it a step further: if the status of the eunuch renders him unable to procreate, he is not disabled, but perfectly prepared for the ideal Christian life, both in the present and in the world to come. The eunuch's body is the one that is healed, or already whole, the body for which Christians should aim (Baden and Moss 2015: 212). If sex is eliminated in the afterlife, as is the claim in Mark 12: 25, then the barren body or celibate person is prepared for the afterlife (Doering 2009). Sexual desire and behaviour are disabling physical and spiritual forces which can keep a person from their true goal. Sexuality is not a blessing, but a sign of corruption.

Disability in general can be understood as something 'taken away' from the whole, some physical or medical defect, something lacking or missing, or harmed or made less than it should be (Baden and Moss 2015: 221). This notion of 'defect' fits the Syriac Christian understanding of sexuality, with one important proviso: in Syriac Christianity disability will be seen as something added to our nature, which could be called a 'corruption' of our true nature instead of a defect, though both terms can be employed. Though the defect might not be visible, it is real and located in the fallen body, something which must be conquered, either today in this world by the celibate, or at the end when it will be healed in the eschaton.

The concept of sexuality as disability would not be discussed overtly in ancient Syriac Christianity (Laes *et al.* 2013a: 5–6). The language used has more to do with 'war', 'contest' and 'struggle'. Who perceives the reality as a disability: the modern scholar imposing his beliefs on Antiquity, or the ancients, who do not use this language to define sexuality? It is an important question, and one which must be considered carefully, but it is the case that in using the language of disability we do unravel a particular strand of belief about the function of sexuality in the Syriac Christian tradition. While the disability is located in each person, the construction of sexuality is not simply a personal idiosyncrasy, but a widely shared social belief in the broad Syriac Christian culture.

Sexuality as disability in Syriac Christianity

What is remarkable about Syriac Christianity is that celibacy and singleness remained essential to the Christian life to a much greater extent in late Antiquity than in other branches of Christianity (Vööbus 1951: 26). The asceticism at the heart of Syriac Christianity is evident in the *GTh*, *AJT*, the *Liber Graduum* and Aphrahat.

There are numerous other texts which could be examined in this context, but for the limits of this chapter these will be sufficient to show how virginity (*btuluta*) and holiness (*qaddishuta*), the latter indicating sexual continence after marriage, were essential for the Christian life. Indeed, 'prior to the fourth century, celibacy was a requirement for baptism in the Syriac Church', and though by the time of Aphrahat in the 4th century this requirement had passed, 'the ideal of celibacy as a necessary step on the road to perfection for the elite among the spiritual pilgrims continued as a fundamental tenet of Syriac spirituality' (Kitchen and Parmentier 2004: pp. xv–xvi). Syriac Christians of all types agreed that asceticism was at the heart of the Christian life and that two distinct categories of Christians existed: those who were willing to combat sexual desire and root it out completely and those who had to have accommodations made for their weakness (Vööbus 1958: 5). The sexual drive or impulse was throughout Syriac Christianity understood as a disabling force for the holy life (Vööbus 1958: 7).

Gospel of Thomas

The *GTh* does not give a systematic examination of any particular sexual issue, but in its *logia* certain sexual themes emerge. Among these is that Jesus' disciples should transcend sexuality and become like children, a basic concept of Greco-Roman thought in this period (Herter 1961). In *GTh* 21 Jesus describes his disciples as 'children living in a plot of land that is not theirs', and further on Jesus compares nursing infants to 'those who enter the kingdom':

> They said to Him, 'Shall we enter the kingdom by being little ones?' Jesus said to them, 'When you (plur.) make the two one, and when make the inside like the outside and the outside like the inside and the above like the below, and that you might make the male and the female be one and the same, so that the male might not be male nor the female be female (…) then will you enter [the kingdom]'.
>
> *(GTh 22)*

In *GTh* 37 Jesus tells the disciples that he will be revealed 'when you strip naked without being ashamed and take your garments and put them under your feet like little children and tread upon them, then [you] will see the child of the living'. While there is an opaqueness in many of the *GTh logia*, there is also a clear sense that Jesus' disciples by becoming children renounce sexuality and gender (Layton 1987: 384; all translations of *GTh* are from Layton 1987: 380–99).

GTh 114 might also fit in this genderless context when Simon Peter dismisses Mary:

> for females are not worthy of Life. Jesus said, 'See, I am going to attract her to make her male so that she too might become a living spirit that resembles you males. For every female who will make herself male will enter the kingdom of heavens'.

While there might be an element here of common ancient misogyny, 'male' might also be understood as moving beyond gender categories in order to achieve salvation (cf. Solevåg in this volume on misogyny; Horn 2013b: 131, n. 56).

GTh 27, which in Bentley Layton's translation reads, 'If you (plur.) do not abstain from the world you will not find the kingdom' offers an interesting possibility in the Syriac Christian context. Vööbus translates it, 'If you do not *fast* to the world, you will not find the kingdom' (Vööbus 1958: 14, n. 43). Vööbus connects this passage to the developed thought world of the *Liber Graduum*, in which 'fasting to the world' is essential to the Perfect Christian and which comprises in the first place celibacy. Layton does note that his 'abstain from' is literally 'fast unto', so Vööbus's insight is important (Layton 1987: 385, note e). It is not that Vööbus is arguing that the *GTh* contains the entire thought world of the *Liber Graduum*, only that both texts reflect a common religious worldview regarding sexuality.

The argument is not that a 'Thomasine community' underlies Syriac Christianity, but that the texts represent certain streams of thought common in Syriac Christianity. Philip Sellew says, 'no doubt the *Gospel of Thomas*, the *Book of Thomas*, and the *AJTh* do share a strongly negative attitude toward the physical world, and, in the latter two books, a special hatred of sexuality' (Sellew 2001: 11, 28). While Sellew would not see the sexual attitudes in *GTh* to be as sharp and thoroughgoing as the other Thomas texts, he acknowledges that Jesus makes disparaging remarks about sex and birth in the *Gospel of Thomas* which would be 'read by an encratite Christian with pleasure' and that such 'similar attitudes' regarding sex 'are notably visible in Syrian Christianity' (Sellew 2001: 28) This is the key point: the sexual milieu of preference for celibacy and even rejection of marriage presented in Syriac Christianity develops from its earliest stages and 'can be traced through the *Gospel of Thomas* (early to mid second century), the *Diatessaron of Tatian* (late second century), and the *Acts of Judas Thomas* (early third century)' (Lehto 2001: 194–5; Brown 1988: 87–102). Our focus moving forward, however, will be on the *Odes of Solomon* and the *AJTh*.

Odes of Solomon and Acts of Judah Thomas

Michael Lattke dates the *Odes of Solomon* to the first quarter of the 2nd century, making the text an early witness to sexual understandings in Syriac Christianity (Lattke 2009: 6–14). Love is presented not in the context of marital union, but the union of God and believer, which leads to salvation. A focus on Lover and Beloved in the divine–human union is found in numerous places, such as *Ode* 3.4–5, 7, 8.22 and 42.7–9. In *Ode* 42.7–9, God speaks, saying that God's love is 'like a bridal tent, pitched in the house of the bridal pair, so my love is over those who believe in me' (Lattke 2009: 582; see also *Ode* 16.2–3).

There are also passages which cast the relationship with sin in marital and erotic terms, speaking of the 'Archcorruptor (corruptor of all)', 'the Bride who brings corruption' and 'the Bridegroom who is corrupting and corrupted'. The narrator asks 'Truth':

> 'Who are these?' And she said to me: 'This is the Deceiver and Error, and they imitate the Beloved and his Bride, and they lead the world astray and corrupt it. And

they invite the many to the wedding feast, and give them to drink, the wine of their intoxication, so that they vomit up their knowledges and their thoughts, and make them foolish/senseless, and then they throw them out/abandon them. But they go about raving and corrupting/ corrupted.

(Ode 38.9–14; Lattke 2009: 510)

In *Ode* 33, the 'Perfect Virgin' stood up against 'Corruption' exhorting the 'Sons of men' and 'their daughters' to 'leave the ways of this Corruption and draw near to me; then I will enter into you and bring you out from destruction and make you wise in the ways of truth. You will not be corrupted or perish' (*Ode* 33.1–9; Lattke 2009: 448).

Sexuality itself must be Corruption. Harris and Mingana note that 'there are some unexplained allusions and unrecognized references, e.g. there is the "Corruptor" who is twice referred to, who will turn up again in Ode xxxviii in just as perplexing a form' (Harris and Mingana 1920: 377). Lattke does note that the Greek underlying the Syriac for 'corruption' is probably *phthora/phtheirô*, a word and lexical set which has at its root sexual corruption and destruction (Lattke 2009: 451–4; see Martens 2009 on the Greek roots). The Perfect Virgin in *Ode* 33 (Greek: *parthenos*; Syriac: *btulta*) is also the force which conquers sexual corruption and draws the believers away from human sexuality.

Apart from these allusions to sexuality there are passages which connect salvation with casting off the human body, primarily the corrupting force of sexuality. We find these in *Ode* 11 and *Ode* 25. *Ode* 11.10–12 says, 'I left folly behind lying on the earth, and I stripped it off and cast it from me. And the Lord renewed me by his garment and gained me by his light and from above he gave me imperishable rest' (Lattke 2009: 150–1). Lattke says, 'The speaking "I" now fixes on the protological *Urzeit* of biblical humankind and connects the eschatological *Endzeit* of the Spirit with the vocabulary of the Psalms and soteriology in general' (Lattke 2009: 362). A key element of the *Endzeit* in Syriac Christianity is the casting off of sexuality and becoming like a child.

Sebastian Brock speaks of a fourfold scenario, known throughout the Syriac tradition, in which Adam and Eve lost the glory of their incarnation. He says,

the 'robe of glory' which Adam and Eve lost in Paradise at the Fall is thus recovered by the Christian at Baptism in the font. Baptism is indeed reentry into Paradise, but this is not just Paradise at the beginning of time, but also an eschatological Paradise. There is a certain tension here, for at baptism the robe of glory is regained in potential, but not yet fully in reality, for this will only happen at the end of time, at the general resurrection. The final reality can, however, to some extent be anticipated in this life by the saints, who preserve their robe 'unspotted'.

(Brock 1982: 13)

This sense of the 'new' person who emerges from salvation is found in *Odes* 17.4, 39.1–6 and 13.3–4. In *Ode* 17.4, for instance, the speaker says, 'I receive the face and figure of a new person. And I walked in it and was saved' (Lattke 2009: 233).

Finally, there are the questions of 'war' which run through the *Odes*. Vööbus says that 'the Odes of Solomon depict the "saints" as those whose life is not an ordinary one but is characterized by "war"' (1958: 8). This is the 'war' of asceticism conducted against the body, particularly sexuality. Those who are engaged in the 'war' and who persevere in this 'war' gain spiritual victory as we see in *Odes* 8.7, 9.6–12, 28.4–7 and 29.9.

This brings us to the *AJTh*, which in the 2nd to 3rd century documents offers the most relentless presentation of sexuality as a disabling force. As Vööbus says, 'in the Acts of Thomas, the chief characteristic of the Christian life is the "contest,"' which 'embraces all aspects of asceticism – privation, mortification, but above all, virginity' (1958: 8). This continues the theme of 'war' against the fallen body, but is much more direct about the disability of sexuality. The following passage is striking for the way in which it presents the disabling force of sexuality and its result, children:

> Remember, my children, what my brother spoke with you, and know to whom he committed you; and know that as soon as you preserve yourselves from this filthy intercourse, you become pure temples, and are saved from afflictions manifest and hidden, and from the heavy care of children, the end of whom is bitter sorrow. And if you have children, for their sakes you will become oppressors and robbers and smiters of orphans and wringers of widows, and you will be grievously tortured for their injuries. For the greatest part of children are the cause of many pains; for either the king falls upon them, or a demon lays hold of them, or paralysis befalls them. And if they be healthy, they come to ill either by adultery or theft, or fornication, or covetousness, or vain-glory; and through their wickedness you will be tortured by them. But if you will be persuaded by me, and keep yourselves purely to God, you shall have living children, to whom not one of these blemishes and hurts comes near; and you shall be without grief and without sorrow; and you shall be hoping (for the time) when you shall see the true wedding feast; and you shall be in it praisers (of God), and shall be numbered with those who enter into the bridal chamber.
>
> *(AJTh 12; Klijn 2003: 52–3)*

Sexual intercourse itself is a category of spiritual disability, but intercourse also leads to 'afflictions manifest and hidden', which might indicate spiritual disabilities, physical maladies or that children themselves are afflictions, a disabling burden brought through sexual intercourse. For children are a 'heavy care' which leads to 'bitter sorrow'. Even more, for reasons which are not explained, children lead people to become 'oppressors and robbers and smiters of orphans and wringers of widows', a developed theme also found in John Chrysostom's *De virginitate* 57 and throughout early Christian texts (Horn and Martens 2009: 110–13). It is not explained why this is the case, but the suggestion is that, to support children, parents will do anything that is necessary, including harming others or lawbreaking. Yet, if you are not breaking the law for them or oppressing others, children cause pain, through the abuse they suffer from political leaders, spiritual oppression or physical ailments. And in the off chance that they are healthy or free of physical, spiritual or political oppression, they are sinful, which itself will torture the parents. There seems to be no possibility of having a child who creates joy, who is free from oppression and who leads a virtuous life.

This theme is constant in the *AJTh*. In *AJTh* 51 sex is described again as 'filthy intercourse' and a male kills his adulterous lover (Klijn 2003: 127). In *AJTh* 52, Thomas says:

> O corrupt love, that has no shame, how it has incited this man to do these things! O the companion of corruption, how this man has not been able to bear up against it! O lascivious intercourse, how it corrupts the minds of men (and turns them away) from the purity of the Messiah! O work of deception, how it rears itself up exceedingly on its own!
>
> *(Klijn 2003: 128)*[1]

In *AJTh* 53, Thomas and the boy (or man) go to find the woman and it turns out she is a girl; they ask Jesus to raise her up. In *AJTh* 54, Thomas makes the sign of the cross on the boy and tells him to take the girl's hand. When he does, the girl comes to life. She has had a horrible vision of hell, destined for those 'which change the union of intercourse that has been appointed by God; and other (souls) are destined to come into this torment, which have not preserved their virginity, and have given themselves up to the deed of shame' (*AJTh* 55) (Klijn 2003: 132).

In *AJTh* 56, a vision is presented of another pit of hell, for men who leave their wives and have sex with someone else's wife, for women who sleep with someone other than their husband, for youths who sleep around with everyone and anyone, and for girls who do not preserve their virginity. The way to be free of this disability is to reject sexuality.

Liber Graduum

We see the development of such teaching in the *Liber Graduum*, in which two sorts of Christians are presented: the 'Upright', ordinary Christians who marry, and the 'Perfect', who renounce family ties and marriage (Vööbus 1958: 11–12; *Mēmrā* 11, col. 475, 7–10; 30, col. 920, 22). The Perfect are 'fasting to the world' by rejecting marriage and sexuality and see themselves as living in the spiritual realm with God even while bodily still on earth (Vööbus 1958: 14–15; *Mēmrā* 15, 16, col. 373, 18–19; 11, 18, col. 382).

The Perfect, or 'solitary' (*iḥidaya*), have become like Adam before his fall and 'reached a status like the angels' (Vööbus 1958: 16; *Mēmrā* 12, 4, cols 293, 296). The disability of sexuality has been excised, for the Perfect have 'made the city into a desert by living in the realized eschaton of the original Eden, while Adam "had not yet sinned"' (Kitchen and Parmentier 2004: p. xxxviii). This encapsulates the view that sexuality is a disability which keeps us from the true life for which we were intended and which the perfect ones have conquered or overcome.

These views seem counterintuitive to human bodiliness and naturalness of sexuality, but in the *Liber Graduum*, the author reflects that 'if all people had earnestly desired holiness/ celibacy, God would have created children for them just as God had made a daughter (Eve) for Adam without marriage or lust' (Kitchen and Parmentier 2004: p. lvix). How can sex be unnatural to the human being?

God did not intend for human beings to engage in sexual intercourse and before Adam and Eve sinned they were without lust (*Mēmrā* 15, col. 340, 2). Once they desired sex, they became like animals instead of like angels (*Mēmrā* 21, col. 613, 10). According to the *Liber Graduum*, sexual desire came to Adam through the teaching of Satan, who had plotted to make him fall from the sanctity of the angels and imitate wild beasts (*Mēmrā* 15, col. 336, 1; Kitchen and Parmentier 2004: 139–40). The sexual organs might be considered an argument for the naturalness of sexuality, but they initially had a different purpose and lust was a defect or corruption of their original purpose. God would have made for people children apart from sexual intercourse, just as Adam and Eve were made, 'or if he had wanted he could have made children by the hairs of their heads or by their finger nails, and the people would have become the images of angels' (*Mēmrā* 21, cols 601, 7–604, 3; Kitchen and Parmentier 2004: 144).

But how might sexual desire 'be removed from his children' (*Mēmrā* 15, col. 336, 1)? If people will turn to God, 'God will command that lust be removed from the heart and the instinct from the body completely. Then they will become "holy" like children' (*Mēmrā* 15, col. 341, 3; Kitchen and Parmentier 2004: 141). The sexual disability was 'planted' in Adam before he sinned and must be 'rooted out' to gain salvation (*Mēmrā* 20, col. 532, 3). Indeed, Christ came to restore to us our true nature, free of disability (*Mēmrā* 23, col. 692, 1). One can only dig out this evil root by not taking wives or husbands, for 'the wounds of Adam and of his children are healed by this when they enter spiritually that Paradise from which their father [Adam] had departed' (*Mēmrā* 25, col. 741, 5; 29, col. 856, 19; Kitchen and Parmentier 2004: 294). There is no wound which disables more than that of sexuality.

Aphrahat, Demonstrations

Aphrahat's *Demonstrations* brings us to the culmination of our study, in which the major issue is the life of virginity, which he describes as 'the heavenly lot, the fellowship of the angels of heaven for there is nothing that is like unto it' (*Dem.* 6.15; Vööbus 1958: 21). Those who truly want to be disciples of Jesus forego marriage and imitate Jesus' life in order to participate in the heavenly life now (*Dem.* 6.8; 18.10). Aphrahat speaks of these people as 'solitaries, ascetics and saints', utilizing the Syriac words *iḥidaye* and *qaddishe*, people we might think of as monks and nuns, though not necessarily living in community (*Dem.* 7.11; Vööbus 1958: 19). While it is not essential for Aphrahat that every baptized Christian be celibate, 'only those who have chosen perfection are given the glorious outlook that will take place in the final resurrection – all those who have grieved the spirit of Christ, however, will at that time remain naked, retaining only their psychic body' (Vööbus 1958: 22). The body is indeed a stumbling block that must be overcome for those who would seek salvation (Koltun-Fromm 2010: 129).

Aphrahat describes sexual renunciation as found among a Christian elite, the *bnay qyama* (members of the covenant), who he will also refer to as *iḥidaye* (single-minded ones), *qaddishe* (holy ones or celibates) and *btule* (virgins) (Koltun-Fromm 2010: 132). Those who renounce their sexuality share in 'a foretaste of heaven' (Koltun-Fromm 2010: 132). Cornelia Horn has stated with respect to Aphrahat and disability that 'Jesus' divinity was the effective cause that worked healing miracles for the benefit of humankind', and the truly healed in body and soul are the *iḥidaye*, who already share in the life in heaven and model Jesus for the rest of humanity (Horn 2013a: 78).

The lives of the celibate are described in *Demonstrations* 7, 18 and 20 in which all of the postulants are asked to turn away from families and wives and property. The *iḥidaye* are prepared either as women betrothed to the Bridegroom Messiah or as men functioning as virginal bridesmaids and wedding guests. The pure virgins 'are betrothed to the Messiah' and so they 'separate themselves from the punishment on the head of the daughters of Eve' (*Dem.* 6.6; 269.6–14; translation Lehto 2001: 199–200; Koltun-Fromm 2010: 142. Vööbus 1958: 21). However they are named, *iḥidaye*, *qaddishe* or *btule*, they are a healed womanhood, unlike the daughters of Eve. For Aphrahat a woman is either 'a virginal bride of the Messiah or a sexually tainted daughter of Eve' (Koltun-Fromm 2010: 143). The healing through celibacy allows one to put on the wedding garments, and brings humanity to wholeness (*Dem.* 6.14/293.24–296.7; Koltun-Fromm 2010: 147).

Those who remain celibate are not just watched and served by the angels (*Dem.* 6.6), but they have also become like the angels, indeed like Christ, in their asexual lives by anticipating and sharing in the life of heaven. In Aphrahat's thought celibacy is regaining the lost 'garments of glory', or bringing the body to its fullness by putting on Christ and becoming like him. Virginity is 'the heavenly lot, the fellowship of the angels of heaven – for there is nothing that is like unto it' (*Dem.* 6.15; Vööbus 1958: 21). It was because Christ took on a body that our bodies can be healed, for Christ's perfect body has mastered the disability for humanity (*Dem.* 6.10; Lehto 2001: 199, n. 25). 'The weak body became strong, and received a glory which was greater and more wondrous than that which Adam stripped off in his fall' (*Dem.* 23.51; Lehto 2001: 197–8). His perfect body allows us to heal our disabled bodies.

Conclusions

Literary Syriac Christianity throughout late Antiquity takes sexuality as a disability at the heart of human existence. Some will be conquered by the disability, some will only manage the disability, with the healing to come in the eschaton. But the fact that Christ has mastered the disability for humanity by his incarnation, allowing the celibate to heal the wounded, corrupt body of Adam, means that the body can be healed even in this life. The disability model presented here moves 'beyond understanding disability as a personal struggle on an individual level as opposed to a structural or systemic one' (Moss and Schipper 2011: 2). There is nothing more structural or systemic than the bodies with which we are born, even if the battle resides in each individual body. Kate Cooper cites Mary Douglas, who says 'the human body is never seen as a body without being treated as an image of society' (Cooper 1996: 57).

Here we see precisely the socially constructed nature of disability, even when it is a theologically idealized view of humanity (Moss and Schipper 2011: 3). This theological sexual disability is universally embedded in human beings as a flaw or bad code in the system, but the reality was that most Syriac Christians accepted the flaw and chose to marry and raise families. There are data that support our intuition that most people married, as 'we know from the tombstones of countless chaste wives throughout the Roman empire that such duties to past and future generations were valued as much by Christians as by pagans' (Cooper 1996: 55). Cooper asks the ancient question of Christian sexual ascetics: 'if chastity (avoidance of fornication) is good, is not continence (avoidance of sex altogether) better?' (Cooper 1996: 56). In practice most Syriac Christians answered: no. They rejected this socially constructed notion of disability in practice, even if it influenced them theologically. It is true that in 'the cultural model descriptions of disability become one way by which we create or shape culture' (Moss and Schipper 2011: 4), but this study also shows the limits of such creation. Historically most Christians did not act as if sexuality was a corruption or a defect.

As an example, a fascinating study waits to be written on these same themes in Armenian Christianity. We know that between the 2nd and 4th centuries it was Syriac Christianity not the Cappadocian Greeks who first brought Christianity to Armenia, even if the Greek tradition finally gained the upper hand (Taft 1997: 177, 179). The number of Syriac Christian texts which survive in Armenian today are many, some surviving only in an Armenian corpus. The Armenian translation of the *Srboyn Ephremi Matenagrowthiwnikh*, for instance, maintains the Christianity of two paths, one of the Perfect, the other of the Upright. It speaks of a spiritual battle or war. In Vööbus's translation, 'whosoever expresses the desire to be enlisted, and inscribes himself in the ranks on the role of the warriors here in this world, in advance he sets this in his mind – to go forth from his home and his relationships, to depart into other regions and to plunge himself into the contest of the war unto death' (Vööbus 1958: 315–19). This asceticism is also found in Ephrem's Armenian *Prayers*, which have 'a very decidedly monastic, even ascetic, flavor' and which depict Ephrem, rather unhistorically, 'as such an extreme ascetic and hermit' (Mathews 2006: 169). This ascetic quality is presented regarding Ephrem even though the *Prayers* are not genuinely Ephrem's and emerge from the Armenian tradition (Mathews 2006: 170). Yet, this literary and theological path of sexual renunciation borrowed from the Syriac tradition did not take hold the same way in the socio-theological milieu of Armenia.

The phrase *bnay kyama* (members of the covenant) survives in Armenian, but not as a description of the elite spiritual warriors, who took on celibacy, but of the whole church as 'Alliance' (Armenian: *uxt*) (Zekiyan 2006: 266). Ascetic rigour was manifested within Armenian Christianity more often in martyrdom than in the rejection of sexuality and family (Zekiyan 2006: 268). In the Armenian context, we might consider that martyrdom valued the human body to a greater degree than Manichaean dualism, as manifested in Syriac spirituality (Cooper 1996: 117). Armenian spirituality certainly shares 'the basic and common trends' of all patristic spirituality, and anachoretism and eremitism did exist in Armenia, but 'the most unusual manifestations of early Christian eremitism, such as stylitism and similar affiliated practices which are frequent and typical, indeed, in the Syriac area especially' were not common in Armenia (Zekiyan 2006: 265–6).

Yet, it is not so much an Armenian rejection of the Syriac view of sexuality as disability that must be offered, but rather the Syrian enthusiasm for it that needs explanation. General answers, even if not definitive, might be suggested. In the sexual model of disability, the defect or corruption is within all of us, planted by an enemy, and the only way to overcome it or defeat it, is to uproot it through celibacy. To conquer the disability, to become perfect, is to become whole again, but most late antique Christians, men and women, yearned rather to engage in sexuality, create families and to have children. As powerful as the impulse to celibacy was in Syriac Christianity, it was in the end an elitist or limited disability, which only those who accepted it as such chose to have. The vast majority of people saw sexuality and children as a desirable gift and barrenness as a disability, regardless of the theological narrative.

As Cornelia Horn shows us, the sexual ascetics in Syriac Christianity, and elsewhere, were used by ordinary Christians as a means to heal more mundane and ordinary physical disabilities, not necessarily as models to emulate (Horn 2013a, 2013b: 121). Even more, it is often the case that those who chose sexual renunciation did so against the wishes of their parents, such as Thecla who refused to marry Thamyris, against her mother's and her fiancé's wishes (Horn and Martens 2009: 318–19; Cooper 1996: 50–3). As we see in the story of Thamyris and Thecla, and as with the Mygdonia cycle in the *AJTh*, sexuality is no longer a part of social continuity and cohesion, but sexual renunciation is 'in the service of a challenge to the establishment' (Cooper 1996: 55). Parents often rejected the ascetic life for children, as they saw 'in asceticism a competing system of social ranking' (Cooper 1996: 82).

On other occasions it could be parents who supported virginity in their children, while the children rejected that life for them, or even the parents who left behind their families for a life of sexual renunciation (Horn and Martens 2009c: 339–45). Ecdicia, for instance, gave away her inheritance to wandering ascetics, even though she had children and a spouse (to whom she had nevertheless made a vow of chastity) (Cooper 1996: 107). While some these texts reflect fictional literary situations, they reflect the reality of the dissonance between the theological claims of celibacy and the desire of most people to marry.

Basically, only a minority even in Syriac Christianity ever saw sexual renunciation as essential to the Christian life, but asceticism creates a genuine possibility for social disorder by presenting to the established order 'an outsider who is patently superior in moral and ethical terms' (Cooper 1996: 57). Ascetic behaviour makes claims designed to create a new identity and new culture, in which power and prestige belong to the spiritual elite (Cooper 1996: 58).

What sort of power, social prestige and self-definition and identity did sexual renunciation grant? In the Syriac Christian context, it was that all others remained in their physically and spiritually disabled states. Only those who had renounced sexuality were a part of a new humanity. Kate Cooper casts this generally as a dispute 'between two very different conceptions of the body social. One, the separatist view, sees religious ideals as a means of distinguishing the chosen few from the unenlightened masses', while the other sees the religion as a means to unite the whole society (Cooper 1996: 93).

For those few, it did not matter that the rest of the society accepted sexuality as a natural part of their lives, as long as within their own tightly woven communities or individual lives they accepted the narrative of the inherent corruption of sexuality. In many ways, in fact, it was the very creation of sexual desire as a disability which allowed the Perfect to make the sorts of sacrifices they felt were essential to their salvation. They named themselves spiritual warriors, in battle against the disabling force of sexuality. In its place they substituted marriage to Christ or some other role in the heavenly nuptial drama, creating an additional, spiritual sexuality in which they were now participating or would participate in the future. No longer flawed like the rest of humanity, they now lived with the angels, even here on earth.

Note

1 Klijn 2003: 128. See also Solevåg 2015 for particular reflections on women, sexuality and disability.

Bibliography

AbouZayd, Shafiq, *Ihidayutha: A Study of the Life of Singleness in the Syrian Orient: From Ignatius of Antioch to Chalcedon 451 A.D.* (Oxford, 1993).
Baden, Joel, and Moss, Candida, *Reconceiving Infertility: Biblical Perspectives on Procreation and Childlessness* (Princeton, NJ, 2015).
Brock, Sebastian, 'Early Syrian Asceticism', *Numen* 20/1 (1973), 1–19.
Brock, Sebastian, 'Clothing Metaphors as a Means of Theological Expression in Syriac Tradition', in M. Schmidt and C.-F. Geyer (eds), *Typus, Symbol, Allegorie bei den östlichen Vätern und ihren Parallelen im Mittelalter: Internationales Kolloquium, Eichstätt 1981* (Regensburg, 1982), 11–38.
Brock, Sebastian, *Studies in Syriac Christianity: History, Literature and Theology* (Aldershot, 1992).
Brown, Peter, *The Body and Society: Men, Women, and Sexual Renunciation in Early Christianity* (New York, 1988).
Cooper, Kate, *The Virgin and the Bride: Idealized Womanhood in Late Antiquity* (Cambridge, MA, 1996).
DeConick, April D., *Holy Misogyny: Why the Sex and Gender Conflicts in the Early Church Still Matter* (New York, 2011).
Deming, Will, 'Mark 9.42–10.42, Matthew 5.27–32, and B. Nid. 13b: A First Century Discussion of Male Sexuality', *New Testament Studies* 36 (1990), 130–41.
Deming, Will, *Paul on Marriage and Celibacy* (Grand Rapids MI, 2004).
Doering, Lutz, 'Marriage and Creation in Mark 10 and CD 4–5', in F. García Martinez (ed.), *Echoes from the Caves: Qumran and the New Testament* (Leiden, 2009), 133–63.
Doering, Lutz, '*Urzeit-Endzeit* in the Dead Sea Scrolls and Pseudepigrapha', in H.-J. Eckstein, C. Landmesser and H. Lichtenberger (eds), *Eschatologie – Eschatology: The Sixth Durham-Tübingen Research Symposium: Eschatology in Old Testament, Ancient Judaism and Early Christianity (Tübingen, September, 2009)* (Tübingen, 2011), 19–58.
Griffith, Sidney H., 'Asceticism in the Church of Syria: The Hermeneutics of Early Syrian Monasticism', in V. L. Wimbush and R. Valantasis (eds), *Asceticism* (New York, 1995), 220–45.
Harris, James Rendel, and Mingana, Alphonse, *The Odes and Psalms of Solomon* (Manchester, 1920).
Harvey, Susan Ashbrook, *Asceticism and Society in Crisis: John of Ephesus and the Lives of the Eastern Saints* (Berkeley, CA, 1990).
Herter, Herman, 'Das Unschuldige Kind', *Jahrbuch für Antike und Christentum* 4 (1961), 146–62.
Horn, Cornelia B., 'Approaches to the Study of Sick Children and their Healing: Christian Apocryphal Acts, Gospels, and Cognate Literatures', in C. B. Horn and R. R. Phenix (eds), *Children in Late Ancient Christianity* (Tübingen, 2009a), 171–98.
Horn, Cornelia B., 'Raising Martyrs and Ascetics: A Diachronic Comparison of Educational Role-Models for Early Christian Children', in C. B. Horn and R. R. Phenix (eds), *Children in Late Ancient Christianity* (Tübingen, 2009b), 293–316.
Horn, Cornelia B., 'Jesus' Healing Miracles as Proof of Divine Agency and Identity: The Early Syriac Trajectory', in C. B. Horn (ed.), *The Bible, the Qur'an, and their Interpretation: Syriac Perspectives* (Warwick, RI, 2013a), 71–100.
Horn, Cornelia B., 'A Nexus of Disability in Ancient Greek Miracle Stories: A Comparison of Accounts of Blindness from the Askleipeion in Epidauros and the Shrine of Thecla in Seleucia', in C. Laes *et al.* (eds), *Disabilities in Roman Antiquity* (Leiden, 2013b), 115–43.
Horn, Cornelia B., and Martens, John W., *'Let the little children come to me': Childhood and Children in Early Christianity* (Washington, DC, 2009).
Horn, Cornelia B., and Phenix, Robert R. (eds), *Children in Late Ancient Christianity* (Tübingen, 2009b).
Kitchen, Robert A., and Parmenier, Martien F. G., *The Book of Steps: The Syriac Liber Graduum* (Kalamazoo, MI, 2004).
Klauck, Hans-Josef, *The Apocryphal Acts of the Apostles: An Introduction* (Waco, TX, 2008).
Klijn, Albertus F. J., *The Acts of Thomas: Introduction, Text, and Commentary* (Leiden, 2003).
Koester, Helmut, *Introduction to the New Testament*, II. *History and Literature of Early Christianity* (New York, 2000).

Koltun-Fromm, Naomi, 'Sexuality and Holiness: Semitic Christian and Jewish Conceptualizations of Sexual Behavior', *Vigiliae Christianae* 54 (2000), 375–95.

Koltun-Fromm, Naomi, *Hermeneutics of Holiness: Ancient Jewish and Christian Notions of Sexuality and Religious Community* (Oxford, 2010).

Laes, Christian, Goodey, Chris F., and Rose, Martha Lynn, 'Approaching Disabilities *a Capite ad Calcem*: Hidden Themes in Roman Antiquity', in C. Laes *et al.* (eds), *Disabilities in Roman Antiquity* (Leiden, 2013a), 1–15.

Laes, Christian, Goodey, Chris F., and Rose, Martha Lynn (eds), *Disabilities in Roman Antiquity: Disparate Bodies* A Capite ad Calcem (Leiden, 2013b).

Lattke, Michael, *Odes of Solomon: A Commentary* (Minneapolis, MN, 2009).

Layton, Bentley, *The Gnostic Scriptures: A New Translation with Annotations and Introductions* (New York, 1987).

Lehto, Adam, 'Women in Aphrahat: Some Observations', *Hugoye: Journal of Syriac Studies* 4/2 (2001), 187–207.

Martens, John W., '"Do Not Sexually Abuse Children": The Language of Early Christian Sexual Ethics', in C. B. Horn and R. R. Phenix (eds), *Children in Late Ancient Christianity* (Tübingen, 2009), 227–54.

Martens, John W., '(Why) Was Jesus Single?', in S. Huebner and C. Laes (eds), *Singles and the Single Life in the Roman and the Late Ancient Worlds* (forthcoming).

Mathews, Edward G., Jr., 'A First Glance at the Armenian *Prayers* Attributed to Surb Ep̄rem Xorin Asorwoy', in R. R. Ervine (ed.) *Worship Traditions in Armenia and the Neighboring Christian East: An International Symposium in Honor of the 40th Anniversary of St Nersess Armenian Seminary* (Crestwood, NY, 2006), 161–74.

Moss, Candida, and Schipper, Jeremy, *Disability Studies and Biblical Literature* (Basingstoke, 2011).

Murray, Robert, 'The Exhortation to Candidates for Ascetical Vows at Baptism in the Ancient Syriac Church', *New Testament Studies* 21 (1975), 58–79.

Murray, Robert, *Symbols of Church and Kingdom: A Study in Early Syriac Tradition* (Piscataway, NJ, 2004).

Sellew, Philip, 'Death, the Body, and the World in the Coptic Gospel of Thomas', *Studia Patristica* 31 (1997), 530–4.

Sellew, Philip, 'Thomas Christianity: Scholars in Quest of a Community', in J. N. Bremmer (ed.), *The Apocryphal Acts of Thomas* (Leuven, 2001), 11–35.

Solevåg, Anna Rebecca, *Birthing Salvation: Gender and Class in Early Christian Childbearing Discourse* (Leiden, 2013).

Taft, Robert, 'The Armenian Holy Sacrifice (*Surb Patarag*)', in R. Taft (ed.), *The Armenian Christian Tradition: Scholarly Symposium in Honor of the Visit to the Pontifical Oriental Institute, Rome, of His Holiness Karekin I, Supreme Patriarch and Catholicos of All Armenians: December 12, 1996* (Rome, 1997), 175–97.

Vööbus, Arthur, *Celibacy: A Requirement for Admission to Baptism in the Early Syrian Church* (Stockholm, 1951).

Vööbus, Arthur, *History of Asceticism in the Syrian Orient: A Contribution to the History of Culture in the Near East*, III (Leuven, 1958).

Yong, Amos, *The Bible, Disability, and the Church: A New Vision of the People of God* (Grand Rapids, MI, 2011).

Zekiyan, Boghos Levon, 'Armenian Spirituality: Some Main Features and Inner Dynamics', in R. R. Ervine (ed.), *Worship Traditions in Armenia and the Neighboring Christian East: An International Symposium in Honor of the 40th Anniversary of St Nersess Armenian Seminary* (Crestwood, NY, 2006), 263–84.

27

THE DISABLED IN THE BYZANTINE EMPIRE

Stephanos Efthymiadis

Byzantine narrative and iconographical sources offer rich and varied material for investigating the history of disabled people in the period from the fourth to the fifteenth century, i.e. the 1,100 years that span the existence of the eastern Roman Empire (330–1453). No doubt as a result of the influence that Christianity exerted on mores, mentalities and institutions, Byzantine authors and artists were less neglectful of this category of vulnerable people than their Greek and Roman predecessors had been. In the first place, suffering people seeking a cure figure prominently in collections of miracles, accounts of miracles included in saints' biographies and, to a lesser extent, in edifying stories, all subgenres of the overarching category of hagiography (Efthymiadis 2014: 1–15, 105–6). In narrative sources of a secular orientation such as historiography and chronicles disability is presented in more matter of fact and less emotional terms, that is, as reports of events involving people who were either born with some serious impairment or disfigurement or who have fallen victim to serious accidents which caused them infirmity or led to their deaths.

In addition to narrative sources and the large number of people with chronic diseases they attest, the history of disabled people in Byzantium can also be reconstructed by recourse to texts of a 'theoretical' nature. By the term 'theoretical' I mean that in these texts the delicate question of disability is treated in general terms with no reference to particular individuals. For instance, several theological discourses of the Church Fathers, writings of spiritual edification and monastic charters (*Typika*), systematically or incidentally, raise the issue of caring about and coping with people suffering from chronic illnesses. Moreover, similar evidence can be culled from Byzantine medical authors who, though heavily dependent on their classical and post-classical counterparts, provide additional information on diseases and their treatment. The absence of references to particular patients and medical cases does not necessarily preclude the possibility that some information was derived from personal 'clinical' experience. Two practising medical doctors, who were at the same time theoreticians, Paul of Nicaea, whose *floruit* can be tentatively placed in the period from the seventh to the ninth century (Ieraci 1995: 15–16), and John Aktouarios (c.1275–post 1328) (Bouras-Vallianatos 2015: 107–8), are cases in point. Finally, a source of equally 'theoretical' character, and one that this time seems most likely to be based on a largely imaginary perception of the disabled, is the *oneirocritica*, i.e. dreambooks, which offer us interesting glimpses into how auspiciously or inauspiciously appearances of figures with impairments in dreams should be interpreted.

Defining and contextualizing the disabled in Byzantium

Nowadays disability is interpreted in broad terms that may entail not only a physical impairment or a sensory imperfection but a mental disorder, emotional instability, retardation in a person's development or some combination of these conditions. In the Byzantine mind, all these categories of people qualified as 'disabled' in the sense that they had some physical (i.e. external) and/or psychic (i.e. internal) defect. To be sure, pride of place was given to those bearing the marks of what might be called extreme disability, namely people who were grossly deformed and disfigured, e.g. monstrous births, dwarfs, lepers and others. In response to this 'embarrassing' challenge, theologians and scientific theoreticians had to provide definitions and seek explanations, which could be used as 'guidelines' for legislation. In sum, both the reception and treatment of the disabled in Byzantine society and law were basically governed by a standard negative attitude based on repulsion and rejection. Nonetheless, a more philanthropic tendency can also be glimpsed, chiefly in response to the teachings of Christianity about social welfare and the humanitarian services that had to be provided for the needy.

All in all, the idea that impairment, imperfection or defectiveness should be easily discernible by others was no doubt often crucial in determining who should be deemed and treated as disabled. Yet this should not be taken to imply that disability was confined to conditions that were obvious and visible. For example, though quite out of step with modern beliefs, albeit in conformity with biblical traditions and a deeply rooted mentality prevailing in pre-modern societies especially in the Mediterranean, the Byzantines considered a woman's inability to conceive a disability. Besides being a curse and cause of social stigma, it was regarded as a serious and chronic illness that required a cure. Byzantine hagiography is teeming with stories relating the miraculous deliverance of women from barrenness. Several saints were said to be the offspring of such miracles, usually following a divine revelation, and cases of barren women going on pilgrimage to a healing shrine or a healer saint are well attested. The *Life of St Nicholas of Sion* relates the story of a woman who, unable to bear a child for no less than twenty-eight years, came to venerate the saint and was told that she would give birth to a boy (ed. I. and N. Ševčenko, 106-109). The miraculous activity of Euphrosyna the Younger, an enigmatic saint from the reign of Leo VI the Wise (886–912), involved the cure of barren women, three of whom were Byzantine empresses. Deliverance from the bonds of barrenness was the result of prayer and/or holding the saint's relic against a women's waist. Nonetheless, in instances where infertility was taken to be the result of demonic possession, the saint had to perform some sort of exorcism. In the long list of miracles found in the *Life of St Symeon the Younger* we hear of a woman from Cilicia who, after twenty years of infertility, managed to conceive a child once the saint had expelled the demon inside her and directed her to return home to live again by her husband's side (ch. 118).

Conversely, another case which contrasts Byzantine with modern ethics concerns a group of people who were particularly prominent in public life throughout a large part of the Byzantine period (i.e. the seventh to eleventh centuries) and who, though they would nowadays be considered 'disabled', were not treated as such in Byzantium. I am referring to the eunuchs. Unlike their marginalization in other societies and cultures, eunuchs in Byzantium formed part of the political and ecclesiastical establishment and some of them came to be venerated as saints. At least two of these saints were subjected by their parents to castration in their early youth (St Metrios: *Synaxarium of Constantinople* 721; St Niketas Patrikios, ed. Papachryssanthou, 325). This act, dictated by the desire for social advancement, is a clear proof of the tolerance with which Byzantine society regarded this particular kind of bodily mutilation, despite the fact that castration was condemned in legislation and penalized in canon law. Evidently, in the case of eunuchs physical disability was not always seen as a defect but was taken as an additional qualification, especially for pursuing certain careers in the imperial administration. Although different views have been put forward as to how they were regarded by Byzantine society at large, for instance, as a third, distinctive gender or as people of fluid identity depending on the context in which they appeared, it is generally accepted that eunuchs obviously shared characteristics that could result in their being labelled as 'disabled' (Ringrose 2003; Tougher 2008; Messis 2014: 361–8.

A more complex problem than that of physical defectiveness was that of defining spiritual, mental or intellectual disability, especially in view of the prevailing mentality that associated these things with evil spirits and demons. The history of mental illness in Byzantium has yet to be written, but it could be argued that its association with the 'demonic' and the 'powers of the Adversary' came about as a result of the establishment of Christianity in the fourth century and society's overall reluctance to totally discard superstition. As a 'disease', demonic possession far outnumbers all other cases of illness that seem to have afflicted people, at least to judge from Byzantine hagiographical accounts, the narrative sources that most commonly refer to patients in search of a cure. Though based on a purely token sample, a survey comparing them with Latin medieval texts of a similar kind shows that demons were much more of a problem in the East than in the West (Moorhead 1981). Two of the most often quoted Byzantine saints' *Lives*, those of Nicholas of Sion and Theodore of Sykeon, are full of cases of cures of demonic possession, most of which are set in rural areas. Yet it is unlikely that different beliefs would have prevailed in the urban domain. The seventh-century collection of the Miracles of St Artemios alludes to a church of St Panteleemon in Constantinople that welcomed demonically possessed people who, apparently, came there to seek a cure through exorcism. The same passage also informs us that in one particular year there were a very large number of the possessed visiting many churches (ed. Papadopoulos-Kerameus, 20; cf.ed. Crisafulli and Nesbitt, 114–55). Evidence drawn from two other hagiographic texts, the *Lives* of Andrew the Fool and Irene of Chrysobalanton, dateable to the tenth and eleventh centuries respectively (ed. Rydén, 18–21, and ed. Rosenqvist, 66–9), shows that similar rituals took place in the Church of Saint Anastasia in the Byzantine capital where people described as having 'drifted' into insanity were led in bound in chains.

The late antique desert fathers meticulously classified demons in different kinds according to the temptations they inflicted on their victims. In eleventh-century Constantinople, an age which was culturally far distant from the deserts of late Antiquity, an erudite intellectual such as Michael Psellos took an interest in popular demonology and on several occasions wrote about it as a scientific subject (Joannou 1971). We must bear in mind that in Byzantium, very much in line with what happened in Greco-Roman Antiquity, the borderline between medicine and superstition was not always clear, with the former frequently overlapping with religion and philosophy (Marx-Wolf and Upson-Saia 2015: 269). Over and above theoretical attitudes, however, the association of madness with demonic possession left its mark on canon law, while civil law was content to strip the insane of their civil rights, rights which in any case were not extended to such categories of 'sane people' as women, small children, slaves, prodigals, etc. (Trenchard-Smith 2010). Echoing this widespread mentality, the *Ecloga*, a collection of laws dating from the mid-eighth century, a period sometimes referred to as the Dark Age(s), introduced demonology into civil legislation, while nonetheless specifying that a spouse who is visited by a demon is no cause for divorce (*Ecloga* 2.9.4).

In setting out the causes and symptoms of demonic possession, authors tend to avoid being as explicit as we might hope. Rather they are content to state whether it was a chronic problem or one due to a temporary aberration or periodic visits from unclean spirits. In a sense, this perception, which indiscriminately and randomly identified any kind of mental disorder with demonic possession, left open the possibility of relief and cure. If it was a devil who entered and dwelt in a person, there was a chance that one day it could be expelled and the captive set free.

Attempting to define the terms that denote physically disabled people collectively produces little in the way of results other than confusion. Indeed, no particular term appears to have been strictly reserved for them rather than indiscriminately referring to sick people at large. For instance, in his description of the Sampson Hospital in Constantinople the historian Prokopios specifies that the establishment was intended for curing the ills of 'ever-suffering' (or troubled) people (ἐς ἀεὶ ταλαιπωρουμένοις ἀνθρώποις, *On Buildings* 1.2.16); his use of a mild term in this context is noteworthy. By contrast, an old man suffering from a hernia and undergoing treatment in another Constantinopolitan hospital is quoted in the collection of miracles of St Artemios as having – in his despair – spat out the following words against the saints, whom he considered his protectors: 'Indeed, St John and St Artemios and St Febronia, have I served you thus from the age of ten right up to the present, that I might become disabled in my old age?' (ed. Papadopoulos-Kerameus, 29; cf. ed. Crisafulli and Nesbitt, 132–3). The word translated here as 'disabled' is ἀνάπηρος, a term, needless to say, with a negative connotation suggesting here some sort of handicap to mobility. As in modern Greek, the use of this term was generalizing, yet exclusively denoted physically disabled people. Sometimes confusion was inevitable. St Philaretos the Merciful is said to have gathered at his mansion a hundred lepers (λωβοί), cripples (κυλλοί), lame (χωλοί), and mutilated (ἀνάπηροι) people whom he had found begging in the porticoes of Constantinople (ed. Rydén, pp. 92-94, vv. 540–1). The citation of these terms one after another is meant to create a cumulative effect and the word ἀνάπηρος, as used here, could equally well designate the 'maimed' as much as the disabled in a more general sense. The late tenth-century *Lexicon of Souda* translates the same word as χωλός, lame, and as applying to one who is exceedingly incapacitated in a limb (ed. Adler 2015). We may thus conclude that, as in Greco-Roman Antiquity (Laes 2008: 89–91), the Byzantine vocabulary of disability was rich but 'flexible', thus lacking in precision and coherence.

Another question arising from our attempt to pinpoint and define cases of disability in Byzantium is whether physical traits that were not consistent with the norm and, as such, provoked mockery and derision, should be reckoned among the social diacritics of disability or rather should not, at least in principle, be viewed from this perspective at all. In keeping with Roman historiographical tradition, physical descriptions, especially of men in positions of power, are a *Lieblingsthema* in narrative sources which, by paying attention to the idiosyncratic traits of such men, aim to convey an implicit message about their character, public image and disposition *vis-à-vis* those they rule. In chronological order, we may single out as examples the emperor Anastasios I (491–518), nicknamed 'Dikoros' (i.e. with irises of two different colours), John, a general of Justinian who had the sobriquet 'the Hunchback' (Prokopios, *Anecdota* 6.5), emperor Michael II (821–9) who was dubbed 'the Stammerer' for his speech impediment and two ill-fated figures in the context of the Sack of Constantinople by the Crusaders in 1204: John Komnenos, surnamed 'the Fat', and the emperor Alexios V Doukas, labelled 'Mourtzouphlos', referring to his overhanging brows and sullen look. These designations must have had some derogatory weight, as they were evocative of commonly held views on what was ugly and abnormal, yet they do not involve any serious hint at disability. Significantly, none of these characteristics would have been an impediment to ascending to the imperial throne or taking up high military office. A similar consideration applies to the most striking example of disability in association with a Byzantine ruler. Emperor Justinian II's first reign (685–95) ended with the cutting off of his nose and tongue followed by a public defamation in the Hippodrome of Constantinople. A western but hardly reliable source, the chronicler Agnellus of Ravenna, later makes mention of a golden nose that must have subsequently covered the missing part (ed. Waitz, 367). Moreover, despite the slitting of his tongue, the main Byzantine sources for his second reign describe him as a talkative person and pay little heed to this handicap. Apparently, to the disappointment of his opponents, his disfigurement did not obstruct his resumption of the imperial dignity some, ten years later (705–11) (Laes 2016).

The case of the violently disfigured Justinian II justifies a brief reference to corporal punishments, first as practised in the public sphere and second as a novelty in Roman law. Historical and hagiographical accounts provide us with numerous instances of corporal punishments imposed on people involved in various capacities in public life. Punitive violence in Byzantium was occasioned by criminal offences related to politics such as plots, perjury, treason and vengeance taken on powerful figures or merely as an abuse of power. Essentially this involved blinding, first as a means of getting rid of one's political enemies and then as a substitute for execution. In a sense, it implied a latent sense of compassion on the part of the powerful and in response called for forgiveness on the part of the 'criminal'. Victims might be members of the family or the entourage of the emperor, his military and ecclesiastical opponents or even captives of a foreign army and other groups of victimized people (Herrin 2000). By the same token, in the eighth century, bodily mutilation, not an unknown means of punishment in Greco-Roman and Oriental practices (Laes 2014: 109–10), has a prominent place in the aforementioned brief law corpus, the *Ecloga*, and in the so-called *Farmer's Law*, a short collection of laws that regulated matters of rural life. As has been argued, despite their cruel character, the introduction of such penalties as blinding or the cutting off of hands or noses for crimes such as sacrilege, robbery, theft, rape and adultery was also meant as a mark of clemency in that mutilation came to largely replace capital punishment (Patlagean 1984).

Judging by the popularity that the *Acts* and *Passions* of the Christian martyrs enjoyed in Byzantium, descriptions of ordeals and tortures were far from being unfamiliar and repulsive to the Byzantines. In these texts the cruel sufferings of the martyrs at the hands of their pagan, Persian or other persecutors were related in the sort of naturalistic detail that must have provoked a highly emotional response from their audience or readership. The effects produced on the Byzantine spectators of scenes of dismemberment and violent martyrdom as represented on church frescoes and in the miniatures of illuminated manuscripts must have been quite similar. Moreover, occurrences of illness and disability were often associated with the idea of suffering and mortification that loomed large in ascetic practice and was variously highlighted in monastic literature, especially of an edifying character (Crislip 2013: 81–108). Overall, in everyday life, the intimate connection that must have developed between people and pain points to a high degree of acceptance of the disturbing, if not awe-inspiring, aspects of disability. This is vividly illustrated in a well-known letter of Synesios of Cyrene (c.370–c.413), which provides a description of a sea-voyage which put his life in jeopardy. Apart from some Jews, the ship's crew consisted of farmers who had had no previous experience of seamanship and were called not by their names but by their misfortunes (οὐκ ἀπὸ ὀνομάτων ἀλλὰ ἀπὸ ἀτυχημάτων): the lame (ὁ χωλός), the hernia (ὁ κηλήτης), the left-hander (ὁ ἀριστερόχειρ), the squint-eyed (ὁ παραβλώψ). 'Each one of them', Synesios adds, 'had a distinctive mark and this was not pleasing at all' (*Ep.* 5.30–4; ed. Garzya, p. 8).

Treating the disabled in society

The continuation in the Byzantine era of a medical tradition and practice that originated in Greco-Roman Antiquity, as can be observed in medical treatises, the tools and instruments used for simple and complicated operations, and the high esteem that physicians enjoyed in society is testimony to the overall care and attention that Byzantine society gave to sick people (Scarborough 1985). However alien to the modern rational mind, the practice of magic and folk medicine, employed especially in rural areas, must be interpreted as a further expression of the same concern. What is more, under the influence of Christian philanthropy and the teaching of the Church Fathers, the Byzantine state and society established and developed a remarkable system of institutional care for the sick and suffering, which was quite elaborate for the infrastructure and expectations of a pre-modern society. Treating patients in charitable foundations sponsored by the state, the church or a monastery formed part of an overall concern for social welfare which also embraced other categories of the population such as the poor and the elderly. As a matter of fact, in all fairness the eastern Roman Empire must be credited with the creation of the hospital as an institution in a form broadly similar to that of modern times, i.e. as a continuously functioning unit providing treatment by trained medical personnel using specialist equipment (Miller 1985; Horden 2005). Hospitals repeatedly appear in the sources in a remarkable line of continuity (from the fourth century to at least the Sack of Constantinople in 1204) and in different corners of the empire outside the major urban centres (Constantinople, Antioch, Alexandria, Thessaloniki). The most famous among them was the aforementioned Sampson hospital in Constantinople situated on the north side of Hagia Sophia and which seems to have gone on functioning until the last centuries of Byzantium (Stathakopoulos 2006). Another remarkable example of a well-organized and well-equipped hospital, about which we know a good deal thanks to its extant regulatory charter (*Typikon*), was the one attached to the imperial monastery of Christ Pantokrator in Constantinople. Founded by Emperor Ioannes II Komnenos (1118–43), it could accommodate fifty bedridden sick people, divided according to the conditions from which they were suffering (e.g. a wound, a fracture, ophthalmia, etc.) and their gender, twelve of the beds being reserved for sick women. Moreover, if from time to time there were vacancies, empty beds would be available to 'other sick people afflicted with simply any disease whatever'. Yet the whole formulation of this provision gives little support to the notion that this astonishing institution was open to serving those suffering from a chronic disability (*Typikon* 83–5; tr. Jordan, 757). At any rate, judging from this example alone, the per capita supply of hospital beds in Constantinople would hardly meet the needs of the most-populated medieval city in Europe.

All in all, we are poorly informed about the flow and the number of sick people receiving treatment in leprosaria and other health-care foundations, and the same holds for the circumstances under which people could find a place in them, let alone the potential duration of their stay. Another episode, concerning the same old man mentioned above who appears in the *Miracles of St Artemios*, testifies to a period of at least ten months in the Constantinopolitan hospital of *Christodote* to which he had turned for a sore in the thorax that risked developing into dropsy. His admission to a hospital was effected by the intervention of the manager of the hospital himself, a person well acquainted with the Patriarch of Constantinople and who pitied the man for living all alone. This last detail leaves room for assuming that a severe or chronic illness did not necessarily entail the transfer of a patient to a hospital if treatment and daily assistance could be provided by the family. Moreover, as follows from this story, admission to a hospital was not a self-evident and recurrent reality for every sick person. Not surprisingly, favouritism and social patronage played a key role. Members of the higher clergy were no doubt expected to get involved in determining the fate of the sick or injured. In the *Life of St Daniel the Stylite* (d. 493) we meet a man travelling from the East who fell victim to robbers in the area of Ankara in Galatia. Passers-by brought him to the town's bishop who had him treated in the local hospital. His wounds healed but he was unable to walk and thus asked the bishop if he could be taken to Constantinople to find a cure through the intercession of the saint. To this end, the bishop provided two assistants and a beast of burden (ch. 87).

Short-term hospitalization was not what was needed for those admitted to the Byzantine leprosaria, hospices providing care for lepers (λεπροκομεῖα). Like St Sampson's hospital, the most famous leprosarium in the City was named after its saintly founder, Zotikos, and was situated on the far shore of the Golden Horn. We know that it was still functioning in the thirteenth–fourteenth century when the hagiographer Constantine Akropolites composed a new text in praise of St Zotikos adding three new miracle tales, two of which concerned two Jewish Khazars who happened to live in the Byzantine capital (ed. Miller, 364–6). We cannot be sure whether foundations actually provided some nursing care to their patients or were chiefly meant as places for keeping them apart from society, for the sake of the 'healthy'. Nonetheless, the fact that we may struggle to answer certain questions pertaining to the actual function of these hospitals hardly invalidates their pioneering character and their witness to a new perception of social philanthropy (Miller and Nesbitt 2014).

Leprosy and epilepsy were the two chronic diseases to which Byzantine theologians, hagiographers and other *literati* constantly turned their attention. Whereas epilepsy had been the disease euphemistically called 'sacred' in Antiquity, it was leprosy that came to be labelled as such in the Byzantine millennium (Makris 1995: 398–401). When discussing epilepsy authors tended to focus on the symptoms and evoke interpretations with regard to its causes. Whether laymen, churchmen, monks or emperors, the record of persons attested in the sources as being tormented by this 'enigmatic' disease is noteworthy. Moreover, setting aside medical authors, eminent Byzantine scholars such as Patriarch Photios (c.810–post 893) and Michael Psellos (1016–post 1073) addressed the subject theoretically, without, however, treating it in a fashion that would challenge the firmly rooted misconception that regularly confused it with mental insanity. The disease spared neither spiritual fathers in the desert nor men of standing (Makris 1995; Leven 1995). The long list of well-known epileptics in Byzantium is headed by the emperors Michael IV (1034–41), John III Vatatzes (1222–54) and his son Theodore II Laskaris (1254–8). At least in the cases of Michael IV and Theodore II the disease was a serious cause of neurosis and depression before turning fatal. Moreover, it must be stressed that suffering from epilepsy was a cause for moral stigmatization and as such was, for instance, a condition attributed by Byzantine chroniclers to Muhammad, the prophet of Islam (Theophanes the Confessor, ed. de Boor, 334; George the Monk, ed. de Boor, II. 698).

Conversely, though there are plenty of references to leprosy, a general label encompassing different skin diseases (Marx-Wolf and Upson-Saia 2015: 266–7), they tend to avoid physical descriptions and merely highlight the plight of sufferers. Nikephoros Xanthopoulos, a fourteenth-century hagiographer, stands out as an exception. In his fourteenth-century collection of the *Miracles of the Virgin of the Source*, he provides us with some explicit details about the appearance of two lepers who benefited from the healing properties of the water and mud that had made this shrine situated outside the walls of Constantinople famous (ed. Pamperis, 70–1, 72–3). All in all, in their homilies the Church Fathers speak of lepers a good deal and provide evidence of their presence in groups (or bands) in urban centres. Gregory of Nyssa urges his audience to feel compassion and look after those human beings who have become like four-footed animals, but who, instead of hooves and claws, support themselves on pieces of wood (*De pauperibus amandis* 2.114). In one of his festal letters pertaining to the celebration of Easter, Cyril of Alexandria (412–44) admonished his flock to visit the lepers and in another he urged them to comfort them by providing the appropriate care (ed. Evieux *et al.*, 398–9, 328–9). The numerous mentions in literary texts and papyri allow us to infer that leprosy, known as *elephantiasis* ('elephant disease'), was endemic to Egypt in that period (Gascou 2005). Moreover, a palaeopathological study has detected traces of the disease in human skeletons found in the Judaean desert, thereby implying its wider dissemination in other regions of the empire (Stathakopoulos 2006: 111).

It was no doubt the conflict between the fear of contagion and infection and the need for compassion and sympathy that led Christian believers to address questions about the treatment of lepers to authoritative spiritual fathers such as the famous recluse ascetic Barsanuphios, who lived in the area of Gaza in Palestine. When asked by someone whether a servant afflicted with leprosy should be released from service or not, the ascetic gave a rather austere reply: 'You need not keep him in your home since not all can put up with living with him ... you should rather take him into a hospice for lepers and offer him food, the necessary clothes and a mattress so that he may not be charged with such expenses' (*Question* 765, ed. Neyt, de Angelis-Noah, 208–10).

Several decades later, at the end of the seventh century, when the empire was shrinking in the face of the rapid advance of the Arabs, we encounter a no less delicate but universal question in the collection of *Questions and Answers* by Anastasios of Sinai, an author active in Cyprus and the Middle East. 'Why is it that among us Christians, rather than among other unbelieving nations, there are often far more maimed people, and lepers, and those crippled with gout, and epileptics, and those in the grip of other complaints?' Quite unexpectedly, in interpreting this imbalance between Christian populations and those of other religions, Anastasios takes a materialistic stance. For him, race and climate and, aside from them, excessive wine-drinking and eating were the significant factors causing an increase in the number of disabled people. He makes comparisons with Jews and Arabs, opining that the former were marked by the same high numbers of invalids as the Christians on account of their rich diet and that the latter benefited from the drier diet and climate of the areas in which they lived (*Question* 26, ed. Munitiz, 106–8).

Agency and the perspective of the disabled

For all the wealth of information to be drawn from this rich variety of sources, we know surprisingly little about the *Sitz im Leben* of disabled people in Byzantium. In fact, we are left very much in the dark about the real conditions in which they lived, the care they received within the family or elsewhere and, last but not least, their integration into society or rejection from it. More often than not, miraculous accounts start with a description of their problematic condition and thereafter put the emphasis on the process of their treatment and final cure. Granted, disability in hagiography plays the same role as any other disease that is simply there for the purpose of making manifest the healing powers of the glorified saint. As a result, any reference to the 'abnormal' status of the disabled is fleeting and interest in their previous way of life is minimal, in most cases the major concern being to denounce the failure of physicians to provide a cure. Exceptions arise to serve the purpose of measuring the extent of the healing saint's capacity against the complications of the sores and other ailments his/her beneficiaries suffered from. Yet in such cases too, it cannot always be ascertained whether it was reality or rhetoric that prompted an author to depict the condition of a sufferer at length and the way they and their household and friends experienced the disability. For instance, in his collection of the miracles of Eugenios, patron-saint of Trebizond in the Pontos, John Xiphilinos (c.1010–75) treats the case of a Scythian deaf-mute (κωφός) soldier (a Varangian mercenary in the Byzantine army) who, on seeing from a distance the shrine of St Eugenios, burst into tears and 'with the lips of his soul', as the text has it, beseeched the saint for his mercy. To be sure, his lengthy account makes up for the lack of concrete information he gives about this particular man. Nonetheless, even in his use of rhetorical phraseology, the hagiographer cannot hide his prejudice as to the status of this 'weak' person: 'the saint must not permit him to be further subdued by the unbreakable and indissoluble fetters, being in no way better than an animal although he was born with reason' (ed. Rosenqvist, 184–7). This dismissive attitude, which was no doubt widely shared, finds a self-reflective turn in a different miracle story in the *Life of St Peter of Atroa* (d. 837), founder of a monastery on Mt Olympus in Bithynia. Having found no remedy in medical doctors, the mother of a boy born with rickets implores the saint to give relief to her 5-year-old malformed son, who had been supported by his bones and nerves alone, deprived as he was of flesh since birth. The woman, who was of senatorial rank, confessed that the cause of this disability was the multitude of her sins and is said to have sought the intercession of the saint because she was unable to bear seeing the living death of her child (ed. Laurent, 169–70).

This story is of real significance from a number of perspectives. To begin with, it confirms that the family was the primary and apparently continual caregiver for its disabled members. The picture of a disabled person escorted by their father or mother makes frequent appearances in miraculous accounts. For instance, the mother of a young man named Stephanos, who was tormented by a demon, is said to have taken him to St Hypatios, founder of a monastery in fifth-century Constantinople. Her demoniac son was so strong as to be able to trounce ten men and break his chains as if they were pieces of wood (ch. 40.8). His case suggests that, in addition to his mother, he must have been cared for by a group of people, including the family's servants or others, of whom, however, we hardly hear a word in the sources. A second example is provided by Sophronios of Jerusalem in the *Miracula* of Sts Cyrus and John whose shrine was in late antique Alexandria. Sixteen servants, we are told, were the successive bearers carrying a certain Menas, who turns up suffering from dropsy (ed. Fernandez Marcos, 250).

In his homily on the paralytics of the Gospels, the one who was bedridden for thirty-eight years and the other at Capernaum, John Chrysostom praises their relentless efforts to reach the source of their cure. 'There are quite a few pusillanimous and peevish people', he adds, 'who would prefer to suffer from their disease instead of being treated by the application of aiding devices' (*PG* 51, col. 56/2). The passage suggests that in reality many people took their disability for granted, and, as a result, neglected the opportunities to seek help from either medical doctors or healing saints. We imagine that those living within a family were 'sequestered' within the safe domestic space, kept hidden from public sight, whereas those living without a family would be lying in the street as marginalized outcasts.

The story of the child born with rickets offers a rare attestation of a cure of a person with a birth defect. As a rule, whether referring to a blind, lame or deaf person, hagiographers are silent as to the origins of their disability and avoid specifying whether the defect was congenital or acquired after birth. In essence, a delicate concern must have lain behind this reticence: the sense that the healing of someone disabled from birth was the province of the Lord alone, and not something to be attempted by just any saint whose healing power had its own limits. St Photeine, who on account of her name (derived from the Greek word *phos* meaning 'light'), was the patron saint of the blind and those with eye troubles in Byzantium, is presented as restoring the vision of people who suffered from afflictions caused by accidents or air pollution. There are no noteworthy examples of saints healing those who had been blind from birth and the few exceptions refer to new-born babies (e.g. *Life of St Symeon the Younger*, ch. 117).

The cure of the man born blind as narrated in St John's Gospel (9: 1–34) raises another issue. Christ's admonition to his disciples that it was neither the blind man who had sinned nor his parents, but 'this happened so that the word of God might be displayed in his life' (John 9: 1–3) targeted an apparently prevailing mentality that was not unknown in the Greco-Roman world and continued to have some force in the Christian community (Horn 2013: 139–40). The case of the woman who considered her child's disability the result of her own sin is just one of many. In Christian Byzantium, disability was associated with the burden of sin that weighed either on the suffering person himself/herself or their parents. The biblical belief that the disabled had in some way fallen away from God never lost its force among the Christian fathers and simple believers alike (Kelley 2009).

By contrast, the Greek belief that a physical imperfection was an appropriate vehicle through which someone might possess or acquire a particular spiritual gift (as in the case of Teiresias) or an extraordinary mental or physical skill (e.g. Hephaestus) seems to have lost its force in the Christian world. Didymos the Blind (c.313–c.398), an erudite and prolific theologian, who was said never to have attended school, may be singled out as an exception. This view can be further supported by the fact that disability, even when it was taken as a blessing, was not greatly valued even when it applied to the saints themselves. Born voiceless, Andrew of Crete (c.660–740), a significant homilist and hymnographer, is referred to as having acquired the power of speech at the age of 8 after taking his first communion. For his biographer this physical imperfection merely prefigured the saint's inclination for quietude and silence, and was not viewed as something that made him spiritually distinctive (ed. Papadopoulos-Kerameus, 170–1). In a similar fashion, the biographer of Elias Spelaiotes (c.864–960), a South Italian monastic saint who lost his fingers after a serious childhood injury and was nicknamed Monocheir (the 'One-Handed'), presents this disability as a cause of his subject's fleeing the world later in life (*Acta Sanctorum* Sep. III, ch. 10, p. 852).

Disability as a literary device

People who were unable to walk or speak like the majority, or men and women who by their impairment or their disfigurement did not look like other human beings, would always incite both positive and negative reactions such as compassion, contempt and laughter. Across societies and cultures, all these emotions have provided fertile ground for different kinds of literary inspiration (dramatic, realistic or satirical) and in this respect Byzantine literature, throughout the period of the empire, was no exception. From the type and number of texts cited thus far, it will have become obvious that literary interest in the disabled in Byzantium was overwhelmingly prompted by an endeavour to pass on an edifying message which, on the one hand, echoed the teaching and miracles of Jesus Christ in the Gospels and, on the other, reaffirmed the overall concern of Christians for the weak.

For all their interest in disability and their differentiation from their pagan predecessors, Christian authors in Byzantium rarely made a leper or a blind, mute, or lame man, let alone a woman, the main, or even the second most important, character in their narrative. In his *Historia Lausiaca* Palladios, Bishop of Helenopolis, relates the story of Eulogios, a former lawyer, who abandoned the world for the desert. Reluctant either to join a community or to live alone, Eulogios picked up a leper from the market who had no hands or feet and decided to look after him for life. Fifteen years went by before the leper, tempted by a demon, started insulting his companion. Eulogios was then counselled to take him to St Antony, the famous ascetic of Egypt. After the latter had severely castigated the demoniac, he admonished them both to live together for the rest of their life. Eulogios died forty days later and the leper three days after that (ed. Bartelink, 104–14). For similar reasons of mortification and humiliation, Daniel of Sketis, an ascetic from the reign of Justinian (527–65), took on the task of caring for a leper in order to redeem himself from a major sin (he thought himself to be the cause of his barbarian captor's death) (ed. Dahlman, 114–19). Another edifying story found in the same corpus of tales associated with Daniel of Sketis elaborates on the theme of hidden sainthood, a topic that dominates late antique hagiography. It is exemplified by a blind man sitting naked in a street in Alexandria, Egypt, begging for a living. As it turned out, whatever he received as charity, he would use to buy food and have it distributed on Sundays to the sick people in the hospitals (ed. Dahlman, 126–9).

Spiritual edification through handicapped people takes a different character in the novel-like hagiographical story of *Barlaam and Ioasaph*, which retells the story of Buddha's awakening from a Christian perspective. When, on one occasion, Ioasaph, the teenage prince of the story, evades the attention of his servants, he meets in the street two sick men, of whom the first was a leper and the second a blind man. The questions prompted by the appalling sight of these two persons were the first steps to his liberation from the bonds of illusion (ed. Volk, 43). In another instance, the literary exploitation of the disabled for edification intersects with satire in the anecdote of the paralysed man and the mute woman, a text which must have had a wide circulation in late Antiquity. It can now be found included in the *Miracula* of Sts Kosmas and Damian (mir. 24, ed. Deubner, 162–4) and of St Menas (mir. 5, ed. Pomjalovskij, 73–5) as a miracle story concerning two patients practising incubation. Incited by a dreamed vision to sleep with the mute woman, the paralysed man crawled into her sleeping quarters for what was taken to be an immoral purpose. The screams prompted by this shocking experience gave the mute woman back her voice, whereas the man was forced to flee in order to escape his pursuers. Interestingly, this kind of paradigmatic tale in which one disabled person proves useful to another looms large in a set pattern that we can pinpoint in three epigrams listed in sequence in the ninth book of the *Greek Anthology*. By being carried on the shoulders of a blind man, a lame man acquires mobility and is able to guide his bearer around. As the poets have it, their imperfections were brought together so that they could complement one another (9.11, 9.12 and 9.13b).

A certain satirical twist is also discernible in the *Description of a Little Man*, a short rhetorical composition by Constantine Manasses, an important intellectual and a prolific writer of the twelfth century. The subject is a dwarf who lived in the imperial palace for the sole purpose of entertaining the court. Upon his arrival at Constantinople, the little man became an object of public display and as such he was noticed by the author who gives a minute description of his bodily appearance and physical traits (Messis and Nilsson 2015).

In paying attention to someone he calls at one point a 'monster' (τέρας) Manasses is in line with a literary tradition of showcasing examples of monstrosity usually with reference to births and appearances of sinister human creatures (Laes 2011: 931–6). In historical narratives this tradition usually takes the form of a digression, intended to put across to readers/listeners the curiosity and excitement experienced by those who had witnessed for themselves or heard about the existence of these odd people. In late antique historiography, what Manasses depicted as a mere portrait without assigning any deeper meaning to it assumes different weight and larger dimensions. Incidents that may refer to teratogeneseis of any kind (monsters, dwarfs, conjoined twins) and that seem to have some basis in historical reality have some political context, in that they are included in the account as portents of evil, an ominous development for emperors and the empire alike. An example cited in the seventh-century historian Theophylact Simocatta is a case in point (Efthymiadis 2010: 181–2). This tradition continued through later historians such as Leo the Deacon in the tenth century (who reports the monstrous prodigy of Siamese twins, ed. Hase, 165; tr. Talbot and Sullivan, 207) and Michael Attaleiates in the eleventh (who tells of a monstrous child put on public display, ed. Tsolakis: 162; tr. Kaldellis, Krallis, 385) who likewise aspire to achieve a twofold purpose: to intrigue the imagination of their audience and to point metaphorically to the intersection of fate with historical developments in the political sphere (Messis 2012: 172–7).

Finally, the ominous or rather portentous aspect of disability is further revealed in a group of texts that it would not be proper to qualify as 'literature'. Byzantine dreambooks were built up from excerpts from collections dating back to Roman times and amalgamated material from Arabic and/or other sources of unidentified provenance. Depending on the collection, the reference to a disability in a dream may vary in terms of length and can unfold in two distinct versions. In the first type, the dreamer sees himself/herself either transformed into a disabled person or suffering an accident causing partial or total disablement. In the second, more exceptional type, the dreamer encounters a disabled person in his/her dream. In either case, the auspicious or inauspicious character of the dream is far from obvious or expected. What is more, a detail may be critical in determining one interpretation or the other. Thus, 'being blind is altogether good in every respect', but 'being led around like a blind man, [is] very inauspicious' or 'exceedingly auspicious'; or, 'if someone dreams that a blind man was walking in his (i.e., the dreamer's) house, let him know that a hidden secret is being wrought in (that house)' (tr. Oberhelman, 150, 129–30, 164, 196). As can be deduced from this cursory glance at a few dreambooks and regardless of whether the affliction is seen in a positive or negative light, it is clear that the imaginary grip of a physical defect should not pass unnoticed and must be seen as a potential fate for everyone.

Conclusions

The texts and references discussed above, a small but hopefully representative sample mostly derived from written sources, confront us with various issues of a theoretical and practical nature. The blind, the lame, the deformed and the 'monstrous' pervade the history of mankind and their silent denunciation of the way they were treated exemplifies a society's failure to accept the Other on its own terms. By virtue of the overall attention that Christianity as a religion paid to the suffering body, disability came to be seen as a call for both divine and human intervention. Leaving disabled people to their fate was no longer regarded as permissible, as it had been in Greek and Roman Antiquity. We have come a long way from cruel practices such as killing disfigured and maimed new-borns in the name of eugenics. A concern for social welfare, as manifested in the functioning of philanthropic institutions in Byzantium, represented a significant change in the treatment of the sick and disabled in human history. What is more, for various reasons the Byzantines were increasingly reconciled to the existence of the suffering and their diseases, making them much more visible than they had been in the Greco-Roman past. All in all, the increased care afforded to these 'special' people was born of a spirit of emulation, modelled on the paradigms of healing and treatment found in the Gospels.

This distinctive tone, however, should not lead us to pass too favourable a judgement on popular attitudes and overestimate what was actually taking place in real life. Even learned writers cannot conceal their superstitions and their misperception of the disabled as barely worthy of being called human. In conformity with the expectations of their readers/listeners, they were ready to caricature them and, in some extreme cases, conspicuously overemphasize their 'universally' negative impact, as if their birth and existence were a phenomenon implying communal fear and guilt. Once again, and not altogether unlike the modern day, we are confronted with people's inherent inability to see disabled people for what they are and to treat them as they deserve.

Bibliography

Primary sources

Agnellus of Ravenna, *Liber Pontificalis Ecclesiae Ravennatis*, in *Monumenta Germaniae Historica. Scriptores rerum Langobardicarum et Italicarum saec. VI-IX*, ed. Georg Waitz (Berlin, 1878).

Anastasii Sinaitae, *Questiones et Responsiones*, ed. M. Richard and J. A. Munitiz (Turnhout, 2006); English tr. Joseph A. Munitiz, *Anastasios of Sinai, Questions and Answers* (Turnhout, 2011).

Anthologia Graeca, ed. H. Beckby, III (Munich, 1968).

Attaleiates, Michael, *Historia*, ed. E. T. Tsolakis, *Michaelis Attaliatae, Historia*, Corpus Fontium Historiae Byzantinae 50 (Athens, 2011); English tr. A. Kaldellis and D. Krallis (Washington, DC, 2012).

Life of Barlaam and Joasaph, ed. R. Volk, *Die Schriften des Johannes von Damaskos*, VI/2. *Historia animae utilis de Barlaam et Ioasaph (spuria)*. Text und zehn Appendices. Patristische Texte und Studien 62 (Berlin, 2009).

Barsanuphios and Jean de Gaza, *Correspondance*, III. *Aux laïcs et aux évêques, Lettres 617–848*, ed. François Neyt and Paola de Angelis-Noah, Sources Chrétiennes 468 (Paris, 2002).

Cyril of Alexandria, *Letters,* ed. Pierre Evieux, William H. Burns, *et al., Cyrille d'Alexandrie, Lettres festales,* Sources Chrétiennes 372 (Paris, 1991).

Daniel of Sketis, *Narrationes,* ed. B. Dahlman, *Saint Daniel of Sketis: A Group of Hagiographic Texts,* Acta Universitatis Upsaliensis-Studia Byzantina Upsaliensia 10 (Uppsala, 2007).

Ecloga, ed. Ludwig Burgmann, *Ecloga: Das Gesetzbuch Leons III. und Konstantinos' V.,* Forschungen zur byzantinischen Rechtsgeschichte 10 (Frankfurt am Main, 1983).

Farmer's Law, ed. Walter Ashburner, 'The Farmer's Law', *Journal of Hellenic Studies* 30 (1910), 85–108.

Georgii Monachi Chronicon, ed. C. de Boor, I–II (Leipzig, 1904).

Gregory of Nyssa, *De pauperibus amandis II,* ed. A. Van Heck, *Gregorii Nysseni opera IX: Sermones* (Leiden, 1967), 111–27.

John Chrysostom, *In paralyticum demissum per tectum* (CPG 4370), *PG* 51, cols 47–64.

Leonis Diaconi, Historia, ed. C. B. Hase (Bonn, 1828); English tr. A.-M. Talbot and D. Sullivan (Washington, DC, 2005).

Life of Daniel the Stylite (BHG 489): ed. H. Delehaye, *Les saints stylites,* Subsidia Hagiographica 14 (Brussels, 1923), 1–94; English tr. E. Dawes and N. H. Baynes, *Three Byzantine Saints* (Crestwood, NY, 1977).

Life of Nicholas of Sion, ed. I. and N. Ševčenko, *The Life of Saint Nicholas of Sion* (Brookline, MA, 1984); ed. and German tr. H. Blum, *Die Vita Nicolai Sionitae* (Bonn, 1997).

Life of Niketas Patrikios, ed. D. Papachryssanthou, 'Un confesseur du second iconoclasme: la Vie du patrice Nicétas (+ 836)', *Travaux et Mémoires* 3 (1968), 309–54.

Life of St Andrew the Fool, ed. L. Rydén, *The Life of St Andrew the Fool (BHG* 117), I–II (Uppsala, 1995).

Life of St Elias Speleotes: Acta Sanctorum Sep. III, 848–87.

Life of Euphrosyne the Younger by Nikephoros Xanthopoulos: *Acta Sanctorum Nov.* III, 861–77.

Life of St Hypatios by Callinicos: ed. G. J. M. Bartelink, *Callinicos: Vie d'Hypatios* (Paris, 1971).

Life of St Irene of Chrysobalanton: ed. and English tr. J. O. Rosenqvist, *The Life of St Irene Abbess of Chrysobalanton: A Critical Edition with Introduction, Translation, Notes and Indices* (Uppsala, 1986).

Life of St Peter of Atroa (BHG 2364): ed. and French tr. V. Laurent, *La Vie merveilleuse de saint Pierre d'Atroa* (Brussels, 1956).

Life of St Philaretos the Merciful by Niketas of Amnia: ed. and English tr. L. Rydén, *The Life of St Philaretos the Merciful Written by his Grandson Niketas* (Uppsala, 2002).

Life of St Symeon Stylites the Younger (BHG 1689): ed. and French tr. P. van den Ven, *La Vie ancienne de S. Symeon stylite le jeune* (Brussels, 1962).

Miracles of St Artemios: ed. A. Papadopoulos-Kerameus, in *Varia Graeca Sacra* (St Petersburg, 1909), 1–75; English tr. V. S. Crisafulli and J. W. Nesbitt, *The Miracles of St Artemios: A Collection of Miracle Stories by an Anonymous Author of Seventh-Century Byzantium* (Leiden, 1997).

Miracles of St Eugenios of Trebizond (BHG 610): ed. and English tr. J. O. Rosenqvist, *The Hagiographic Dossier of St Eugenios of Trebizond in Codex Athous Dionysiou 154* (Uppsala, 1996), 170–203.

Miracles of St Menas by Timotheos Patriarch of Alexandria: ed. N. Pomjalovskij, *Žitije prepodovnago Paisija velikago i Timotheja part. Aleks. povestvovanie o čudesah sv. velikomučenika Miny* (St Petersburg, 1900), 62–89.

Miracles of St Photeine (BHG 1541m): ed. F. Halkin, *Hagiographica inedita decem* (Turnhout and Leuven, 1989), 111–25; English tr. A. M. Talbot, 'The Posthumous Miracles of St. Photeine', *Analecta Bollandiana* 112 (1994), 85–105.

Miracles of St Zotikos: ed. T. S. Miller, 'The Legend of Saint Zotikos according to Constantine Akropolites', *Analecta Bollandiana* 112 (1994), 339–76.

Miracles of Sts Kosmas and Damian (BHG 391): partial ed. L. Deubner, *Kosmas und Damian: Texte und Einleitung* (Leipzig and Berlin, 1907), 193–206.

Miracles of Sts Kyros and John by Sophronios of Jerusalem: ed. N. Fernandez Marcos, *Los 'Thaumata' de Sofronio, Contribucion al estudio de la 'Incubatio Cristiana'* (Madrid, 1975); French tr. J. Gascou, *Miracles des saints Cyr et Jean (BHG* 477–9) (Paris, 2006).

Miracles of Zoodochos Pege: ed. Ambrosios Pamperis, Νικηφόρου Καλλίστου τοῦ Ξανθοπούλου Περὶ συστάσεως τοῦ σεβασμίου οἴκου τῆς ἐν Κωνσταντινουπόλει Ζωοδόχου Πηγῆς, καὶ τῶν ἐν αὐτῷ ὑπερφυῶς τελεσθέντων θαυμάτων καὶ ὁ Βίος τοῦ ἐν ἁγίοις Κλήμεντος . . . (Leipzig, 1802), 1–99.

Palladios of Helenopolis, *Historia Lausiaca: Palladio, la Storia Lausiaca,* ed. G. J. M. Bartelink (Milan, 1998⁵).

Paul of Nicaea: ed. A. M. Ieraci Bio, *Paolo di Nicea, Manuale medico,* Hellenica et byzantina neapolitana 16 (Naples, 1996).

Procopii Caesariensis opera omnia, ed. J. Haury; rev. G. Wirth, I–III (Leipzig, 1962–4).

Suidae Lexicon, ed. A. Adler, I–V (Leipzig, 1928–38).

Synaxarium Ecclesiae Constantinopolitanae, Acta Sanctorum, Propylaeum ad Acta Sanctorum Novembris, ed. H. Delehaye (Brussels, 1902).

Synesios of Cyrene, *Correspondence*: ed. A. Garzya, *Synésios de Cyrène*, II. *Correspondance, Lettres I–LXIII*, tr. and commentary D. Roques (Paris, 2000).

Typikon of the Monastery of Pantocrator: ed. P. Gautier, 'Le typikon du Christ Sauveur Pantocrator', *Revue des Études Byzantines* 32 (1974), 1–145; English tr. R. Jordan, in J. Thomas and A. Constantinides Hero (eds), *Byzantine Monastic Foundations Documents: A Complete Translation of the Surviving Founders' Typika and Testaments* (Washington, DC, 2000), 725–81.

Theophanis Chronographia, ed. C. de Boor, I (Leipzig, 1883).

Secondary sources

Bouras-Vallianatos, Petros, 'Contextualizing the Art of Healing by Byzantine Physicians', in Brigitte Pitarakis (ed.), *Hayta Kısa, Sanat Uzun: Bizans'ta Şifa Sanatı – Life is Short, Art Long: The Art of Healing in Byzantium* Pera Müzesi (Istanbul, 2015), 105–22.

Crislip, Andrew, *Thorns in the Flesh: Illness and Sanctity in Late Ancient Christianity* (Philadelphia, PA, 2013).

Efthymiadis, Stephanos, 'A Historian and his Tragic Hero: A Literary Reading of Theophylaktos Simokattes' *Ecumenical History*', in R. Macrides (ed.), *Byzantine History as Literature* (Farnham and Burlington, VT, 2010), 167–83.

Efthymiadis, Stephanos (ed.), *Ashgate Research Companion to Byzantine Hagiography*, II. *Genres and Contexts* (Farnham and Burlington, VT, 2014).

Gascou, Jean, 'L'éléphantiasis en Égypte gréco-romaine (Faits, représentations, institutions)', *Mélanges Jean-Pierre Sodini, Travaux et Mémoires* 15 (2005), 261–85.

Herrin, Judith, 'Blinding in Byzantium', in C. Scholz and G. Makris (eds), *ΠΟΛΥΠΛΕΥΡΟΣ ΝΟΥΣ: Miscellanea für Peter Schreiner zu seinem 60. Geburtstag* (Leipzig, 2000), 56–68.

Horden, Peregrine, 'The Earliest Hospitals in Byzantium, Western Europe, and Islam', *Journal of Interdisciplinary History* 35 (2005), 361–89.

Horn, Cornelia B., 'A Nexus of Disability in Greek Miracle Stories: A Comparison of Accounts of Blindness from the Asklepeion in Epidauros and the Shrine of Thecla in Seleucia', in C. Laes, C. F. Goodey and M. L. Rose (eds), *Disabilities in Roman Antiquity: Disparate Bodies* A Capite ad Calcem (Leiden, 2013), 115–43.

Joannou, Pericles Petros, *Démonologie populaire – démonologie critique au XIe siècle: La Vie inédite de S. Auxence par Michel Psellos* (Wiesbaden, 1971)

Kelley, N., 'The Deformed Child in Ancient Christianity', in C. B. Horn and R. R. Phenix (eds), *Children in Late Ancient Christianity* (Tübingen, 2009), 199–216.

Laes, Christian, 'Learning from Silence: Disabled Children in Roman Antiquity', *Arctos* 42 (2008), 85–122.

Laes, Christian, 'How Does One Do the History of Disability in Antiquity? One Thousand Years of Case Studies', *Medicina nei Secoli* 23 (2011), 915–46.

Laes, Christian, *Beperkt? Gehandicapten in het Romeinse Rijk* (Leuven, 2014).

Laes, Christian, 'Disability at Court: Byzantine Emperors', in C. Nolte, B. Frohne, U. Halle and S. Kerth (eds), *Handbuch der Dis/ability History* (Affalterbach, 2016) forthcoming.

Leven, Karl-Heinz, 'Die "unheilige" Krankheit – Epilepsia, Mondsucht und Besessenheit in Byzanz', *Würzburger medizinhistorische Mitteilungen* 13 (1995), 17–57.

Makris, Georgios, 'Zur Epilepsie in Byzanz', *Byzantinische Zeitschrift* 88 (1995), 363–404.

Marx-Wolf, Heidi, and Upson-Saia, Kristi, 'The State of the Question: Religion, Medicine, Disability and Health in Late Antiquity', *Journal of Late Antiquity* 8 (2015), 257–72.

Messis, Charis, 'L'impureté corporelle suprême: La monstruosité à Byzance, ses perceptions et ses élaborations littéraires', in F. Mosetti Casaretto (ed.), *Il corpo impuro e le sue rappresentazioni nelle letterature medievali* (Alessandria, 2012), 183–98.

Messis, Charis, *Les eunuques à Byzance, entre réalité et imaginaire* (Paris, 2014).

Messis, Charis, and Nilsson, Ingela, 'Constantin Manassès, La *Description d'un petit homme*: Introduction, texte, traduction et commentaires', *Jahrbuch der Oesterreichischen Byzantinistik* 65 (2015), 169–94.

Miller, S. Timothy, *The Birth of the Hospital in the Byzantine Empire* (Baltimore, MD, 1985).

Miller, S. Timothy, and Nesbitt, John W., *Walking Corpses: Leprosy in Byzantium and the Medieval West* (Ithaca, NY, 2014).

Moorhead, John, 'Thoughts on Some Early Medieval Miracles', in E. Jeffreys, M. Jeffreys and A. Moffat (eds), *Byzantine Papers Proceedings of the First Australian Byzantine Studies Conference, 17–19 May 1978* (Canberra, 1981), 1–11.

Oberhelman, Steven M., *Dreambooks in Byzantium: Six Oneirocritica in Translation with Commentary and Introduction* (Aldershot and Burlington, VT, 2008).

Patlagean, Evelyne, 'Byzance et le blason pénal du corps', in Y. Thomas (ed.), *Du châtiment dans la cité: Supplices corporels et peine de mort dans le monde antique. Table ronde de Rome (9–11 novembre 1982)* (Rome, 1984), 405–26.

Ringrose, M. Kathryn, *The Perfect Servant: Eunuchs and the Social Construction of Gender in Byzantium* (Chicago, IL, and London, 2003).

Scarborough, John (ed.), *Symposium on Byzantine Medicine* (Baltimore, MD, 1985).

Stathakopoulos, Dionysios, 'Discovering a Military Order of the Crusades: The Hospital of St. Sampson of Constantinople', *Viator* 37 (2006), 255–73.

Stathakopoulos, Dionysios, 'Death in the Countryside: Some Effects of Famine and Epidemics', *Antiquité tardive* 20 (2012), 105–14.

Tougher, Shaun, *The Eunuch in Byzantine History and Society* (Abingdon and New York, 2008).

Trenchard-Smith, Margaret, 'Insanity, Exculpation and Disempowerment in Byzantine Law', in W. J. Turner (ed.), *Madness in Law and Custom* (Leiden, 2010), 39–55.

28

WHAT DIFFERENCE DID ISLAM MAKE?

Disease and disability in early medieval North Africa

Matthew Alan Gaumer

Historical backdrop: prelude to a public health and social crisis

No other region of the Roman world changed so inexorably as northern Africa at the end of Antiquity. What was at one time a prosperous breadbasket for the Roman Empire retained only the shell of its former glory in the centuries after the sack of Carthage in 439 CE. Economic output plummeted, trade throughput dried up, urban centres emptied in favour of greener pastures to the north and east, and material culture reached a low ebb. What caused these changes? As with all changes in global order, there are those who gain and those who lose. North Africa of this period was condemned as much by its geography and natural nemeses as by invading armies. Military and economic marginalization of this part of the former empire was often accompanied by the scourge of acute infectious diseases such as plague, smallpox, and other ailments found in urban and agricultural settlements, along with the physical disabilities often found in tandem, all of which played a somewhat unacknowledged role in ushering in the end of a Roman and Byzantine North Africa and the rise of a wholly Islamic civilization. This chapter analyzes the effect of infectious disease and physical disability in this social transition and shows how the everyday realities of sickness and death and the medicine to treat the former spanned and shaped these two distinct cultural epochs. Was the way in which early medieval Muslims viewed disease and disability in historical continuity with pre-Islamic Antiquity or was it a form of rupture with the past?

Any discussion of contagious disease and disability in ancient North Africa, the present-day Maghreb (from western Libya to Morocco), can hardly be undertaken without looking back to the period starting with the Vandal invasion of the Roman provinces in 429 and the capitulation of Carthage to the Vandal general Genseric in 439 (Merrills and Miles 2007). The question of who was in control (first the Romans, then the Vandals, and later the Byzantines and Umayyad Arabs) is less important than the underlying factors influencing North Africa in this period. The Roman annexation of Africa after 146 BCE, stitched the region into the economic fabric of the empire as it developed into a major agricultural area, as well as a nexus for commercial maritime hubs and inland routes connecting the Mediterranean with the Sahel and Sub-Saharan African (Lockhard 2011), all of which sustained the garrison posts stretching across the expansive distances of the southern imperial *limes*. The following factors provided nearly all that was required to place a society within the grasp of ravaging disease: (1) intensive agricultural activities, (2) rotations of Roman legions throughout northern Africa and (3) easy maritime transport, provided nearly all that is required to place a society within the grasp of abundant disease (Cartwright and Biddiss 2014; Clark 2010). The lynchpin, (4), for ensuring Roman Africa would share the same pestilence-filled future as the rest of the empire was the proliferation of Roman *castellae, coloniae* and cities. Where there was once only Punic Carthage, in the centuries after Roman dominance well-connected settlements such as Caesarea (Chercell, Algeria), Tipasa (Tipaza, Algeria), Cirta (Constantine, Algeria), Hadramentum (Sousia, Tunisia), Hippo Regius (Annaba, Algeria), Leptis Magna (Libya), Sala Colonia (Chella, Morocco), Thamugadi (Timgad, Algeria), Thysdrus (El Djem, Tunisia) and Volubilis (northern Morocco) emerged from the planning and labouring of Roman soldiers throughout the region (Southern 2007). This web of Roman urbanizations created the backbone of the richest western provinces: Numidia, Byzacena, Africa Proconsularis, Cyrenaica and Tripolitania (Heather 2010). As Roman settlements, they boasted engineering feats that would not be bested till the mid-19th century: water piping, sewage systems, flush toilets and hot baths (Cartwright and Biddiss 2014). While this went far towards improving the living standards and life-expectancy of Roman citizens, the inescapable reality of thousands of humans living in close proximity with each other, and with domesticated animals, ensured that this civilization too would share the same microbial destiny as other ancient societies throughout the world, past and present (Hays 2007; Diamond 1999).

These new urban agglomerations, juxtaposed against the historical spatial pattern of sparsely placed Berber pastoral settlements, were deeply connected through trade and military rotations with north-east Africa, Asia Minor and the northern Mediterranean. On a quantitative level, the induced risk of this interconnected ancient world is visible in the numbers of soldiers that would have served in the Roman legions: upwards of 645,000 by the year 430 (Bachrach 2005). Throughout the late imperial period, 200–400s, various tribal groups (*peregrini*) would have made up the majority (90 per cent) of the force: Alans (steppe peoples), Germans and Sarmatians (from southern Russia). Within North Africa itself, a semi-permanent force level would have stood at almost 30,000 personnel, again a composite force from throughout the Roman world (Southern 2007). This was a significant presence in the African provinces, including Egypt, where a combined population stood at five million at its peak (Russell 1958).

Romanization, urbanization and disease proliferation

So what was the outcome of social restructuring from dispersed pastoral settlements to networked urbanizations in North Africa? The answer is two-fold: (1) increased economic development and further expansion of human population densities close to the coast, and (2) permanent integration of the hinterland by way of carriage roads (Linard *et al.* 2012). Both of these changes created a context that would shape the future of North Africa, in terms of infectious disease communicability as well as the resultant impact of postnatal disability on group identity and social constitution.

Endemic human diseases, such as smallpox, typhus, cholera, diphtheria, meningitis, dysentery, tuberculosis, influenza and measles (Stannard 1999), emerged as epizootic strains with the advent of agrarian settlements in the ancient Nile and Mesopotamia, and as humans began living in close quarters with domesticated animals (Kinnear-Wilson 1967). Key to the survival of these endemic diseases, as opposed to zoonotic diseases (e.g. malaria, anthrax or

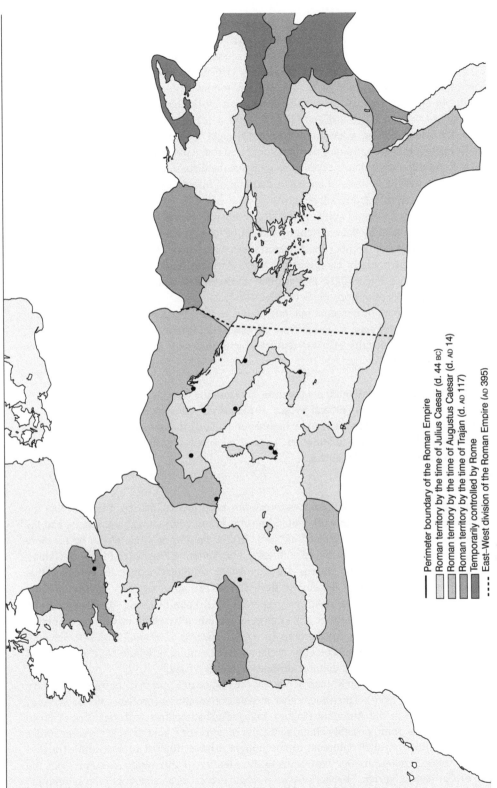

Perimeter boundary of the Roman Empire
Roman territory by the time of Julius Caesar (d. 44 BC)
Roman territory by the time of Augustus Caesar (d. AD 14)
Roman territory by the time of Trajan (d. AD 117)
Temporarily controlled by Rome
East-West division of the Roman Empire (AD 395)

Figure 28.1 The Roman Empire. Source: Logos Software

modern ebola which depend on non-human animal species for transmission and hosting), is a stable and critical level of human population in order for a bacterium or virus to recur through subsequent generations (Clark 2010). Such diseases require human population concentrations large enough to sustain them: to provide enough critical mass in terms of bodies, but at the same time not to be so fatal as to kill off hosts too swiftly, preventing their spread and continuity. In epidemiological terms, this is measured by the basic reproduction number, or R_0 (pronounced "r nought") (Cliff and Haggett 1990; Diekmann et al. 1990). This factor is essential for understanding what Romanization brought to western North Africa: enough people living together and communities interconnected that a disease would not die out from a lack of new potential hosts, but spaced out enough that the disease would not kill off the human population too swiftly (R_0 = rate of contact + duration of infectivity + probability of pathogen transmission from an infected to a fresh host).

Roman North Africa would suffer virtually all epidemic events that occurred elsewhere in the Imperium, facilitated by the constant exchanges of Roman soldiers and frequent maritime throughput from ports throughout the Mediterranean Sea (Hays 2007; Kohn 2008). Several cases stand out as particularly egregious for North Africans, both in cities and inland rural settlements, but more importantly that display a discernible uptick in the regularity and frequency of outbreaks of various kinds (Patrick 1967).

The very first account of potential bubonic plague in the Mediterranean region is found in a 4th-century Greek-language fragment from the physician Rufus of Syria (who lived during the reign of Trajan) that tells of a 1st-century plague outbreak in Libya (though this was smallpox; Hopkins 2002):

> The buboes termed pestilential are the most fatal and the most acute, especially those that are seen in Libya, Egypt, and Syria ... which occurred especially in Libya. They have said that it was characterized by high fever, pain, disturbance of the entire body and buboes, hard and non-suppurating. They develop not only in the ordinary places but also in the groins and the neck.
>
> *(Oribasius, Collectiones medicae 44.14.2)*

Though the impact of that particular outbreak has been lost to history, it is clear that the trans-Mediterranean shipping network would transmit future communicable diseases; and the next time a contagious disease surfaced in North Africa, the implications would be far more sobering in terms of the pattern of future outbreaks. The Antonine Plague (or Plague of Galen), named after the famed emperor Marcus Aurelius, was a smallpox or measles epidemic that affected all principal regions of the empire from 164 to 189 approximately (Cartwright and Biddiss 2014). The frequency of death was reported by Roman historian Dio Cassius to be approximately 2,000 per day in Rome at its pinnacle, including two famous victims: emperors Lucius Verus (d. 169) and Marcus Aurelius (d. 180) (*Historia Romana* 72.14.3–4; Scheidel 2013). The next time a sustained epidemic surfaced in the empire, it would have a permanent effect on the social make-up and cultural attitudes of North Africa.

The first epidemic centred on Roman Africa was the Plague of Cyprian in the mid-3rd century (251–70) (Scourfield 1996). This time, either measles or smallpox (probably the opposite of that which occurred in the Antonine Plague), ravaged urban centres with fatalities of up to 5,000 per day at one point, possibly claiming the life of emperor Claudius in 270 (Kohn 2008). Postnatal disability from such outbreaks can be thought to have affected a considerable fraction of the surviving population. Our best clues to the identity of this outbreak come from the Bishop of Carthage, Cyprian. His work *De mortalitate* preserves an account of the symptoms:

This trial, that now affects the bowels, relaxed into a constant flux, discharge the bodily strength (severe diarrhoea); that a fire originated in the marrow fermented into wounds of the throat; that the intestines are shaken with a continual vomiting; the eyes are on fire with the infected blood; that in some cases the feet or some parts of the limbs are taken off by the contagion of diseased putrefaction.

(Cyprian, De mortalitate 7.14)

Whether this epidemic was smallpox or measles is ancillary to the fact that densely packed cities became powder-kegs of deadly infectious disease, ensured by the omnipresence of human waste and the lack of uncontaminated drinking water (Garland 2010). When combined with the constant inflows of soldiers and trade throughput at port cities, this ensured that the outbreak would be shared throughout the empire (Cartwright and Biddiss 2014). A distinctive feature of the Plague of Cyprian, which had potential influences on the arrival of the Umayyad Arabs in the late 600s, is the reaction of the survivors to the epidemic. In brief, there is some basis in surviving sources for identifying a permanently altered perspective amongst the populace concerning disease. As North Africans were starting to convert in large numbers to Christianity in the mid-200s, the disease broke out and North African Christians would retain a unique group identity from this formative period.

The writings of Cyprian attest to various responses to the epidemic: almsgiving for the relief of the suffering, the goodness of assuaging disability, of likening death from disease to martyrdom (Scourfield 1996), of some Christians abandoning this new faith in favour of the time-tested imperial *cultus* and then reverting back after the subsiding of the outbreak, and of a sense of contamination from outsiders with purity coming only from God (Dunn 2004, 2006). In fact, some of Cyprian's most famous lines come from his summation of this disease-triggered social chaos: lapsed believers are 'pests and plagues of the faith, snake-tongued deceivers, skilled corrupters of the truth, spewing venom from their poisonous fangs' (*De unitate* 10) and their separation from the church begets their exclusion from God's salvation, '*extra ecclesiam nulla salus*' (*Epistula* 73.21). Interestingly, we see in this scenario the materialisation of what would become a uniquely African Christian perspective in the 4th-century Donatist controversy: that unfaithful Christians are worse than the unbaptized and it is because of both lapsed Christians and pagans that the outbreak is justified. Cyprian condemns both in *De mortalitate*: 'how necessary is this plague and pestilence … the just are called to refreshment, the unjust are carried to torture' (7.16). For Cyprian and other contemporary Christians, disease is divine justice.

For Cyprian, and the Donatist Christianity that carried forth his authority (Lancel 2002), infectious disease and its contamination is a physical incarnation of sin and this threat is to be taken with deathly seriousness. Those baptized into the church who sinned risked 'polluting' and deforming its purity and needed to be rebaptized (Scourfield 1996). This fear of sin spreading through the church developed into an obsession about ritual pollution and a critical part of the African Christian identity in later centuries (Burns 2005). This belief formed a core aspect of African theology and manifested itself in a vast array of biblical typologies: a 'dove', 'enclosed garden' or 'paradise', 'without spot or wrinkle', 'wheat amongst tares', an 'orchard of pomegranates', 'the Ark of Noah' and the '*collecta* of Israel' (Tilley 1997). Confronting infectious disease and its resultant disabilities therefore became the underlying reality of Cyprian's career as a bishop and an indelible dimension of religion in North Africa thenceforth.

Out of Africa: vermin and the demon

The horrific experience of the Plague of Cyprian never completely disappeared from the outlook and theological make-up of Christians in North Africa. Donatist Christians held fast to an identity as a *collecta* of Israel, defended against the contagion and filth of the world (*sæculum*), and even saw the Catholic Church in the 4th and 5th centuries as an infestation and imposter (Gaumer 2008). But the story does not end there. The boldest elements of the way infectious disease shaped the history of North Africa as it morphed from a largely Christian to an overwhelmingly Muslim region appear when the Roman world started to become unhinged.

In the 6th century, the former Roman Empire, long since divided into eastern (Greek-speaking) and western (Latin/Germanic) zones of influence, had changed into a Byzantine empire based out of Constantinople. Battered by wars, famine and climate change, former hubs of imperial control, such as the old capital city Rome, retained only vestiges of their former glory (Ward-Perkins 2005). North Africa was the target of Byzantine military campaigns to reunite Roman civilization and impose orthodoxy, and was slowly bleeding out in terms of economic and demographic mass (Davis 1999). Centuries of Vandal rule and the marked decline in agricultural activity and manufacturing resulting from a constant drop in demand from elsewhere in the Mediterranean meant Latin-speaking Africans with means often emigrated to Sicily and Italy (Cuoq 1984). Although the invasion provided a short period of financial stimulus for North Africa, the Byzantine campaign to retake the area in the 530s severely depleted Byzantium's treasury and manpower and it became unable to sustain such a widely dispersed theatre of operations (Bachrach 2005; Naylor 2009).

Despite the man-made hollowing out of Roman Africa, it would be nature that would usher in the social transformation of North Africa from its former identity to an Islamic one. The first event occurred in the mid-530s when the eruption of Krakatoa (in modern Indonesia) sent temperatures plummeting throughout Asia, Africa and Europe (Laes 2015; Arjava 2005; Wohletz 2000). In Africa, the historian Procopius described the climatic event in apocalyptic terms: 'the sun gave forth its light without brightness, like the moon during the whole year, and it seemed exceedingly like the sun in eclipse, for the beams it shed were not clear nor such as it is accustomed to shed' (*De bellis* 3.14.4–10). The dense acidic fog that blocked the sun devastated agriculture in the Mediterranean world; drought and famine paved the way for an even greater scourge (Fagan 2004). Then came the Justinian Plague (542–90), the first known bubonic pandemic in the world, which eviscerated the Byzantine Empire and emptied its zones of influence (Cartwright and Biddiss 2014). This plague, entering the Mediterranean world via Clysma on the Red Sea and via Pelusium in Egypt (Tsiamis *et al.* 2014; Sallares 2007), was caused by the bacterium *Yersinia pestis*, which is genomically similar to, yet independent of, the Black Death *Y. pestis* strain that would become a pandemic between 1346 and 1353 (Wagner *et al.* 2014; Carmichael 1999). Symptoms included quick-onset fever, dark buboes in the groin and armpit areas, coma, delirium and death. With a 40 per cent fatality rate that killed somewhere between 15 and 30 million humans throughout Europe, North Africa, the Middle East and Asia Minor (though Procopius, d. 560, set the total fatalities at 100 million), those who survived lived only to see the horror of a shattered economy and vast numbers of disabled. This was one of the most catastrophic pandemics in human history, and it shook the Byzantine Empire and the Mediterranean world to its foundations (Rosen 2007).

The Plague of Justinian, *Y. pestis*, had the ancient Roman transportation network as a conduit for its spread. While the black rat (*Rattus rattus*), which is the *Y. pestis* host (though recent research is questioning the specific vector, proposing instead the Mongolian gerbil (Xu *et al.*, 2015), originated in southern Asia and likely arrived in North Africa via the ancient Indian Ocean and Nile link that was a major East–West conduit, the *Xenopsylla cheopis* flea that transmits the plague to rats and to humans was indigenous to north-eastern Africa (Sallares 2007; Carmichael 1999)). Patient Zero for *Y. pestis* was at Pelusium in the Nile Delta in 540, and was in Carthage by 543 (Rosen 2007). As was characteristic of disease outbreaks in centuries before, *Y. pestis* made short shrift of the Mediterranean's network of seaports, land-routes, urban concentrations and invading armies. Within a few short decades, cities throughout the ancient Roman world emptied as survivors of the 'Demon' plague sought refuge in the countryside (McCormick 2007). The plague's most pronounced effects were seen in its aftermath: societal breakdown, lost generations, abandoned cities and farms, commonplace disability and malnutrition, and a desensitized population in what had been the most advanced civilization in the world for centuries (Little 2007). Adding to this overall malaise was the persistent virulence of endemic diseases in North Africa and other parts of the former Roman world, especially malaria. Those not stricken by *Y. pestis* were probably at risk of this mosquito-borne disease (Sallares and Gomzi 2001; Sallares *et al.* 2004; Scheidel 2013). This was a period of life in the history of the human species that was nasty, brutish and short.

But not everything was lost to the Justinian Plague. Human civilization remained resilient enough to survive and to flourish again. In this case, another group would fill the vacuum left by the pestilence-stricken Byzantine world; they would come from the east: Mecca (Naylor 2009). However, this would not be a complete transformation; the ancient thought and cultural elements of the Greeks and Romans would endure, both in terms of prejudice and compassionate care. In early medieval North Africa a distinctive fusion of Islamic society blended with an inherited *romanitas*.

Disease and disability across deities: from Apollo to Allah

The Umayyad invasion brought an infusion of new life into post-plague North Africa. Starting from Arabia, the Prophet Mohammed's successors, the caliphs, dispersed. They entered North Africa at Egypt in 640–2 and Cyrenaica and Tripolitania (modern Libya) by 642–7 (Naylor 2009). Their first attempt at conquering Carthage and modern Tunisia, Algeria and Morocco, or what was to be called *Jazîrat al-Maghrib* (the 'island of the setting sun') started in 670–83, but was repelled in a last stand of weakened Byzantine and indigenous Berber forces. Carthage, the great southern pearl of the Romans, was taken in 698, and by 705 Islam would be the dominant religion from Egypt to Morocco under the control of the Umayyad dynasty (McEvedy 1995). But does this radical paradigm shift in political and religious power indicate an absolute form of historical discontinuity with the previous Greco-Roman and Byzantine world as envisaged by Phillip Naylor (2009)? An Islamic North Africa would be shaped just as profoundly by its axis-position on the Mediterranean as the terminus for trans-Saharan trade routes (McNeill 1998). Indeed, geography, as much as biology, ensured the Maghreb would remain as transculturally infused as it had been historically. Disease and disability remained realities with great daily bearing in newly Muslim North Africa. Methods of treatment and ways to intellectually conceptualize disease and disability were heavily influenced by the Greco-Roman tradition, yet at the same time signalled a fusion of the tradition with the later spiritualist orientation of Christianity.

Early Islam and disability

An account of the effects of infectious disease in Roman North Africa has already been stitched together. But what must now be ascertained is how this transferred, if it did at all, into the early medieval Islamic civilization that had taken root in North Africa. Did early Muslim scholars and physicians essentially assume the Greco-Roman traditions and views of disease and disability? Given the unparalleled loss of life and crippling economic retraction during the Justinian Plague, would the new Umayyad North Africa experience significant contraction as well? As post-Roman Europe entered into its 'dark age', how did infectious disease and medicine shape the new Muslim culture in North Africa?

From a very early stage, outlooks on disease (*'adwā*) and disability (*adhā*) were articulated in the most important sources of Islamic theology: the *Qur'ān* and *hadīth* (oral traditions of the Prophet Mohammed) (Panzac 2012). However, it was when the new faith began its geographic expansion across Asia and Africa that 'Islamic medicine' as such began to take form (Gallagher 1999). First, the Umayyads and then the Abbasid caliphs (a caliphate centred on present-day Iraq and Iran, which eventually absorbed the Umayyads to the west) sponsored translation of Greek medical works into Arabic and Syriac as early as the 7th century; this continued unabated for the better half of a millennium throughout the Muslim world. Early Muslim physicians and philosophers respected Greek medical thought and appropriated it into Islamic thought. This synergistic development, of burgeoning Islamic thought combined with ancient Greco-Roman medical knowledge, profoundly shaped the course and flavour of Islamic culture and history (Ullmann 1978).

The Prophet's Medicine in the greater Muslim world and in North Africa

The Muslim assimilation of Greek medicine forged a sort of Greco-Islamic school of medical thought (in Arabic this came to be called *fiqh*, or 'understanding', 'jurisprudence', 'intelligence', Ghaly 2010): part naturalistic, part theological, part doctrinal, part scientific, but entirely legalistic (Katz 2005). Disease and disability were seen through the lens of Galen and his forebears: cold, hot, moist, dry humours in imbalance caused human disease, not divine intervention (Gallagher 1999). While not uniform in regional placement or theological disposition, a steady procession of great physicians and medical scholars emerged in the first centuries of Islam: Yuhanna ibn-Masawaiyh (Latinized as Mesue, c.770s–850s, Assyrian, Nestorian), Hunayn ibn-Ishaq (Lat.: Joannitus, c.810s–870s, Assyrian, Nestorian), Ali ibn Sahl Rabban al-Tabari (c.830s–870s, Persian, Muslim), Qusta ibn-Luqa al-Balabakki (Lat.: Constabulus, 820–912, Greco-Lebanese, Melkite Christian), Muhammad ibn Zakariya Razi (Lat.: Rhazes, 854–925, Persian, Muslim), Ali ibn al-Abbas al-Majusi (Lat.: Haly Abbas, d. 994, Persian, Muslim), Ali ibn-Sina (Lat.: Avicenna, c.980s–1037, Persian, Muslim), Musa ibn Mayum (Lat.: Moses Maimonides, 1130s–1204, Almoravid-Spanish, Sephardic Jew), Ahmad ibn-Rusd (Lat.: Averroes, 1126–98, Berber-Moroccan, Muslim), Abd al-Latif al-Baghdadi (1160s–1232, Arab-Iraqi, Muslim) and Ibn Abi Usaybia (1230s–1270s, Arab-Iraqi, Muslim) (Ghaly 2010; Prioreschi 2001; Gallagher 1999; Selin 1997; Ullmann 1978). One of the most spectacular aspects of this host of medical thinkers is the diversity of religious (Christian, Jewish, Shi'i and Sunni Islam) and cultural backgrounds that early Islam garnered into a corpus of thought. This seems to be in stark contrast to the insularity of Christian awareness towards other faiths and sciences in the same period (Ohlig 2013).

This is not to say that Islamic medicine was purely naturalistic in orientation; on the contrary, medical thought within early medieval Islam assumed some of the same diversity found within pre-Christian Greco-Roman thought, as well as in late antique Christianity. Expressions of local superstitions, mystical beliefs and magical hermeneutics affected the shape of early Islamic medical thought too, in time leading to the evolution of the influential *ulamā* (elite religious authorities) and the *sufis* (mystics deriving the cause of illnesses from spiritual sources, finding cures through prayer) within most Muslim societies of the era.

Islamic medical *fiqh* instituted in North Africa

The *ulamā* had the most pronounced long-term impact on the shape of Islamic medical *fiqh* in medieval North Africa. Whilst the Umayyad rulers were key in deposing the Byzantine armies and imposing a new Arab and Islamic regime throughout the new *Ifrîkiyah* province (northern Africa), it was the emergence of the Abbasid caliphate in the 800s and parallel ascendance of the vassal Aghlabid dynasty (a century-long period, roughly 800–900) that assured the region would be a powerhouse of Muslim thought concerning disease and disability. Under this dynasty, two prominent centres of Islamic thought emerged: Kairouan (modern Tunisia) and Fez (modern Morocco). Both locations feature prominently in world history, Kairouan (al-Qayrawan) as a mosque and school that was second only in stature and popularity to Mecca and Medina, and Fez (University of al-Qarawiyyin founded in 859) as one of the oldest universities in the world (Knapp and Barbour 1977; Sebag 1963).

While both locations were bastions of Muslim *fiqh* regarding medicine, disease and disability, it was Kairouan that emerged as the centre of controversy once the Sunni Malikite school emerged as a force within Muslim jurisprudence and as the predominant version of Sunni Islam in most of northern Africa (Nasir 1990). Malikite Sunni Islam focused on a strict interpretation of only the Qur'an, al-ḥadīth and rulings of the early caliphs. While this movement gradually declined in relative importance, it still remains a strong force within Sunni Islam. By contrast, the university or madrassa at Fez was renowned for its Athens-like eclectic gathering of thought concerning medicine based on the Qur'an and Greco-Roman sources. The difference between Kairouan and Fez, displaying two distinct expressions of early Islamic thought, is perhaps symbolized in the masculine military and financial power (Kairouan) on the one hand, and the soft-power education centre that was founded by a woman, Fatima al-Fihri, on the other (Esposito 2003: 328). The influence of the moderate Islam found in Fez is seen perhaps most intensely in two of the greatest sons and daughters to leave Africa and later influence Islamic medical thought: the Berber Ummul Banin Najmaj (mother of the influential Sufi leader Ali ibn Musa al-Rida), herself a notable Islamic scholar of the 8th century (Rizvi 1988); and one of the most well-known Islamic physician-scholars, Ahmad ibn-Rusd (Averroes) a few centuries later.

Islamic medical *fiqh*, based on a Greco-Roman heritage, remained an enduring force throughout subsequent history. For example, the Greco-Roman theory of the four humours

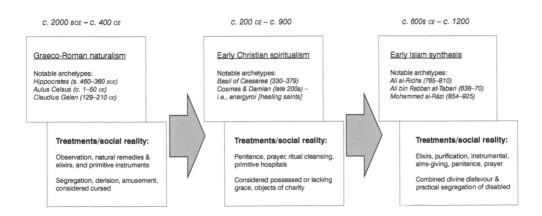

Figure 28.2 Methods of medical treatment of disease and disability in antiquity. Source: author

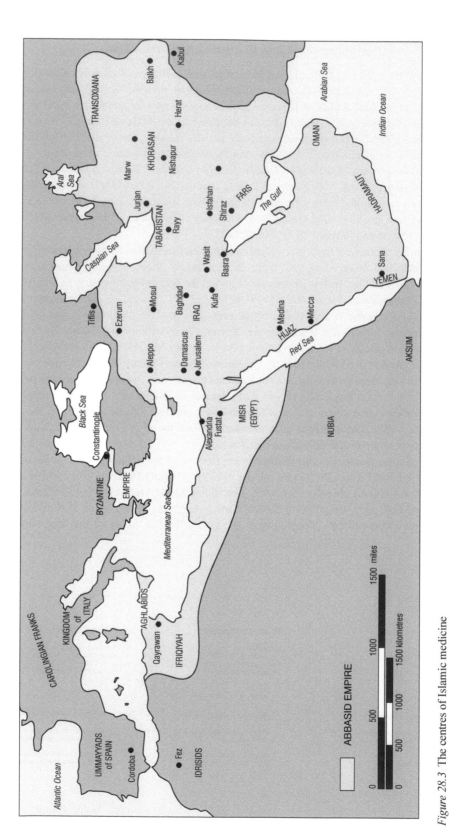

Figure 28.3 The centres of Islamic medicine

endured within Islamic medicine until as recently as the 19th century (Scalenghe 2014). But it is not enough to merely lay out the historical significance of Islamic medicine, one must also gain an assessment of its structure and characteristics in order to see its enduring impact on Islamic theology and sciences.

Ṭibb

One of the best researched realms of Islamic medicine is that of medical care and treatment methods, *ṭibb*. The pluralistic context of medicine in this period is very clearly evidenced in the prevalent practices: mixing Greco-Roman, Christian, Jewish, Mazdaean, Sabian, Zoroastrian and Hindu traditions into a fusion-type Islamic medical style that had matured by the 800s (Savage-Smith, Klein-Frank and Zhu 2012; Carra de Vaux 2012). This fusion style made inroads in North Africa, especially in the royal power centres. Amongst the hallmarks of this new style was the treatment of all forms of maladies, ranging from fevers, illnesses, physical injuries, disabilities and mood disorders. Even a form of veterinary medicine was developed due to the close proximity of animals with their human masters (Carra de Vaux 2012). Throughout Abbasid domains, hospital complexes were erected that were rather more elaborate than the earlier Christian versions. These often served as convalescent centres, insane asylums, retirement homes, paediatric clinics and prototypical 'day-care centres'. These multi-generational *loci* were also melting pots where one could find folkloric practices alongside the most learned Greek approaches to treatment. One particularly resilient form, practised then and today, is *al-ṭibb al-nabawī*, or prophetic medicine, that was rooted in pre-Islamic Arabia and heralded as a spiritualist alternative to the non-Muslim Greek school of medicine (Savage-Smith, Klein-Frank and Zhu 2012; Ghaly 2010). In a sense, medicine in that context is not completely different from what is seen in cosmopoles today.

Wabā'

The medical treatments and theories of disease, *wabā'*, put forth by scholars in these early centuries of the new religion were complex schemas (Renhart 2005). Perhaps the most famous was Ali ibn-Sina's principles of medicine, *kullīyāt*, which covered topics including anatomy, hygiene, disease symptoms and treatment, tumours and fractures, remedies and pharmaceutics (*akrabadhin*) (Panzac 2012). Because of the prominence of infectious disease throughout history, and the Greco-Roman influence, it stands as no surprise that the tomes and encyclopedia of early Muslim scholars frequently concerned scourges such as smallpox, malaria, leprosy and syphilis (Savage-Smith, Klein-Frank and Zhu 2012; Hopkins 2002). Again, understanding of these diseases revolved round the Greek humours theory, with therapies ranging from prayer intercessions, 'sweat-therapies', bloodletting and pharaceutical remedies. The most powerful display of medicinal knowledge in that time was in two areas: the connection between poor hygiene and disease, and quarantine as a method of disease and vector control (McNeill 1998). In the first instance, a northern Egyptian in the early 1000s, Ali bin Riḍwan, composed a breakthrough discourse on the relation between climate, topography, geography and disease (especially outbreaks) (Savage-Smith, Klein-Frank and Zhu, 2012). In the second instance, various early sources insisted on distance from the sick, most prominently *hadith*: 'When you learn that epidemic disease exists in a county, do not go there; but if it breaks out in the county where you are, do not leave' (Ullman 1978). This sense of quarantine also applied to neighbours within the community suffering from leprosy, *djudhām*. This disease was considered divine punishment for immoral behaviour, requiring isolation and legal exclusion from society. The divine dimension of this punishment is clear. In the Qur'an, leprosy is the only physical illness Allah cures and he does so through Jesus (Q 3.48 and 5.110) (Dols 2012). Interestingly, while *hadith* provide a rich source for disease topics, the Qur'an only contains a description of five plagues in the Moses story (see book 7: The Heights / *Al-A'raf*). Qu'rānic silence on the other four traditional plagues led some early Muslim exegetes to propose that Moses' hand, staff, and tongue (and the Red Sea) were the others. In this case, Moses' disfigured hand and speech disability symbolized divine affliction (Lowin 2005).

A number of well-recognized disciplines brought Islamic medicine renown in late medieval Europe, including anatomy, ophthalmology and pharmacology. Ophthalmology presents a particularly interesting case study as it had direct theological cross-over in that physical seeing (and hearing) had symbolic importance as the faculties of perceiving faith in Allah (seeing) and in receiving faith (hearing). More will follow on this in the last section of this chapter.

Tahāra

The last component of *fiqh* is ritual purity, *tahāra*. Of the pillars of *fiqh*, *tahāra* is the most obviously legalistic in the sense evinced in other Semitic traditions, notably the First (Old) Testament accounts of ancient Judaism. The legalism surrounding ritual purity was put into sharp focus at the learning centres of Kairouan and Fez. On one level, purification of bodily extremities through *wuḍū'*, ablution (washing and wiping), is identified as being necessary for those who have been contaminated by minor impurities before prayers: excrement and other bodily functions (*hadath*), sexual fluids or touching women (*aw lāmastum al- nisā'a*), intoxication (*sukārā*) and menstruation (*al-maḥīḍ*; which was considered a temporary disability) (Lowry 2005).

This physical sense of purity surfaces throughout the Qur'ān, notably 2.232; 7.82; 11.78; 27.56; and 33.53. In addition, almsgiving, *zakāt*, etymologically 'to be pure', is used in the Qur'ān in 9.103 and 58.12 to denote the purifying effect of almsgiving (Ghaly 2010). There is a primal identification, shared throughout many religions and cultures, of dirt and fluids as a vector of disease, passed between animals and humans, which must be neutralized to ensure health (this entered Muslim thought via pre-Islam Bedouin poetry (Stearns 2010)). While this idea is deeply engrained in the human psyche, it is also relevant today as new purification rituals emerge to combat the proliferation of food-borne and inter-species bacteria and viruses (especially zoonotic and RNA viruses) such as SARS and ebola.

On a more symbolic level, *tahāra* regards internal purification, *ghusl*, as protection from major substantive and moral pollution. This is where Islamic thought intersects with other systems such as Christian ethics. Moral pollution is categorized as *tayyib/khabīth,* a classical good/evil distinction (Katz 2005). This symbolic type of contamination is described in the Qur'ān as *najas* (unclean), *rijs* (filthy), *rijz* (abomination) and *rujz* (incurring divine wrath). Those falling into this level of defilement include: impious polytheists, idol-worshippers, and those engaged in sinful conduct and sacrificing unclean foods to false gods (e.g. blood and pork). This good/evil dichotomy is even further elaborated in physical terms: *harām*, denoting that which is taboo, and *halāl*, denoting that which is free from this ban (Lowry 2005). A final dimension of major pollution concerns *rujz*. Christian and Jewish references to occasions of divine wrath are understood within the context of a covenantal construction; in this regard early Islamic theology was no different. Much like the Donatist Christians mentioned earlier, early North African Muslims understood themselves as a community set apart by Allah with strict boundaries and purity requirements. Within this framework personal and social *khabīth* invite divine wrath in the form of famine, natural disasters and pestilence (Q 2.59; 7.134–5 and 162; 29.34).

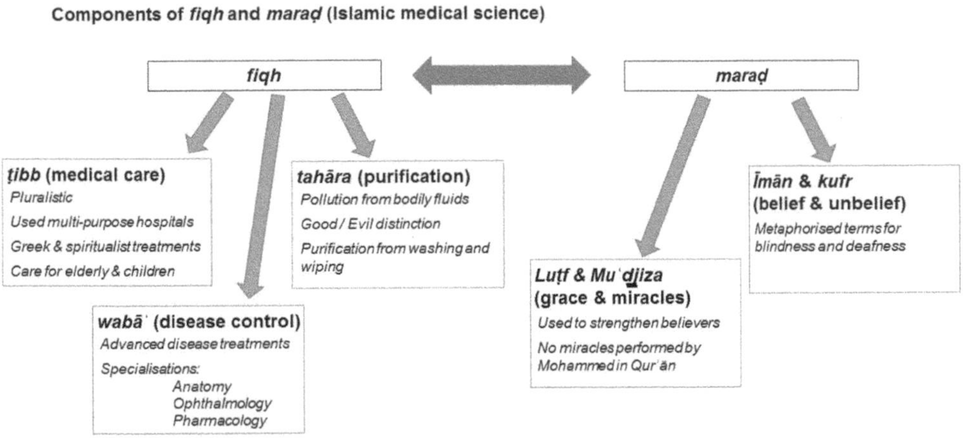

Components of *fiqh* and *maraḍ* (Islamic medical science)

Figure 28.4 Components of *fiqh* and *maraḍ* (Islamic medical science)

Final excursus: maraḍ

A discussion of the shape of medicine and medical thought in early medieval Islam is incomplete without looking at the meaning of illness of the 'heart', *maraḍ*. It is important to note that the Qur'ān places more emphasis on moral illness than the physical type (Zayd 2005). This topic is divided into two tracks: literal illnesses and metaphorical illnesses.

The response to literal illnesses demonstrates the diversity of thought and traditions in early Islam. Alongside the dominant Greco-Islamic tradition was the use of prophetic medicine in diagnosing illnesses. In this school of thought, Allah is the source and cure of all illnesses: both physical and psychological. It is Allah's divine will that illness reminds humans of the fires of hell and also his generosity in creating cures for illnesses. Terminal diseases were trials for the faithful and death meant martyrdom. In the prophetic school, Allah alone (*tawakkul*) it is beginning and end of all health matters (Perho 2005). Treatments were considered relevant in all matters of the body and soul with divine medicaments (*adwiya ilāhiyya*) of prayer (*ṣalāt*), patience (*ṣabr*), fasting (*ṣawm*), jihād, the Qur'ān itself and chanting (*ruqan*). All of these methods were used to provide spiritual and bodily health and restore a believer to covenant with Allah (Perho 2005).

A final component of literal illness is the role of grace, *luṭf*, and miracles, *mu'djiza*, in strengthening believers. Much as in the Christian scriptures, miracles are used frequently in the Qur'ān (Gril 2005). The Prophet Mohammed never performed miracles, but in their stead performed signs, *āyāt*, to prove his legitimacy to his followers (Wensinck 2012). In later theological developments, especially in various *ḥadīth*, both miracles and signs are associated with the Prophet's life to explicate Allah's strengthening of believers to weather afflictions, disabilities and diseases through grace and blessed examples (Leaman 2012). The most profound effect that miracles and signs are supposed to elicit is a deeper faith in Allah through their eschatological import.

Metaphorical illness provides a rich assortment of typological themes in the early Islamic tradition. Seeing, hearing and belief are synonymous with faith in Allah, whilst blindness, deafness, and unbelief mark the absence thereof. *Īmān* (belief) and *kufr* (unbelief) are central tenets of Islam, with *īmān* being closely affiliated with the verb *islām*. Belief allows the adherent *mu'min* to see the 'unseen things' and grants him gratitude, awe, repentance, submission, chastity, modesty, humility, forgiveness, and truthfulness, respect for contracts and covenants (see Q 8.2–4 and 74; 9.112; 13.20–3; 23.1–6, 8–11, 57–61; 24.36–9; 25.63–8, 72–4; 28.54–5; 32.15–17;

33.35–6; 42.36–43; 48.29; 70.22–35; 76.7–10) (Adang 2005). Opposed to this, the disbelieving, blind and deaf *kāfir* is denoted for his iniquity, hypocrisy, sinfulness, arrogance, ingratitude and denial (see Q 2.152; 16.55, 83 and 122–4; 17.27; 26.18–19; 29.66; 30.24; 43.15).

Seeing in the Qur'ān is primarily concerned with faith or 'vision of the heart'. For this reason, blind people (without the ability to see) are able to have profound spiritual vision, such as the blind man the Prophet Mohammed turned away and later regretted in Q 80.1–6 (Kugle 2005). Seeing is connected with *nūr*, 'light', which is guidance (*hudan*), revelation (*mubīn*) and proof (*burhān*). The verb *absara*, seeing, is better classified as knowing, understanding or learning. Seeing is further paired with *nazara* (to behold) and *ra'ā* (thinking). The opposite of *absara* is blindness: doubt, error, illness, disability, ignorance and darkness (Rippin 2005; Elias 2005).

Hearing and deafness follow in parallel with seeing and blindness. In this case as well, hearing takes on a spiritual character as a metaphor for knowledge and obedience, with the phrase *sami 'nā wa-aṭa 'nā* ('we heard and obeyed') appearing in Q 2.285; 4.46; 5.7; 24.47 and 51 (van Gelder 2005). It follows that deafness is equated with blindness, darkness, ingratitude, disbelief and ignorance, with the phrase *ṣummun bukmun 'umyun* ('deaf, dumb, blind') appearing 2.18 and 171; 6.39 and 17.97.

What difference did Islam make? Conclusions

While the assimilation of Greco-Roman medical thought into early Islam is clear enough at this point, what remains to be seen is the historical endurance of this synergy. In the centuries after the formation of medieval Muslim North Africa, complex methodologies emerged with regard to disease and disability. Rules and practices concerning the dignity of the disabled and sick, their medical treatment, employability and financial relief for the poor, all assumed form in the *fiqh* that developed after the late first millennium (Ghaly 2010). While there are today diverse schools of thought concerning such rules and practices, what this research has shown is that this is nothing new within Islam, nor something novel in the history of Muslim North Africa.

A critical review of disease and disability in North African history demonstrates the pronounced effect that morbidity played in both pre-Christian and Christian late Antiquity. North Africa was a place constantly under siege from pestilence and warfare. It also remained a synergy hotspot for thought and culture across different eras. The state of research would profit from an analysis of further documentary and archaeological evidence about disease and disability in the early medieval period. The brevity of this chapter excludes a thorough reckoning of all of the most significant figures and their works in the history of medicine in medieval North Africa, but such an effort would be beneficial in the future. Alongside this, what sort of picture would emerge if research was conducted into Christian sources or influences in early and medieval Muslim scientific texts? Would only Hellenistic sources be discernible?

But perhaps the most felicitous conclusion from this historical assessment is not the commonality of the affliction of disease and disabilities throughout history, or that people can improve life and survivability for themselves and societies. Instead, this research shows something that is often tossed aside in modern discourse: the inter-reliance of all of the world's religions, philosophies and practices. In this regard, it seems fortuitous to quote an overlooked section of the Qur'ān (*Al-Baqara* 2.62):

> The (Muslim) Believers, the Jews, the Christians, and the Sabians – all those who believe in God and the Last Day and do good – will have their rewards with their Lord. No fear for them, nor will they grieve.

In the end, between humans, there is more in common than not, and disease and disability do not discriminate. As the human race enters a period of global interconnection, issues of disease and disability will only become more pressing (Holmes 2009). Hopefully the sharing of scientific knowledge and best-practices of care will be the norm, a precedent well established in the history covered here.

Bibliography

Adang, Camilla, 'Belief and Unbelief', in J. D. McAuliffe (ed.), *Encyclopaedia of the Qur'ān* (Leiden, 2005). <http://referenceworks.brillonline.com/entries/encyclopaedia-of-the-quran/belief-and-unbelief-EQCOM_00025>

Allen, Peter Lewis, *The Wages of Sin: Sex and Disease, Past and Present* (Chicago, IL, 2002).

Arjava, Antti, 'The Mystery Cloud of 536 CE in the Mediterranean Sources', *Dumbarton Oaks Papers* 59 (2005), 73–94.

Arnott, R., 'Healers and Medicines in the Mycenaean Greek Texts', in D. Michaelides (ed.), *Medicine and Healing in the Ancient Mediterranean World* (Oakville, CT, 2014), 44–53.

Bachrach, B. S., 'On Roman Ramparts', in G. Parker (ed.), *The Cambridge History of Warfare* (New York, 2005), 64–91.

Benedictow, Ole, *The Black Death, 1346–1353: The Complete History* (Woodbridge, 2006).

Brothwell, Don, and Sandison, A.T. (eds), *Disease in Antiquity: A Survey of Diseases, Injuries and Surgery of Early Populations* (Springfield, IL, 1967).

Burns, J. Patout, 'Appropriating Augustine Appropriating Cyprian', *Augustinian Studies* 36/1 (2005), 113–30.

Carmichael, A. G., 'Bubonic Plague', in K. F. Kiple (ed.), *The Cambridge World History of Human Disease* (Cambridge, 1999), 628–30.

Carra de Vaux, B., 'Ṭibb', in M. T. Houtsma, T. W. Arnold, R. Basset and R. Hartmann (eds), *Encyclopaedia of Islam* (Leiden, 2012; 1st edn 1913–36). <http://referenceworks.brillonline.com/entries/encyclopaedia-of-islam-1/t-ibb-SIM_5758>.

Cartwright, Frederick, and Biddiss, Michael, *Disease and History* (London, 2014).

Clark, David, *Germs, Genes, and Civilization: How Epidemics Shaped Who we are Today* (Upper Saddle River, NJ, 2010).

Cliff, A. D., Haggett P., 'Epidemic Control and Critical Community Size: Spatial Aspects of Eliminating Communicable Diseases in Human Populations', in R. W. Thomas (ed.), *Spatial Epidemiology* (London, 1990), 93–110.

Crawley Quinn, Josephine, '"Roman Africa?", "Romanization"?', *Digressus Supplement* 1 (2003), 7–34.

Crislip, Andrew, *From Monastery to Hospital: Christian Monasticism and the Transformation of Health Care in Late Antiquity* (Ann Arbor, MI, 2005).

Cuoq, Joseph, *L'Église d'Afrique du Nord à IIᵉ au XIIᵉ siècle* (Paris, 1984).

Davis, Paul, *100 Decisive Battles from Ancient Times to the Present: The World's Major Battles and How they Shaped History* (New York, 1999).

Diamond, Jared, *Guns, Germs, and Steel: The Fates of Human Societies* (New York, 1999).

Diekmann, O., Heesterbeek J. A. P., and Metz, J. A. J., 'On the Definition and the Computation of the Basic Reproduction Ratio R_0 in Models for Infectious Diseases in Heterogeneous Populations', *Journal of Mathematical Biology* 28/4 (1990), 365–82.

Dols, Michael W., 'Djudhām', in P. Bearman, T. Bianquis, C. E. Bosworth, E. van Donzel and W. P. Heinrichs (eds), *Encyclopaedia of Islam*, 2nd edn (Leiden, 2012). <http://referenceworks.brillonline.com/entries/encyclopaedia-of-islam-2/d-j-ud-h-a-m-SIM_8513>.

Dols, Michael W., 'Leprosy in Medieval Arabic Medicine', *Journal of the History of Medicine and Allied Sciences* 34 (1979), 314–33.

Dossey, Leslie, *Peasant and Empire in Christian North Africa* (Los Angeles, CA, 2010).

Dunn, Geoffrey, 'The White Crown of Works: Cyprian's Early Pastoral Ministry of Almsgiving in Carthage', *Church History* 73/4 (2004), 715–40.

Dunn, Geoffrey, 'Validity of Baptism and Ordination in the African response to the "Rebaptism" Crisis: Cyprian of Carthage's Synod of Spring 256', *Theological Studies* 67 (2006), 257–74.

Elias, Jamal J., 'Light', in J. D. McAuliffe (ed.), *Encyclopaedia of the Qur'ān* (Leiden, 2005). <http://referenceworks.brillonline.com/entries/encyclopaedia-of-the-quran/light-EQSIM_00261>.

Esposito, John (ed.), *The Oxford Dictionary of Islam* (New York, 2003).

Fagan, Brian, *The Long Summer: How Climate Changed Civilization* (New York, 2004).

Gallagher, Nancy, 'Islamic and Indian Medicine', in K. F. Kiple (ed.), *The Cambridge World History of Human Disease* (Cambridge, 1999), 27–34.

Garland, Robert, *The Eye of the Beholder: Deformity and Disability in the Graeco-Roman World* (London, 2010[2]).

Gaumer, Matthew, 'The Evolution of Donatist Theology as Response to a Changing Late Antique Milieu', *Augustiniana* 58/3–4 (2008), 171–203.

Ghaly, Mohammed, *Islam and Disability: Perspectives in Theology and Jurisprudence* (London and New York, 2010).

Gleeson, Brendan, *Geographies of Disability* (London and New York, 2006).

Gril, Denis, 'Miracles', in J. D. McAuliffe (ed.), *Encyclopaedia of the Qur'ān* (Leiden, 2005). <http://referenceworks.brillonline.com/entries/encyclopaedia-of-the-quran/miracles-EQCOM_00122>.

Hays, Jo N., 'Historians and Epidemics: Simple Questions, Complex Answers', in L. K. Little (ed.), *Plague and the End of Antiquity: The Pandemic of 541–750* (New York, 2007), 33–58.

Hays, Jo N., *The Burdens of Disease: Epidemics and Human Response in Western History* (New Brunswick, NJ, 2009).

Heather, Peter, *Empires and Barbarians: The Fall of Rome and the Birth of Europe* (New York, 2010).

Holmes, Edward, *The Evolution and Emergence of RNA Viruses* (New York, 2009).

Hopkins, Donald, *The Greatest Killer: Smallpox in History* (Chicago, IL, 2002).

Katouzian-Safadi, M., and Bonmatin, Jean-Marc, 'Du diagnostic différentiel aux thérapies prudentes: *Le traité de la rougeole et de la variole* de Râzî', in D. Michaelides (ed.), *Medicine and Healing in the Ancient Mediterranean World* (Oakville, CT, 2014), 338–49.

Katz, Marion Holmes, 'Cleanliness and Ablution', in J. D. McAuliffe (ed.), *Encyclopaedia of the Qur'ān* (Leiden, 2005). <http://referenceworks.brillonline.com/entries/encyclopaedia-of-the-quran/cleanliness-and-ablution-EQSIM_00081>.

Kinnear-Wilson, J. V., 'Organic Diseases of Ancient Mesopotamia', in D. Brothwell and A.T. Sandison (eds), *Disease in Antiquity: A Survey of Diseases, Injuries and Surgery of Early Populations* (Springfield, IL, 1967), 191–208.

Knapp, Wilfrid, and Barbour, Nevill, *North West Africa: A Political and Economic Survey* (Oxford, 1977).

Kohn, George, *Encyclopedia of Plague and Pestilence: From Ancient Times to the Present* (New York, 2008).

Kugle, S., 'Vision and Blindness', in J. D. McAuliffe (ed.), *Encyclopaedia of the Qur'ān* (Leiden, 2005). <http://referenceworks.brillonline.com/entries/encyclopaedia-of-the-quran/vision-and-blindness-EQCOM_00213>.

Laes, Christian, 'Children and their Occupations in the City of Rome (300–700 CE)', in C. Laes, K. Mustakallio and V. Vuolanto (eds), *Children and Family in Roman Antiquity: Life, Death and Interaction* (Leuven, 2015), 79–109.

Lancel, Serge, *Saint Augustine* (London, 2002).

Leaman, O.N.H., 'Luṭf', in P. Bearman, T. Bianquis, C. E. Bosworth, E. van Donzel and W. P. Heinrichs (eds), *Encyclopaedia of Islam*, 2nd edn (Leiden, 2012). <http://referenceworks.brillonline.com/entries/encyclopaedia-of-islam-2/lut-f-SIM_4701>.

Linard, Catherine, Gilbert, Marius, Snow, Robert W., Noor, Abdisalan M., and Tatem, Andrew J. 'Population Distribution, Settlement Patterns and Accessibility across Africa in 2010', *PLOS ONE Journal* 7/2 (2012), 1–8. <http://journals.plos.org/plosone/article?id=10.1371/journal.pone.0031743>.

Little, Lester K., 'Life and Afterlife of the First Plague Pandemic', in L. K. Little (ed.), *Plague and the End of Antiquity: The Pandemic of 541–750* (New York, 2007), 3–32.

Lockhard, Craig, *Societies, Networks, and Transitions: A Global History* (Boston, MA, 2011).

Lowin, Shari, 'Plagues', in J. D. McAuliffe (ed.), *Encyclopaedia of the Qur'ān* (Leiden, 2005). <http://referenceworks.brillonline.com/entries/encyclopaedia-of-the-quran/plagues-EQSIM_00330>.

Lowry, Joseph, 'Ritual Purity', in J. D. McAuliffe (ed.), *Encyclopaedia of the Qur'ān* (Leiden, 2005). <http://referenceworks.brillonline.com/entries/encyclopaedia-of-the-quran/ritual-purity-EQCOM_00178?s.num=1&s.f.s2_parent=s.f.book.encyclopaedia-of-the-quran&s.q=disability>.

McCormick, Michael, 'Toward a Molecular History of the Justinianic Pandemic', in L. K. Little (ed.), *Plague and the End of Antiquity: The Pandemic of 541–750* (New York, 2007), 290–312.

McEvedy, Colin, *The Penguin Atlas of African History* (London, 1995).

McNeill, William, *Plagues and Peoples* (New York, 1998).

Mermann, Alan, *Some Chose to Stay: Faith and Ethics in a Time of Plague* (Atlantic Highlands, NJ, 1997).

Merrills, Andrew, and Richard Miles, *The Vandals* (London, 2007).

Morris, C., and Alan Peatfield, 'Health and Healing on Cretan Bronze Age Peak Sanctuaries', in D. Michaelides (ed.), *Medicine and Healing in the Ancient Mediterranean World* (Oakville, CT, 2014), 54–63.

Nasir, Jamal, *The Islamic Law of Personal Status* (Leiden, 1990).

Naylor, Phillip, *North Africa: A History from Antiquity to the Present* (Austin, TX, 2009).

Ohlig, Karl-Heinz, 'Evidence of a New Religion in Christian Literature "Under Islamic Rule"', in K.-H. Ohlig (ed.), *Early Islam: A Critical Reconstruction Based on Contemporary Sources* (Amherst, MA, 2013), 251–307.

Panzac, D., 'Wabā', in P. Bearman, T. Bianquis, C. E. Bosworth, E. van Donzel and W. P. Heinrichs (eds), *Encyclopaedia of Islam*, 2nd edn (Leiden, 2012). <http://referenceworks.brillonline.com/entries/encyclopaedia-of-islam-2/waba-COM_1320>.

Patrick, Adam, 'Disease in Antiquity: Ancient Greece and Rome', in D. Brothwell and A. T. Sandison (eds), *Disease in Antiquity: A Survey of Diseases, Injuries and Surgery of Early Populations* (Springfield, IL, 1967), 238–46.

Perho, Irmeli, 'Medicine and the Qur'an', in J. D. McAuliffe (ed.), *Encyclopaedia of the Qur'ān* (Leiden, 2005). <http://referenceworks.brillonline.com/entries/encyclopaedia-of-the-quran/medicine-and-the-qur-a-n-EQCOM_00118>.

Prioreschi, Plinio, *A History of Medicine: Byzantine and Islamic Medicine* (Omaha, NE, 2001).

Renhart, Kevin, 'Contamination', in J. D. McAuliffe (ed.), *Encyclopaedia of the Qur'ān* (Leiden, 2005). <http://referenceworks.brillonline.com/entries/encyclopaedia-of-the-quran/contamination-EQSIM_00091>.

Rippin, Andrew, 'Seeing and Hearing', in J. D. McAuliffe (ed.), *Encyclopaedia of the Qur'ān* (Leiden, 2005). <http://referenceworks.brillonline.com/entries/encyclopaedia-of-the-quran/seeing-and-hearing-EQSIM_00379>.

Risse, Günter, 'History of Western Medicine from Hippocrates to Germ Theory', in K. F. Kiple (ed.), *The Cambridge World History of Human Disease* (Cambridge, 1999), 11–19.

Rizvi, Sayyid, *Slavery from Islamic and Christian Perspectives* (Richmond, 1987).

Rosen, William, *Justinian's Flea: The First Great Plague and the End of the Roman Empire* (New York, 2007).

Russell, Josiah Cox, *Late Ancient and Medieval Population* (Philadelphia, PA, 1958).

Sallares, Robert, 'Ecology, Evolution, and Epidemiology of Plague', in L. K. Little (ed.), *Plague and the End of Antiquity: The Pandemic of 541–750* (New York, 2007), 231–89.

Sallares, Robert, and Gomzi, Susan, 'Biomolecular Archaeology of Malaria', *Ancient Biomolecules* 3 (2001), 195–213.

Sallares, Robert, Bouwman, Abigail, and Anderung, Cecilia, 'The Spread of Malaria to Southern Europe in Antiquity: New Approaches to Old Problems', *Medical History* 48 (2004), 311–28.

Savage-Smith, Emilie, Klein-Franke, F., and Zhu Ming, 'Ṭibb', in P. Bearman, T. Bianquis, C. E. Bosworth, E. van Donzel and W. P. Heinrichs (eds), *Encyclopaedia of Islam*, 2nd edn (Leiden, 2012) <http://referenceworks.brillonline.com/entries/encyclopaedia-of-islam-2/t-ibb-COM_1216>.

Scalenghe, Sara, *Disability in the Ottoman Arab World, 1500–1800* (New York, 2014).

Scheidel, Walter, *Death on the Nile: Disease and the Demography of Roman Egypt* (Leiden, 2001).

Scheidel, Walter, 'Disease and Death in the Ancient City of Rome', in P. Erdkamp (ed.), *The Cambridge Companion to Ancient Rome* (New York, 2013), 45–59.

Scourfield, J. H. D., 'The *De Mortalitate* of Cyprian: Consolation and Context', *Vigiliae Christianae* 50 (1996), 12–41.

Sebag, Paul, *La Grande Mosquée de Kairouan* (Paris, 1963).

Selin, Helaine, *Encyclopaedia of the History of Science, Technology, and Medicine in Non-Western Cultures* (Dordrecht, 1997).

Shelmerdine, Cynthia W., *The Perfume Industry at Pylos* (Göteborg, 1985).

Southern, Pat, *The Roman Army: A Social and Institutional History* (Oxford, 2007).

Stannard, Jerry, 'Diseases in Western Antiquity', in K. F. Kiple (ed.), *The Cambridge World History of Human Disease* (Cambridge, 1999), 262–9.

Stearns, Justin K., 'Contagion', in K. Fleet, G. Krämer, D. Matringe, J. Nawas and E. Rowson (eds), *Encyclopaedia of Islam, Three* (Leiden, 2010) .<http://referenceworks.brillonline.com/entries/encyclopaedia-of-islam-3/contagion-COM_23480>.

Thomas, Richard, 'The Role of Trade in Transmitting the Black Death in the Middle Ages', *TED Case Studies* 7/2 (1997) <http://www1.american.edu/ted/bubonic.htm>.

Tilley, Maureen, 'Sustaining Donatist Self-Identity: From the Church of the Martyrs to the Collecta of the Desert', *Journal of Early Christian Studies* 5/1 (1997), 21–35.

Tsiamis, Costas, Poulakou-Rebelakou, Effie, and Androutsos, George, 'The Role of the Egyptian Sea and Land Routes in the Justinian Plague: The Case of Pelusium', in D. Michaelides (ed.), *Medicine and Healing in the Ancient Mediterranean World* (Oakville, CT, 2014), 334–7.

Ullmann, Manfred, *Islamic Medicine* (Edinburgh, 1978).

Upson-Saia, Kristi, 'Resurrecting Deformity: Augustine on Wounded and Scarred Bodies in the Heavenly Realm', in D. Schumm and M. Stoltzfus (eds), *Disability in Judaism, Christianity, and Islam: Sacred Texts, Historical Traditions, and Social Analysis* (New York, 2011), 93–122.

van Gelder, Geert Jan H., 'Hearing and Deafness', in J. D. McAuliffe (ed.), *Encyclopaedia of the Qur'ān* (Leiden, 2005). <http://referenceworks.brillonline.com/entries/encyclopaedia-of-the-quran/hearing-and-deafness-EQSIM_00187>.

Wagner, David, Klunk, Jennifer, Harbeck, Michaela, Devault, Alisoon, *et al.*, '*Yersinia pestis* and the Plague of Justinian 541–543 AD: A Genomic Analysis', *The Lancet Infectious Diseases* 14/4 (2014), 1–8.

Ward-Perkins, Bryan, *The Fall of Rome and the End of Civilization* (Oxford, 2005).

Wensinck, A. J., 'Muʿdjiza', in P. Bearman, T. Bianquis, C. E. Bosworth, E. van Donzel and W. P. Heinrichs (eds), *Encyclopaedia of Islam* (Leiden, 2012; 1st edn 1913–16) <http://referenceworks.brillonline.com/entries/encyclopaedia-of-islam-2/mu-d-j-iza-SIM_5309>.

Wohletz, Ken, 'Were the Dark Ages Triggered by Volcano-Related Climate Changes in the 6th Century? (If so, was Krakatau Volcano the Culprit?)' (2000). <http://www.ees.lanl.gov/geodynamics/Wohletz/Krakatau.htm>.

Xu, Lei, Schmid, Boris, Liu Jun, Xiaoyan Si, Nils, C., Stenseth, Nils C., and Zhang Zhibin, 'The Trophic Responses of Two Different Rodent-Vector-Plague Systems to Climate Change', *Proceedings of the Royal Society B: Biological Sciences* 282/1800 (2015) <http://www.ncbi.nlm.nih.gov/pubmed/25540277>.

Zayd, Nasr Hamid Abu, 'Illness and Health', in J. D. McAuliffe (ed.), *Encyclopaedia of the Qur'ān* (Leiden, 2005). <http://referenceworks.brillonline.com/entries/encyclopaedia-of-the-quran/illness-and-health-EQSIM_00214>.

29

IMPOTENT HUSBANDS, EUNUCHS AND FLAWED WOMEN IN EARLY ISLAMIC LAW

Hocine Benkheira

Introduction

To the modern readers' eyes, Roman marriage was strikingly informal. If two people decided to live together as man and wife, man and wife they were. There was no state registration, and mutual consent from both partners was the crucial point that determined the validity of a marriage. Divorce was legally as easy and informal as contracting the marriage (Treggiari 1991 is the starting point for any study on Roman marriage). Compared to the Greco-Roman tradition, Jewish and Christian views and practices of marriages were more stringent. Sexuality and fertility came to play a crucial role. Marriage became a religious duty towards God and mankind, unless one chose a celibate existence out of religious motives (Cooper 2007). For those who for some reason or another could not comply with these expectations of marriage, some of the consequences were disabling (cf. Watts Belser and Lehmhaus in this volume on the Jewish tradition, Metzler on Christianity). Born in the same late ancient Mediterranean world, early Islam also had its specific views and expectations of marriage. This contribution will deal with men and women who somehow fell away from these expectations – specifically, they are reported to have been impotent men, eunuchs and sterile women. Were they 'disabled' within this new Islamic context?

The Qur'an is completely silent on these issues. In other Islamic source material, the information is very sparse. The Islamic legal tradition, however, is much more abundant and developed. I will focus on this tradition, especially in its earliest stage, towards the end of the 8th century and the beginning of the 9th century. In addition to legal compilations, there are some treatises from the same period. From a variety of authors, I selected Malik (d. 795), who lived at Medina and al-Šāfi'ī (d. 820) and who, after having taught in Baghdad, moved to al-Fusṭāṭ, a town near the site of the future city of Cairo (which was not founded until the following century). These two lawyers lived under the successful rule of the Abbasids.

A compilation of traditions, al-*Muwaṭṭaʾ*, authoritative within the Maliki school up to the present, is attributed to Mālik, but this is not the book that will be considered here. There is a book that explains Mālik's teaching in more detail and much more directly, even though the book is not his own writing: the *Mudawwana*, the author of which is Sahnun (d. 856), a Maġribī. This book shows the oldest known state of the Maliki legal doctrine (Calder 1993: 1–19). It is presented as a dialogue between Sahnun and Ibn al-Qasim (d. 806), an Egyptian who was one of the great disciples of Mālik. He was enriched by traditions generally transmitted on the authority of 'Abd Allāh b. Wahb (d. 812), another Egyptian, also a disciple of Mālik. Mālik's teaching was also transmitted by other scholars; unfortunately, their compilations have rarely survived.

Two books are attributed to al-Šāfi'ī: *al-Risāla* and *Kitāb al-umm*. The first is a treaty, which has long been exemplified as the first presentation of 'legal theory' (*uṣūl al-fiqh*), although it is actually a defence of the Sunna and prophetic authority. I will not discuss this book in this chapter, but instead I will focus on the *Kitāb al-umm*, our second major source, which is a massive compilation of several thousand pages. Šāfi'ī's pupils, particularly al-Rabī' b. Sulaymān (d. 884), compiled his teachings, sometimes adding their own observations. The current state of the book – in its division into sections and chapters – dates from the late fourteenth century.

The jurists themselves make the link between impotence and castration: the case of the married eunuch and that of the impotent husband are often mentioned together. It is also relevant to mention the case of defects ('*uyūb*) that affect women, to the extent that the jurists discuss it (see Rispler-Chaim 2007; Ghaly 2010; Scalenghe 2014).

The husband's impotence

In Islamic law, the marital relationship is asymmetrical. The husband takes the initiative to marry, and he also has the power to end it whenever it suits him. No one can oppose him, except for the judge, and then only in specific situations. Sexual impotence is one such condition. Even early Islamic law specified that impotence could be submitted to the judge as grounds for divorce or annulment of marriage at the request of the woman herself (Benkheira 2014). Marriage was defined by two primary goals: satisfaction of the sexual appetite of both spouses and procreation. Sexual impotence can prevent the realization of these goals, especially the second. In the 8th century, one doctrine became dominant: in the case of marital impotence ('*unna*) the judge subjected the marriage to a probation period of one year. If the marriage was not consummated after this year, the judge would pronounce divorce, but only if the wife wanted it. This is a rare case where the wife may invoke separation, through the judge, since usually the power of repudiation was a marital privilege of the male partner.

Legally, sex could take place in two distinct situations: in the context of marriage (*nikāḥ*), or as part of the domination that characterizes the relationship between master and slave. This situation was, however, limited to the male master and the female slave. A woman was not allowed have sex with her slave, male or female, and a master could not do so with his male slave. A woman could not have sex with her male slave because she was a free woman and thus the superior of the slave. In sexual relations, the male always prevailed over the female. But in a social context, free men (or women) always dominated slaves. So if a free woman had sex with a male slave, her privilege would be subjected to slavery. This situation contradicted the social norms. When a man took his slave-girl as a sexual partner, this evidently did not go against social norms. But slavery could never make lawful what was forbidden by religious law: a man could not have sex with his male slave because male homosexuality was considered a crime. Moreover, in the relationship between a master and his slave-girl, the latter had, unlike the legal wife, no rights. Therefore, she could not ever complain about the master's impotence.

Jurists examine the question of impotence in the section on 'tares' ('*uyūb*) of both spouses that can lead to marriage annulment. Either spouse could claim an annulment due to dementia, leprosy and elephantiasis. Men could also request an annulment in cases of malformation in the genitals, women in cases of impotence or amputation of the male organ, whether entire or partial. Spouses could file an action in court for other reasons, for example if one spouse had concealed his/her servile condition or had lied about his\her roots. Such cases will not be discussed here.

Mālik (d. 795).

The earliest authorities of Islam – the Companions and Successors – recognized the need to set a time limit of one year for the man whose wife complained about impotence. On the basis of this doctrine, which was shared by almost all, one wonders from which moment the probation period began for the husband: from the celebration of the marriage or from the time the case was first submitted to the judge? Only the latter possibility is considered by the legalists. This means that if a woman waited some time to bring the case to the court, the time she had already spent with her husband would not be included in the one-year probation period granted to the allegedly impotent husband. When a woman eventually divorced her husband because of impotence, the question of the nature of the separation was necessarily discussed. Could it be treated as a repudiation (*ṭalāq*)? The jurists were divided into two 'parties'. According to the first 'party', presumably also the oldest and that which was related to Mālik, separation needed to be treated as repudiation (Saḥnūn, *al-Mudawwana* 2.265) which meant that it had the same consequences. The second 'party', related to al-Šāfi'ī, argued that it is nothing more than a cancellation.

If the wife chose divorce, after the failure of the masculinity test and the probationary period, she was bound to observe the obligations of divorced women, in particular, a period of abstinence (*'idda*). Unfortunately, there is no evidence in the sources about the nature of this test. The period of sexual continence was originally meant to prevent the problem of illegal offspring when at the time of separation the woman would be pregnant without realizing it, or realizing it but hiding the fact. The period of continence – about three months – was enough to reveal a hidden or unperceived pregnancy. One may ask why a wife who divorced a proven impotent husband had to observe such period of continence, since the marriage had apparently never been consummated. This is in fact a matter of legal formalism: since the separation was considered a case of repudiation, all effects of repudiation applied. Usually, during the period of abstinence, the husband retained his pre-emptive right: the option to resume cohabitation with his wife. Mālik refuses to recognize such a right in the cases of the husband's impotence.

Another point of controversy was the nuptial gift. In normal circumstances, a man gave one half of the bridal gift at the moment of the marriage celebration and the other half after the consummation of marriage.

> If the impotent cannot consummate the union during the waiting period which is prescribed to him, that is after one year, and if consequently both spouses are separated, is she entitled to the entire wedding gift or just a half of it? – She is entitled to the full nuptial gift if he shared his life for a year because he is responsible for the separation, not to mention that he cohabited with her in privacy (*ḫalā bihā*) for a long time, and as she undressed in his presence, her state has changed (*taġayyara ṣibġuhā*), as they lost the initial modesty (*taġayyara ǧihāzuhumā 'an ḥālihi*). My opinion is that he has no right over her (*lā arā lahu 'alayhā šay '*). However, if the separation takes place soon after marriage, he should pay her half the nuptial gift. There are people who argue that [in any case] she is entitled to only half of the nuptial gift. My opinion is that if the cohabitation has been long, he has taken pleasure from her [even without consuming] (*talaḏḏada minhā*) and if they were intimate, she is entitled to the full nuptial gift.
>
> (*Saḥnūn, al-Mudawwana 2.264*)

Therefore, according to Mālik, if after a one-year waiting period, the husband is still unable to consummate the union, the wife is entitled to the full nuptial gift.

In case of disagreement between spouses about the consummation of marriage, how do they resolve the dispute?

> And if the husband says that he consummated while his wife denies the fact (*mā ğāma'anī*)? – I asked about it Mālik. This same question was asked in our country and the Governor also asked me about it. But I did not know the answer. People say that other women have to be put with her,[1] others that one has to put in her vagina (*qubul*) a yellow dye (*ṣufra*).[2] I do not know what to say. Ibn al-Qāsim added: Except that I know that Mālik's opinion is that the husband must take an oath; I heard the expression many times. It is also my opinion.
>
> *(Saḥnūn, al-Mudawwana 2.263)*

Tricks and cheating are usually left out of the 'classical' doctrine, which became hegemonic from the 9th century on. It was preferable to use the oath. Perhaps it was also recommended to examine the woman immediately after reports by married women, who were deemed sufficiently expert in the field. In the case of a virgin bride, the fact that she had lost her virginity meant that the marriage was consummated. In the case of a bride who was not a virgin, one had to examine the vagina to explore the presence of semen. However, all this was not the doctrine of Mālik, who preferred the oath. However, spouses can refuse to take the oath:

> If the impotent man refuses to swear the oath? – We should ask the woman to take the oath. If she does, they will be divorced; if she refuses, she will remain his wife. This is my opinion (*haḏa ra'yī*).
>
> *(Saḥnūn, al-Mudawwana 2.265)*

Thus, the judge will decide in favour of the partner who agreed to take the oath. But nothing is said about the case when both spouses refuse to take the oath.

According to Muslim jurists, impotence is neither irreversible nor absolute, and they take into account that a man may be simultaneously impotent with one woman but not with another (surely in cases of polygyny or polygamy):

> If this man has other wives and slave-girls, and if he has sex with all of them except with one wife, will he also be subject to a period of one year according to Malik? – Yes. He is subject to a waiting period even if he had children with others. It was the view of Malik.
>
> *(Saḥnūn, al-Mudawwana, 2.265)*

It is safe to assume that impotence was not envisaged as a permanent condition, taking place on every single occasion. To the legalists, it was not important to strictly determine the impotence of the husband concerned, but rather to ensure the rights of the wife. When she or one of her relatives contracted a marriage, the goal was having sexual intercourse and children. Living with an impotent husband meant having neither. For her, this situation was to be avoided. That is why the jurists considered the possibility that impotence could occur in one specific relationship and not others.

On the other hand, if after having consummated the marriage, the husband became impotent, the judge should not consider the complaint of the unsatisfied wife (Saḥnūn, *al-Mudawwana*, 2.265). For as he has proven his potency once, he does not need to be put to the test again.

al-Šāfiʿī (m. 820).

Like Mālik, al-Šāfiʿī argues that the husband accused of impotence by his wife shall observe a probationary period of one year. If he does not consummate the marriage within this period, the judge will ask the bride to choose between remaining with her husband or to divorce. The delay of one year was necessary, since the defect was not always irreversible, and could have been caused by incidental reasons (Al-Šāfiʿī, *Kitāb al-umm* 5.40).

Again, one of the problems which turns up in the discussion relates to whether or not impotence was absolute. Who should be regarded as impotent? Only men who cannot have sex with any woman, or also the ones who cannot manage to have sex with a particular woman? This question has been discussed in a collection of early traditions, though admittedly sometimes in a way that might seem strange to the modern reader. The founder of the Umayyad dynasty, Muʿāwiya (d. 680), is credited with the idea that if one wants to check whether or not a man is impotent, that man must be married subsequently to another woman. After this other wedding night the result would be clear: if he does not consummate the union, he is actually impotent. But if he consummates it, his impotence was either the result of a passing disorder or was perceived or fabricated by his wife who complained. In this case, the man who proved his potency in an alternate scenario could not be considered impotent (Benkheira 2014: 24).

This is the solution that al-Šāfiʿī chooses. He discusses the case of a man who had several wives, or who had both wives and slave-girls. Then he assumes that the man is unable to consummate the union with his most recent wife. Should we consider him impotent? Can a man indeed be impotent with some women and not with others? Al-Šāfiʿī radically excludes such a possibility (Al-Šāfiʿī, *Kitāb al-umm* 5.40). Though not void of consistency and logic, this solution was rejected by his disciples and by most jurists who succeeded him. They preferred to opt for a pragmatic approach, which was evident in the doctrine attributed to Mālik (see above).

If a wife notices her husband's impotence, she should bring the matter to a judge:

> If she asks the judge for a divorce, the latter will submit the union to the test during one year from the day the case was submitted. If during this period, the husband has intercourse with her *once* [my emphasis], she is his wife; but if he does not have sexual intercourse with her, the judge will give the woman a choice between separation and remaining with her husband.
>
> If he once had, in a union, sexual intercourse with his wife and if she asks the judge to submit her husband to a probation period of a year, the judge has to refuse. Such a case is different from that of the husband who has no relations with one wife, but does have with others, because by fulfilling his duties towards them, he does not fulfill his duty to the first (*li-anna adāʾahu ilā ġayrihā ḥaqq laysa bi-adāʾ ilayhā*).
>
> (*Al-Šāfiʿī, Kitāb al-umm 5.40*)

Thus, in order to be valid, a marriage does not need regular sexual intercourse. If a man consummates the marriage, then his wife cannot claim the grounds for separation, even when he becomes impotent or observes permanent continence. Such a clause considerably limits the rule that the husband's impotence can be grounds for breaking the marital bond.

One of the most significant differences between al-Šāfiʿī and his predecessors is linked with the nature of legal divorce, when the wife opts for this possibility. Divorce cannot be, according to him, repudiation (*ṭalāq*), but only cancellation (*fasḫ*) (Al-Šāfiʿī, *Kitāb al-umm* 5.40). The reason for this restriction is that the cancellation is initiated by the wife. Therefore, it can never have the legal effects of repudiation.

If a man is separated from his wife because of his impotence but marries her a second time, she is entitled to request a new test by the judge Al-Šāfiʿī, *Kitāb al-umm* 5.40)

In the case where the judge sets a one-year period for the husband accused by his wife of sexual impotence, a dispute could arise between spouses regarding the consummation. Indeed, in the case of non-consummation, the wife was entitled to ask for divorce. But what if the husband says that he consummated the union, while she denies it?

> If the allegedly impotent man submitted to the test of a year and [at the end of this period,] there is a disagreement between the spouses, the husband proclaiming that he had intercourse during the year with his wife when she says the opposite, if she was not a virgin [at the time of marriage], the judge has to take in account the words of the husband, because it is she who seeks to annul the union; however, the husband will take the oath. If he takes an oath, the marriage will be confirmed, but if he refuses, the judge does not separate them until she has sworn that they had no sexual intercourse. If she takes the oath, she will have to choose between separation and remaining with her husband; but if she does not, she will remain his lawful wife. If, instead, she is a virgin, the judge will order her examination by four honourable women. If they confirm her statements, their testimony will be a proof of her sincerity (*dalīl ʿalā ṣidqihā*). In case of disagreement between the spouses, the husband can also choose to oblige his wife to take an oath. If under oath, she states she had no sexual intercourse with him, the judge will declare the divorce. If she does not take an oath while he, under oath, swears he had intercourse with her, she will remain with him and will not have any other choice.
> (Al-Šāfiʿī, *Kitāb al-umm* 5.40)

So, in case of a dispute regarding consummation, one must distinguish the virgin from the other women. The case of the virgin is simple. If there was consummation, the disappearance of the hymen is enough evidence. Therefore, she must be examined by four female experts. But in the case of the woman who was not a virgin when married, one cannot use the review of the state of the hymen. In such a situation, the husband's statement will prevail over that of the spouse, provided he confirms his statements with an oath. It was expected that severe punishment awaited the perjurer after death – a threat which was considered sufficient to dissuade husbands who might be tempted to resort to perjury.

However, a bit further on we read:

> If the man claims to have consummated the union and the woman disputes his statement, she is entitled to only half the nuptial gift and is not required to observe the waiting period.
> (Al-Šāfiʿī, *Kitāb al-umm* 5.41)

On the occasion of this discussion, al-Šāfiʿī tells us that the hymen can recover, as a result of prolonged sexual abstinence:

> According to experts in this field, the hymen can recover if there is no continuous sexual intercourse (*al-ʾuḏra qad taʿūdu fīmā zaʿama ahl al-ḥibra bihā iḏa lam yubāliġ fī-l-iṣāba*).
> (Al-Šāfiʿī, *Kitāb al-umm* 5.41)

He does not, however, draw any legal consequences from this belief.

The legalists also asked what form of penetration dismissed the accusation of impotence. The only permitted form was vaginal penetration. Anal intercourse could not remove the accusation of impotence, because it was not a permissible method of intercourse. However, full penetration was not required: the penetration by the glans or prepuce was sufficient. It was not required, either, that there be semen emission. If vaginal penetration occurred at a time when sex was forbidden (sacred periods, fasting, menses) it nevertheless had the same legal effect as it would had it occurred during periods when it was permitted. What mattered was not the husband's respect for certain prohibitions, but only whether or not he was able to fulfil his marital duties (Al-Šāfiʿī, *Kitāb al-umm* 5.41).

Impotence could surely pose a problem, and so did cases of individuals who had undergone genital mutilation. We must distinguish, in this case, between those who still had a penis from those who did not. For the former category, the judge could again impose a probation period; for the latter, obviously not, since they were totally emasculated (*maǧbūb al-ḍakar*) (Al-Šāfiʿī, *Kitāb al-umm* 5.40).

Also, one must distinguish the impotent husband from the sterile husband.[3] Though a woman can request cancellation of marriage due to impotence, she cannot do so on grounds of infertility.

> A man may have difficulty begetting a child as he is young, while he can father him when he is at an advanced age (*walad al-raǧul yubtā'u lahu šābban wa yūladu lahu šayḫan*). But in the absence of children, there is no reason to choose [for the woman]. The judge gives the wife the opportunity to choose in the case of her husband's inability to have sex, not when there are no children (*al-taḫyīr fī faqd al-ǧimāʿ lā al-walad*). Do not you see that a eunuch is not submitted to a probation period, if he is able to have sexual intercourse, while in most situations, he cannot have children? If it happens that a part of his penis has been cut, the judge will submit him to a probation period as he does for the sexual impotent, because in this case he may have sexual intercourse.
>
> *(Al-Šāfiʿī, Kitāb al-umm 5.40)*

However, it was recognized that the man who was aware of his own sterility had to inform the woman he was about to marry (Al-Šāfiʿī, *Kitāb al-umm* 5.40, on which see Benkheira 2014: 18).

Al-Šāfiʿī also considers the issue of hermaphroditism from the perspective of the male spouse (see also Benkheira 2008):

> If a man marries a hermaphrodite who identifies as a woman and who is confirmed female (because the urine comes out through the female organ) or if he marries a problematic hermaphrodite [in which the sex is not confirmed] who has never married as a male, the marriage is valid and the male spouse has no choice. But if the hermaphrodite who identified as a man marries [a woman], but urine comes through the female organ [i.e. he must be considered female] or if he was married as a woman but urine comes through the male organ, the marriage is canceled (*mafsūḫ*), because one is allowed to marry, as a man or a woman, according to the organ through which one urinates.
>
> *(Al-Šāfiʿī, Kitāb al-umm 5.40)*

It appears that the man who marries a hermaphrodite cannot claim the annulment. However, in the case of the non-problematic hermaphrodite whose gender is determined by the organ with which he or she urinates, that person (i.e. the hermaphrodite) cannot decide to identify as the gender that corresponds to the opposite organ. If such a person enters marriage on that basis (i.e. while identifying as a gender contrary to the urinary organ), the marriage is not legal. In other words: when the gender of the hermaphrodite is defined, he/she cannot decide to choose the opposite gender. So when a hermaphrodite is defined as a female, she cannot decide to become a male; if she does anyway, it is forbidden for her to marry as a male. Only the hermaphrodite in which we cannot determine the sex may choose annulment.

Like all Muslim jurists, al-Šāfi'ī estimated that impotence is not irreversible in every case:

> No man knows in advance that he is impotent as long as he has not experienced sex. Indeed, a man can be sexually powerful, and become powerless and become potent again.
>
> *(Al-Šāfi'ī, Kitāb al-umm 5.40)*

All these remarks on impotence may be based on practical everyday life experience or on medical writings. Indeed, sexual impotence was a major concern of medicine in the Islamic world. Many medical treatises devote an important place to remedies to treat it. Among them, we can cite the treatise of Abu Bakr al-Razi (d. 925) titled *Kitab al- Bah*, especially chapter 10: 'Ointments that improve erection and treatment of the powerless.' The treaty was published in a series on the same subject written by Mu'ayyid al-Dīn Abū al- Naṣr Samwaʾāl al-Magribi (d. 1175), *Nuzhat al- aṣḥāb fī muʾāšarat fī al- Ahbâb*, p. 363.

Eunuchs

Castration in general (let alone emasculation) is prohibited in Islamic law, including in the case of horses. This is why eunuchs had to come from non-Muslim countries. According to several accounts, at the end of the 8th century, one could distinguish only two cases: *ḥaṣiyy* (or *ḥaṣī*) and *maġbūb*. The *ḥaṣiyy* is one who had been mutilated in his testicles, the *maġbūb* is one who had been emasculated. Al-Šaybānī (d. 805) follows this line of thought. According to him, the *ḥaṣiyy* can be prosecuted for adultery, the *maġbūb* cannot (vol. 10.254).

We find the same distinction in the writings of al-Šāfi'ī (*Kitāb al-umm*, 6.111). But he argues that the *ḥaṣiyy* is usually sterile (*wa-l-aġlab annahu lā yūlad lahu*). This is why he says that a woman cannot bring up this incapacity as grounds to divorce her eunuch husband: 'the wife is given the choice in case of marital impotence, not in case of infertility' (Al-Šāfi'ī, *Kitāb al-umm* 6.112).

Al-Šāfi'ī considers another case too: a man whose penis was only partly amputated. Such a person is treated as one who has full sexual power (Al-Šāfi'ī, *Kitāb al-umm* 6.111).

The distinction between *ḥaṣiyy* and *maġbūb* is also characteristic of the thinking of Malik. Thus, at the end of the 8th century and the beginning of the 9th century, one could distinguish only two cases: *ḥaṣiyy*, 'eunuch', and *maġbūb*, '[man] emasculated'.

Whatever the situation, the eunuch could marry. This is, for example, the doctrine of Mālik:

> I asked: Marriage and the repudiation of a eunuch (*ḥaṣiyy*): are they allowed in the doctrine of Mālik? – Mālik claimed that both his marriage and his repudiation were valid (*ǧā'iz*). He added: 'Umar b. al-Ḥaṭṭāb (second Caliph, d. 644) had a eunuch neighbor (*ḥaṣiyy*). 'Umar heard the voice of his wife and her screams [when he struck]. The same 'Umar would, according to Ibn Wahb, have divorced Ibn Sandar, who was a eunuch, from his wife, because he had married her without informing her about his condition.
>
> *(Saḥnūn, al-Mudawwana, 2.198–9)*

Observe that Sahnun cautiously distinguishes the *maǧbūb* from the *ḥaṣiyy*.

> I asked: The marriage of man emasculated (*maǧbūb*): is it also allowed in the doctrine of Mālik? – Mālik replied affirmatively because, he said, he also needs [desires?] women (*li-annahu yaḥtāǧ min amr al-nisā›*). According to 'Aṭā› b. Abi Rabah (d. 732), if a woman marries an emasculated man knowing that he cannot have sex (*annahu lā ya'tī al-nisā'*), she cannot complain about him.
>
> *(Saḥnūn, al-Mudawwana, 2.199)*

Here too the answer is interesting. The man who has been emasculated does not possess a male member, but nevertheless could retain his libido and desire for women. However, one must be aware of the legal difficulty: the purpose of marriage is both sexual satisfaction and procreation. But if a man is emasculated, he cannot procreate. Moreover, in satisfying his partner he has to use non-standard methods. This is why a eunuch was not to hide his condition from the woman he wanted to marry. Only when she received full disclosure and still agreed was the marriage valid. This is the meaning of the remark ascribed to the Meccan 'Aṭā› (d. 732).

> I asked: What do you think if she marries a man emasculated (*maǧbūb*) or a eunuch (*ḥaṣiyy*), ignorant of his condition, and if she finds out later, has she a choice? – Mālik argued that if a woman marries a man while unaware that he is a eunuch and if she finds out later, she has a choice. She may, if she wishes, decide to stay with him or to leave. The case of the emasculated is more serious. – If she marries a eunuch or an emasculated man and is ignorant of his condition and if, discovering the fact, she elects the dissolution of marriage, is she required to observe a period of abstinence (*'idda*)? – If he had sex with her (*yaṭa›*), yes, otherwise she is not required to. – And if she chooses the triple repudiation? – This is not one of her prerogatives. She can choose separation, which shall be final (*bā'ina*) ... – If she marries a man who has been emasculated (*maǧbūb al-ḏakar*) but still possesses testicles (*qā'im al-ḥuṣy*), and if she chooses separation after they have been intimate (*daḥala bihā*), is she required to observe the period of abstinence (*'idda*)? – If the person in this state is able to procreate (*in kāna miṯluhu yūladu lahu*), then she must observe the period of continence. Ibn al-Qāsim said: If such a man may be the author of a pregnancy, the child will be linked to him, otherwise one cannot ascribe to him the newborn.[4]
>
> *(Saḥnūn, al-Mudawwana 2.213)*

The doctrine of Mālik is repeated: if a woman marries a eunuch or an emasculated man, she cannot go to court if she knew about his disability. If she did not know, she can ask for divorce. After recalling this doctrine, Ibn al-Qasim added:

> I have not heard from Mālik about the woman who marries an impotent man knowingly, but this is my opinion (*haḏā ra›yī*): if a woman knows that the man she married is impotent, definitely unable to have sex (*lā yaqdir 'alā al-ǧimā' ra'san*) and if he has informed her, she has no choice if she marries him knowing this.
>
> *(Saḥnūn, al-Mudawwana 2.213)*

Mālik distinguished the case of the eunuchs from that of impotent men. He states that if a woman discovers that her husband is a eunuch and accepts his condition, she loses the right of appeal to the judge to dissolve her marriage if she wishes to do so later on.

What is your opinion (*ara'ayt*) about the wife of the impotent (*'innīn*), the eunuch or emasculated man who after discovering the disability of her spouse, does not submit the dispute to the judge (*sulṭān*) and allows her husband to enjoy his body (*amkanathu min nafsihā*), but after that she decided to bring the case to court (*rafa'athu ilā al-sulṭān*), what about her? – As for the woman of the eunuch or the emasculated man, she has no choice if she lived with her husband and has accepted his disability, according to Malik. ... As for the separation, it will be a repudiation (*taṭlīqa*).

(Saḥnūn, al-Mudawwana, 2.214)

So the consent of the wife must be taken into account in the case of such unions, even if such consent is only implicit. Having known and accepted the state of her husband, she must stay with him.

Flawed women

Men also had the power to end the marriage on grounds of defects and flaws in their partners. This allowed them to return their wives to their families, without paying the nuptial gift. Here's what Mālik states about this:

– Consider a man who married and realizes that his wife has a defect. What are the defects that give him the opportunity to return her (*yarudduhā*) according to Mālik? – According to him, he can give her back if she's suffering from madness (*ǧunūn*), leprosy (*ǧuḏām*), elephantiasis (*baraṣ*) or malformation of the vagina (*al-'ayb al-laḏī fī-l-farǧ*). – If he marries a woman but he has never seen her, and if he discovers after that she is blind (*'amyā'*), one-eyed (*'awrā'*), with a member amputated (*qaṭ'ā'*), one-armed (*šallā'*) or she is sick or she has given birth to a child as a result of illegitimate relations (*min al-zinā*)? – Mālik argued that no one cannot return a woman back to her parents except for defects that I have listed.

(Saḥnūn, al-Mudawwana 2.211)

Thus, according to Mālik, the only defects that allowed the cancellation of the marriage to the husband's benefit are four: insanity, leprosy, elephantiasis and malformation in the genitals. Al-Šāfi'ī (d. 820) defended the same point of view as Mālik: if a man marries a woman believing she is beautiful, young, wealthy, physically well and a virgin, and he realizes after having seen her that she is old, ugly, poor, amputated, deflowered, blind or suffering from any evil, he has no choice (*lā ḫiyār lahu*). Al-Šāfi'ī adds: 'Marriage is not like selling. There is no choice [possible for the husband] [who observes] a physical defect in his wife' (Al-Šāfi'ī, *Kitāb al-umm* 6.215 (§ 8 *Fī-l-'ayb bi-l-mankūḥa*)). This passage indicates that families did not hesitate to deceive contenders by marrying them to women, some of whom could be unsightly or morally questionable. The law did not prohibit such conduct. The text sharply contrasts with the remark by St Jerome on parents sending their unmarriageable daughter to monasteries (cf. Kuuliala in this volume), an option which for Islamic families obviously did not exist. At the same time, we learn that the absence of hymen cannot be a ground for annulment of marriage – this is remarkable, to say the least, for a society which attached so much importance to the virginity of women.

Surely, a man could arbitrarily divorce his wife. But if he did so, he had to pay the full nuptial gift. However, when he returned her to her family because of one of the four recognized defects mentioned above, he was not required to pay the nuptial gift. So one must remember that a man could not, according to Mālik, return the woman he had just married and keep the nuptial gift for himself even if she were blind, one-eyed, one-armed, ill or because she had given birth to a child resulting from an illegitimate union.

On another occasion, the discussion returns to the malformation in the genitals:

> – If the woman has a defect in the genitals that comes from a malformation, or that is a result of a fire, or which is not serious, and all this does not hinder sexual intercourse (*ǧimā*), do these defects permit marriage annulment according to Mālik? Or is such the case if she has defects that render sexual intercourse impossible? – Mālik quoted 'Umar: I said that a man can give a woman back because of insanity, leprosy and elephantiasis. He added: As for me, I think that vaginal illness has the same effects. As for defects that scientists define as vaginal illness, a man can give the woman back for that reason, even if such a failure does not prevent sexual intercourse. Do you not see that a man can have sexual intercourse with the woman who suffers from insanity, and with a wife who is affected by leprosy, or elephantiasis? But in such cases, a man can give her back. So it is the same for the malformation of the genitals.
>
> *(Saḥnūn, al-Mudawwana 2.211–12)*

Thus, according to Mālik, malformation of the genitals is not taken into account simply because it would prevent normal sexual intercourse; that is to say, if malformation were to make sexual intercourse impossible, this alone did not constitute a motive for legal separation. On this point, the doctrine of al-Šāfi'ī took the opposite view (*Kitāb al-umm 6.215–16*).

The following discussion is logically linked with what has been said above. If a man was not allowed to return a woman who had serious defects to her family, could he nevertheless impose conditions at the moment the wedding contract was made?

> – Consider a man who marries a woman but states the requirement that she has to be physically healthy (*ṣaḥīḥa*); he realized afterwards that she is blind, one-armed or sick. Can he give her back because of one of these reasons? – Yes, he stipulated such a condition to the one who has married him. He is also not required to provide the nuptial gift if there was no consummation. If there was consummation, she is entitled to the gift of equivalence (*mahr miṯlihā*), due to sexual intercourse (*bi-l-masīs*). In the latter case, he may accuse him who has married her off, if he had insisted she was neither blind nor amputated or in a similar state and he has married in accepting such a condition ... He added: Mālik argued about the one who married a Negress (*sawdā*), a one-eyed or a blind woman, he could not return her. Because you cannot give a woman back, except because of four specific flaws – insanity, leprosy, elephantiasis, and vaginal malformation. The husband should check in advance on his behalf. If he put faith in a man who turns out to be a liar, the latter [i.e. the guardian who is the liar] is not bound to anything unless he had given him warning that the woman was not consistent with the description that he had made to him (*in kānat al-ǧāriya 'alā ḫilāf mā ankaḥahu 'alayhi*).
>
> *(Saḥnūn, al-Mudawwana 2.212)*

Thus, we have to distinguish two situations: one in which the man stipulated nothing and another in which he made stipulations concerning the physical and mental state of his future wife. Only in the latter situation can he take action against the one who gave him the woman for marriage. The provider may even deliberately lie about the future bride in an attempt to protect her. This is of no consequence to him, since he was not formally instructed on the physical and mental state of the bride. It was in fact the bridegroom's task to take care of this legal aspect.

Conclusions

In Islamic law, marriage is a contract, just like any business transaction. To be valid, there should not be any contractual flaw, such as a lack of willingness to fulfil the contract, or fraud or failure by either party to fulfil the contractual obligations. One of the most significant contractual obligations is sexual intercourse. If one spouse is unable to take on his/her share of this obligation, he/she violates the contract to which he/she has subscribed. This is why the proposed solution, initially, is automatic divorce, later replaced by chosen separation.

Sexual impotence or, equivalently, emasculation are grounds to void a union, if the woman wants. The reason is the double purpose of marriage: to satisfy the sexual appetite of both spouses and to produce offspring. From the 9th century, however, Muslim scholars begin to admit that one can do without children and can even observe complete sexual abstinence (Benkheira 2013, 2016).

Other legal grounds for breaking the marriage bond are leprosy, elephantiasis or madness. These states were defined early on, since their formulation is attributed to the second Caliph, but it may be an apocryphal tradition. Leprosy and elephantiasis are particularly loathsome diseases, and frightening. Those affected in Antiquity and the Middle Ages were banned from society (Dols 1983). Madness was not considered to be good for a married couple, which is why a marriage could be broken in this case (Dols 1992 and cf. Toohey in this volume; note that there is no study about madness in Islamic legal literature). In all cases, these flaws are grounds for breaking the marriage bond if the flawed spouse concealed his/her state when the marriage was contracted.

Sexual impotence is probably considered the worst defect for a man. This is why, if a man is impotent, he will never discuss the topic, nor will others ever mention it, unless it is legal information in the case of separation or divorce. Infertility for women is similar, although female infertility is probably less serious than male impotence. But if impotence is a sign of weakness, sterility is a sign of danger: a woman who is not fertile, for example, might be viewed as a witch. But the Muslim jurists do not discuss infertility because it cannot be established in advance. It can only be deduced after many months, if not years, of engaging in sexual intercourse (see Edwards 1998 for the Greek dossier).

Acknowledgements

I wish to thank Christian Laes and Lynn Rose for the careful revision of my English text.

Notes

1 This is the choice of al-Awzāʿī (d. 768), a Syrian jurist: see Benkheira 2014: 39.
2 This is the choice of a al-Layt b. Saʿd (d. 791), an Egyptian jurist: see Benkheira 2014: 39.
3 Before marrying, a man cannot know his sterility. But the question here is restricted: may a woman claim an annulment for sterility? The answer is: she cannot.
4 If a man has testicles, he can be fertile: the semen can be introduced into the vagina by other means than the male organ.

Bibliography

Primary sources

Al-Šāfiʿī, *Kitāb al-umm*, ed. Al-Naǧǧār, 5 vols (Beirut : Dār al-maʿrifa, n.d.).
Al-Šaybānī, *Kitāb al-aṣl*, ed. Būyinūkālin, 12 vols (Beirut: Dār Ibn Ḥazm, 2012).

Saḥnūn, *al-Mudawwana*, 8 vols (Beirut: Dār Ṣādir, n.d. [offset reprint of the 1st edn, Cairo, 1905]).
Mu'ayyid al-Dīn Abū al-Naṣr Samwaʾāl al-Magribi, *Nuzhat al- aṣḥāb fī mu'āšarat fī al- Ahbâb*, ed. Farīd Aḥmad al-Mazidi (Cairo, Dār al-Afaq al-'arabiyya, 2007).

Secondary sources

Benkheira, Mohammed Hocine, 'Homme ou femme? Les juristes musulmans face à l'hermaphrodisme', in A. Caiozzo and A.-E.Demartini (eds), *Monstre et imaginaire social: Approches historiques* (Paris, 2008), 163–85.
Benkheira, Mohammed Hocine, 'Jouir sans enfanter? Concubines, filiation et coït interrompu au début de l'islam', *Der Islam* 90/2 (2013), 238–98.
Benkheira, Mohammed Hocine, 'L'impuissance sexuelle, motif légal de rupture du lien matrimonial: Genèse d'une doctrine', *Islamic Law and Society* 21/1 (2014), 1–48.
Benkheira, Mohammed Hocine, *La maîtrise de la concupiscence: Mariage, célibat et continence sexuelle en islam des origines au 16ᵉ siècle* (Paris, 2016).
Calder, Norman, *Studies in Early Islamic Jurisprudence* (Oxford, 1993).
Cooper, Kate, *The Fall of the Roman Household* (Cambridge, 2007).
Dols, Michael W. 'The Leper in Medieval Islamic Society', *Speculum* 54 (1983), 891–916.
Dols, Michael W., Majnūn: *The Madman in Medieval Islamic Society* (Oxford, 1992).
Ghaly, Mohammed, *Islam and Disability: Perspectives in Theology and Jurisprudence* (London and New York, 2010).
Edwards, Martha L., 'Women and Physical Disability in Ancient Greece', *The Ancient World* 29/1 (1998), 1–9.
Rispler-Chaim, Vardit, *Disability in Islamic Law* (Dordrecht, 2007).
Scalenghe, Sara, *Disability in the Ottoman Arab World, 1500–1800* (Cambridge, 2014).
Treggiari, Susan, *Roman Marriage. "Iusti coniuges" from the Time of Cicero to the Time of Ulpian* (Oxford, 1991).

30

DISABILITY IN RABBINIC JUDAISM

Julia Watts Belser and Lennart Lehmhaus

Dedicated to the memory of Judith Abrams, z'l

This chapter examines disability in the sources and traditions of rabbinic Judaism, a period that begins after the Roman destruction of the Second Temple in Jerusalem in 70 CE and extends to encompass the redaction of the Babylonian Talmud in the 6th or 7th century. During the rabbinic period, a small cadre of scholars and sages developed the foundational and formative sources of rabbinic Judaism, developing texts and traditions that remain central to most contemporary forms of Jewish practice. In its textual approach, rabbinic literature reveals both conservative and innovative impulses. Rabbinic texts are often framed as exegesis and interpretation of the Hebrew Bible, and rabbinic literature operates in large part through the citation and interpretation of the oral traditions of earlier generations. Though rabbinic texts constantly situate themselves in relation to earlier sources of authority, rabbinic interpretation is often profoundly innovative – articulating novel approaches to law and ritual that adapt tradition to new circumstances, as well as expressing through narrative and story a range of complex and often contradictory approaches to religious thought and ethics.

Disability is a well-represented presence within the rabbinic corpus. Rabbinic texts often engage disability as a legal subject, focusing especially on the degree to which physical, sensory and mental impairments represent grounds for excluding an individual from the performance of religious rituals and commandments. Disability also appears in rabbinic narrative: in traditions that speculate about the etiology of different disabilities, in texts that use disability as a religious symbol or metaphor, and in stories that feature characters with disabilities. In the first portion of this chapter, Julia Watts Belser assesses disability in rabbinic literature from a social and cultural perspective. Drawing on contemporary theoretical work in disability studies, Belser examines how rabbinic sources construct disability as a social category, while tracing the cultural and religious consequences of disability in rabbinic society. In the second half of the chapter, Lennart Lehmhaus examines medical approaches to disability in rabbinic sources, tracing the social and discursive ways the rabbis use medical knowledge to identify and understand various impairments, as well as how these medical perspectives shape rabbinic responses to distinct forms of disability in Late Antiquity.

Disability in rabbinic culture

Identifying disability in rabbinic sources

Julia Watts Belser

Disability studies theorists have challenged the 'naturalness' of disability as a category, emphasizing that notions of disablement and bodily difference are neither straightforward nor stable over time (Davis 1995; Garland-Thomson 1997). Rather than treating disability as a fixed category, a historically sensitive assessment of disability within Jewish Late Antiquity must probe the ways that ancient Jewish sources conceptualize and stigmatize mental, physical and sensory difference (Schipper 2006). Neither biblical nor rabbinic texts possess a single term that aligns precisely with the modern concept of disability. Perhaps the closest term is *mum* (blemish), which biblical and rabbinic authors use to categorize a variety of physical and sensory impairments. Used primarily to enumerate the physical characteristics that render an animal unfit for sacrifice (Lev. 22: 17–25) or that make a priest ineligible to offer sacrifices at the altar (Lev. 21: 16–24), the biblical *mum* reveals key differences between ancient and modern notions of disability. According to the Hebrew Bible, a priest with a once-broken arm possesses a permanent *mum*, a condition few moderns would regard as an enduring disability. Deafness, while significantly stigmatized in other biblical contexts, does not register as a *mum*. Neither does intellectual disability or mental illness (Abrams 1998; Olyan 2008; Raphael 2008). Rabbinic texts continue to use the term *mum* to refer to physical and sensory impairments, though they significantly expand the range of what constitutes a blemish (Rosen-Zvi 2005–6; Belser 2015a).

While the term *mum* signals particular physical characteristics of non-normative bodies, biblical and rabbinic sources also use certain disabilities as identity categories, most notably singling out individuals who are blind (*'ivver*), lame (*piseah*), deaf-mute (*heresh*) and mentally disabled (*shoteh*). Rabbinic sources describe the *heresh* as a person who can neither hear nor speak, a condition that was tantamount in the rabbinic mind to being entirely unable to communicate. The category *shoteh* indicates a wide range of mental disabilities; it can signal disabilities that affect a person's intellectual cognition, as well as mental illness or other psychiatric disabilities. Rabbinic sources most frequently use the classification *shoteh* to describe a person who displays disordered and destructive behaviour, perhaps approximating the modern diagnostic category of psychosis (Strous 2004). Rabbinic legal texts frequently appeal to the triad of 'the deaf-mute (*heresh*), the mentally disabled (*shoteh*), and the young person (*qatan*)' to identify individuals who are exempt from the performance of certain *mitzvot* (religious obligations); Roman law similarly excludes those who are deaf-mute, mentally disturbed or minors from serving as judges, while also limiting their legal autonomy (Laes 2011: 466–7). This legal framework suggests an implicit category of 'disabled persons', a set of stigmatized identities constructed through real or perceived impairments – and classified, along with children, as individuals who are considered unable to exercise reason or understanding. Within the highly intellectual and oral cultures of rabbinic Judaism, deafness and mental disability are highly stigmatized disabilities. The *heresh* and the *shoteh* remain profoundly marginalized in rabbinic circles; their disabilities largely prevent them from participating in the highly privileged institution of Torah study and the oral transmission of rabbinic traditions. Judith Abrams (1998) has argued that, within rabbinic culture, disabilities of hearing, speech and cognition represent a 'master-status' that limited a deaf or mentally disabled person's (perceived) ability to exercise agency in virtually all legal situations.

In contrast to deafness and intellectual disability, blindness and physical disability become relevant in rabbinic legal thought only in limited instances when an individual impairment limits a person's ability to perform a specific religious obligation. Rabbinic law disqualifies a blind person from serving as a witness, for example, for the law assumes sight to be an essential qualification for perception and legal testimony. Yet in most cases, rabbinic sources treat blindness as no obstacle to the performance of other *mitzvot* (Steinberg 2002; Nevins 2003). The Mishnah permits a Jewish man who is blind to lead the congregation in prayer, for example, allowing him to recite the Sh'ma, a central declaration that calls the congregation to affirm God's unity (mMegillah 4:6).[1] Rabbinic literature likewise testifies to the fact that blind people held positions of authority and prestige within rabbinic communities, including the blind Babylonian rabbis Rav Sheshet and Rav Yosef. Rabbinic texts frequently present blind rabbis as exemplary scholars, whose loss of physical sight often affords them deeper religious insight (Neis 2013: 72–82; Belser 2011). Rabbinic sources suggest that people with vision disabilities participated in many aspects of Jewish ritual – and could participate fully in the intellectual life of the rabbinic study house.

Disability and the discourse of ritual exemption: power, authority and difference in rabbinic culture

Disability most commonly surfaces in rabbinic legal thought when it affects (or is perceived to affect) an individual's capacity to perform *mitzvot*. Consider an example drawn from the Mishnah, one of the earliest rabbinic texts of law and ritual practice, redacted in Palestine in 200 CE. Introducing the religious obligation to appear at the Jerusalem Temple for the three annual pilgrimage festivals, Mishnah Ḥagigah 1:1 begins:

> All are obligated regarding the appearance offering, except for the deaf-mute (*ḥeresh*), the mentally disabled (*shoteh*), the young (*qatan*), the gender-indeterminate *(tumtum)*, the double-sexed (*androgynous*), women, slaves who have not been set free, the lame, the blind, the sick, the old, and anyone who is not able to ascend upon his feet.
>
> Who is young? One who is not able to ride upon the shoulders of his father to ascend to Jerusalem to the Temple Mount – these are the words of the House of Shammai. The House of Hillel says: One who is not able to grasp his father's hand and ascend to Jerusalem to the Temple Mount, as it says: *Three walking-pilgrimages (shalosh regalim)*
>
> *(Exodus 23: 17)*

The Mishnah's discussion of who is obligated to make pilgrimage and perform the sacrifices serves as a striking example of the role disability plays in rabbinic legal reasoning (Belser 2011). The first portion of the text identifies the people who are exempt from the pilgrimage offering, beginning with the familiar triad of *ḥeresh, shotesh*, and *qatan* – but also expands the notion of disablement to encompass a wide range of other individuals who are distinguished by particular markers of social or physical difference. By the conclusion of the list, the category 'all' has shrunk considerably: free, healthy men of stable gender status, who can hear, speak, reason, walk and see, and who are neither too young nor too old.

The Mishnah's approach underscores the physicality of the commandment to make pilgrimage to Jerusalem, releasing from obligation 'anyone who is not able to ascend upon his feet'. Appealing to the biblical language used for the three pilgrimage festivals, the Mishnah stresses that the journey is meant to be a 'walking pilgrimage', a commandment performed by means of the legs and feet. A man who cannot walk is released from the obligation to make pilgrimage, for his disability presents an obstacle in the fulfilment of this commandment (Abrams 1998). Later rabbinic discussion of this passage makes the logic of exemption explicit: a lame man is exempt because he cannot walk, a sick man because he cannot rejoice and an old man because he cannot come by foot (yḤagigah 1:1, 76a). The language of exemption is often understood as a form of rabbinic 'accommodation' to the impairments of the population in question. But such a framework misses an important dimension of exemption. Disability-based exemptions from *mitzvot* are not simply straightforward responses to bio-physical impairment. Some of the individuals in the Mishnah's list are indeed exempt from pilgrimage because of difficulty walking, whether due to disability, youth or advanced age. Yet the ability to walk is not required in all cases. The House of Shammai maintains that a young child – old enough to be carried on his father's back but presumably not yet able to walk the distance on his own feet – is still be obligated to make pilgrimage. Other figures have no mobility impairments, but are nonetheless exempt from obligation. Women and people of indeterminate gender status are both exempt, as are enslaved men. Rabbinic texts commonly exempt women, slaves and children from the performance of certain *mitzvot*, a practice which Judith Hauptman (1988) argues reflects a rabbinic claim that observance is linked with social status, that individuals who are socially subordinate to others cannot fully and freely accept religious obligations because of their social obligations to a husband, master or patriarch.[2] Examined from a disability studies perspective, such claims suggest that rabbinic texts conceptualize certain forms of disability as a critical sign of dependency, a marker of social difference that renders a person unable to fully embody rabbinic masculinity.

Exemption from *mitzvot* has significant social and religious implications in rabbinic culture. As rabbinic legal thought developed, exemption became translated into exclusion. To track the implications of this shift, consider the following text, attributed to the blind Babylonian rabbi, Rav Yosef:

> Rav Yosef said: At first, I would have said – someone who taught the law according to Rabbi Yehudah, who said, 'the blind are exempt from the *mitzvot*,' I would make a feast for the rabbis. What is the reason? Because I am not commanded, and yet I perform the *mitzvot*. But now I have heard that which Rabbi Hanina said, 'Greater is the one who is commanded and who does it, than one who is not commanded and who does it.' The one who says to me that the law is not like Rabbi Yehudah, I will make a feast for the rabbis. What is the reason? If I am commanded, then I will have a greater reward.
>
> *(Babylonian Talmud, Baba Kamma 87a)*

Rav Yosef's account reveals a critical shift in the nature of rabbinic thought regarding obligation and exemption. Rav Yosef had originally assumed that exemption would prove advantageous, for it would allow him to express his devotion through voluntary performance of the *mitzvot* – an act he considers even more meritorious than obligatory actions. Yet such a position proves to be untenable. Rav Yosef learns instead that certain rabbis maintain that it is superior to perform *mitzvot* in response to an explicit obligation. According to this framework, the fact of being commanded conveys higher religious status and brings greater merit. Rabbinic Judaism eventually came to link exemption with exclusion, arguing that only a person who was commanded to perform a ritual act could fulfil that duty on behalf of the community (Alexander 2013). The rabbis frequently prohibited an exempt person from undertaking even a *voluntary* performance of a particular action. While exemption may have originated as a benevolent impulse, its development in rabbinic legal thought is deeply intertwined with social power and authority, as elites structure and circumscribe the religious practice available to those they have exempted.

As Mishnah Ḥagigah 1:1 makes plain, the identification of disability in rabbinic thought straddles the line between identities that impair a person's social status and those that impair a person's physical or sensory capacity. While the logic of exemption may seem sensible or compassionate in the case of disability, the culture-bound specificity of exemptions is more evident in the case of exemptions made on the basis of gender. In both cases, the presumed 'facts' of physical or social difference are scripted upon people's bodies. In many respects, then, we might argue that rabbinic texts treat women and enslaved persons as people with (social) disabilities. Though such comparisons can help illuminate the way that rabbinic social and cultural dynamics treat women, slaves and people with disabilities as 'dependent' bodies, I ultimately argue against treating women and slaves as *de facto* disabled. Collapsing the notion of 'social' disability with 'organic' disabilities based on sensory, mental or biophysical impairment risks obscuring the material reality of disability in rabbinic sources. The claim that women and slaves are always already disabled can veil the ways that disability intersects with gender, class and enslavement in rabbinic thought. Disability studies offers a vantage point for considering the way that impairment affects marginalized peoples differently, considering, for example, the experiences of enslaved persons who sustain physical injury or examining how the perception of a bodily blemish affects a woman in rabbinic marriage law (Belser 2015a, b).

Disability and deafness in rabbinic sources: recognizing the multivocality of law

While rabbinic sources articulate broad legal principles that assess the status of people with various disabilities, such overarching principles rarely offer a full and conclusive account of the available textual evidence – nor do they fully encompass the complexity of rabbinic thought about disability, impairment and bodily difference. Though rabbinic texts occasionally present settled legal rulings, the discourse of most rabbinic literature is profoundly multivocal, emphasizing dispute and argumentation about the law. One of the most influential rabbinic sources is the Babylonian Talmud (Bavli), an expansive and wide-ranging rabbinic commentary on the Mishnah redacted in Sassanian Persia in the 6th or 7th centuries CE. The Babylonian Talmud constructs rabbinic legal thought through the dialectical adjudication of many different legal opinions and explicitly values the preservation of minority opinions. Rabbinic legal thought is largely casuistic in nature; argumentation from specific cases plays an important role in rabbinic literature. Rabbinic sources reveal important differences between these broad principles and individual cases, suggesting that rabbinic responses to disability were not, in fact, a matter of settled law. Instead, these texts suggest that bodily difference and disability were ongoing subjects of cultural and legal reflection.

Consider rabbinic traditions about deafness. As we have seen, rabbinic law profoundly stigmatizes the deaf-mute (*heresh*) and categorically excludes a person who cannot speak or hear from the performance of *mitzvot*. Rabbinic texts generally distinguish between a 'true *heresh*,' who can neither hear nor speak, and a person who cannot hear but who can speak or otherwise communicate (bHagigah 2b). Yet certain rabbinic sources contest the claim that an inability to speak is tantamount to an inability to learn. Challenging the exclusion of those who cannot speak, the Babylonian Talmud reports that the mute sons of Rabbi Yoḥanan ben Gudgada took part in rabbinic education, sitting and learning at the feet of the great authority Rabbi Judah the Patriarch; they were eventually revealed to have expert knowledge of Jewish scripture and law (bHagigah 3a). Despite their tendency to privilege orality, rabbinic sources do recognize that communication need not rely on speech (Gracer 2003; Barmash 2011). The Mishnah rules that a *heresh* can transact business via sign language or by lip-reading (mGittin 5:7, mTerumot 1:2, mYevamot 14:1). Rabbinic law affirms that a person who is deaf may contract a marriage or divorce by means of gesture, though Pamela Barmash argues that, in such cases, the deaf individual remains dependent on a hearing person to affirm his language and intent. In the case of the *ḥeresh*, classical rabbinic thought simultaneously constructs a category of profound ritual exclusion and works to limit its effects. While rabbinic law denies legal standing to a person who can neither speak nor hear, it affirms (with certain limitations) the ritual and legal competence of deaf individuals who can communicate by voice or gesture. In the modern era, great advances in deaf education have spurred a profound reappraisal of deafness in Jewish law. Most contemporary rabbinic authorities now recognize the cognitive and communicative capacity of deaf people and regard them as fully bound by the *mitzvot*, except for specific *mitzvot* that require hearing (Taub 2012).

Rabbinic sources themselves also show change over time, as shifting circumstances and social attitudes led rabbis to re-evaluate and reinterpret earlier traditions. Rabbinic interpretation of the priestly prohibitions in Leviticus 21, which forbid priests with blemishes from serving at the altar, illuminates the way rabbinic approaches to biblical texts simultaneously conserve and transform earlier legal traditions. The legal context of the Leviticus 21 prohibitions is itself strikingly different in the rabbinic era. Since the Roman destruction of the Jerusalem Temple in 70 CE, a date that is often used as a symbolic marker of the rise of the rabbis in Jewish historiography, Jewish religious practice no longer centres around the authority of the priest or the rituals of temple sacrifice. After the destruction of the Second Temple, priestly duties shift to the emerging site of the synagogue, where priests are charged with offering the priestly blessing to the community. In language resonant of the levitical prohibitions, Mishnah Megillah 4:7 asserts that the presence of certain blemishes (*mumim*) disqualifies a priest from 'lifting up his hands' to give this blessing:

> A priest whose hands are blemished may not lift up his hands. Rabbi Yehudah says: Also one whose hands are stained by woad or madder may not lift up his hands because the people might gaze at him.

The logic of the Mishnah's prohibition reflects the centrality of the hands in the priestly blessing practice. To convey the blessing, the priest spreads his fingers in a particular gesture and lifts up his hands. Despite the significance of the hands themselves, the ritual gesture is meant to remain unseen. Those who receive the blessing are forbidden from looking at the priests while they bless, while the priests customarily draw their prayer shawls over their heads and hands, veiling themselves at this intimate moment. As I have discussed elsewhere (Belser 2011), the Mishnah's discourse suggests that the blemish becomes a cultural problem not because of an organic, functional defect in the hands themselves – but because bodily difference causes the people to stare. The problem lies not in the hands, but in the act of looking. The congregation's misplaced gaze threatens to undermine the appropriate ritual conveyance of the blessing (cf. Metzler in this volume on the canonical dossier).

While the Mishnah uses this risk to prohibit the blemished priest from giving the blessing, the Babylonian Talmud takes a different approach. After affirming a ruling that prevents a priest from performing the blessing if he has a blemish on his hands, face or feet, the text acknowledges a series of situations that contradict the principle:

> Rav Ḥuna said: A man with bleary eyes shall not lift up his hands. But there was a man like this in Rav Ḥuna's neighborhood – and he spread his hands! He was familiar in his town. Likewise it was taught: A man with bleary eyes shall not lift up his hands, but if he is familiar in his town it is permitted.
>
> Rabbi Yoḥanan said: A man who is blind in one eye may not lift up his hands. But there was a man like this in Rabbi Yoḥanan's neighborhood – and he spread his hands! He was familiar in his town.

Likewise it was taught: A man who is blind in one eye may not lift up his hands, but if he is familiar in his town it is permitted. Rabbi Yehudah said: He whose hands have stains shall not lift up his hands. It was taught: If most of the people of the town work in that way, it is permitted.

(bMegillah 24b)

In each of these cases, the Babylonian Talmud asserts that a priest who is well-known in a particular town is not subject to the prohibition. If a priest's condition is commonplace or already familiar to the community, the Bavli maintains that his hands will not startle the congregation or cause them to stare. By highlighting the problem of the stare, the Bavli's discourse echoes a critical claim made by disability studies scholarship: that being 'disabled' is not simply a straightforward fact of bodily difference, but also a product of the way bodies are seen and treated by others. Disability is produced not only by organic bodily difference, but also by social attitudes: by the act of staring that reinforces social otherness, by cultural disdain that generates stigma. Significantly, the Bavli asserts that familiarity can defuse the dynamics of stigma – and it rules therefore that, when a disabled priest is familiar in his place, he is allowed to bless (Belser 2011). This principle of familiarity (*dash beiro*) remains an important legal concept in later Jewish rulings about the status of people with disabilities. The Shulkhan Arukh, a 16th-century code of law that remains highly influential to this day, follows the talmudic principle of familiarity in its rulings on priestly blessings. According to the Shulkhan Arukh, it takes only thirty days in a place to become familiar, as long the person intends to stay for a while (Marx 2002).

Medical approaches to disability in rabbinic traditions

'Healing the blemish': disability and medicine in rabbinic sources

Lennart Lehmhaus

Though disability frequently appears in rabbinic sources that address ritual and legal practice, medical discourse represents another important site for examining disability in rabbinic texts. Julius Preuss's foundational work on biblical and talmudic medicine (Preuss 1909; translation in Preuss and Rosner 1978) is marked by a positivistic 19th-century medical approach to disability. He collects bits and pieces of relevant information in various chapters (on 'injuries and malformations', 'ophthalmology', 'otorhinolaryngology', 'neurological dysfunctions' and 'madness') without much attention to layers of tradition, literary history and discursive or cultural context. Preuss's approach was shared by most of his contemporaries in classics or history of medicine, who showed little or no interest in physical impairments, speech and hearing impediments, or intellectual disabilities. This absence of attention is a phenomenon endemic to the sources. Greek and Latin authors, especially medical writers, paid little attention to impairments/disabilities. Except for miraculous or divine curing (Vlahogiannis 2005), disability was not considered to be the 'business' of doctors, who focused instead on healing healthy persons with temporary illnesses (cf. Garland 2010: 123–125; Laes *et al.* 2013b). By contrast, rabbinic texts refer quite frequently to various forms of disability, both in their socio-religious discourses (cf. Abrams 1998; Marx 2002) and as a medical subject.

In his comparative study on Greece, ancient Israel and Mesopotamia, Hector Avalos identifies three basic aspects of ancient medical discourses about 'health care-systems': etiology of illness, consultative options available and attitudes towards the patient in society

(Avalos 2013: 238). Drawing upon Avalos' three pillars, I will discuss three aspects of rabbinic medical discourse that reveal rabbinic notions of impairment and disability:

1 explanations regarding the origin of disabilities;
2 medical and technical aids, remedies or cures for disabled persons;
3 attitudes toward disabled people expressed in rabbinic society or culture.

These categories help us grasp the rabbis' own medical understandings of disability, which undergird their discussions of disability in legal, ethical or theological contexts. Further, I will argue that physiological, anatomical and psychological medical knowledge shapes rabbinic perceptions and definitions of disabilities. A comparative cultural analysis reveals both similarities and striking differences with corresponding medical concepts in the rabbis' cultural surroundings.

Bodily perfection and etiologies of disabilities

Rabbinic sources frequently voice the idea, also prevalent in non-rabbinic Jewish traditions (e.g. Targum Pseudo-Jonathan to Gen. 1: 27), that there is a close correspondence between the perfect micro-cosmic human body and the divine or macro-cosmic creation (Cf. mOholot 1:8; bMakkot 23b). Such traditions echo a common motif in the ancient Mediterranean world. In Greek myths, descriptions of deities without any blemish establish a threshold of bodily perfection for religious offices (priests/vestals) and for sacrificial animals (Garland 2010: 63–5). Similar concerns animate rabbinic texts that require physical perfection, or even beauty, of the priests performing sacrifices (mBekhorot 7) and animals to be sacrificed in the Jerusalem Temple (mBekhorot 6; mHulin/bHulin). These discussions about ritualistic fitness, while not being medical discourses, utilize detailed anatomic and physiological knowledge in their definition of 'common/fit' and 'deviating/unfit' bodies (cf. Abrams 1998: 16–70; Belser 2011; Fishbane 2007: 103–6).

Rabbinic sources do not engage in systematic discussion about the causes of certain disabilities, but they do interject etiological opinions about disability into discussions of sexual behaviour, marriage or moral and healthy ways of living. Certain rabbinic traditions about conception parallel Greek 'two-seed' theory (Kessler 2009; Kiperwasser 2009). The rabbinic teaching that there are 'three partners in a person's creation/conception' asserts that the contributions of male seed (white: bones, sinews, nails, brain) and female seed (red: blood, flesh, skin, hair) are complemented by the vital parts coming from the divine (breath, soul, intellect, understanding and an 'able' body).[3] Such recognition that the parents contributed vital elements to the formation of their children leads the Talmud to argue that children born to a couple of very large or small stature most likely will be even taller or dwarf sized (bBekh 45b; for dwarfs in other ancient texts, see Dasen 2013). However, elsewhere the Talmud asserts that children of disabled persons will not necessarily be disabled (for Greek medicine, see Garland 2010: 146–8), since physical abilities and mental faculties ultimately come from God.

Rabbinic sources also articulate concepts prevailing in ancient teratologies (Hippocrates, Plato, Aristotle, Empedocles, Soranos), theories that seek to explain how external circumstances or sensual impacts affecting the mother during conception or pregnancy shape as well the physical appearance and/or character of the unborn child (Bien 1997: 79–84; Garland 2010: 141–58, also 87–104; Laes 2013: 127–9; Wyszynski 2001). According a well-known rabbinic story, Elisha ben Abuya (famously called *aher*) allegedly became an apostate in his later years because his mother was tempted during pregnancy by the smell of idolatrous shrines, particularly the wine and meat offerings therein (yHagigah 2:1, 77b–c). Elsewhere, the Bavli claims that maternal actions can affect the physical stature of children, such as a passage in bKetubot 60b–61a (cf. bPesahim 112b) that discusses the positive and negative effects of sexual habits (cf. also bGittin 70a), nutrition and contact with certain substances:

> A woman who couples in a [public] mill will have **epileptic children** (cf. also *Leviticus Rabba 16,1/ Kalla Rabbati* 1). One who couples on the ground will have **children with long necks**. [A woman] who treads on the blood of an ass will have **scabby children**. One who eats mustard will have **intemperate children**. One who eats cress will have **bleary-eyed children**. One who eats fish brine will have children with blinking eyes. One who eats clay will have **ugly children**. One who drinks intoxicating liquor will have **ungainly children**. One who eats meat and drinks wine will have children of a robust constitution. One who eats eggs will have children with big eyes. One who eats fish will have graceful children. One who eats parsley will have beautiful children. One who eats coriander will have stout children. One who eats etrog will have fragrant children.

Another Talmudic account claims that immodest sexuality causes specific impairments, each of which are directly linked via their location in the body (legs, mouth, ears, eyes) to the respective lewd/lecherous behaviour:

> R. Yoḥanan b. Dahabai said: The Ministering Angels told me four things: People are **born lame** because [their parents] 'turned their table' [i.e. practised some other position/ sort of cohabitation]; **mute**, because they kiss 'that place' [i.e. the sexual organs]; **deaf**, because they talk [lewdly] during cohabitation; **blind**, because they look at 'that place'.
>
> *(bNedarim 20a)*

Similar ideas can also be found Greco-Roman culture and cults, as well as in Greek myths that link the anomalous bodies of the Minotaur or Hephaistos to the illegitimate sexual practices of their parents. The birth of children with a different morphology was conceived as divine punishment for religious transgressions like the breaking of an oath, or for criminal and unethical acts. Regardless of whether the parents were actually subject to socio-religious exclusion or stigmatization, abnormal births were certainly interpreted as a warning (*monstrum à monere*, 'to admonish') that someone caused the gods' anger (Garland 2010: 58–63, 67–72). Similarly, ancient Mesopotamia 'sex-omina' connected specific settings or behaviours during intercourse to illness, appearance and character of parents and child (Guinan 1997 and Kellenberger in this volume)

Some rabbinic traditions attribute the presence of disabilities to rather fanciful natural causes. Becoming blind, the rabbis claim, stems from 'the salt of Sodom' (bEruvin 17b), bile of a hornet (bSota 36b) or some undefined herbs (Lev. Rabba 12,4/ Num. Rabba 18,22). Yet rabbinic traditions more commonly attribute disabilities to disease or accident (Lev. Rabba 31,4). Though rabbinic texts sometimes use congenital disability as an occasion for moralizing, they also frequently describe such impairments as natural phenomena that occur during the conception and development of the embryo.

Mitigating and curing disabilities: therapeutic approaches to impairments

Prostheses/technical aids

Prostheses or corrective aids are known already in ancient Mesopotamia, Egypt and Greco-Roman cultures (Blisquez 1996; Reeves 1999). The Mishnah also discusses walking aids or prosthesis used by people with different mobility impairments, mainly in the case of congenital deformation or amputations (mShabbat 6:8). The *Qav ha-kite'a* (lit. 'cavity of the amputee') was most probably a (hollowed out) wooden leg or foot, often equipped with pads or rags on which to place the remaining limb (mShabbat 6:8; bYoma 78b). Other devices for legs or arms called *samokhot/semukhot* (lit. 'support') were cushions made of fabric or leather, at times used in combination with a small stool (*kisse*). Other passages mention artificial teeth (mShabbat 6:5/b Shabbat 65a), eyes made of gold or silver (yNedarim 9 (41c); bNedarim 66a–b), and rather extraordinary aids for animals, such as an artificial leg for a hen or a reed to allow a lamb with a perforated windpipe to breathe (bChulin 57b). None of these texts contain information about the actual production, usage or treatment of medical problems resulting from the prosthesis or aid. Instead, the discussions remain focused on technical-halakhic issues, relating to whether using such an aid violates the commandments regarding Shabbat and the Day of Atonement or whether the device can transmit (ritual) impurity. On the social level, persons with wooden aids are exempt from the pilgrimage to Jerusalem (bHagigah 3a), but included in the performance of certain rituals like the ceremony of release from levirate marriage, *halitzah* (bYeb 103a).

Sexual disabilities

Detailed medical and anatomical information appears in rabbinic sources about family law, marriage and the obligation to procreate, as well as texts that serve to define the gender identity of a person in the context of Jewish rituals and religious rules. The unambiguous sexual/gender status of a person and physical integrity of the (male) genitals were of crucial importance for halakhic rulings (cf. Benkheira in this volume for striking parallels with early Islam). People of indeterminate gender status (*tumtum*), those who possess both male and female genital characteristics (*androgynos*), and those who experience sterility/infertility combined with developmental disorders of their sexual characteristics (*saris ḥama* and *aylonit*) were regarded as 'disabled' in relation to the sharp male/female dichotomy in everyday Jewish rituals, liturgy and law. In ancient Greece and the Roman Republic, hermaphrodites were regarded as despicable 'monsters' and a bad omen (*prodigium*). In later times, Roman culture became inclined to look at the *androgyni* as an exotic and curious fallacy of nature.[4] In contrast to these Roman religious and cultural attitudes, many rabbinic discussions on sex/gender ambiguity appear to utilize medical knowledge that circulated in their surroundings (Bien 1997) for the purpose of a more balanced discourse (Fonrobert 2006, 2007; Levinson 2000). Most strikingly, the strict binary scheme of halakhic discussion resembles the Roman juridical treatment of people with ambiguous gender/sex (Graumann 2013: 196–7). The Bavli (bYeb 83a) offers a surgical therapy for a person of unspecified sex (*tumtum*) whose sexual organs are described as concealed, either covered by a slight skin or inside the body. In order to enable this person to procreate and become a fully respected male member of Jewish society, some rabbis suggest a surgical extrication of the sexual organs. Other sages demur that this dangerous procedure might be useless if it becomes apparent that the person is a congenitally infertile or a woman.

More frequent and therefore more severe for the rabbis were cases of injured (male) genitals. Following Deuteronomy 23: 2, rabbinic law forbids a man with crushed testes (*petzu'a daka*), softened testicle (*meroah eshek/me-ushkan*), a mutilated penis or a mutilated urinary and spermatic duct (*kerut shophkhah*) from marrying a Jewish woman (mYevamot 8:2). Both the Babylonian and the Palestinian Talmuds (yYevamot 8,2 9b//bYevamot76a) discuss the anatomical details that make a person subject to this exclusion. Which degree, place (right or left testicle), shape (e.g. perforation) and type (man-made/congenital) of the mutilations render someone fit or unfit (*pasul/kasher*)? In these cases, rabbinic sources again include instructions for surgical 'corrections', even in the case of a perforated membrum that would ordinarily prevent a man from impregnating a woman. The text counsels that the physical intactness of the penis, especially the spermatic duct, can be restored to a degree sufficient for impregnation – with the help of a giant ant that serves as butterfly stitches/clip/plaster. While this proposed surgery may well have been a rabbinic medical fiction, it exemplifies the twofold rhetorical tendency of the text towards enabling allegedly (sexually) disabled persons. First, rabbinic sources commonly advocate surgery (mutilated penis/extrication of the *tumtum*'s genitals) in order to reintegrate impaired persons within the common binary gender scheme. This strategy corresponds to tendencies found also in Greco-Roman culture, where the medical discourse on disabilities was overly concerned with medically curing or repairing bodily defects (Jackson 2005; Garland 2010: 128–34). Second, rabbinic sources also 'rehabilitate' some individuals through discursive strategies that create manifold exceptional cases (e.g. one who is born with injured testes, or whose penis has the shape of a reed or a spout), thereby narrowing down the number of individuals who fit within the original, discriminatory category.

Intellectual disabilities/mental disorders

As Judith Abrams has observed, rabbinic categorization of disabilities shifted from the biblical or priestly focus on physical blemish to disabilities that excluded a person from participation in the intellectual culture of the rabbis (Abrams 1998: 123–51, 168–97). Rabbinic sources, in a way similar to Greek concepts (Ahonen 2014; Harris 2013) are particularly concerned with conditions that cause a lack of *da'at* (knowledge, intellectual ability and/or intention), which is crucial for halakhic actions, liturgy and study (Fishbane 2007: 106–20).

THE SHOTEH

Similar to Greco-Roman culture (Laes *et al.* 2013a), the rabbinic designation *shoteh* – besides being used as a metaphor (the 'fool'/bSotah 3a: foolishness of every transgression) – was an umbrella term comprising very different manifestations of mental illnesses and disabilities (like schizophrenia, bipolar disorders, mentally unstable persons; demonic possession or maniac obsession; intellectual/learning disabilities). Rabbinic sources distinguish these conditions from temporary states of disorientation called *sha'amumit* (*amum* = blurred/obfuscated), which the rabbis thought were induced either by idleness or by wearing filthy clothes (cf. bBaba Metzia 80a; bKetubot 59b; bNedarim 81a).

In some rabbinic texts, one can trace a gradual application of medical concepts in order to identify the *shoteh*. This is all the more striking since even in ancient medical traditions no subfield of psychiatry/psychology whatsoever existed and, thus, many divergent or even contradicting explanations and treatments of mental disorders or impairments were developed (Harris 2013). While the earliest tradition (Mishnah) offer no further exemplifications, other early Palestinian rabbinic sources already define the *shoteh by* 'diagnosing' certain strange behaviours. The Tosefta, an early Palestinian rabbinic text, asks 'who [can be considered] a *shoteh*?' (tTerumot 1:3) and lists four definite behavioural patterns:

1 who goes alone out at night
2 who spends the night at cemeteries/graveyards
3 who tears up his cloths
4 who forfeits what is given to him

If those behaviours are absent and the person behaves well/sanely (*ḥalum*), the Tosefta does not consider the individual impaired by any means. The Palestinian Talmud (yTerumot 1:1) debates whether all four or only one behavioural type – called the 'signs/symptoms of the mentally disabled (*simanei shoteh*)' – are necessary conditions. Moreover, the rabbis provide a narrower definition by linking the different behaviours, mentioned in Tosefta, to more specific mental disorders known from the Greco-Roman cultural context:

1 'who goes alone out at night' = *Kanitrochos/Kanitropos* (Kynanthropos). *Kynanthropia/ Lycanthropia* is described in contemporary Greek sources (e.g. Aetius *Tetrabibloi* 6.11, Galen 19.719 Kühn) as a kind of curable melancholia with dog-like human behaviour induced by delusions (Metzger 2011).
2 'who spends the night at cemeteries' = one burning incense for demons/ foreign deities. While this practice was closely related to religious Greco-Roman cults, the Gospels (cf. Luke 8: 27-33; Mark 5: 2-13) and other sources link the presence in graveyards to madness or demonic possession (Sorensen 2002; Metzger 2013).
3 'who tears up his clothes' = *Cholikos* (yTer). This might refer to melancholia, a depression induced by a dominance of black-bile (*mela/chole*), at times manifested in an outburst of anger (Gr. *cholos*) and aggression, usually associated with the choleric type in humoral theory (cf. Flashar 1966). Roman medical encyclopedists like Celsus described the connection between melancholic depression and a type of insanity or rage that was deemed curable by starvation, shackling and other therapeutic approaches.
4 'who forfeits what is given to him' = yTerumot: *Qodiakos* (MS Leiden/ed.p.)/*Qiniqum* (MS Vatican)//yGittin: *Qinoqos-Qoniqos/Kynikos.* The mental disorder of *Qordiaqos* (see below) is explicitly excluded by the Talmudic discussion itself: 'in the case of the *Qordiaqos*, one does not find any of all these symptoms'. There might be a connection with the already mentioned choleric type or with rage (cf. Num. Rabba 19,8/yYoma 8 (45b)). The Talmudic reference to *qinoqos*/cynic (Luz 1989) might point to Greek sources contemporary with rabbinic traditions. Several authors mention common notions that describe adherents to the philosophical school of Cynics as mad or insane due to their offensive behaviour, including tearing one's clothes, eating raw meat, masturbating and defecating in public (Krueger 1996a: 72–107; Ahonen 2014: 103–23; Krueger 1996b; Navia 1996: 37–118).

In this text, the Palestinian Talmud adopts a cautious, discursive strategy of specification that seems to recognize – and strive to mitigate – the severe consequences and socio-religious exclusion that follow from a broad definition of the category *shoteh*. By linking the characteristics of the rabbinic *shoteh* with mental disorders that were commonly known in Hellenistic societies, the passage actually softens the 'diagnosis' and releases affected individuals from a life-long social blemish or stigma. In contrast to the totally disabling status of the *shoteh*, these other disorders were regarded by contemporary physicians as temporary and partly curable by medical means.

The parallel tradition in the Babylonian Talmud (bḤagigah 3b–4a) employs a similar strategy of rationalization, though it largely appeals to Mesopotamian medical concepts, instead of Greek medicine. The Bavli modifies or eliminates references to certain behavioural patterns that are distinctively Greek, such as the Kynikos. The Greek term Kynanthropos was likewise apparently no longer known to the Babylonian rabbis. In the Bavli's discussion, the one staying at night in the cemetery is understood not as one who burns incense, but as a person who is possessed by a spirit of uncleanness (cf. bNiddah 17a). The one who 'tears up his clothes' is no longer described as a *Cholikos,* but as one who 'is lost in thought'.

In contrast to the discussions in Tosefta and Yerushalmi, the Bavli's discussion introduces a striking innovation. Instead of using behavioural patterns alone to diagnose a person as a *shoteh,* the Bavli argues that the manner of performing the behaviour is crucial. If one cannot discern an 'insane manner' (*derekh shtut*), then even the presence of all these symptoms together do not determine a *shoteh*. The introduction of this flexible condition serves as a deliberate complication to stigmatizing a person with this negative label, particularly since the assessment of an 'insane manner' was especially subject to interpretation. The Bavli's innovative category of 'insane manner' appears as a deliberate inversion that counters the idea of a lack of *da'at* (intention/reason) commonly alleged to our triad of the 'deaf-mute (*ḥeresh*), the mentally disabled (*shoteh*), and the young person (*qatan*)'. As in the case of sexual disabilities, rabbinic medical discourse follows the trend to narrow down the scope of people who would fall into this discriminatory category.

The difficult term *Qordiaqos,* mentioned above in the discussion of the *shoteh,* was probably a seizure or a state of (alcohol induced?) delirium accompanied by temporary mental disorder. Thus, one who is 'seized by *Qordiaqos*' cannot request a writ of divorce (*get*) or annul such a document (*mGittin* 7:1). The term itself is somewhat odd. Although it seems to be of Greek origin, one cannot find a clear correspondence in Greek medical terminology.[5] In the Yerushalmi it is explained as 'a state of delirium or a temporary mental disorientation' (see yGittin 7, 48c–d = yTerumot 1:1, 40b) which can be cured by a special diet (broiled red meat/diluted wine). The Bavli (bGitttin 67b/70b) exploits two etiologies of the ambiguous term (cf. Freeman 1999; Lehmhaus 2015). First, such a condition might arise in one who is 'bitten by new wine from the vat (*de-nakhtei hahamra hadata de-meatzarta*)'. Mental distortions or incompetencies induced by strong wine or alcohol abuse were also known in Greek and Roman culture and were often linked to madness, disability and premature death (Gourevitch 2013; Garland 2010: 138) Alternatively, one might be seized by a (evil) spirit or demon whose name (*Qordiaqos*) is crucial for a charm or amulet used as a remedy (see Naveh and Shaked 1998; Bohak 2008, esp. 374).

Although the symptoms were regarded as disabling through confusion and cognitive incompetence (and therefore also legal incompetence), the *Qordiaqos* is clearly distinguished from similar disorders. On the one hand, the symptoms were described as being different from seizures of an epileptic person, called *nikpeh* ('to be forced'). This 'sacred disease' of the Greeks and Babylonians (cf. Temkin 1971; Longrigg 2000; Laskaris 2002) was considered by the rabbis as a stable 'hidden blemish' (cf. Preuss 1911: 341–50: mBekhorot 7; bKetubot 77a; bBaba Metzia 80a; tBaba Batra 4.5) with a genetic disposition (bYevamot 64b/bBaba Metzia 80a). Epilepsy resembled the Babylonian etiology of *Qordiaqos* in being regarded as demonic possession in Egyptian, Mesopotamian (Stol 1993) and Jewish/Christian traditions (Matt. 4: 24; Mark 9: 14–29; Weissenrieder 2003: 267–83; Sorensen 2002: 118–221). Another similarity is the use of amulets as the most effective remedy (Lev. Rabba 26.5; bShabbat 67a/tShabbat 4:9). On the other hand, the temporary nature and the curability of *Qordiaqos* distinguished it substantially from chronic mental illnesses or the state of a mentally or intellectually disabled person (Hankoff 1972 and above).

Conclusion

Disability appears most frequently in rabbinic texts when its presence complicates (or is perceived to complicate) rabbinic legal and ritual practice. Rabbinic discussion of disability centres primarily around the question of impairment in terms of its implications for halakhic issues. If, in the eyes of the rabbis, a certain impairment constituted an obstacle to the performance of the commandments (*mitzvot*), or other legal acts, the rabbis frequently discussed the exclusion of persons with such disabilities – and often developed strategies for managing or mitigating individual limitations. By contrast, bodily or mental differences deemed to have no particular consequences for halakhic affairs receive little attention in rabbinic sources. Such cases are usually mentioned only in passing, without any further discussion.

Disability discourse serves not only as a potent site for the production and expression of medical knowledge, but also the articulation of cultural values about gender, sexual propriety and morality. Rabbinic approaches to disability oscillate between a position of moral judgement and a stance of openness and inclusivity (cf. Abrams 1998: 118–22). Many texts give an explicitly moral account of the etiology of impairments, an approach that is evident in the blessing of the 'true judge' (*dayyan ha-emet*):

> [One who sees] an amputee, or a lame person, or a blind person, or a person afflicted with boils says, 'Blessed [are you Lord our God, Ruler of the Universe], the True Judge.'
>
> *(tBerakhot 6:3)*

Because rabbinic sources call for this blessing to be recited when hearing bad tidings (mBerakhot 9:2), this tradition interprets the disabilities and illnesses it mentions as a (justified) divine punishment or judgement. The authors of the later Talmuds (y.Ber 9:1/bBer 58b) took pains to emphasize that this assumption pertains only to non-congenital conditions.

By contrast, an attitude demonstrating an awareness and acceptance of physical and behavioural disparity is expressed in the very same Tosefta passage:

> One who sees an Ethiopian, or an albino, or a [man] red-spotted in the face, or [a man] white spotted in the face, or a hunchback, or a dwarf (or a *ḥeresh* or a *shoteh* or a drunk person) says, 'Blessed [are you Lord our God, Ruler of the Universe who creates such] varied creatures.'
>
> *(tBerakhot 6:3)*

This blessing offers a more appreciative reading of bodily difference. Both the Palestinian and the Babylonian Talmuds specify that this blessing is to be recited upon seeing those whose disabilities are congenital and incurable. This blessing treats the presence of disability in a strikingly different fashion, affirming that physical and mental difference is part of the divine design (cf. Dupont in this volume for similar thoughts in Augustine). Yet it nonetheless reveals a clear privileging of what Rosemarie Garland-Thomson has called 'the normate' body. The dominant rabbinic subject who recites this blessing possesses an unremarkable body – and holds sufficient cultural and corporeal capital to mark out the bodies of others as a source of spectacle. Disability, like ethnic difference, is simultaneously celebrated as a wondrous dimension of creation and set apart as a source of strangeness.

Within halakhic frameworks, rabbinic discussion of disability are characterized first and foremost by an impulse to categorize and define impairment, as it relates to ritual and legal concerns. In some instances, the rabbinic penchant for categorization and definition brings about an expansion of those affected, such as the expansive rabbinic lists of blemishes (*mumim*). Rabbinic discussions of halakhic obligation and exemption often result into a *de facto* exclusion of disabled persons. Yet in some cases, rabbinic interest in detail and definition serves to narrow the scope of excluded categories. A deeper understanding of the nature of impairments leads the rabbis to make fine distinctions between congenital impairments and such caused later by accidents or disease. At times, they point to surgical techniques and cures that would promote bodily restoration or recovery. However, such medical or technical attempts to 'cure or correct' disabilities strive only to rehabilitate or accommodate individuals; their presence leaves in place the basic mechanisms of ascribing inferiority, dependency and difference in rabbinic culture. Rabbinic texts also deploy discursive and exegetical strategies for dealing with physical and mental impairments, strategies that often prove to be more effective and more embedded in their own culture. The rabbis' thorough discussions of bodily, behavioural and cultural features of disability served to 'rehabilitate' affected individuals through discourse, sometimes by creating many exceptional cases and sub-categories (e.g. *heresh*), by emphasizing a narrow definition (e.g. *shoteh/qordiaqos*), or by taking into account cultural or contextual factors that could be used to mitigate stigma and exclusion (e.g. the principle of familiarity).

Rabbinic efforts to limit the number of people stigmatized by the law might certainly be read as an ethical impulse, a legal principle that emerges out of rabbinic desire to ease or erase the burden of bodily disparity or imperfection. Yet this discourse might also be a consequence of rabbinic self-awareness regarding the proper application of halakhah. In many cases – not simply in matters related to disability – the rabbis sought to balance the strict application of the law with the needs of the community and the specifics of each individual case. Rabbinic discussions of disability reveal a creativity and flexibility inherent to rabbinic legal thought, a system of law that reflects a deep engagement with biblical texts and traditions, while also engaging seriously with rabbinic medical knowledge and grappling with the social implications of law in practice. Rabbinic texts thus reveal the profound interrelationship between medical and social discourses of disability, illuminating the diverse ways in which physical and mental difference come to bear medical, religious and cultural meaning.

Notes

1 This position was not without controversy in early rabbinic sources. Because one of the blessings surrounding the Sh'ma praises God as the creator of the heavenly lights, Rabbi Yehudah argues that someone who has never seen the sun with his own eyes should not praise God for its creation. In bBaba Kamma 87a, discussed more fully below, Rabbi Yehudah rules conservatively that a blind man is exempt from all the *mitzvot*. The Tosafot, medieval commentators on the Talmud, point out a logical contradiction with these traditions, arguing that if Rabbi Yehudah exempted the blind from all the mitzvot elsewhere, he surely need not specify that people who are blind are exempt from reciting these blessings on behalf of the congregation. Ultimately the Tosafot use this logical inconsistency to conclude that Rabbi Yehudah must have actually considered blind Jews obligated to keep most commandments, except those that specifically require vision (Nevins 2003).
2 Certain rabbinic texts articulate the claim that women are generally exempt from positive, time-bound commandments, a ruling often explained by commentators as a reflection of the competing claims that children and family life place upon a woman's time. According to this logic, a woman is freed from time-sensitive commandments because she has a prior obligation to nurse an infant or care for children. Hauptman 1998 provides a compelling analysis of the insufficiency of this and other apologetic explanations. For an incisive discussion of the origins of this principle, its inability to account for all rabbinic sources, and its eventual elevation by the late redactors of the Babylonian Talmud, see Alexander 2013.
3 While yKilayim 8,4 (31c) mentions only the animate elements ('And the breath, spirit and soul come from the Holy One, Blessed be He. And all three are partners in his creation'), the Bavli in bNiddah 31a adds other elements, namely the senses and motor skills ('And the Holy One, blessed be He, gives him the spirit, and breath, the features of the face, knowledge, understanding and wisdom, eyesight, the hearing of the ear, the speaking of the lips and the walking of the feet.'). Later midrashic sources (Kohelet Rabba 5:10) add other features of an ideal or 'normate' body, such as the strength to raise one's hands.

4 Garland 2010: 68–72 mentions the expiation and expulsion of hermaphrodites as victims or sacrifices by the Romans, while babies were drowned in the sea accompanied in a ritualistic procession. See also Graumann 2013 on the image of the hermaphrodite as changing from 'monster' to a curiosity in Roman culture.

5 See Rosner 1995: 60–4, who surveys all earlier scholarly attempts to make sense of this wording. Cf. also Kottek 1996: 2924–6. The new proposal offered by Jesse John Rainbow (2008) in a recent article seems to add to the confusion rather than resolving it. He relies fully on one singular translation (καρδιόω) in the Septuagint for Solomon's madness and the interpretation of *Qordiaqos* in the Babylonian Talmud as a demon. This argument does not pay attention to the usage in the Mishnah and the Palestinian Talmud, where such a demonic explanation is missing.

Bibliography

References to rabbinic sources have been abbreviated as follows: mBerakhot = Mishnah; tBerakhot = Tosefta; yBerakhot = Yerushalmi/Jerusalem or Palestinian Talmud; bBerakhot = Babylonian Talmud/Bavli.

Abrams, Judith, *Judaism and Disability: Portrayals in Ancient Texts from the Tanach through the Bavli* (Washington, DC, 1998).

Ahonen, Marke, *Mental Disorders in Ancient Philosophy* (Heidelberg and New York, 2014).

Alexander, Elizabeth Shanks, *Gender and Timebound Commandments in Judaism* (Cambridge, 2013).

Avalos, Hector, *Illness and Health Care in the Ancient Near East: The Role of the Temple in Greece, Mesopotamia, and Israel* (Atlanta, GA, 2013).

Barmash, Pamela, 'The Status of the Ḥeresh and of Sign Language', *Committee on Jewish Law and Standards of the Rabbinical Assembly,* 24 May 2011. <http://www.rabbinicalassembly.org/sites/default/files/public/halakhah/teshuvot/2011-2020/Status%20of%20the%20Heresh6.2011.pdf>.

Belser, Julia Watts, 'Reading Talmudic Bodies: Disability, Narrative, and the Gaze in Rabbinic Judaism', in D. Schumm and M. Stolzfus (eds), *Disability in Judaism, Christianity and Islam: Sacred Texts, Historical Traditions and Social Analysis* (New York, 2011), 5–27.

Belser, Julia Watts, 'Brides and Blemishes: Queering Women's Disability in Rabbinic Marriage Law', *Journal of the American Academy of Religion* (2015a), 1–29.

Belser, Julia Watts, 'Disability, Animality, and Enslavement in Rabbinic Narratives of Bodily Restoration and Resurrection', *Journal of Late Antiquity* 8/2 (2015b), 288–305.

Bien, Christian G., *Erklärungen zur Entstehung von Mißbildungen im physiologischen und medizinischen Schrifttum der Antike* (Stuttgart, 1997).

Blisquez, Lawrence, 'Prosthetics in Classical Antiquity: Greek, Etruscan, and Roman Prosthetics', *ANRW* 2/37/3 (1996), 2640–76.

Bohak, Gideon, *Ancient Jewish Magic: A History* (Cambridge, 2008).

Dasen, Véronique, *Dwarfs in Ancient Egypt and Greece* (Oxford, 2013).

Davis, Lennard, *Enforcing Normalcy: Disability, Deafness, and the Body* (New York, 1995).

Fishbane, Simcha, *Deviancy in Early Rabbinic Literature: A Collection of Socio-Anthropologica* (Leiden, 2007).

Flashar, Helmut, *Melancholie und Melancholiker in den medizinischen Theorien der Antike* (Berlin, 1966).

Fonrobert, Charlotte, 'The Semiotics of the Sexed Body in Early Halakhic Discourse', in M. A. Kraus (ed.), *Closed and Open: Readings of Rabbinic Texts* (Atlanta, GA, 2006), 69–96.

Fonrobert, Charlotte, 'Regulating the Human Body: Rabbinic Legal Discourse and the Making of Jewish Gender', in C. Fonrobert and M. Jaffee (eds), *Cambridge Companion to Rabbinic Literature* (Cambridge, 2007), 270–294.

Freeman, D., 'The Gittin "Book of Remedies"', *Korot* 13 (1999), 151–64.

Garland, Robert, *The Eye of the Beholder: Deformity and Disability in the Graeco-Roman World* (London, 2010²).

Garland-Thomson, Rosemarie, *Extraordinary Bodies: Figuring Disability in Popular Culture* (New York, 1997).

Gourevitch, Danielle, 'Two Historical Case Histories of Acute Alcoholism in the Roman Empire', in C. Laes *et al.* (eds), *Disabilities in Roman Antiquity* (Leiden, 2013), 73–87.

Gracer, Bonnie, 'What the Rabbis Heard: Deafness in the Mishnah', *Disability Studies Quarterly* 23/2 (2003), 192–205.

Graumann, Lutz Alexander, 'Monstrous Births and Retrospective Diagnosis: The Case of Hermaphrodites in Antiquity', in C. Laes *et al.* (eds), *Disabilities in Roman Antiquity* (Leiden, 2013), 181–209.

Guinan, Ann K., 'Auguries of Hegemony. The Sex Omens of Mesopotamia', *Gender and History* 9/3 (1997), 462–79.

Hankoff, Leon D., 'Ancient Descriptions of Organic Brain Syndrome: The "Kordiakos" of the Talmud', *American Journal of Psychology* 129/2 (1972), 233–6.

Harris, William V. (ed.), *Mental Disorders in the Classical World* (Leiden, 2013).

Hauptman, Judith, *Rereading the Rabbis: A Woman's Voice* (Boulder, CO, 1998).

Jackson, Ralph, 'Circumcision, De-circumcision and Self-Image: Celsus's "Operations on the Penis"', in A. Hopkins and M. Wyke (eds), *Roman Bodies: Antiquity to the Eighteenth Century* (London, 2005), 23–32.

Kessler, Gwynn, *Conceiving Israel: The Fetus in Rabbinic Narratives* (Philadelphia, PA, 2009)

Kiperwasser, Reuven, '"Three Partners in a Person": The Genesis and Development of Embryological Theory in Biblical and Rabbinic Judaism', *Lectio Difficilior: European Electronic Journal for Feminist Exegesis* 2 (2009). <http://www.lectio.unibe.ch/09_2/kiperwasser.html>.

Kottek, Samuel S., 'Selected Elements of Talmudic Medical Terminology, with Special Consideration to Graeco-Latin Influences and Sources', *ANRW II*, 37, 3 (1996) 2912–2932.

Krueger, Derek, *Symeon the Holy Fool: Leontius' Life and the Late Antique City* (Berkeley, CA, 1996a).

Krueger, Derek, 'The Bawdy and Society: The Shamelessness of Diogenes in Roman Imperial Culture', in R. B. Branham and M.-O. Goulet-Cazé (eds), *The Cynics: The Cynic Movement in Antiquity and its Legacy* (Berkeley, CA, 1996b), 222–39.

Laes, Christian, 'Silent Witnesses: Deaf-Mutes in Graeco-Roman Antiquity', *Classical World* 104/4 (2011), 451–73.

Laes, Christian, 'Raising a Disabled Child', in J. Evans Grubbs, T. Parkin with R. Bell (eds), *The Oxford Handbook of Childhood and Education in the Classical World* (Oxford, 2013), 125–44.

Laes, Christian, Goodey, Chris F., and Rose, Martha Lynn (eds), *Disabilities in Roman Antiquity: Disparate Bodies A Capite ad Calcem* (Leiden, 2013a).

Laes, Christian, Goodey, Chris F., and Rose, Martha Lynn, 'Approaching Disabilities *a capite ad calcem*: Hidden Themes in Roman Antiquity', in Laes *et al.* (eds), *Disabilities in Roman Antiquity* (Leiden, 2013b), 1–15.

Laskaris, Julie, *The Art is Long: On the Sacred Disease and the Scientific Tradition* (Leiden, 2002).

Lehmhaus, Lennart, 'Listenwissenschaft and the Encyclopedic Hermeneutics of Knowledge in Talmud and Midrash', in J. Cale Johnson (ed.), *In the Wake of the Compendia: Infrastructural Contexts and the Licensing of Empiricism in Ancient and Medieval Mesopotamia* (Berlin, 2015).

Levinson, Joshua, 'Cultural Androgyny in Rabbinic Literature', in S. Kottek *et al.* (eds), *From Athens to Jerusalem: Medicine in Hellenized Jewish Lore and in Early Christian Literature* (Rotterdam, 2000), 119–40.

Longrigg, James, 'Epilepsy in Ancient Greek Medicine: The Vital Step', *Seizure* 9 (2000), 12–21.

Luz, Menachem, 'A Description of the Greek Cynic in the Jerusalem Talmud', *Journal for the Study of Judaism* 20 (1989), 49–60.

Marx, Tsvi C., *Disability in Jewish Law* (New York, 2002).

Metzger, Nadine, *Wolfsmenschen und nächtliche Heimsuchungen: Zur kulturhistorischen Verortung vormoderner Konzepte von Lykanthropie und Ephialtes* (Remscheid, 2011).

Metzger, Nadine, 'Battling Demons with Medical Authority: Werewolves, Physicians and Rationalization', *History of Psychiatry* 24 (2013), 341–355.

Naveh, Joseph, and Shaked, Shaul, *Amulets and Magic Bowls: Aramaic Incantations of Late Antiquity* (Jerusalem, 1998).

Navia, Luis E., *Classical Cynicism: A Critical Study* (Westport, CT, 1996).

Neis, Rachel, *The Sense of Sight in Rabbinic Culture* (Cambridge, 2013).

Neumann, Josef N., 'Die Mißgestalt des Menschen – ihre Deutungim Weltbild von Antike und Frühmittelalter', *SudhoffsArchiv* 76/2 (1992), 214–31.

Nevins, Daniel, 'The Participation of Jews who are Blind in the Torah Service', Committee on Jewish Law and Standards of the Rabbinical Assembly, 15 January 2003. Repr. in J. Z. Abrams and W. C. Gaventa (eds.), *Jewish Perspectives on Theology and the Human Experience of Disability* (Binghamton, NY, 2006), 27–52.

Olyan, Saul, *Disability in the Hebrew Bible: Interpreting Mental and Physical Differences* (Cambridge, 2008).

Preuss, Julius, *Biblisch-talmudischeMedizin: Beiträge zur Geschichte der Heilkunde und der Kulturüberhaupt* (Berlin, 1911).

Preuss, Julius, and Rosner, Fred, *Biblical and Talmudic Medicine,* tr. and ed. F. Rosner (New York, 1978).

Rainbow, Jesse, 'The Derivation of Kordiakos: A New Proposal', *Journal for the Study of Judaism in the Persian, Hellenistic, and Roman Periods* 39 (2008), 255–66.

Raphael, Rebecca, *Biblical Corpora: Representations of Disability in Hebrew Biblical Literature* (New York, 2008).

Reeves, Nicholas, 'New Light on Ancient Egyptian Prosthetic Medicine', *Studies in Egyptian Antiquities: A Tribute to T. G. H. James* (London, 1999), 73–7.

Rose, Martha L., *The Staff of Oedipus: Transforming Disability in Ancient Greece* (Ann Arbor, MI, 2003).

Rosen-Zvi, Ishay, 'The Body and the Book: The List of Blemishes in Mishnah Tractate Bekhorot and the Place of the Temple and its Worship in the Tannaitic Beit Ha-Midrash' [Hebrew], *Mada'ei Hayahadut* 43 (2005–6), 49–87.

Rosner, Fred, *Medicine in the Bible and Talmud: Selections from Classical Jewish Sources* (Hoboken, NJ, 1995).

Schipper, Jeremy, *Disability Studies and the Hebrew Bible: Figuring Mephibosheth in the David Story* (New York, 2006).

Sorensen, Eric, *Possession and Exorcism in the New Testament and Early Christianity* (Tübingen, 2002).

Steinberg, Abraham, 'The Blind in the Light of Jewish Thought and Law', in J. Sacks (ed.), *Tradition and Transition: Essays Presented to Chief Rabbi Sir Immanuel Jakobovits* (London, 2002), 283–93.

Stol, Marten, *Epilepsy in Babylonia* (Leiden, 1993).

Strous, Racl, 'The Shoteh and Psychosis in Halakhah with Contemporary Clinical Application', *The Torah u-Madda Journal* (Dec. 2004), 158–78.

Taub, Moshe, 'Deafness in Halacha: A Reappraisal', *Journal of Halacha and Contemporary Society* 14/1 (2012), 5–30.

Temkin, Owsei, *The Falling Sickness: A History of Epilepsy from the Greeks to the Beginnings of Modern Neurology* (Baltimore, MD, 1971).

Vlahogiannis, Nicholas, '"Curing" Disability', in H. King (ed.), *Health in Antiquity* (London and New York, 2005), 180–91.

Weissenrieder, Annette, *Images of Illness in the Gospel of Luke: Insights of Ancient Medical Texts* (Tübingen, 2003).

Wyszynski, Diego F.,'Dysmorphology in the Bible and the Talmud', *Teratology* 64 (2001), 221–5.

V

The endurance of tradition

31

THEN AND NOW

Canon law on disabilities

Irina Metzler

Introduction

In simplest terms, canon law forbids the ordination of 'disabled' men to the priesthood. It is worth pointing out that the issue of impaired persons in holy orders is still not satisfactorily resolved in the modern Catholic Church. In 1995 the Vatican 'provoked fury by issuing a decree banning men who suffer from an allergy to gluten from becoming priests' (Bunting 1995). The Vatican insisted on communion wafers containing gluten as the only suitable kind of wafers; gluten can trigger the debilitating coeliac disease. This episode highlights the cultural and socio-economic consequences of what happens when impairments (the underlying medical phenomenon) are loaded with disabilities (the imposition of cultural construction).[1]

Canon law (from the Greek *kanon*, 'rule') refers to the rules, regulations and laws of the church, as opposed to secular or, as it was termed in western Christianity, Roman law. Canonical law defined certain features or qualities perceived negatively in ways that are reminiscent of 'disabilities' in the modern sense, in that these personal features prevent a person from acting in a specific role – as priest. In its fully fledged form, canon law was a medieval phenomenon, but the antecedents, the ideas, religious notions and social concepts leading to the formation of canon law can be traced all the way back to Greco-Roman Antiquity, and in turn even further back to roots ultimately in the ancient Near East – which of course includes the cultural environs of the Old Testament.

Canon law relates almost exclusively to what we now term 'disabilities' amongst just one group, the medieval clergy, with virtually no interest in 'disabilities' amongst the secular rest of the population (the one exception being impediments to marriage, discussed below). This chapter examines what the theoretical underpinnings were for the concept of physical and mental integrity of the Christian clergy, a concept termed priestly idoneity. Members of the Catholic priesthood were, and still are, subject to an examination for physical and mental 'fitness for work'. One can explore the opposite of idoneity, i.e. cases of clerical unsuitability on physical or mental grounds, to gain an understanding of what culturally specific notions of idoneity were held in that period – the high and later Middle Ages – when canon law had reached sufficient levels of development to warrant interest in regulating idoneity. Thus one can ask what were the consequences of health, illness and disability as reflected in ecclesiastical records in western Europe between the 13th and 15th centuries. By studying such material we can gain a better understanding of why particular groups of people – the clergy – were considered to be physically and mentally ill or disabled in the pre-modern, pre-Reformation past. We can also use these records to tell us which illnesses or disabilities were seen to be more detrimental than others, and which permitted or prohibited a career in the church. Of practical concern was the further question whether physically or mentally incapacitated medieval clergy actually continued acting in their roles. This chapter will present the hypothesis that practical solutions to incapacitated clergy balanced the theoretical stipulations against 'defects' inherent in the concept of idoneity.

Origins

A recent addition to previous disability models (medical, social, cultural) has been Edward Wheatley's 'religious model' of disability (Wheatley 2013). At first glance this constitutes an attractive proposition for the medievalist looking at medieval disability, since religion obviously plays a major role in medieval culture. One hypothesis to be examined by this chapter is to test the applicability of the 'religious model' of disability as proposed by Wheatley. There seems to be some confusion between his application of his model to a single phenomenon, namely blindness, and to a variety of phenomena, namely different disabilities in the plural. With this in mind it is worth citing in full the relevant text from John de Burgh's *Pupilla oculi* on the idoneity of priests from 1384:

On the Age and Quality of Those to be Ordained

9. Anyone who in any way mutilates himself or another by his own hand and without just cause, either out of anger, pride, or frustration, may not be ordained. Those who castrate themselves for the sake of continence and who think they are making themselves a gift to the Lord, should be barred from ordination and, if ordained, deposed. The same applies to one who loses an entire limb or a large enough part of one that he is unable to carry out the office of his order or gives rise to scandal. If one removes a part of his body for good reason, such as leprosy, or has some part of his body amputated to avoid infection in the rest, whether obvious or hidden, even if it be a finger (so long as it is not used in making the sign of the cross), he should not be rejected or deposed ...

10. Also, if a priest loses part of a finger in some conflict in defense of his own rights, as long as he can officiate with the missing part without causing scandal and provided that no one's murder or mutilation came about as a result of the fight, he may officiate with the dispensation of his bishop.

11. A cripple may be ordained so long as he does not need a crutch to get to the altar. There is no right or custom allowing a blind person to be ordained or any person with a visual defect that could develop into a deformity and a scandal.

12. Lepers, when they are expelled from common cohabitation, are absolutely prohibited from ordination. If, however, a priest should become leprous, he shall cease his ministry with those who are well; but he may celebrate the divine ministries among lepers or celebrate mass on his own in private.

13. A hump-backed person should not be rejected from orders unless his deformity is severe and causes disability. Those who have more or less toes than are usual for human beings are to be rejected.

14. But those who have six fingers or two fingers fused together, as long as there be no impediments in the use of the fingers, should not be rejected.

15. Madmen, lunatics, epileptics, and those who are possessed are not to be ordained even if they should be freed completely from their condition. But if they are ordained first and then suffer such diseases, they should abstain from celebrating the sacraments for a full year after their complete recovery.

16. Those who cannot drink wine should not be ordained to the priesthood since those who celebrate need to take communion.

(John de Burgh, Pupilla Oculi 7.3.4)

Thus blind priests were considered definitely unacceptable, which does indicate something special about blindness – but crippled priests, hump-backed priests and even amputees were considered acceptable.

The types and incidences of illness and disability as they are encountered in the sources can therefore be used to draw conclusions as to the relative 'weighting' or severity of different pathologized conditions. The historical context, despite being considered 'medieval' in the pejorative sense as a dark, pre-modern or alien ('the past is a foreign country') kind of culture may nevertheless intrude upon contemporary debates about policy and practice, precisely by being challenging of popularly accepted stereotypes. Such considerations might allow for interesting contemporary debates at a public level into the relative importance or weighting given to different diseases or disabilities in contemporary societies. The historical context demonstrates that notions of what is deemed 'diseased', 'sick' or 'disabled' are socially and culturally constructed, and hence subject to change over time and place. The approaches of the medieval church in how to deal with its 'members of staff', i.e. the priesthood, in cases of incapacity or retirement might contribute to considerations of similar matters in contemporary society, but certainly highlight how cultural, religious and socio-economic factors impact on what is defined as incapacity, disability or 'being old'. Further research into concepts of idoneity could lead to questions as to whether there are certain situations when physical or mental integrity might matter more than equal opportunity. For instance, is it acceptable to bar someone from a certain occupation on the grounds of a specific disease, and if so, why? A modern example would be the case of a visually impaired pilot. A blind pilot guiding a passenger plane would be deemed an unacceptable risk to the lives of all concerned, and in that sense a blind pilot would not possess idoneity for performance of the task. In similar fashion, a medieval priest was responsible for the *spiritual* lives of his parishioners, and an unsuitable priest, one not possessing idoneity, endangered the spiritual health not just of himself, but of those others he was responsible for.

Pollution and purity were linked in many ways (Douglas 1966). In early Christian times, the church father Dionysius, Bishop of Alexandria (r. 247/8–264/5), advised on a number of topics relating to the ritual impurity of sexuality, always a matter of concern, and of far greater import than physical disability. For example, 'menstruating women were to be banned from approaching the Eucharist, as they would defile the purity of the place of God. Not all Christians agreed, but Dionysius's ruling lies at the root of a lasting tradition in the Eastern Church' (Fox 1986: 543). In general, concerns over ritual (im)purity were focused on the proper conduct of sexuality, among the laity too (Angenendt 1997: 406–8), but since the laity were only receiving and not performing the sacraments the requirements were less stringent than for the clergy.

In the Bible, the Old Testament books of Deuteronomy and Leviticus contain the most relevant passages with regard to impairments becoming disabilities (cf. Kellenberger in this volume). Among general injunctions concerning proper sacrifice and worship, Deuteronomy 17:1 stipulates against the offering up of any animal in sacrifice that has a 'blemish'; a passage similar to Leviticus 22:22, where blind, broken or maimed animals are also mentioned. The concept of ritual purity surfaces in Deuteronomy 23:1, which forbids a man who is 'wounded in the stones' or 'hath his privy member cut off' from entering 'into the congregation of the Lord' (cf. Watts Belser, Lehmhaus and Benkheira in this volume for similar concern on the amputated *membrum virile* in Judaism and Islamic thought). Furthermore, Deuteronomy 28 has verses connecting the character of a person, sin and physical imperfection, in that those who disobey the divine law are afflicted with various illnesses and impairments, such as blindness (Deut. 28: 29) and leg ailments (Deut. 28: 61). Just to make sure and to keep all eventualities covered, the sinner or enemy of Israel is further threatened with 'every sickness, and every plague, which is not written in the book of this law' (Deut. 28: 61). The book of Leviticus treats illness and impairment after a more precise fashion, listing very specific ailments. There are some protective injunctions, such as leaving part of the harvest for the poor to glean (Lev. 19: 9–10, repeated at 23: 22), and not cursing the deaf or deliberately tripping up the blind (Lev. 19: 14). The most (in)famous passage, however, relates to proscriptions regarding the priesthood, on who is allowed to become a priest and who not, and is worth quoting in full:

> Whosoever he be of thy seed in their generations that hath any blemish, let him not approach to offer the bread of his God. For whatsoever man he be that hath a blemish, he shall not approach: a blind man, or a lame, or he that hath a flat nose, or any thing superfluous, or a man that is brokenfooted, or brokenhanded, or crookbackt, or a dwarf, or that hath a blemish in his eye, or be scurvy, or be scabbed, or hath his stones broken.
>
> *(Leviticus 21: 17–20)*

A manuscript illumination from the Bible of King Wenceslas, dating from around 1400, neatly illustrates the scene where Moses prohibits the priesthood to some of the impaired persons mentioned in this passage (Vienna, Österreichische Nationalbibliothek, MS Codex Vindobonensis 2759, fo. 121ʳ). This passage relates purely to prospective priests, and on its own does not imply any negative attitudes to disabled persons in general, though it has often been cited to emphasize the supposed disadvantaging of the impaired in ancient Jewish society by modern scholars. The 'blemishes' mentioned in Leviticus could be considered to be 'canonical irregularities' and, as modern commentators point out, 'The persons affected were not unclean and therefore were not excluded from a share of the sacred offerings' (Orchard *et al.*, 1953: 241), so that the injunctions against impaired people can be interpreted to mean only that the impaired should not approach the sanctuary, not that they are excluded from *all* sacred ritual, let alone cast out from society altogether (even if the prohibition against becoming priests means they cannot join the elite of society).

Notions of pollution and purity are deeply connected with ritual acts and the efficacy of ritual. The sacraments of the medieval church possessed divine power – but only if they were performed correctly, which also meant performed by the correct person. The idea of ritual purity entailed that all those who were involved in preparation of the eucharist had to be 'clean', for which reason every polluting action was to be avoided otherwise the celebrant could not act. This was a cross-cultural phenomenon amongst the religions of the ancient Mediterranean world, found in similar forms in Greek, Roman and Hebrew religious practice (Angenendt 1997: 453–4). But sexual purity and literal washing of hands was not enough; the whole body of the celebrant had to be 'pure' and 'intact'. Ambrose of Milan (d. 397), in whose time it was already practice to hold a daily mass, demanded that his clergy were not only 'clean' in a behavioural or spiritual-internal sense, but also in body (*De officiis* 1.50.248; see Angenendt 1997: 454). One consequence of the belief in the efficacy of ritual only under conditions of purity of the celebrant was that, at times of crisis, reform or renewal of the church, purity became more rigorously enforced. This happened, for example, in the late 11th century, when various malpractices among the clergy (incontinence, simony, plurality of office) came under scrutiny not just by the ecclesiastical leadership, but were enthusiastically endorsed by the laity – the Patari of Milan are a prime example, as are the somewhat later Waldensians and other so-called heretical groups (Angenendt 1997: 459–60). One consequence of the challenge heretical movements posed to the established church was that requirements among the clergy for purity, in all its shapes and forms, were of concern, and raised among both laity and theologians the question of the validity of sacraments such as baptism or absolution by 'polluted' priests. Amongst the reforming orders, the Franciscan and Dominican friars, with the latter especially keen on combating heresy in all its permutations, similar 'health and fitness' requirements existed. So for instance an amendment of 1239 to the Franciscan statutes made it clear that any candidate who 'had any sort of incapacity in addition to mutilation' (*si infirmitatem aliquem habeat vel praevam corporis qualitatem propter quam foret postea onerosus si membrum aliquod mutilatum habeat vel inefficax quoquomodo*) (cited in Montford 2002: 103 n. 35) would not be received into the order. And a Franciscan statute from the French province ordered in 1337: 'Novices must publicly acknowledge and witness that they are not concealing any latent illness they have, otherwise the Order shall not have any obligations to them' (Montford 2002: 95). The earliest constitution of the Dominican order prescribed that a panel of three friars should examine potential novices concerning their health, character, legitimacy and education, with the question on health specifically asking whether the candidate had any 'hidden infirmity (*occultam habeat infirmitatem*)' (Montford 2002: 98). But if a friar did not disclose disabilities on application to join the order which however were discovered later, the friar should not be ejected from the order against his will (Montford 2002: 103–4; 2004: 30–3). Ostensibly such screening of potential recruits to the orders was intended to reduce the burden on money and resources, but there is an undertone of more general notions of bodily perfection expected of those who were to set spiritual as well as practical examples to the wider Christian community (cf. Kuuliala in this volume on early monastic communities). It is against this background that one should view the canonical injunctions against physically impaired priests.

Canon law

Theoretically, canon law is based on the Old and New Testaments, but this was not enough, so that the first known collection of rules, the *Didache* or *Doctrine of the Twelve Apostles*, already came into being around the turn of the 1st to 2nd century (Brundage 2008: 40). From those disparate sources that fed into canon law, church councils and synods attended by bishops and the higher clergy, together with papal decisions known as decretals, were the most important. The vast and expanding body of regulations, opinions and advice rapidly became unwieldy and unmanageable, so that already from the 5th and 6th centuries onwards collections of passages from the various canonical authorities were made to aid legal administration of the church. 'The Church had the beginnings of canon law, but some of it was not forged until the Carolingian period, when it was "forged" in both senses. The Ps.-Isidorian decretals contain the Ps.-decrees of Ps.-popes' (Evans 2002: 49, 56; see also Brundage 1995: 26–7). These highly influential *Decretals* of Pseudo-Isidore were a complex collection of material incorporating fragments of the church fathers, notably Augustine, as well as texts of spurious papal authority; the exact origin, compilation and transmission of the *Decretals* remains unclear but may have been associated with the monastery of Corbie (Brundage 2008: 64–6). In the 11th century, further use was made of Pseudo-Isidore by compilers such as Burchard of Worms and Ivo of Chartres, and by the twelfth century such burgeoning canonists were faced with a mass of material requiring an equally massive task to make sense of it all and to codify it.

In short, while canon law had developed gradually from late Antiquity through the early Middle Ages, it was substantially collected and systematized around 1140 in Gratian's *Decretum*. The full title of this work attributed to Gratian was *Concordia discordantium canonum*, and it 'marked the most important turning point in the maturation of medieval canon law' (Brundage 2008: 96). By the middle of the 13th century even this collection had been further added to by various papal decrees, and came to be called the *Corpus iuris canonici*. Thus by the 13th century canon law emerged in more or less fully developed form, and legal scholars, canon lawyers and proctors became ever more essential to the bureaucracy of the church. For instance, in the very early 13th century the former lawyer-turned-pope Innocent III embodied the apogee of this development. Finally, one must bear in mind that canon law, in contrast to medieval secular laws, 'emerged as a working and often quite effective international law' (Brundage 1995: 3).

The passage from Leviticus relating to the prohibition on 'blemished' men becoming priests has always been overemphasized, in that there has been an assumption by scholars that this prohibition against disabled people was always strictly adhered to throughout the Middle Ages. Theoretically, of course, such a ban existed, but in practice medieval priests would have been able to obtain a dispensation, though it may have been rarely applied for. Most of these dispensations date from the 13th century, and there is also some interesting canon law material which effectively cancels out the prohibition in Leviticus. Some earlier material also exists. The *Apostolic Constitutions*, dated to the 4th and 5th centuries, include a passage stating that bishops must not be prevented from holding their office because of physical impairment or deformity (Donaldson 1880: 267, section 8, paragraphs 77–9; see Bredberg 1999: 193). The implication seems to be, perhaps, that people who had an impairment prior to applying for the priesthood were discouraged from doing so, but if someone became impaired after they had become a priest, they should not be prevented from carrying out their duties. In the Middle Ages proper, the *Liber extra*, a collection of canonical documents promulgated in 1234 by pope Gregory IX, and which was designed to be authoritative throughout the church, contained an entire *titulus* on the subject of physical intactness and perfection, with rules for the opposite, namely impediments to the ordination of priests in cases of physical impairment. *Titulus* xx, chapters I to VII, was titled 'Corpore vitiatis ordinandis vel non', and summarized various rulings on the subject, by previous popes as well as archbishops and bishops. Chapter I states the case of a priest who lacked parts of his fingers but could still be ordained, provided that he could celebrate solemnly without scandal (*quin ipse sine scandalo possit solenniter celebrare*); while chapter II deals with the visual impairment of a cleric from the see of Canterbury who was nevertheless permitted to be promoted to the episcopate (*in promotione tua ex multa dispensatione procedat*); Chapters III, IV and V concern those clerics who were 'eunuchs', either by accident or from birth (*eunuchus, si per insidias hominum factus, vel ita natus sit*) but could also be ordained; chapter VI provides for dispensation for an abbot with mutilated hands (*Mutilatus manu, si promotus fuerit in abbatem*); and chapter VII concerns the monk Thomas of Brixen, who in his childhood had suffered an accident involving injury to his right thumb (*in annis puerilibus esset constitutus, quaedam barra ferrea super dextrae suae pollicem fortuito casu cadens*) but could still be ordained as a priest (see *Corpus Iuris Canonicis*, vol. II, cols 144–6).

Most decretals included therein dealing with bodily defects and mutilations dated from the twelfth century, and six decretals confirmed that physical deformity, mutilations and serious blemishes morally disqualified a person as a candidate for *higher orders*. One may surmise that lower orders, in contrast, did not warrant such disqualifications. In cases where a physical or mental illness or impairment rendered medieval clerics unsuitable for office, a dispensation was required, and commonly received. Such dispensations were applied for by clergy from dioceses across the community of western Christendom. The records of dispensations in the papal curia exist in their thousands. However, frequent dispensation did not diminish the overall significance of these prohibitions (Mellinkoff 1993: I. 114).

With regard to dispensations, one may look at just two kinds of sources, which are however copiously extant. These sources are the records of the papal curia and those of regional episcopal registers, letters and acta (see bibliography for samples of edited printed sources). The papal curia from the 13th century onwards regarded dispensations not just as an essential requirement to ensure idoneity of the clergy, but also as a convenient cash income. Supplications were received, evaluated and if successful issued with a confirming letter. Records were therefore carefully kept, most originals still being located in the Vatican archives. The medieval records of the papal penitentiary, instigated under Innocent III, were not rediscovered until 1913. Over the past century, however, various national historical institutions have transcribed, edited and published these documents held by the Vatican. For instance, the case studies of supplications to the papal curia for the German dioceses have been fully edited by now in a series of volumes which are easily accessible online (although with an inadequate search facility for the purposes of disability history) and in major libraries. The English and Irish series of entries in the papal registers with regard to papal correspondence in general have been printed in calendar form. Papal correspondence with French dioceses from the 13th century onwards is covered by a similar series published by the École Française de Rome. The records of the papal penitentiary, at least as far as records from the medieval period to the later 16th century are concerned (those more recent are still covered by confidentiality), have been opened up to researchers since 1983. In addition to records stemming from the papal curia, one may consult the equally well-edited series of (archi)episcopal visitation records, letters and acta, especially those for English and German dioceses between, again, the 13th and 15th centuries. Bishops would tour the area in their jurisdiction and note items of concern or in need of improvement, thus these records contain numerous references to physically impaired or chronically ill clergy, especially with regard to elderly priests whose physical or mental debilities forced them into retirement. Episcopal registers, acta and letters have been edited by various historical and local societies (for both England and Germany) and are widely available in libraries.

In theory such dispensation then permitted continuation as clergy in higher orders, that is from parish priest on upwards via bishop to cardinal. Arising from developments in the late twelfth to early 13th centuries, canon law came to distinguish between two types of irregularities: *irregularitas ex defectu*, that is, 'defects' of mind or body, derived from the 'blemishes' in the book of Leviticus (21: 17–20), and *irregularitas ex delictu*, that is, delinquent acts such as homicide or heresy. Physical illness and impairment, e.g. skin diseases, blindness, deafness and lame or missing limbs, as well as mental disorders such as insanity or senile dementia, were categorized under the former and made a priest unsuitable. It is these health-related issues that can be encountered in the source material. Underpinned by a theology of relaxing the rules in individual circumstances if in the general or best interest, canon law decretals confirmed that physical deformity, mutilations and serious 'blemishes' morally disqualified a person as a candidate for higher orders and required dispensations as a way of exempting individuals from the normal operations of the law. Dispensations 'exempt some person or group from legal obligations binding on the rest of the population or class to which they belong' (Brundage 1995: 161).

What does become apparent is that there is evidence that physically impaired people *can* have been in holy orders during the medieval period. An individual case of eye injury concerning a 15th-century priest who asked for dispensation due to canonical irregularity has come down to us: the priest was soldering the handle of his knife with lead (a clumsy do-it-yourself attempt at repair?) when a drop of lead splashed into his left eye, with which he no longer saw anything at the time of supplication, but emphasized that this injury was not obvious to others (Esch 2010: 48; see Schmugge 2005: case no. 3225). Another priest was decorating the altar of St Dorothy with fresh leaves from trees but while whittling a branch something flew into his eye (Esch 2010: 48; Schmugge 2008: case no. 2327). The question of physical integrity as a requirement for the priesthood goes beyond the scope of this present volume, but it suffices to draw attention to a single issue: visibility to others of an impairment. Humbert of Romans, Master General of the Dominicans during the 13th century, had argued that

> people who are disfigured in this way are debarred from the Lord's service in Leviticus [21: 17] and similarly the church has banned them from public office for fear of popular scandal and ridicule
>
> *Ecclesia removit huismodi a solemniter officiis propter derisionem et scandalum populare*
> *(Cited by Montford 2004: 30; see Opera de vita regulari, ed. J. J. Berthier*
> *(Rome, 1888–9, repr. Turin, 1950), II. 406.)*

Also in the 13th century Thomas of Chobham had commented on the public aspect of scandal as the defining criterion:

> When the apostolic rule says 'a bishop must be without fault,' the word 'fault' here means something deserving blame and condemnation; in other words, something that would cause scandal if it were made public.
> *(Summa confessorum, article 1, Thomas of Chobham 1968: 79–85)*

This emphasizes in/visibility as a measure by which people were judged fit, or not, to be a priest, something which the priest with his unfortunate molten lead incident was also keen to point out. Visibility of one's impairment had also been of concern to King Alfred: according to his biographer Asser, Alfred was afflicted by an unspecified illness for many years, so that at one point he entered a church and prayed that his present malady might be changed for some lesser infirmity which should not appear outwardly in the body lest it should render him useless and despised (Asser, *Life of Alfred*, ch. 74, see discussion of this episode by Kershaw 2001).

Practical considerations concerning disabled priests

In the high and later Middle Ages, that is, the period approximately from the twelfth to the fifteenth centuries, there is an apparent gulf between theory and practice. The theory, as in the canonical law texts outlined above, stated that ordained priests had to possess physical idoneity. Legal texts tend to be theoretical texts, that is, they do not necessarily reflect an actual, 'real' situation, but instead prescribe an ideal state. In practice, things may well be different. The registers of bishops, with their visitations records, paint far more of a 'real' picture of what condition – physically, mentally and materially – the clergy in a locality presented. One can study the actual practice, as evidenced by individual case-histories in the bishops' registers, acta and letters and, from the 15th century onwards, the supplications to the papal curia. By looking at such records in detail, one may consider what effect a certain health status had on the continued employability of the medieval priesthood, and question how much of an issue age-related retirement and incapacity were. The problem of a priest incapable of saying the mass or of elevating the host for the congregation to view, with its associated quasi-medicinal properties, went beyond just personal incapacity and questions of financial support (e.g. lack of employment as chaplains or chantry priests) to touch on the belief in the efficacy of liturgical ceremonial. By the later medieval period, institutional care may often have been offered to blind, aged and disabled priests (Rawcliffe 1999: 27–8; for further cases of deaf clergy see Lincoln Archives Office, Episcopal Register iii, fos 366^v–367^r; for generally 'decrepit' priests see Storey 1999: no. 431).

What to do with elderly and hence often impaired priests was a problem to the extent that already by the later 13th century a number of English and French hospitals were founded specifically to cater for elderly disabled, especially blind, priests. For instance, the hospital of St Saviour at Bury St Edmunds looked after aged and infirm priests from the later 13th century onwards, and by the 1240s a hospital for aged clerics had been established at Tournai. Specialist institutions for the mentally incapacitated did not yet exist. An abortive attempt was made in the 14th century, by the chaplain Robert Denton, to found a hospital at All Hallows, Barking, specifically for priests and others who 'suddenly fell into a frenzy and lost their memories', but the project failed due to lack of funding (Talbot 1967: 183). Therefore, mentally ill or senile clergy were neither confined nor treated any differently from clerics whose incompetence might be caused by other, more physical reasons (King 2010).

The intriguing case of Thomas de Capella, rector of Bletchingdon in Oxfordshire, has all the elements of a modern whodunit. Thomas's disappearance while in a state of 'temporary insanity', reports of his wanderings around the countryside, and subsequent reappearance a year and half later in 1293, apparently then of sound mind, was gleaned from the episcopal records of the vast diocese of Lincoln, to which Oxford belonged at the time (King 2010). With regard to attitudes toward the mentally ill, this story provides an illuminating aspect. What emerges strongly from analysis of the memoranda rolls of Bishop Sutton of Lincoln, for instance, with regard to the mentally ill vicar Hugh of St Martin, who appeared to have been taken advantage of by his parishioners (whose stealing from Hugh left him destitute), is that the bishop's prime concern was for the wellbeing of his diocesan clergy – an exemplary attitude for any modern manager who should take an interest in the health and safety of their staff. And to continue the modern analogy, the return to work after prolonged illness is gradually phased in again, with initial periods of supervision, so Bishop Sutton kept an eye on Hugh once he had regained his mental competence and checked on his progress. It was most unlikely that the church had to concern itself with so-called 'idiots' or natural fools, as the congenitally intellectually disabled were then termed, since people with such disabilities would not have been able to embark on an ecclesiastical career in the first place.

Another modern parallel also springs to mind when looking at the medieval role of coadjutor. Coadjutors were appointed in cases where the cleric in question was deemed incapable of doing the work he was responsible for, but where it was not possible to remove the cleric from his benefice – this is very similar to the situation regarding civil servants in many modern states, who cannot be 'sacked' simply for not doing their job effectively but only in extreme cases of (criminal) misdemeanour. The *Decretales* of Gregory IX had enshrined the principle that a benefice could not be removed in cases of physical illness and/or disability. It seems a logical step to grant the same right to the mentally ill and cognitively disabled too, and one must remember the 13th century was the era of the great lawyer-popes (and even bishops at local level more often than not had an academic background) who would have been keen exponents of strictly logical reasoning. The further cases from episcopal records of coadjutor appointments to clerics who were incurably ill, had become blind or were suffering from the deteriorations of old age (a possible case of senile dementia is particularly interesting) are in keeping with what one would expect as a demographic trend among a well-fed, low-risk occupational group, to use modern parlance (King 2010). Being relatively secure in terms of income and food supply and having little or no high-risk physical work (e.g. no fighting, no industrial accidents), it is the overall effects of ageing and specifically low-level degenerative diseases that cause problems for the clergy. Interestingly, this is corroborated by archaeological investigations, where palaeopathological examinations frequently indicate that monastic burial sites, and burials within confirmed ecclesiastical contexts, show higher levels of degenerative diseases caused by 'easy living' (well-fed rich diet, little physical exertion, greater age at death) than other contemporary burials. Most likely the real-life model for Friar Tuck really was fat (Patrick 2014).

Cultural constructions of disability

Physical impairment under medieval canon law was, as was described above, an irregularity that prevented the attainment of priesthood – or at least entry into higher orders – unless a special case was made and a dispensation granted. The impediments were called *debilitas corporis* and *defectus scientiae* in the *Decretalium collectiones* (*Liber extra* 1.9.10 and 3.6.1–6). But in general, canon law was more concerned about preventing people from marrying who could not fulfil their duty to 'multiply', i.e. those who were frigid, impotent or infertile (cf. Benkheira in this volume for similar concerns in early Islamic law). In contrast to most modern thinking on the matter, for medieval theologians and canonists, such as Gratian's *Decretum*, these were 'disabilities' and impediments to marriage. Opinions were reinforced by the early 13th-century *Decretals*, which contained a section 'The Frigid and the Hexed (*Maleficiatis*), and Inability to Copulate' (*Decretales* 4.15). As may be explained further, the 'title dealt with physical disabilities to the contracting of a valid marriage' (Noonan 1966: 289), but not with impediments pertaining to the priesthood. Canonists and theologians had explored various conditions which provided physical impediments to marriage, e.g. congenital bodily defects relating to the genitalia, mutilation and sorcery (see Dalla 1978 for Roman law on the matter of impotence). Robert of Courson (d. 1219) had said that the impossibility of intercourse was an impediment, which was sometimes caused by frigidity, sometimes by sorcery, sometimes by defect or vice (i.e. fault) of members and sometimes by poisonous abuse (i.e. homosexual practices):

> Sequitur de alio impedimento matrimonii quod est impossiblitas coeundi que provenit multiplici de causa quia quandoque provenit ex frig[id]itate, quandoque ex malefico, quandoque ex defectu vel ex vicio membrorum, quandoque ex infectione abusionis (...)
> *(Paris, Bibliothèque nationale, MS lat. 14524, Summa, XLII, 16, fo. 142[rb], cited in Baldwin 1994: 96, 294 n. 34)*

The medieval notion of what constituted a 'disability' was, in this sense then, a far more extended one than the commonly held modern European definition, which tends not to view infertility as a disability.

With regard to canonical law and disability, one may further investigate how medieval ecclesiastical decisions were justified, by asking what were the medical or canonical reasons for questioning idoneity of the clergy in the detailed records of the dioceses and the papacy. Such research might usefully pinpoint what types of health status typically attracted successful dispensations, and what meaning health, illness or impairment had with regard to enabling or disabling someone. Generally, minor impairments tended to escape the notice of ecclesiastical superiors, or were issued with a dispensation. Candidates for ordination were to possess physical idoneity, 'but minor disabilities could be overlooked as was the case with a man who had lost a finger in a battle. Such dispensations for physical disabilities were secured fairly easily, so long as the flaw did not interfere with the proper exercise of ministry' (Shinners and Dohar 1998: 52–3). The crucial test was whether a priest was able to celebrate mass, and if so, whether he could do so without arousing *scandalum*, i.e. causing his parishioners to remark on his demeanour, appearance or somatic condition, important aspects of sacerdotal idoneity that all the commentators, John de Burgh (*Pupilla Oculi* 7.3.4), Thomas of Chobham (*Summa confessorum* article 1) and the *Liber extra* (*titulus* xx) had remarked on in the passages quoted above.

In this discussion, one cannot escape addressing the apparent medieval link between illness and sin, a link that, it must be emphasized, has greater appeal to the modern view of the medieval period as one inherently 'dark', 'superstitious' or 'primitive' than is shaped by medieval sources themselves. The Fourth Lateran Council of 1215 did enact a canon, no. 22, with the incipit *Cum infirmitas* (sometimes also known as *Quum infirmitas*), which soon after became part of Gregory IX's codification of canon law, the *Decretales*, and hence acquired official status in the church. In *Cum infirmitas* is stated with regards to the apparent link between sin and illness: 'Since bodily infirmity is *sometimes* [my emphasis] caused by sin', the physician ought to ensure a patient hears confession before the physician then applies medical treatment, so that the soul is 'cured' prior to the body (cited in Amundsen 1996: 266). The canon does not, however, present an invariable causal link between sin and illness, it is only *sometimes* the case. One could argue that asking the physician to refrain from treatment until after confession is a way of hedging one's bets (in case the patient died, it would at least be with absolution), not a statement of immutable certainty.

Practically every believer in the Christian Middle Ages accepted that human beings in general were sinners, that sin therefore was something not just endemic to but part and parcel of the human condition – at least the post-lapsarian one – so that in the grand scheme of things physical disability, whether among the clergy or the laity, paled into insignificance.

Note

1 The matter was settled in a Circular Letter of 24 July 2003. While showing understanding for priests and lay persons not able to ingest gluten bread or wine and allowing the use of low-gluten hosts and mustum for both categories, the letter also states under C 3: 'A priest unable to receive Communion under the species of bread, including low-gluten hosts, may not celebrate the Eucharist individually, nor may he preside at a concelebration'. See <http://www.vatican.va/roman_curia/congregations/cfaith/documents/rc_con_cfaith_doc_20030724_pane-senza-glutine_en.html#top>.

Bibliography

Primary sources

Alfred the Great: Asser's Life of King Alfred and Other Contemporary Sources, ed. and tr. Simon Keynes and Michael Lapidge (London, 1983).
Corpus Iuris Canonici, ed. Emil Friedberg, 2 vols (Leipzig, 1879; repr. Graz, 1959).
Donaldson, Alexander (tr.), *The Clementine Homilies, with The Apostolical Constitutions*, Ante-Nicene Christian Library 17 (Edinburgh, 1880).
Gratian, *Decretum Gratiani*, ed. Emil Friedberg, 2 vols (Leipzig, 1879; repr. Graz, 1959).
Liber extra (= *Decretales Gregorii IX*), ed. Emil Friedberg, 2 vols (Leipzig, 1879; repr. Graz, 1959).
John de Burgh, *Pupilla Oculi* (London, 1515).
Storey, R. L. (ed.), *The Register of Gilbert Welton, Bishop of Carlisle, 1353–1362* (Woodbridge, 1999).
Thomas of Chobham, *Summa confessorum*, ed. F. Broomfield, Analecta mediaevalia Namurcensia 25 (Louvain, 1968).

Dispensation records

Calendar of Entries in the Papal Registers Relating to Great Britain and Ireland: Papal Letters, 17 vols (Dublin and London, 1893–1994) [registers cover period 1198–1503].

English Episcopal Acta, to date 42 vols (Oxford University Press for the British Academy, 1980–)

English episcopal registers: editions of many medieval rolls, letters and registers of dioceses are available in print, mainly in the *Lincoln Record Society* and *Canterbury and York Society* volumes (both publications managed by the publishers Boydell & Brewer), and are too numerous to list fully here; as examples one may cite *The Rolls and Register of Bishop Oliver Sutton, 1280–1299*, ed. Rosalind Hill, 8 vols (Hereford: Lincoln Record Society, 1942–86), which detail the case of the 'Mad Rector' in 1292; other local record societies have produced registers pertaining to their region, e.g. the Sussex Record Society or the Somerset Record Society.

German episcopal registers, letters and acta: in progress is the supra-regional series *Regesta Pontificum Romanorum. Germania Pontificia*, series ed. Rudolf Hiestand from 1992, ed. Klaus Herbers from 2005.

Registres et lettres des Papes du XIIIe siècle, 32 vols (Rome, 1883–); electronic version via Brepols online database 'Ut per litteras apostolicas'.

Registres et lettres des Papes du XIVe siècle, 48 vols (Rome, 1899–); electronic version via Brepols online database 'Ut per litteras apostolicas'.

Repertorium Germanicum [RG], series published by the Deutsches Historisches Institut in Rom, 9 vols (1916–2004) [calendar of people and places in papal registers pertaining to dioceses in the Holy Roman Empire of German Nations, to date covering period 1378–1484]; online at <http://194.242.233.132/denqRG/index.htm>.

Schmugge, Ludwig (main ed.), *Repertorium Poenitentiariae Germanicum* [RPG], series published by the Deutsches Historisches Institut in Rom (Tübingen/Berlin: De Gruyter, 1998–); online at <http://www.romana-repertoria.net/993.html>; volumes to date: I. *Eugen IV (1431–1447);* II. *Nikolaus V (1447–1455);* III. *Calixt III (1455–1458);* IV. *Pius II (1458–1464);* V *Paul II (1464–1471);* VI *Sixtus IV (1471–1484);* VII. *Innozenz VIII (1484–1492);* VIII *Alexander VI (1492–1503).*

Smith, David M. (ed.), *English Episcopal Acta*, 28 vols (London, 1980–).

Smith, David M., *Guide to Bishops' Registers of England and Wales: A Survey from the Middle Ages to the Abolition of Episcopacy in 1646* (London, 1981).

Smith, David M., *Supplement to the Guide to Bishops' Registers of England and Wales* (York, 2004).

Supplications from England and Wales in the Registers of the Apostolic Penitentiary, 1410–1503, ed. Peter D. Clarke and Patrick N. R. Zutshi, I. *1410–1464* (Woodbridge, 2013); II. *1464–1492* (Woodbridge, 2014); III. *1492–1503* (Woodbridge, 2015).

Secondary literature

Amundsen, Darrel W., *Medicine, Society, and Faith in the Ancient and Medieval Worlds* (Baltimore, MD, and London, 1996).

Angenendt, Arnold, *Geschichte der Religiosität im Mittelalter* (Darmstadt, 1997).

Baldwin, John H., *The Language of Sex: Five Voices from Northern France around 1200* (Chicago, IL, and London, 1994).

Bredberg, Elizabeth, 'Writing Disability History: Problems, Perspectives and Sources', *Disability and Society* 14/2 (1999), 189–201.

Brundage, James A., *Medieval Canon Law* (London and New York, 1995).

Brundage, James A., *The Medieval Origins of the Legal Profession* (Chicago, IL, and London, 2008).

Bunting, Madeleine, 'Wafer Allergy Bars Priests', *Guardian*, 10 Oct. 1995.

Dalla, Danilo, *L'incapacità sessuale in diritto romano* (Milan, 1978).

Douglas, Mary, *Purity and Danger: An Analysis of Concepts of Pollution and Taboo* (New York, 1966).

Esch, Arnold, *Wahre Geschichten aus dem Mittelalter: Kleine Schicksale selbst erzählt in Schreiben an den Papst* (Munich, 2010).

Evans, Gillian Rosemary, *Law and Theology in the Middle Ages* (London and New York, 2002).

Fox, Robin Lane, *Pagans and Christians in the Mediterranean World from the Second Century AD to the Conversion of Constantine* (London, 1986).

Kershaw, Paul, 'Illness, Power and Prayer in Asser's *Life of King Alfred*', *Early Medieval Europe* 10/2 (2001), 201–24.

King, James R., 'The Mysterious Case of the "Mad" Rector of Bletchingdon: The Treatment of Mentally Ill Clergy in Late Thirteenth-Century England', in W. J. Turner (ed.), *Madness in Medieval Law and Custom* (Leiden, 2010), 57–80.

Mellinkoff, Ruth, *Outcasts: Signs of Otherness in Northern European Art of the Late Middle Ages*, 2 vols (Berkeley-Los Angeles, CA, and Oxford, 1993).

Metzler, Irina, *Disability in Medieval Europe: Thinking about Physical Impairment during the High Middle Ages, c.1100–1400* (London and New York, 2006).

Metzler, Irina, *A Social History of Disability in the Middle Ages: Cultural Considerations of Physical Impairment* (London and New York, 2013).

Montford, Angela, 'Fit to Preach and Pray: Considerations of Occupational Health in the Mendicant Orders', in R. N. Swanson (ed.), *The Use and Abuse of Time in Christian History* (Woodbridge, 2002), 95–106.

Montford, Angela, *Health, Sickness, Medicine and the Friars in the Thirteenth and Fourteenth Centuries* (Aldershot, 2004).

Noonan, John T., *Contraception: A History of its Treatment by the Catholic Theologians and Canonists* (Cambridge, MA, 1966).

Orchard, Bernard, Sutcliffe, Edmund F., Fuller, Reginald C., and Russell, Ralph (eds), *A Catholic Commentary on Holy Scripture* (London, 1953).

Patrick, Pip, *The 'Obese Medieval Monk': A Multidisciplinary Study of a Stereotype* (Oxford, 2014).

Rawcliffe, Carole, *Medicine for the Soul: The Life, Death and Resurrection of an English Medieval Hospital* (Stroud, 1999).

Shinners, John, and Dohar, William J. (eds), *Pastors and the Care of Souls in Medieval England* (Notre Dame, IN, 1998).

Talbot, Charles H., *Medicine in Medieval England* (London, 1967).

Wheatley, Edward, *Stumbling Blocks Before the Blind: Medieval Constructions of a Disability* (Ann Arbor, MI, 2013).

32

THE IMPERFECT BODY IN NAZI GERMANY

Ancient concepts, modern technologies

Toon Van Houdt

Adolf Hitler was an inveterate chatterbox and loved to hear his own voice, whether he was dwelling in the private rooms of his office in Berlin or in the gaudy, but still cosy, country house which he had built in the mountains of Obersalzburg; during, and especially after, lunch and before the film which he regularly showed his guests – a select group of his privileged intimates – in the evenings. Later, during the war, the table-talks, or rather monologues, were held in the Führer's military headquarters and there was no time for screening films. Hitler would speak for hours about one or another of his favourite topics. His repertoire was limited and his position was usually well-known in advance. One of his most preferred subjects was the greatness of classical Antiquity; time and again he returned to the topic and could talk about it interminably, even in the middle of the war. Hitler's knowledge of Greek and Roman Antiquity was mediocre, but he nevertheless praised it highly (Demandt 2001: 136–57; Ryback 2008). Perhaps it was because he was the Führer and, as such, wished to found a thousand-year empire which would rival the powerful Roman Empire: first he would take Europe, and then he would conquer the whole world.

Hitler understood very well that such an empire could not be founded on the basis of the vague Germanic mysticism which the Nazi-ideologue Alfred Rosenberg or Heinrich Himmler, the leader of the SS, were trying to propagate, each in his own manner. That a monumental statue was raised in honour of the Germanic warrior Arminius (Hermann in German), who in 9 CE had, in a humiliating manner, wiped out the legion of the Roman general Varus in the Teutoburger Forest (Demandt 2001: 144–5; Benario 2004: 83–94) was good. And praising the Germanic virtues as described in a short work by the Roman writer Tacitus (physical prowess, desire for war, chastity, 'racial purity') was fine, too (Demandt 2001: 136); but exterminating Christianity and substituting a Germanic cult to be celebrated with the meagre leftovers of an equally meagre old-Germanic culture – no, that was going too far, according to Hitler (Chapoutot 2008: 83–8; Pringle 2006; Krebs 2011: 201–8). It would needlessly offend and alienate not only the leaders of the church but also ordinary people and the socio-economic elite of the country. And that must not happen, as he badly needed those groups, to build his thousand-year empire and, first of all, to win the world war which was sure to come, even though as late as in August 1939 Hitler was hoping that the enemy would be too weak, too cowardly and too decadent to check his unbridled urge for expansion. Hitler was mistaken, and the war did indeed break out. The Führer's grand plans to give the capital of his empire-to-be a suitably imperial air were reluctantly put on hold, while the German economy turned into a war economy.

Hitler's architectural plans were surely ambitious, not to say megalomaniac. His new Berlin, which in the future would be given the (Latin) name *Germania*, was not only to overshadow the splendour of Rome which the emperor Augustus had constructed in his lifetime, but also to contrast sharply with contemporary capitals like London and Paris (Hitler 2000: 98). Even when thousands of years had passed Germania's archaeological remains would bear witness to the lost glory of Nazi Germany. Hitler's favourite architect Albert Speer deliberately developed a building style which was calculated to remain beautiful and impressive as it decayed: glass and steel were avoided as far as possible while marble and granite were used in abundance (Hitler 2000: 81; Chapoutot 2008: 455–9).

The gigantic domed building which Speer designed for Germania's political heart was many times higher than Rome's famous Pantheon; at the same time it would be the world's highest building. That edifice would be joined, by means of a broad avenue, several miles long, to the triumphal arch which was to stand ostentatiously in front of the so-called Great Hall. That Hall looked – at least as a model – like an excessively large classical temple, while the 120-metre-high triumphal arch in Hitler's honour was infinitely larger, and thus infinitely more impressive, than the famous Arch of Constantine in Rome or the renowned Arc de Triomphe in Paris. Though at the beginning his explicit intention had been to furnish the centre of the new Berlin with a sober, 'Doric' décor, Speer's drafts, under the Führer's influence, became more and more bombastic. Not until many decades later, in the Spandau prison, did Speer understand the deeper meaning of that development: the architecture of public buildings which Hitler wished to create had to support his imperial and imperialist ambitions in a visual manner. As a result the government buildings which were to be re-erected showed, to a higher and higher degree, extravagance and luxury like that of ancient eastern tyrants and of the Roman emperors of late Antiquity. It was an architecture of decadence, a clear harbinger of the destiny awaiting Hitler and his supposedly thousand-year empire – certain and premature ruin (Speer 2000: 231–2; Chapoutot 2008: 297–316).

Greek Germans and German Greeks

As mentioned, Hitler knew his history to a limited, but sufficient, extent. That is, sufficient to know that the ancient Germans were, on the whole, savage and uncivilized brutes, and had remained so for many centuries while, on the other hand, the Greeks and Romans had built a superior civilization and founded a powerful empire – an empire of a sort which he, for the time being, could only dream of, as his friend and ally Mussolini had kindly reminded him at their first meeting in Venice in June 1934. German scholars liked to represent Italians as a racially impure, and therefore physically and morally inferior, people. Mussolini retaliated: that silly theory was being put forward by representatives of a people which did not even know how to write at a time when Rome had had its Caesar, its Vergil and its Augustus (Losemann 1999: 227; Chapoutot 2008: 88–91).

Hitler did not have much to put forward in response. In a conversation with Himmler he would teasingly repeat Mussolini's comment:

> At a time when other people already had paved roads, we hadn't the slightest evidence of civilisation to show. [...] Those who had remained in Holstein have not changed in two thousand years, whilst those who had emigrated to Greece raised themselves to the level of civilization.
>
> *(Hitler 2000: 289–90)*

Nevertheless, Hitler had a decisive reply to that marked contrast, which fitted in seamlessly with the views of the classical authors which he knew. They had already pointed out the great impact of climate and geographical circumstances on any people. The Führer took over that reasoning in its entirety:

> The Germanic needed a sunny climate to enable his qualities to develop. It was in Greece and Italy that the Germanic spirit found the first terrain favourable to its blossoming. [...] For any Roman, the fact of being sent to *Germania* was regarded as a punishment – rather like what it used to mean to us to be sent to Posen. You can imagine those rainy, grey regions, transformed into quagmires as far as eye could see.
> *(Hitler 2000: 289; Demandt 2001: 144–5; Pringle 2006: 66)*

Those were provocative and offensive words, since Hitler knew all too well that his faithful follower Himmler idolized Germanic prehistory and was wholly convinced that archaeological and (pre)historical investigation would irrefutably reveal the cultural supremacy of the ancient Germans. To that purpose he had founded Ahnenerbe, a scientific group which soon grew into a prestigious and well-staffed research institute, even though the high expectations were never fulfilled. In spite of their assiduous searches, their diligent forgery and their wild fantasies, there was never a trace found of the highly developed and technologically superior civilization which would – among other advantages – provide the Nazis with the revolutionary superweapon of which they were dreaming (Pringle 2006: 80–1 and 281–90).

It is easy to conclude from the table talks quoted above that Hitler took it for granted that the ancient Greeks and Romans were in fact Germans. But the opposite was equally true: in his opinion the Germans were, in essence, Greeks. This is a view which had taken root in Germany as early as the eighteenth century. In his influential work *The Myth of the Twentieth Century* (1930) Rosenberg would give it an explicitly Nazi twist. Following the nineteenth-century German philologist Karl-Otfried Müller, Rosenberg distinguished sharply between two specific ethnic groups which were diametrically opposed in character, mentality, and origin: the 'northern' Dorians and the 'southern' Ionians. The Dorians were characterized by typically northern frugality, moderation, perseverance, rationality and spirit of freedom (it is no coincidence that the same qualities were readily ascribed to the good German Protestant). This was contrasted with the immoderate and luxurious way of life and the impulsive, servile character of the Ionians.

The description of the Dorians as 'northern' must also be taken literally: according to Müller they had indeed originated in the north. In ancient times they had diverged from a people who most likely had moved and spread throughout Europe from northern Germany. To put it simply, the Dorians were in fact Germans, and vice versa. So there was not only a certain cultural similarity between 'real' (that is, Dorian) Greeks and Germans, but also an actual blood relationship. Rosenberg liked to elaborate on this, arguing at length that the Greeks were in fact Aryans. Ancient Greeks who did not live up to the stereotype of the tall, handsome, and athletic Aryan were without further ado 'disqualified' as being impure Greeks. That was especially true of Socrates. According to Rosenberg he belonged to 'the stupid, hairy, negroid-eastern race-type'. Socrates was not only a typical product of mixture of races, he had also, with his 'race-destroying' teaching, contributed to a large extent to this hybridization. With his depraved doctrine about the good he undermined the racially pure and elitist educational ideal of the real, true Greeks and opened the gates for large-scale mixture of races. Greeks and non-Greeks, Aryans and Semites – under the influence of Socrates they all became part of the same worldwide, multi-racial community (Rosenberg 1938: 282–4; Chapoutot 2008: 261–5).

This had disastrous consequences. Rosenberg got his inspiration on this point from the works of Hans F. K. Günther (1891–1968), one of the most popular practitioners of the biology of race in Germany in the 1920s and 1930s, who through his work had ended up in Nazi territory. He had trained as a philologist, but in 1930 he was the first to be appointed professor of social anthropology at the university of Jena – a chair which the Nazi regime had created especially for him. Hitler even took the trouble to be present in person at Günther's inaugural lecture. And on 1 May 1932 Günther himself enlisted as member of the National-Socialist Workers' Party (the NSDAP).

'Social anthropology' simply means 'racial doctrine'. And within the framework of this racial doctrine Günther gives a prominent place to physiognomy as a diagnostic tool. According to Günther the looks of a person reveal in a perfectly trustworthy manner his or her racial origin and also give an instantaneous and unequivocal indication of his or her racially inherited mental features. Günther's physiognomy is partly craniometric: the measures of cranium and face provide evidence of a person's belonging to a certain race. Günther distinguishes various races, and the place of honour is, unsurprisingly, given to the so-called 'nordic' race. He himself does not use the word 'Aryan', but to his readers the two terms were interchangeable:

> The nordic race is tall, long-legged, and slender. The limbs appear very slender [...] The nordic race is dolichocephalic and narrow-faced [...]. The face is narrow with a fairly narrow forehead, narrow, marked nose and a narrow lower jaw with a pronounced chin. The shape of the face of the nordic race makes a characteristically bold impression. The skin [...] is light pink and lets the blood show through, so that it looks particularly lively and moreover, as a rule, somewhat cool or fresh. The skin of the face, at least in the youth, and in the female sex fairly often until middle age, makes an impression of 'milk and blood'. The hair colour is blond [...]. Persons who are light blond in their youth later often become dark blond, fairly often also darkhaired: a phenomenon which is taken as a sign of a nordic streak. Nordic eyes [...] are blue, bluish grey, or grey. Nordic eyes often have a radiant quality, and under the influence of certain emotions also an expression which the Romans experienced as a 'terrifying look' in the Germans.
>
> *(Günther 1935: 21–5)*

The beautiful, radiant looks of a nordic person reveal superior spiritual qualities. Here is a selection of catchwords from Günther's racial psychology: cool, determined, resolute, noble, heroic, coolly judicious, an urge for truthfulness, an inclination to chivalrous justice, visionary leadership, creative power in technology, science and art, calm in movements and words, youthful, vivid feeling for nature, an inclination to physical exercise, walking and trekking, and to cleanliness and a carefully kept appearance (Günther 1935: 59–61).

The most perfect 'realization' of the nordic race is, according to Günther, found in classical Greek man. By means of that blood relationship between today's Germans and the ancient Greeks, the Greek ideal may be presented as an example which must be followed: just as the ancient Greeks did, contemporary Germans should strive for harmonious development of both body and soul. The ancient ideal – a beautiful soul in a beautiful body – at the same time becomes the true 'spirit of the nordic movement'. Typically enough, the incorporation of the ancient Greeks into the nordic race is also carried out by physiognomic reasoning:

> The bodies and heads which ancient artists created freely (that is, not from a live model) show that the Greek could only conceive of the ideal image of handsome and heroic man as embodied in the nordic race. The nordic race is the material from which artists shape gods and heroes.
>
> *(Günther 1929: 25)*

The classical Greek sculptures are a model for the contemporary representatives of the nordic race because those classical Greek sculptures were themselves modelled on excellent representatives of the nordic race. Here, for the sake of convenience, Günther overlooks the high degree of idealization displayed by ancient sculpture.

Contrasted with the superior nordic race are other races which, from physical as well as mental viewpoint, differ from the nordic race and are humiliatingly inferior to it. This applies especially to the Jews who are subjected to an extremely detailed racial-physiognomic description. This is as strange as it is typical. Strange, since the Jews, according to Günther, do not constitute a separate race but are the sad result of a mixture of races. Typical, since the author, with his allegedly scientific-physiognomic description, actively contributes to the stigmatization and criminalization of the Jews which, in Nazi Germany, would soon lead to the so-called *Endlösung* (complete annihilation).

Günther's description of the prototypical Jew certainly leaves nothing to the imagination. Contrasted with the well-proportioned, radiantly white northerner is the dark-skinned Jew with his bandy legs (proof of physical weakness, often ascribed to an appalling lack of body-care and physical training, and at the same time an outspokenly animal characteristic) and his flat feet (traditionally ascribed to black people and already by Cesare Lombroso regarded as an unmistakable sign of criminal tendencies). Contrasted with the refined and straight nose of the northerner is the Jew's typical hook-nose, though Günther readily admits that it is found less frequently than is commonly believed. And at least the Jews who live in Central Europe display, according to the author, negroid characteristics. It is quite obvious, then, that according to Günther the typical Jew does not in any respect meet the classical Greek (read: nordic) ideal of beauty. With the physiognomic principle in mind, Günther can only conclude that the Jew also lacks the high-minded mental features of the pure northerner. And indeed: the description of the Jew's outer appearance seamlessly changes into a summary of typically Jewish criminal behaviour. The criminalization goes as far as the ill-founded claim that the human trafficking of girls in contemporary Germany is an exclusively Jewish phenomenon. Jews assault and kidnap, and in the popular iconography of the 1930s and 1940s this picture is even more accentuated: Jews are not only kidnappers, but even cannibals. In short, Jews are monsters rather than human beings (Blankenburg 1996; Gray 2004: 219–72; Jahn 2010).

Platonic utopia, Nazi dystopia

Günther himself does not take that last step. Nevertheless he, too, regards the Jews as a huge problem – a problem of racial hygiene, that is. All over Europe, and beyond, Jews mix with pure and superior northerners and by doing so they bring about large-scale degeneration. This must be urgently checked. Mixture of races must be avoided at any cost, by elimination of the Jews and sterilization of racially impure Germans. But selecting was easier said than done, for the criteria used by Günther and other German anthropologists often turned out to be too vague or not generally valid. Therefore, in February 1942, Günther's student Bruno Beger, together with the anatomist August Hirt, put together a promising research project: a large-scale comparative physiognomic investigation of Jews from more or less all regions in Europe and Central Asia. The aim was to establish, once and for all and indisputably, the distinctive characteristics of the Jewish race, in order to facilitate further tracing, isolation and liquidation of all Jews in the world. The practical method would be the selection of 'interesting' specimens from the human material which was readily and amply available in the concentration camp of Auschwitz. There the selected 'objects', completely naked, would be subjected to the initial physiognomic examination. They would be measured, photographed or filmed, and there would even be plaster casts made of the more striking heads of certain persons. Thereupon all that study material – both living and lifeless – would be brought by train to the smaller concentration camp of Natzweiler in the Vosges. There the selected Jewish men and women would be subjected to gruesome medical experiments and finally gassed. The bodies would end up in the anatomical institute at the German university of Strasbourg, where they would be immersed in a bath of caustic acid and reduced to clean skeletons, then carefully stored; occasionally they would be exhibited. Himmler, the leader of the SS, was wildly excited about the project when it was presented and immediately authorized it; his belief in the principles of (racial) physiognomics was absolute (Pringle 2006: 239–56).

However, systematic liquidation of Jews was not enough from the viewpoint of racial hygiene. It had to be combined with actual improvement of the nordic race by means of elimination of inferior specimens. Günther was outspoken in his argumentation for detention, and even elimination, of the physically and mentally disabled, and he found support for this in ancient Greece. Like Hitler, Günther was frank about his great admiration for the Spartan state. He called it the first truly 'popular' state – a state which kept its own population racially pure by means of a radical, if fairly primitive, eugenic programme. According to Günther, that programme was based on two cornerstones: avoidance of mixture of races and killing of deformed children (Losemann 1999: 222; Demandt 2001: 143; on Spartan eugenics see Huys 1996). Nevertheless, it was especially in the works of the Greek philosopher Plato that Günther found his inspiration for the authoritarian and eugenically organized *Volksstaat* which he had in mind. In his work *Plato als Hüter des Lebens* (*Plato as the Guardian of Life*), first published in Munich in 1928, Günther interpreted Plato's ideas from the point of view of racial hygiene. The book was a great success and a second enlarged edition was published in 1935. After all, Günther's ideas meshed frighteningly well with the racial politics of the Nazis.

In his extensive work *The Republic* Plato drafted the blueprint of an ideal political community, which, according to him, consists of three classes. The highest class is the class of guardians or philosopher-kings, the embodiment of understanding, who are prepared for their ruling tasks by extensive education in mathematics and philosophy. The second class consists of the auxiliary guardians or soldiers, who ensure the internal and external security of the state. At the bottom is the class of farmers and artisans, who are responsible for the maintenance of the entire community. From this short description it is clear that Plato's utopia is based on the primacy of the spirit; there is absolutely no question of racial division of the population. Nevertheless Günther would, in a fairly forced manner, translate Plato's view into strictly racial terms. The Platonic class of guardians is without hesitation equated with a class of northerners, who are selected on the basis of physical power rather than spiritual characteristics, such as understanding or wisdom. The eugenic programme which Plato unfolds in *The Republic* is thereupon reinterpreted in the racial sense. It is indeed impossible to deny that eugenics are a mainstay of Plato's ideal state: the producing and bringing up of guardians is literally compared to the breeding of purebred animals (Plato, *Republic* 5, 458a–460c).

While Plato devised a eugenic programme to safeguard the relatively limited group of guardians, Günther turned it into a very broad programme for safeguarding and improving an entire race, that is, the nordic race. A state-controlled breeding farm for future guardians in combination with discouragement from breeding for inferior citizens, and state-organized nurturing and upbringing of future leaders in combination with detention of worthless and disturbing elements of the community: this was music to the ears of Günther and certain leading Nazis. And indeed, in this racial reinterpretation Plato's eugenics has suspiciously many features in common with the '*Lebensborn*-project' – which was extremely secret in those days but has since become infamous – which Heinrich Himmler had launched in December 1935 in order to further improve and expand the nordic, or Aryan, race. Racially pure Aryan women were sought – and later even kidnapped – to be impregnated by SS-officers. To Himmler and his companions in spirit women were indeed, from the first to the last, human breeding mares. The children who were the result of such matings were to be raised and educated at the bosom of the SS. Himmler ardently dreamed of (once more) providing Germany with a genetic aristocracy, and classically inspired academics like Günther delivered to him the necessary intellectual ammunition (Joshi 2011).

Günther personally had little or nothing to do with the *Lebensborn*-project, or with other SS-programmes for racial cleansing. He was, and all his life remained, an introverted, somewhat asocial, scholarly recluse. Moreover, it was precisely his ideas on racial biology which in the course of time caused a certain cooling of his relationship with the Nazi regime, which indeed found his opinions much too radical. According to Günther's calculations, no more than 52 per cent of the Germans could claim a nordic origin; 48 per cent of the Germans at that time did not have a single drop of Aryan blood. In fact the situation was even worse: just 6 to 8 per cent of all Germans were racially pure, he wrote, while 45 to 50 per cent were contaminated by foreign blood, and the rest belonged to inferior races. So racial mixture had already occurred on an alarmingly large scale, and with all the disastrous degenerative consequences which could be expected (Pringle 2006: 34-36). This lies behind the urgency with which Günther argued for his Plato-inspired eugenic programme. But it is easy to see how a radical political rendering of that programme would thoroughly disrupt German society, and that was something which the Germans could not afford on the eve of a world war.

Another, pragmatic, reason played a part, too. As has been said, Günther took a fairly static concept of race for granted. That made it very difficult for many confirmed and hardworking Nazis to present themselves as true representatives of the nordic race. And that was hardly acceptable to high-ranking Nazis who wished to reward deserving members of their party and people by granting them – all pure race-biology notwithstanding – a certificate of being *rassisch hochwertig*. A rigorous application of Günther's racial doctrine would even discredit leaders like Hitler and Himmler, whose looks were hardly Aryan, and this was naturally very embarrassing. And so, in Nazi practice, the soup of racial biology may have been served piping hot by Günther and other scientists but it cooled considerably before it was eaten, and for very opportunistic reasons (Stock 2004; Pringle 2006: 41–42).

The perfect body

Hitler called a spade a spade: according to him the Aryan body had in Nazi Germany reached a perfection which had earlier been realized only by the ancient Greeks. And in his eyes the Germans were the modern Greeks – or in any case had to become the modern Greeks as soon as possible. They had to grow into a race of 'supermen' and 'superwomen', and for that a careful application of the elementary principles of classical Greek education was essential. In *Mein Kampf* and in his many table talks Hitler liked to refer to the Spartan variant of that education which, even more than its Athenian counterpart, put extremely strong stress on physical hardening (Weiler 2001: 188). To Hitler a harmonious connection between body and mind was of the utmost importance, but he took the primacy of the body for granted. The well-known phrase 'a sound mind in a sound body' (*mens sana in corpore sano*) took on a very pregnant meaning:

> (Even here) there must be a certain harmony. A decayed body is not made one whit more aesthetic by a brilliant mind, and in fact the highest intellectual training could not be justified at all if its possessors were at the same time physically degenerate and crippled, weak-willed, wavering and cowardly in character. What makes the Greek

ideal of beauty immortal is the marvelous pairing of magnificent bodily beauty with brilliant mind and noble soul.

(Hitler 1939: 395–6; Speer 2000: 150–1; Mosse 1996: 161; Weiler 2001: 171–2)

Hitler's ideal was interpreted in an exemplary manner in the sculptures by Nazi-inspired artists such as Arno Breker and Josef Thorak. They gave actual shape to the aesthetic utopia which Hitler and his fellow party-members had in mind: Aryan sportsmen and warriors of marble or bronze which give an impression of being classical and therefore obtain a timeless, eternal quality; smooth, muscled bodies which evoke steely will-power and aggressive impetuousness; naked bodies which for the most part radiate little or no eroticism – as a rule they are too hard and too stylized. Some of those sculptures got a place at the monumental stadium which was built for the 1936 Olympic Games in Berlin, others were intended for the 1937 World Fair in Paris, where Nazi Germany wanted to demonstrate its self-proclaimed cultural supremacy, while others still were to impress visitors, German as well as foreign, to the new capital of Germania. And they were certainly impressive, but in comparison with their ancient models they were also hopelessly artificial, and therefore lacking both soul and life (Mosse 1996: 170–4; Peeters 2007: 179–96).

The sculptures by Breker, Thorak and other Nazi artists did not have just a decorative function, quite the opposite. Their psychological effect was distinctly phrased by Hans Surén, one of the most prominent German gymnastics pedagogues of the years between the wars:

The contemplation of an exemplary body releases a profound pedagogical influence not only in the physical, but also in the mental sphere. The nakedness of a noble body forms an unusually strong incitement to follow – this the ancient Greeks knew well.

(Surén 1925, quoted in Chapoutot 2008: 228; Möhring 2004)

Continuous and varied contemplation of ideal 'Aryan' beauty would, almost by itself, produce perfect Aryans: that was the essentially very classical (Platonic) reasoning by certain Nazi art connoisseurs. The sight makes sure that the Idea of immaculate beauty is fixed in the mind of the beholder, and that Idea will then animate the matter and change and improve the body (Chapoutot 2008: 229–30). That process, however, also requires a personal effort, as Surén and other gymnastics teachers added. Ordinary people could, and had to, become living sculptures by means of intensive exercise of the body, at school, but especially outside school, in gymnasia and sports complexes and, perhaps even better, in the open air, naked or nearly naked, just as the Greek youth in ancient times hardened their naked bodies – and thereby also their minds – in the gymnasium, without embarrassment or shame (Wildmann 1998; Diehl 2006).

Despite the special importance of body culture in Nazi Germany there was, at the beginning, much scepticism about the Olympic Games: internationalism and pacifism did not mesh with the official doctrine. That attitude changed drastically as soon as the huge propagandist possibilities of the world event became clear. From 1933 everything was done to make sure that the winter and summer games of 1936 would be held in Germany. This was by no means a certainty: several members of the International Olympic Committee raised serious objections. After endless discussions about the treatment of Jews – especially Jewish athletes – in Germany, the request was nevertheless finally granted. On 6 February 1936 the winter games started in Garmisch-Partenkirchen, and on 1 August the same year the summer games were – while the rain was pouring down – solemnly opened in Berlin (Walters 1996: 4–63).

Both events had the same aim. The Nazi leaders wanted to show the new Germany to the world: powerful and efficient, and at the same time civilized and peaceful. Furthermore they wished to place the country as a prominent sports nation on the map: it was time to bring the 'New German

man and woman' into the limelight. Some wanted to go even further and dreamed openly about a thorough 'Nazification' of the Olympic Games. Thus there was a secret plan to have the games organized in Nazi Germany for ever, but the war put a spoke in the wheel. Nevertheless, during the winter and summer games of 1936 Olympic symbolism blended with Nazi symbolism. To a certain extent such a blend was unavoidable, as the games were indeed organized on Nazi territory. Members and leaders of the party were prominently present all the time, flags with the well-known swastika hung everywhere, many athletes enthusiastically (or half-heartedly) made the Nazi salute – or very demonstrably did not. That blend was also the result of the fact that both the modern Olympic movement and Nazi Germany claimed a classical Greek heritage. In any case, during the games of 1936 the tie with ancient Greece was strongly emphasized. For the winter games a new ski stadium was built, with place for an audience of no less than 15,000 persons. The two gates were flanked by enormous pillars on which Greek statues were displayed; one of them held a German eagle in its left hand. And during the summer games Aeschylus' *Oresteia* was staged: a series of classical tragedies which were systematically interpreted as the story of the triumph of the Aryan race (Flashar 1991: 164–8; Walters 1996: 64–5).

That fairly ostentatious recycling of ancient Greece is also found in the double-film *Olympia*, which Leni Riefenstahl (1902–2003) shot at the summer games in Berlin. The question is whether, with this film, she fully subscribed to the ideology of the regime. After the war she strongly denied this, and to save herself she happily presented herself as an independent director who had simply wanted to make an artistic film. She emphatically pointed out that she had not worked on the authority of the minister of propaganda Joseph Goebbels, but of Carl Diem, who chaired the committee which dealt with the organization of the German games, and that, financially and logistically, she was not supported by the Nazi government but by a company called Olympia-Film GmBH, which, moreover, she herself had founded. In any case, she argued, she had never been a member of the NSDAP.

This is contradicted by the fact that when *Olympia* appeared in 1938 it was indeed immediately considered a beautiful sample of Nazi propaganda, and that perception was strengthened by Riefenstahl's very close ties to different Nazi leaders, not least to Hitler himself. Like so many others Riefenstahl was spellbound by the Führer after having heard him speak at a party meeting. Immediately after attending an assembly in March 1932 she asked for a private audience with him, and this was the beginning of a long-lasting friendship – a heartfelt and artistically fruitful friendship (Trimborn 2002: 81).

In September 1933 the *Reichsparteitag des Sieges* was to take place. Already in June that year Hitler asked Riefenstahl to perpetuate the historic event on film and she happily accepted the offer. The result was the sixty-minute propaganda film *Sieg des Glaubens*, the first in a series of three films of party rallies which would be counted to her disadvantage after the war. Hitler was very pleased with her work, which led to more. In 1935 he himself commissioned Riefenstahl to record the summer games in Berlin; Goebbels was simply skipped and Riefenstahl eagerly jumped at the offer. After much labour her double-film *Olympia* had its premiere on 20 April 1938, and on 1 May it received the State Prize, the highest film award of the Third Reich. With the same film and in the same year Riefenstahl carried off first prize at the film festival of Venice. In the United States, too, her film was received with open arms. And in 1939 the International Olympic Committee awarded her a gold medal and a certificate. After the war, Riefenstahl would deftly play the card of that international recognition to prove that her film was no piece of propaganda.

Olympia seamlessly joined in the Nazi glorification of the young and powerful body – a glorification moulded in pictures which were very recognizable to the Nazi regime and which were also systematically employed by that regime. With *Olympia* Riefenstahl testified to her great admiration for physical perfection – an admiration which she may have shared with the Nazis but by no means with them only (Zweiniger-Bargielowska 2006; Blanshard 2007: 336–7). She had displayed that fascination before her first meeting with Hitler – as a skilled dancer, mountain-climbing actress and director of *Das blaue Licht*, a film which was not directly intended to serve as Nazi propaganda.

As we have seen, ancient Greece played a crucial part in the Nazi cult of the perfect, racially pure body. Also in Riefenstahl's film Greece is prominently present. In the long prologue a gradual transition from ancient to modern times is evoked; the two coalesce, as it were. At first the spectator's eye roams over a landscape strewn with ruins of temples and those scenes alternate with pictures of classical sculptures. Those sculptures, in turn, fluidly change into the film's presentation of contemporary athletes. In this manner the picture of Myron's statue of a discus thrower – one of Hitler's favourite classical sculptures – changes into a picture of a real discus thrower who is standing in the same position as the sculpture but – unlike the statue – is in full action (Demandt 2001: 142; O'Mahoney 2013: 707). It looks as though the ancient marble has come to life. A more obvious visualization of the continuity between ancient Greeks and modern Germans is difficult to imagine. And in order to accentuate that continuity even more, Riefenstahl depicts the German athlete as almost naked: like the other male athletes in the prologue all he wears is a thong. The female dancers in the prologue are completely naked.

The close tie between ancient Greece and Nazi Germany is revealed also in the manner in which the Olympic flame appears. First we see how that flame is lit on the fundament of a pillar of an ancient temple. Then follows the relay race to Berlin; this was a completely new feature of the Olympic Games, which was introduced in 1936 (Walters 1996: 142–5 and 192–4). The destination of the race is the brand-new stadium which the Nazis had built especially for the games. A salient detail: the relay race as the film shows it to us is mostly a fake, like the rest of the prologue. After the games the race was – partly in other, better locations – redone to give Riefenstahl the opportunity to make better and more beautiful shots. For exactly the same reason the demanding director asked different athletes to repeat their achievements once again during the games, for the aim of her film was not to reproduce reality – no, it was meant to surpass reality. Therefore athletes who did not live up to her high aesthetic ideals were mercilessly kept out of the film, even if they had won their competition. Riefenstahl was hard: in *Olympia* there was place only for perfect bodies.

Perfect bodies – white or black – included the muscular but supple body of the black American athlete Jesse Owens. To the great frustration of the Nazi bosses he became the indisputable star of the Berlin games: he won no less than four gold medals. American journalists made much use of his outstanding achievements to take the edge off, or even to ridicule, the Nazi myth about the superiority of the Aryan race. This ideological clash was reflected especially in the long-jump contest where the German athlete Luz Long competed against Owens. Long lost but took his defeat in a strikingly sportsmanlike manner – at least much more sportsmanlike than the Nazi leaders who were hard-pressed to hide their anger. Riefenstahl could hardly have shown no interest at all in Owens, but the interest she took seems to have gone much further than strictly necessary. It seems as if she was honestly charmed by the highly photogenic American – just as many ordinary German spectators were (Walters 1996: 166 and 195–6).

Epilogue: modern body fascism

After the Second World War Riefenstahl was taken to court several times, accused of collaboration with the Nazi regime. As a consequence she was not allowed to exercise her profession any more. It was not until 1952 that she was 'de-nazified' and could, in principle, take up her job as director again. Public opinion, however, would stay hostile towards her for a long time to come. That explains why she finally decided to accept new artistic challenges, and from 1956 she was completely enthralled by Africa. She would spend much time on long expeditions there and would take numerous pictures. Those photos were collected in the 1970s into two magnificent books about the Nuba, a fairly isolated warlike mountain people in Sudan (Riefenstahl 1973, 1976).

Those documents make it clear that Riefenstahl still, after all those years, was fascinated by the beautiful, athletic and naked or nearly naked body. That this time her admiration was exclusively focused on men and women of a fairly obscure African tribe did not save her from sharp comments. Riefenstahl's photo-documentary is simply an extension of her *Olympia*-film, according to a biting remark by the American feminist Susan Sontag in 1975. Once again she sings an ode to the perfect body: there are no old, sick or disabled Nuba in her pictures. Other, later critics elaborated, and still elaborate, diligently on this: Riefenstahl's photography testifies to appalling imperialism and blind Eurocentrism. First of all, she constantly plays the boss. Young and healthy tribe members are photographed, but only if they undress and nicely assume the monumental but artificial poses which she commands. And the young and healthy Nuba she has chosen look surprisingly European. They may be black, but for the rest they look as if they have escaped from an art book by Winckelmann or Riefenstahl's own *Olympia*. A mere coincidence? Not at all. According to Sontag and her followers Riefenstahl proves that she is still what she was during all those years, even though she always tried to deny it – a confirmed adherent of the Nazi cult of the perfect body. At the same time the success of her photo-books proves, according to Sontag and followers, how strongly that cult has become rooted in Western culture: in every one of us there is a secret wish for physical perfection. What is beautiful is good, and 'ugly' means 'bad', almost by definition. It is thus perfectly clear: yesterday's fascism is alive again, as a political fringe phenomenon, and also, and much worse, as widespread and deeply rooted 'body fascism'. Riefenstahl subscribed to and spread this body fascism by means of 'inverted racism', glorifying of the body of the black Nuba, 'her' Nuba, noble warriors and heavenly savages, so difficult for the ordinary Westerner to reach, and therefore so attractive (Sontag 1980: 73–105; Trimborn 2002: 280–2; Pronger 2002; Ludewig 2006).[1]

Note

1 Translated from the Dutch by Ingrid Sperber.

Bibliography

Benario, Herbert W., 'Arminius into Hermann: History into Legend', *Greece and Rome* 51 (2004), 83–94.
Blankenburg, Martin, 'Rassistische Physiognomik: Beiträge zu ihrer Geschichte un Struktur', in C. Schmöller (ed.), *Der exzentrische Blik. Gespräch über Physiognomik* (Berlin, 1996), 133–61.
Blanshard, Alastair J. L., 'Gender and Sexuality', in C. W. Kallendorf (ed.), *A Companion to the Classical Tradition* (Malden, MA, and Oxford, 2007), 328–41.
Chapoutot, Johann, *Le national-socialisme et l'Antiquité* (Paris, 2008).
Demandt, Alexander, 'Hitler und die Antike', in B. Seidensticker and M. Vöhler (eds), *Urgeschichten der Moderne: Die Antike im 20. Jahrhundert* (Stuttgart and Weimar, 2001), 136–57.
Diehl, Paula (ed.), *Körper im Nationalsozialismus* (Munich, 2006).
Fitzpatrick, Katie, and Tinning, Richard, 'Health Education's Fascist Tendencies: A Cautionary Exposition', *Critical Public Health* 24 (2014), 132–42.
Flashar, Hellmut, *Inszenierung der Antike: Das griechische Drama auf der Bühne der Neuzeit, 1585–1990* (Munich, 1991).
Gray, Richard T., *About Face: German Physiognomic Thought from Lavater to Auschwitz* (Detroit, MI, 2004).

Günther, Hans F. K., *Rassengeschichte des hellenischen und römischen Volkes* (Munich, 1929).

Günther, Hans F. K., *Kleine Rassenkunde des deutschen Volkes* (Munich, 1935).

Hitler, Adolf, *Mein Kampf*, tr. Ludwig Lore (New York, 1939).

Hitler, Adolf, *Hitler's Table Talk, 1941–1944: His Private Conversations*, tr. N. Cameron and R. H. Stevens (New York, 2000).

Huys, Marc, 'The Spartan Practice of Selective Infanticide and its Parallels in Ancient Utopian Tradition', *Ancient Society* 27 (1996), 47–74.

Jahn, Bernhard, 'Deutsche Physiognomik. Sozial- und mediengeschichtliche Überlegungen zur Rolle der Physiognomik in der Weimarer Republik und im Dritten Reich', in M. Huber and G. Lauer (eds), *Nach der Sozialgeschichte* (Berlin and New York, 2010), 575–592.

Joshi, Vandana, 'Maternalism, Race, Class and Citizenship: Aspects of Illegitimate Motherhood in Nazi Germany', *Journal of Contemporary History* 46 (2011), 832–53.

Krebs, Christopher B., *A Most Dangerous Book: Tacitus's Germania from the Roman Empire to the Third Reich* (New York and London, 2011).

Losemann, Volker, 'The Nazi Concept of Rome', in C. Edwards (ed.), *Roman Presences: Receptions of Rome in European Culture, 1789–1945* (Cambridge, 1999), 221–35.

Ludewig, Alexandra, 'Leni Riefenstahl's Encounter with the Nuba', *Interventions: International Journal of Post-Colonial Studies* 8 (2006), 83–101.

Möhring, Maren, *Marmorleiber: Körperbildung in der deutschen Nacktkultur (1890–1930)* (Cologne, 2004).

Mosse, George L., *The Image of Man: The Creation of Modern Masculinity* (Oxford, 1996).

O'Mahoney, Mike, 'In the Shadow of Myron: The Impact of the Discobolus on Representations of Olympic Sport from Victorian Britain to Contemporary China', *International Journal of the History of Sport* 30 (2013), 693–718.

Peeters, Michel, *Beelden voor de massa: Kunst als wapen in het Derde Rijk* (Antwerp and Amsterdam, 2007).

Pringle, Heather, *The Master Plan: Himmler's Scholars and the Holocaust* (New York, 2006).

Pronger, Brian, *Body Fascism: Salvation in the Technology of Physical Fitness* (Toronto, 2002).

Riefenstahl, Leni, *Die Nuba: Menschen wie von einem anderen Stern* (Munich, 1973).

Riefenstahl, Leni, *Die Nuba von Kau* (Munich, 1976).

Rosenberg, Alfred, *Der Mythus des 20. Jahrhunderts: Eine Wertung der seelisch-geistigen Gestaltenkämpfe unserer Zeit* (Munich, 1938).

Ryback, Timothy W., *Hitler's Private Library: The Books that Shaped his Life* (London, 2008).

Sontag, Susan, 'Fascinating Fascism', *New York Review of Books* 22 (6 Feb. 1975); repr. in Susan Sontag, *Under the Sign of Saturn* (New York, 1980), 73–105.

Speer, Albert, *Inside the Third Reich* (London, 2000).

Stock, Clemens Augustinus, '... das Schöne und Gute in Mensengeschlechtern zu verleiblichen': Hans F. K. Günthers Buch 'Plato als Hüter des Lebens'. Werkkritik und historische Einordnung* (unpublished PhD, Düsseldorf, 2004).

Surén, Hans, *Gymnastik der Deutschen* (Stuttgart, 1925).

Trimborn, Jürgen, *Riefenstahl: Eine deutsche Karriere* (Zurich, 2002).

Walters, Guy, *Berlin Games: How Hitler Stole the Olympic Dream* (London, 1996).

Weiler, Ingomar, 'Zur Rezeption des griechischen Sports im Nationalsozialismus: Kontinuität oder Diskontinuität in der deutschen Ideengeschichte?', in B. Näf and T. Kammasch (eds), *Antike und Altertumswissenschaft in der Zeit von Faschismus und Nationalsozialismus* (Mandelbachtal and Cambridge, 2001), 171–88.

Wildmann, Daniel, *Begehrte Körper: Konstruktion und Inszenierung des 'Arischen Männerkörpers im 'Dritten Reich'* (Würzburg, 1998).

Zweiniger-Bargielowska, Ina, 'Building a British Superman: Physical Culture in Interwar Britain', *Journal of Contemporary History* 41 (2006), 595–610.

INDEX

Milton Keynes UK
Ingram Content Group UK Ltd.
UKHW051848071024
449327UK00025B/1890